AUDITORY DIAGNOSIS

Principles and Applications

AUDITORY DIAGNOSIS
Principles and Applications

Shlomo Silman

Department of Speech, Brooklyn College
City University of New York, Brooklyn, New York

Department of Speech and Hearing Sciences
Graduate School and University Center
City University of New York, New York, New York

Audiology and Speech Pathology Service
Veteran Administration Medical Center
East Orange, New Jersey

Carol A. Silverman

Communication Sciences Program, Hunter College
City University of New York
New York, New York

Academic Press, Inc.
Harcourt Brace Jovanovich, Publishers
San Diego   New York   Boston   London   Sydney   Tokyo   Toronto

Line Drawings by
PierceAxiom™, Brooklyn, New York

This book is printed on acid-free paper. ∞

Copyright © 1991 by ACADEMIC PRESS, INC.
All Rights Reserved.
No part of this publication may be reproduced or transmitted in any form or
by any means, electronic or mechanical, including photocopy, recording, or
any information storage and retrieval system, without permission in writing
from the publisher.

Academic Press, Inc.
San Diego, California 92101

United Kingdom Edition published by
Academic Press Limited
24–28 Oval Road, London NW1 7DX

Library of Congress Cataloging-in-Publication Data

Silman, Shlomo.
    Auditory Diagnosis : principles and applications / Shlomo
Silman, Carol A. Silverman.
        p.   cm.
    Includes bibliographical references and index.
    ISBN 0-12-643451-4
    1. Audiometry.   2. Hearing disorders--Diagnosis.   I. Silverman,
Carol A. (Carol Ann), Date.   II. Title.
    [DNLM: 1. Hearing Disorders--diagnosis.   2. Hearing Tests.   WV
272 S584d]
RF294.S55   1991
617.8'075--dc20
DNLM/DLC
for Library of Congress   90-14465
                                                    CIP

PRINTED IN THE UNITED STATES OF AMERICA
91 92 93 94   9 8 7 6 5 4 3 2 1

This book is dedicated to my son, Benny Silman, whom I love so dearly.
SHLOMO SILMAN

And to my dear parents, Dr. and Mrs. Jerome S. Silverman, who have always
given me their love and support.
CAROL A. SILVERMAN

And to Dr. Maurice H. Miller, our beloved teacher, and our audiology students who inspire us.
SHLOMO SILMAN AND CAROL A. SILVERMAN

CONTENTS

Foreword   *xiii*
Preface   *xv*

CHAPTER ——————— 1

STIMULI COMMONLY EMPLOYED IN AUDIOLOGIC TESTS

I. Filtered Noise   1
    A. Broad-Band Noise   *3*
    B. Narrow-Band Noise   *4*

II. Critical Band   5

III. Masking   5

IV. Short-Duration Stimuli   6
    A. Clicks   *6*
    B. Tonebursts   *7*

V. Speech Noise   8

References   9

CHAPTER ——————— 2

BASIC AUDIOLOGIC TESTING

I. The Auditory System   10

II. Air-Conduction Measurement   10

    A. Conventional Pure-Tone Thresholds   *11*
    B. Discrete-Frequency or Sweep-Frequency Testing by Automatic Audiometry   *13*
    C. Rationale for Frequency Range Used in Audiometric Testing   *14*
    D. Reference Threshold Levels   *15*
    E. Soundfield Testing   *16*
    F. Pediatric Testing   *16*
    G. High-Frequency Audiometry   *18*

III. Bone-Conduction Measurement   18
    A. Mechanism   *19*
    B. Artificial Mastoid   *21*
    C. Bone Vibrator   *21*
    D. Reference Levels   *22*
    E. Vibrator Replacement   *23*
    F. Acoustic Radiation   *23*
    G. Effect of Middle-Ear Pathology on Bone-Conduction Thresholds   *24*
    H. Tactile Bone-Conduction Thresholds   *26*
    I. High-Frequency Bone-Conduction Thresholds   *26*
    J. Procedure   *26*
    K. Tuning-Fork Tests   *26*

IV. Variables Affecting Pure-Tone Air- and Bone-Conduction Measurement   27
    A. Patient Variables   *27*
    B. Instrumentation and Environmental Variables   *28*
    C. Clinician Variables   *29*

V. Speech-Recognition Threshold   29
    A. Terminology   *30*
    B. History of the Development of the SRT Test Materials   *30*
    C. Relation between the SRT and Pure-Tone Average   *32*
    D. The SRT–PTA Agreement   *32*
    E. The Relation between the SRT and SDT   *33*
    F. Recorded versus Live-Voice Presentation   *33*

G. Carrier Phrase   33
H. Response Mode   33
I. Familiarization and Practice   33
J. Procedure   34
K. Considerations for the Pediatric Population   36

VI. Clinical Masking   36

A. Interaural Attenuation   36
B. When to Mask   39
C. Occlusion Effect   40
D. Effective Masking   41
E. Initial Masking   41
F. Overmasking   41
G. Maximum Masking   42
H. Central Masking   42
I. Technique for Clinical Masking   42
J. Masking Dilemma   43
K. Insert Earphones   44

VII. Audiometric Interpretation   44

A. Hypothetical Cases for Masking by Air-
   and Bone-Conduction   44
B. Type of Hearing Loss   48
C. Audiometric Configuration   49
D. Magnitude of Hearing Impairment   51

VIII. Major Etiologies of Auditory
Disorders   52

A. Conductive Hearing Impairment   52
B. Sensorineural Hearing Impairment   55
C. Central Auditory Disorders   62

IX. Case History   63

References   65

C. Amplitude and Shape   88
D. Combining Static-Acoustic Middle-Ear
   Admittance and Tympanometry to Resolve
   Special Cases   102
E. Acoustic-Reflex Testing   103
F. Acoustic Immittance Testing in Infants   120
G. Relation between Otoscopy and Acoustic
   Immittance   124
H. Detecting Middle-Ear Effusion in Children   124
I. Assessment of Eustachian-Tube Function   128
J. Proposed Classification of Acoustic-
   Immittance Results with Respect to
   Middle-Ear Functioning   129
K. Medical Referral in Cases of
   Suspected Middle-Ear Pathology   132

References   132

Chapter _____ 4

FUNCTIONAL HEARING IMPAIRMENT

I. Prevalence   137

A. Adults   137
B. Children   138

II. Behavioral Signs   138

III. Indicators within Routine Audiologic
Tests   138

A. Test–Retest Reliability   138
B. Interaural Attenuation of Air- and
   Bone-Conduction Tones   139
C. Poor Bone-Conduction Threshold Levels   139
D. False-Alarming   140
E. Error Responses during SRT and
   Monosyllabic PB-Word Speech-Recognition
   Assessment   140
F. SRT–PTA Discrepancy   140
G. Speech-Recognition Testing with
   Monosyllabic PB Words   141
H. Audiologic Configuration   141

IV. Special Behavioral Tests   142

A. Sensorineural Acuity Level   142
B. Lombard and Sidetone-Amplification
   Effects   142
C. Doerfler–Stewart Test   143
D. Stenger Test   144
E. Bekesy (Automatic) Audiometry   147
F. Delayed Auditory Feedback Test   148

Chapter _____ 3

ACOUSTIC-IMMITTANCE ASSESSMENT

I. Concept of Immittance   71

A. Impedance   71
B. Admittance   77
C. Acoustic-Immittance Instrumentation   77

II. Clinical Applications of Acoustic
Immittance   79

A. Static-Acoustic Immittance   80
B. Pressure   84

V. Electrophysiologic Tests 150

A. Acoustic-Reflex Thresholds 150
B. Electrodermal Audiometry 150
C. Auditory-Evoked Potentials 151

VI. Uncommonly Employed Tests 153

VII. Counseling 153

VIII. Recommendations 154

References 154

CHAPTER ——————— 5

TRADITIONAL AUDIOLOGIC SITE-OF-LESION TESTS

I. Speech-Recognition Testing 159

A. Development of the CID W-22s 159
B. Binomial Distribution Model 163
C. Speaker Effect 164
D. Development of the NU-6s 164
E. Synthetic Sentence Identification (SSI) Test 166
F. Diagnostic Significance of the Suprathreshold Speech-Recognition Score for a Single Presentation Level 167
G. Diagnostic Significance of Rollover on the Performance-Intensity Function 168
H. Digitized Speech Recordings 170
I. Abbreviated Word Lists 170
J. Pediatric Population 171
K. Masking 171

II. Tests of Auditory Adaptation 172

A. Procedure 173
B. Tonality versus Audibility 176
C. Clinical Populations 176
D. Reliability 177
E. Comparison of the Various Adaptation Procedures 177
F. Temporal Characteristics of Adaptation 178

III. Recruitment Tests 178

A. Alternate Binaural Loudness Balance Test 178
B. Monaural Loudness Balance Test 189
C. Difference-Limen Tests 189
D. Loudness Discomfort Level Test 190
E. Acoustic-Reflex Threshold 190

IV. Short Increment Sensitivity Index 190

A. Intensity Difference Limen for Loudness 190
B. Description of the SISI Test 193

V. Bekesy Testing 200

A. Bekesy Types 200
B. Variables Affecting Bekesy Audiograms 204
C. Modifications of the Bekesy Technique 204
D. Relations among Bekesy Tracings, Auditory Adaptation, and Loudness Recruitment 207
E. Hit and False-Alarm Rates 207

VI. Masking for Suprathreshold Tonal Tests 208

A. Initial Masking 209
B. Overmasking 209
C. Maximum Masking 209

References 209

CHAPTER ——————— 6

CENTRAL AUDITORY SPEECH TESTS

I. Monaural Low-Redundancy Speech Tests 216

A. Low-Pass Filtered 216
B. Time Compressed 216

II. Dichotic Speech Tests 217

A. Model for Contralateral and Ipsilateral Ear Effects 218
B. Digits 220
C. Consonant–Vowel Nonsense Syllables 222
D. Staggered Spondaic Words 225
E. Competing Sentences 232
F. Binaural Fusion 234

III. Other Speech Tests 235

A. Synthethic Sentence Identification Test 235
B. Rapidly Alternating Speech Perception Test 238
C. Masking Level Difference Test 239

IV. Effect of Peripheral Hearing Impairment 241

V. Assessment of Central Auditory Processing
Disorders in the Pediatric Population   243

References   245

CHAPTER ———————————— 7

BRAINSTEM AUDITORY-EVOKED
POTENTIALS

I. Overview of the Auditory-Evoked
Potentials   249

II. Instrumentation and Signal
Processing   252
   A. Amplifier and Filter   253
   B. Common Mode Rejection Ratio   253
   C. Signal Averager   254

III. Effects of Technical and Subject
Parameters   255
   A. Technical Parameters   255
   B. Subject Parameters   262

IV. Normative Data   264
   A. BAEP Components   264
   B. Intensity   264
   C. Latency–Intensity Function   265
   D. Amplitude   265
   E. Replicability   266

V. Generator Sites   266

VI. Prediction of Hearing Threshold Level
from the BAEP Threshold   266

VII. Absent BAEPs   267

VIII. BAEPs Elicited with Bone-Conducted
Signals   267

IX. Frequency Specificity   268
   Conclusions   271

X. Effect of Auditory Pathology on the
BAEP   271
   A. Conductive Hearing Impairment   271
   B. Cochlear Hearing Impairment   273
   C. Retrocochlear Impairment   276

XI. Pitfalls in BAEP Testing and
Interpretation   286

XII. BAEPs in Infants   287
   A. Threshold   287
   B. Peak Latency   287
   C. Interpeak Latency   288
   D. Latency–Intensity Function   288
   E. Recording Techniques   288
   F. BAEP Screening of Infants   289

XIII. Special Applications of BAEP Testing   290
   A. Comatose Population   290
   B. Interaoperative Monitoring   291

References   292

CHAPTER ———————————— 8

ELECTRONYSTAGMOGRAPHY

I. Anatomy and Physiology of the
Vestibular System   298

II. Systems Which Control Horizontal Eye
Movements   301
   A. Vestibulo-Ocular Reflex   301
   B. Saccadic Eye Movement   305
   C. Smooth Pursuit Eye Movements   305
   D. Optokinetic Eye Movements   305

III. Principles Underlying
Electronystagmography Recordings   306

IV. Measurement of Nystagmus Strength   308

V. ENG Procedure   308
   A. Calibration   309
   B. Gaze Testing   311
   C. Pendular Tracking   311
   D. Optokinetic Testing   311

E. *Positional Testing*   312
F. *Dix–Hallpike Test*   312
G. *Caloric Testing*   312
H. *Mental Alerting Tasks*   314

VI. Low-Frequency Sinusoidal Harmonic Acceleration Testing   314

VII. Pediatric ENG Test Modifications   316

VIII. ENG Interpretation   316

A. *Saccadic Testing*   316
B. *Spontaneous Nystagmus*   317
C. *Gaze Nystagmus*   318
D. *Slow-Pursuit Nystagmus*   319
E. *Optokinetic Nystagmus*   320
F. *Positional Nystagmus*   321
G. *Paroxysmal Nystagmus*   323
H. *Caloric Nystagmus*   324
I. *Rotary Nystagmus*   326
J. *Pitfalls in ENG Testing and Interpretation* 327

References   329

CHAPTER _____ 9

PERSPECTIVES ON SITE-OF-LESION TESTS AND CASE STUDIES

I. Criteria for Evaluating Test Performance   332

II. Evaluation of the Performance of the Test Battery   337

III. Application of Cost–Benefit Analysis to Audiologic Tests   341

IV. Proposed Protocol for Detection of Retrocochlear and Central Pathology   342

A. *Retrocochlear*   342
B. *Central*   345

V. Concept of Combined Cochlear and Retrocochlear Sites and the Traditional Site-of-Lesion Test Results   346

VI. Case Illustrations   346

A. *Case 1*   346
B. *Case 2*   350
C. *Case 3*   354
D. *Case 4*   358
E. *Case 5*   358
F. *Case 6*   362
G. *Case 7*   362
H. *Case 8*   365
I. *Case 9*   374
J. *Case 10*   382
K. *Case 11*   382

References   390

APPENDIX _____

STIMULUS CALIBRATION

I. Brainstem Auditory-Evoked Potentials Calibration   391

A. *Intensity*   391
B. *Acoustic Waveform*   392
C. *Acoustic Spectrum*   392
D. *Polarity*   393
E. *Repetition Rate*   393

II. Acoustic-Immittance Calibration   394

III. Audiometric Calibration   394

A. *Air Conduction*   394
B. *Bone Conduction*   396
C. *Speech*   397
D. *Soundfield*   397

References   398

Index   399

FOREWORD

This textbook is both a product of and a stimulant to exciting developments in audiology. A young profession—about 45 years old—audiology's knowledge base has reached noteworthy proportions. Its diagnostic responsibilities are increasingly called for by the public and by other professions, and it has a scope of practice which demands a rigorous educational preparation. This textbook adheres scrupulously to the point of view that audiology education must prepare the practitioner to integrate patient case history and audiologic and vestibular results into a coherent diagnosis.[1] It speaks to an audience of audiologists in professional education programs who are preparing to learn rapidly, but in depth, the complex interrelationship between the pure tone audiogram, acoustic immittance battery, and speech audiometry[2] as well as psychoacoustic concepts such as critical band theory or masking. Its presentation of material matches the rigors of scope of practice realities as articulated by commentators on contemporary audiology practice.[3,4]

Many excellent edited textbooks with multiple contributors are available today. However, this authored text achieves a distinctive internal organization, consistency, and density of information presented in a clear writing style. Although all of these chapters amply illustrate these features, a particularly good example of this tight yet clear presentation of material can be found in Chapter 3, Acoustic-Immittance Assement, which is almost a textbook in its own right. Another particularly good example is the last chapter, which integrates diagnostic procedures discussed in earlier chapters, in the presentation of 11 case histories.

While recognizing our heritage through an extensive review of historical procedures, the authors cover the leading edge of diagnostic procedures in audiology. They integrate theory with practice and provide coherent analyses of unresolved issues. At the same time they give the reader their opinions on these unresolved issues. The considerable experience represented by these two authors and their schol-arly approach to textbook writing is evident in the balance achieved in these analyses. The result is a book suitable for use as a reference by the practitioner after graduation.

This work begins with an introductory chapter on stimuli employed in audiologic tests. In addition there is a chapter on basic audiologic tests. Other chapters introduce their material with basic overviews. The style and content of these introductions are geared to audiology students with a solid preaudiology foundation in science. As a result, students can get on track for text content without wasting their time with repetition of basic concepts. An appendix on stimulus calibration provides a tight compendium of the complex elements in the quantification and calibration used in our diagnostic procedures.

As audiologists assume greater direct responsibilities for the comprehensive diagnosis mentioned earlier and as pressures build to contain spiraling health care costs, it behooves the audiology practitioner to have an evaluation strategy which adheres to cost–benefit realities. No longer is it acceptable simply to do as many tests as possible regardless of cost involved or potential returns in information. Chapter 9 provides a thorough and uniquely effective treatment of diagnostic strategies and cost–benefit outcomes. Nicely woven into this chapter are 11 case illustrations which tie together the information provided throughout the text as well as the test strategy and cost–benefit considerations. Rather than simply theorize, the authors give recommendations based on their own considerable experience.

As audiology grows and matures, new demands are placed on its textbooks. This text, the first authored rather than edited treatise, leads in this transition.

David P. Goldstein
Purdue University
West Lafayette, Indiana

[1] Kileny, P. (1990). Diagnostic audiology. *Audiology Today*. July-August, 23.

[2] Schwartz, D.M. (1990). Clinical perspective: Whatever happened to those bygone days? *Audiology Today,* May-June, 26–27.

[3] Hall, J.W. (1989). Scope of practice in audiology. Annual Convention of the American Academy of Audiology, April, 1989, Kiawah Island, South Carolina.

[4] Roeser, R. (1990). Issues on scope of practice in audiology. *Audiology Today,* September.

PREFACE

Diagnostic audiology has undergone many changes since World War II. At that time, diagnostic audiology consisted essentially of establishing the magnitude and type of hearing impairment. Now, with the advent of sophisticated, noninvasive procedures such as high-frequency probe-tone acoustic immittance and brainstem auditory-evoked potentials, audiologists assist in the diagnosis of etiologies of various types of hearing impairment such as middle-ear effusion, retrocochlear disorders, ossicular discontinuity, and ossicular fixation. Such procedures make possible early medical intervention or early aural habilitation/rehabilitation in children and adults. Procedures based on the acoustic reflex, Stenger phenomenon, and brainstem auditory–evoked potentials enable estimation of hearing sensitivity in the difficult-to-test population, for example infants, the developmentally or mentally disabled, the multiply handicapped, and the functionally hearing impaired. The field of diagnostic audiology has expanded rapidly over the last 40 years, particularly within the past 15 years. A book solely devoted to diagnostic audiology is now a necessity.

This is the first authored (nonedited) graduate text on diagnostic audiology. This book was intended primarily as a graduate text for two or more consecutive courses on basic and advanced diagnostic audiology. We hope that students of diagnostic audiology will find this approach to be of educational value. This approach to the book was necessary for us to convey our more than 30 years combined clinical and academic experiences in diagnostic audiology. Our clinical experiences have been drawn from speech and hearing centers in a variety of settings including hospital, university, developmental, Veterans Administration, and private practice. We look forward to incorporating the responses of colleagues, students, and clinicians in the field in future editions of this book.

We have attempted to provide an honest critical assessment of the audiologic techniques available in diagnostic audiology. We have also attempted to present the theoretical bases underlying the diagnostic audiologic tests. We hope such information will enable the reader to select the most appropriate audiologic procedure, stimulus, and instrumentation so the most accurate and comprehensive audiologic diagnosis can be reached.

In Chapter 1, stimuli commonly employed in audiologic tests are covered comprehensively. We felt that placing this topic as an opening chapter would provide basic scientific foundation for understanding the nature of the stimulus used in diagnostic audiology throughout the book.

Chapter 2, Basic Audiologic Testing, addresses the audiologic test employed in routine audiologic assessment. Hypothetical cases are presented to facilitate understanding of the principles of masking and type and magnitude of hearing impairment. In Chapter 3, Acoustic-Immittance Assessment, the concepts of acoustic immittance, use of acoustic immittance for differential diagnosis of cochlear versus retrocochlear pathology and detection of middle-ear pathology, and acoustic-reflex-based procedures for prediction of hearing impairment are discussed. Case studies are presented to enhance understanding of acoustic immittance. Chapter 4, Functional Hearing Impairment, is critical since site-of-lesion tests should not be employed unless functional hearing impairment has been ruled out. The audiologic tests in Chapter 5, Traditional Audiologic Site-of-Lesion Tests, were the dominant, audiologic site-of-lesion tests in the 1960s and 1970s. Studies on the sensitivity and specificity of these tests have led to a loss of confidence in such tests. Nevertheless, an understanding of these tests provides a historical perspective of diagnostic audiology, and some of these tests still remain in use in many audiologic centers. An understanding of these tests also sheds light on many of the effects of auditory pathology such as recruitment and auditory adaptation. Chapter 6, Central Auditory Speech Tests, critically examines the audiologic speech-recognition tests commonly used for detection of central auditory disorders. Chapters 7 and 8 address brainstem auditory-evoked potentials and electronystagmography, respectively. Because posturography is a relatively new and costly technique which has not been widely adopted nor costly technique which has not been widely adopted nor extensively evaluated, it is not covered in Chapter 8 in this edition. In Chapter 9, Perspectives on the Site-of-Lesion Tests and Case Studies, the principles underlying clinical decision analysis and a comparison of the sensitivities and specificities of the various audiologic tests, singly and in combination, are discussed. Also in this chapter, case studies for ears with cochlear, retrocochlear, and central auditory pathology are presented with the raw data from the various audiologic tests. These case studies include client histories and are analyzed according to the principles developed in earlier chapters. The Appendix, Stimulus Calibration, describes the principles and procedures of calibration of stimuli and equipment used for pure-tone air- and bone-conduction testing, speech-recognition testing, acoustic-immittance testing, and brainstem auditory-evoked potentials testing. Recommendations are given in most chapters based on our clinical experiences and our critical evaluation of related research. These recommendations are only suggestions to assist students and clinicians in marking clinical audiologic decisions and diagnoses.

In this text, no attention is given to the magnitude or latency measures of the acoustic reflex and only cursory attention is given to the middle and late auditory-evoked potentials. The data on such measures from normal and pathologic populations are not sufficient, at this time, to enable critical evaluation of these tools. These topics will probably be included in future editions of this book.

This book was a labor of love. We are indebted to the following individuals for their support, comments, and assistance in the development of this book: James Jerger, Daniel Schwartz, Kristine Olson, Wayne Olsen, Robert Turner, David Miller, Donald Dirks, Paul Kileny, Frank Musiek, Dennis Kisiel, John Jakimetz, Michael Vivion, Adrienne Rubinstein, Rochelle Cherry, Chuck Berlin, Michelle Emmer, Lucy Mendez, Ann Wallin, Alan Richards, B. Todd Troost, and Jackie Spitzer. Special thanks and appreciation go to Stanley A. Gelfand, our dear friend and colleague, who inspired and encouraged us over the years. His guidance and support are gratefully acknowledged. We apologize if we have inadvertently omitted names of persons who have contributed.

Artwork appearing in Chapters 2, 3, 4, 5, 6, part of 7, 8, 9, and part of the Appendix was rendered by Pierce-Axiom™, Brooklyn, New York.

Shlomo Silman
Carol A. Silverman

CHAPTER 1

STIMULI COMMONLY EMPLOYED IN AUDIOLOGIC TESTS

Any acoustic stimulus can be described with reference to time and frequency domains. In the time domain, the waveform of a stimulus represents the instantaneous amplitude of the stimulus as a function of time. The waveform can be electrical or acoustic. To visualize an electrical waveform, the acoustic stimulus is routed from a sound generator directly to an oscilloscope. To visualize an acoustic waveform, the acoustic stimulus is routed from a sound generator through an earphone (coupled with a sound-level meter) into an oscilloscope. In the latter case, the amplitude is modified by the earphone characteristics. Figure 1 shows the electrical waveforms for the simplest acoustic signal, a pure tone, and for the most complex signal, a click.

In the frequency domain, the spectrum of a stimulus represents amplitude as a function of the frequency of a signal. In the case of a pure tone, the average amplitude of the single frequency is shown. In the case of a complex signal, the average amplitude of each of the constituent frequency components is shown. Figure 2 illustrates electrical spectra for a pure tone and click. Figure 3 illustrates an acoustic spectrum for a click. Figures 2B and 3 reveal the absence of a resonance peak (increased amplitude) for the click in the electrical spectrum, in contrast with the presence of a resonance peak at approximately 3000 Hz in the acoustic spectrum. The resonance peak reflects the resonance of the earphone (in this case, the TDH-49). The stimuli employed in audiologic testing vary on a continuum from pure tones to clicks.

The rise time of a signal is the time required for the amplitude of the signal to increase from 10% to 90% of its steady-state value. The fall time of a signal is the time required for the amplitude of the signal to decrease from 90% to 10% of its steady-state value. The plateau of a signal is the time elapsed between the amplitude of the signal reaching 90% of its steady-state value at the end of the rise time and reaching 90% of its steady-state value at the beginning of the fall time. Duration of the signal consists of the rise time from the 10% point, the plateau, and the fall time to the 10% point. As will be discussed later in this chapter, the rise and fall times and duration of a signal affect its spectrum.

A pure-tone signal has tonal quality and contains a single frequency component. The rise and fall times of pure-tone signals employed in clinical audiology range from 15 to 25 ms with a total duration of 1–2 s.

A periodic complex signal is a sound wave which consists of a fundamental (the lowest frequency component) and other frequency components at whole-number multiples of the fundamental. An aperiodic complex signal is a sound wave which contains more than one frequency component; the frequency components are not integral multiples of the fundamental frequency.

I. FILTERED NOISE

Filtering involves the restricted passage of energy from a noise band either above a certain frequency (high-pass filter), below a certain frequency (low-pass filter), or within a frequency range (band-pass filter). Figure 4 illustrates electrical spectra for high-pass filtered noise, low-pass filtered noise, and band-pass filtered noise. The filtering of the noise signal is generally done electrically before it reaches the transducer. (Acoustic filtering can also be done, but it is costly.) The upper and lower cutoff frequencies of the filtered noise are the frequency points on both sides of the center frequency of that noise at which the energy is 3 dB less than that at the center frequency. As will be mentioned in the case of broad-band noise signals, the 3-dB down points represent the half-power points.

The ability of a filter to reject energy below the low-frequency cutoff or above the high-frequency cutoff of the filtered noise is called the rejection rate of the filter. The rejection rate is determined by the reduction in decibels over one octave from the center frequency of the filtered noise. For example, a filtered noise with an intensity of 90 dB at the center frequency of 1000 Hz and an intensity of 60 dB at 2000 Hz has a filter rejection rate of 30 dB (90 dB − 60 dB).

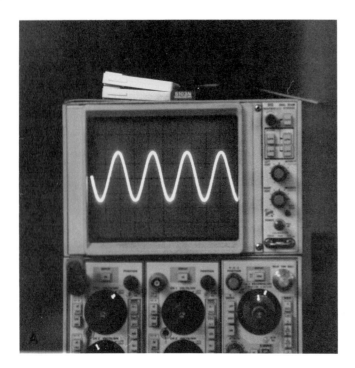

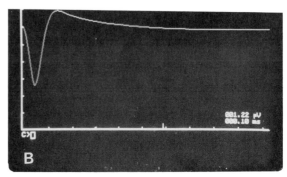

Figure 1 (A) The electrical waveform for a 2000-Hz signal routed from the signal generator of a Coulbourn System through an oscilloscope. (B) The electrical waveform for a click routed from the click generator of a Nicolet Compact Auditory System through an oscilloscope. The abscissa represents time in milliseconds and the ordinate represents the amplitude in millivolts.

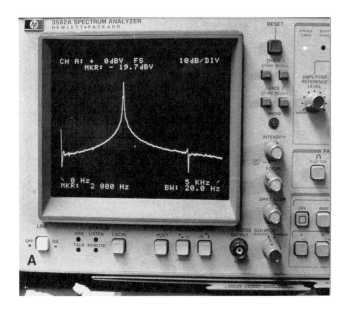

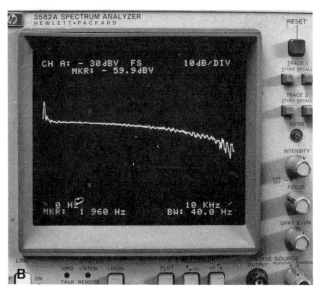

Figure 2 (A) The electrical spectrum for a 2000-Hz pure-tone signal having a rise–fall time of 25 ms and plateau of 950 ms. The electrical spectrum of the pure tone was obtained by routing the signal from the signal generator of a Coulbourn System through a real-time analyzer. (B) The electrical spectrum for a click of 100 μs duration. The electrical spectrum of the click was obtained by routing the signal from the click generator of a Nicolet Compact Auditory System through a real-time analyzer. The abscissa represents frequency in Hertz and the ordinate represents relative amplitude.

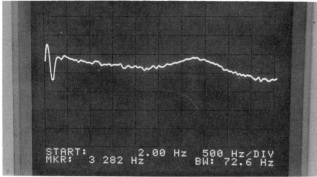

Figure 3 The acoustic spectrum for a click routed from the click generator of a Nicolet Compact Auditory System through a TDH-49 earphone coupled to a sound-level meter. The AC output of the sound-level meter was routed through a real-time analyzer.

The rejection rate of the filter and the bandwidth of the signal are determined by the frequency response of the filter and transducer.

Good examples of band-pass filtered noises are broad-band noise and narrow-band noise signals.

A. BROAD-BAND NOISE

Broad-band noise (BBN) is derived from a white-noise signal. White noise consists of an infinite number of frequencies and has essentially equal power per cycle. Figure 5 illustrates an electrical spectrum for white noise routed from a noise generator into a real-time analyzer. When a white noise signal is routed through a transducer (e.g., earphone, bone oscillator, or speaker), its bandwidth is reduced because of the limitation imposed by the frequency

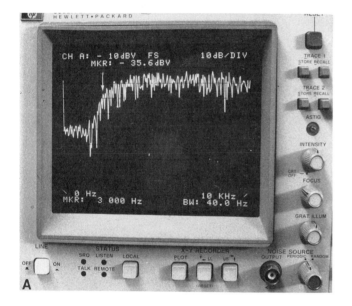

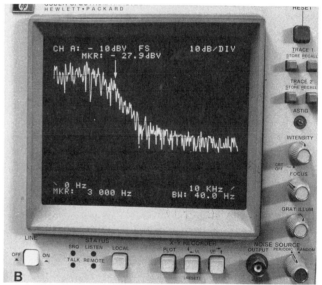

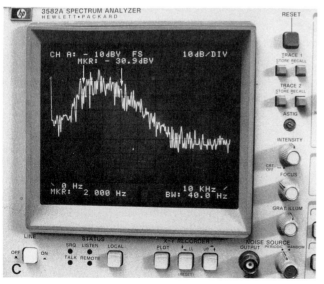

Figure 4 (A) The electrical spectrum for a white-noise signal routed from the white-noise generator of a Coulbourn System through a high-pass filter with a cutoff frequency of 3000 Hz into a real-time analyzer. (B) The electrical spectrum for a white-noise signal routed from the white-noise generator of a Coulbourn System through a low-pass filter with a cutoff frequency of 3000 Hz into a real-time analyzer. (C) The electrical spectrum for a white-noise signal routed from the white-noise generator of the Coulbourn System through a band-pass filter (2000–4000 Hz) into a real-time analyzer. The arrows represent the half-power points. The ordinate represents relative amplitude and the abscissa represents frequency Hz (10 KHz full scale).

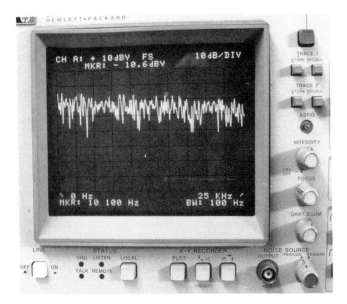

Figure 5 Electrical spectrum for a white-noise signal routed from the white-noise generator of the Coulbourn System to a real-time analyzer. The ordinate represents relative amplitude and the abscissa represents frequency Hz (25 KHz full scale).

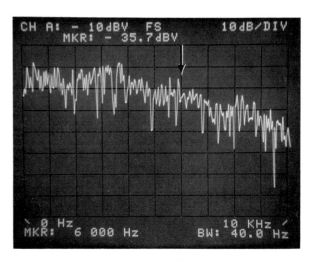

Figure 6 Acoustic spectrum for a broad-band noise signal. The broad-band noise signal was formed by routing the white-noise signal from the white-noise generator of the Coulbourn System through the TDH-49 earphone coupled to a sound-level meter. The AC output of the sound-level meter was routed through a real-time analyzer. The ordinate represents relative amplitude and the abscissa represents frequency Hz (10 KHz full scale).

response of the transducer. White noise shaped by the transducer is called BBN. Figure 6 illustrates the acoustic spectrum of a BBN signal as measured at the output of a TDH-49 earphone. Observe from Figure 6 that the spectrum level is essentially uniform but falls off at the higher frequencies at approximately 6000 Hz.

The energy per cycle of a BBN signal can be determined mathematically by dividing the overall sound-pressure level (SPL) by the number of cycles of the BBN. Since the dB SPL is a logarithmic quantity, whereas the number of cycles in a BBN signal is not a logarithmic quantity, the number of cycles in a BBN signal must first be converted into decibels using the formula $dB = 10 \log(N_1/N_2)$ where N_1 is the number of cycles in the BBN signal and N_2 is the reference number of cycles (1 cycle). Using this formula, a BBN signal with 10,000 cycles will be equal in decibels to $10 \log(10,000/1)$ or 40 dB. The logarithmic equivalent of 10,000 cycles is 40 dB.

To calculate the energy in 1 cycle of this BBN, the total SPL value of the BBN, for example, 100 dB, is divided by 40 dB. Thus, the energy per cycle is 60 dB. (When dividing logarithmic quantities, the denominator quantity is subtracted from the numerator quantity.) Since a white-noise signal is shaped by a transducer such as an earphone, and since transducers differ in their frequency response characteristics, some transducers will pass more of the energy of the white noise than other transducers. To determine the spectrum level or the energy level per cycle, the bandwidth characteristics of the transducer employed at a particular clinic should first be determined.

The bandwidth of a signal is specified by the points at which the power is halved or the intensity is 3 dB down from the maximum output of the stimulus. For example, the TDH earphones have a bandwidth of 6000 Hz (see Figure 6). The number of cycles in decibels of a BBN signal with a bandwidth of 6000 Hz is $10 \log(6000/1)$ or 37.8 dB. The spectrum level associated with 37.8 cycles is the overall dB SPL, 100, divided by 37.8 cycles, which is 62.2 (100 − 37.8) dB SPL per cycle.

B. NARROW-BAND NOISE

Narrow-band noises (NBNs) are used in clinical audiology to mask pure-tone signals or to obtain thresholds in soundfield. To derive the NBNs used in clinical audiology, the filter is set at 3 dB down from the maximum output (the half-power points) to produce a noise bandwidth containing a center frequency at the nominal frequency of the test tone to be masked. Narrow-band noises contain bandwidths narrower than those of BBN (e.g., third-octave, half-octave, and octave bandwidth). The noise generator of a clinical audiometer generates NBNs containing center frequencies at the nominal frequencies of the octave pure-tone signals. Narrow-band noises are generally characterized with reference to their bandwidth (the range in frequencies between the 3-dB-down points), center frequency, and rejection rate. Many commercially available audiometers employ third-octave bandwidths for NBN signals. The bandwidths for the third-octave NBNs used in clinical audiology are (a) 56 Hz for the NBN with a center frequency of 250 Hz, (b) 110 Hz for the NBN with a center frequency of 500 Hz, (c) 220 Hz for the NBN with a center frequency of 1000 Hz, (d) 440 Hz for the NBN with a center frequency of 2000 Hz, (e) 950 Hz for the NBN with a center frequency of 4000 Hz, and (f) 1900 Hz for the NBN with a center frequency of 8000 Hz.

Outside the third-octave band of the NBN, the rejection rate of the filter may vary between 10 and 60 dB per octave. Therefore, in cases with significantly rising or sloping audiograms, threshold responses may be obtained at frequencies outside the third-octave band rather than at the center frequency of the NBN, when using filters with low rejection rates. Therefore, the audiologist should be cautious in interpreting the results of audiometric testing based on NBN signals.

II. CRITICAL BAND

The concept of the critical band was initially introduced by Fletcher and Munson (1937) and substantiated by others (Hawkins & Stevens, 1950; Egan & Hake, 1950). When a pure tone is masked by BBN, only a limited band of noise around the center frequency close to the pure-tone frequency is essential to mask the pure tone. This limited band of frequencies is called the critical band for masking. The critical bandwidths for the audiometric test frequencies are (a) 50 Hz at 250 Hz, (b) 50 Hz at 500 Hz, (c) 56.2 Hz at 750 Hz, (d) 64 Hz at 1000 Hz, (e) 79.4 Hz at 1500 Hz, (f) 100 Hz at 2000 Hz, (g) 158 Hz at 3000 Hz, (h) 200 Hz at 4000 Hz, (i) 376 Hz at 6000 Hz, and (j) 501 Hz at 8000 Hz. The critical band for masking a tone of 1000 Hz, for example, has a bandwidth of 64 Hz with a center frequency of 1000 Hz. Therefore, in a BBN signal with a 10,000 Hz bandwidth, only the energy in the critical band will contribute to the masking of the 1000-Hz pure tone. The rest of the BBN will contribute only to the loudness of the masking noise. Furthermore, when the pure tone is just audible in the presence of a masking noise, the energy of the critical band is equal to the energy of the pure tone. For example, a 1000-Hz pure tone of 40 dB SPL will be masked when the total energy of a critical band of 64 cycles is equal to 40 dB SPL.

As illustrated by the critical band concept, critical band masking is preferable to BBN masking. The overall sound-pressure level of the critical band required to mask a pure tone is less than the overall sound-pressure level of a BBN required to mask a pure tone. For example, as mentioned before, to mask a 1000-Hz tone of 40 dB SPL, a critical band with an overall sound-pressure level of 40 dB is required. Since the critical band for masking a 1000-Hz tone has a 64-Hz bandwidth, the bandwidth in dB is equal to

10 log(64/1) or 2.5 dB. Therefore, the spectrum level per cycle of this critical band is equivalent to (40 dB SPL) (2.5 dB) or 37.5 dB per cycle. If the critical bandwidth is 64 Hz and a BBN masker with a bandwidth of 6000 Hz is employed, the total sound-pressure level of the BBN required to mask the 1000-Hz tone with an intensity 40 dB SPL is equivalent to the number of cycles of the BBN masker in decibels [10 log(6000/1) = 37.8] multiplied by the spectrum level per cycle (37.5 dB for a 64-Hz critical band), which is 75.3 dB SPL. This total sound-pressure level of 75.3 for the BBN to mask a 40 dB SPL tone at 1000 Hz is approximately 35 dB more than the total sound-pressure level of 40 dB SPL for a critical band to mask this tone.

III. MASKING

Figure 7 shows the electrical spectrum of a narrow-band noise signal with a center frequency of 2000 Hz routed from a GSI-10 audiometer through a real-time analyzer. The frequencies to which the arrows point represent the half-power points (3 dB down) from the peak sound-pressure level of the noise. Note the narrowness of the frequency range encompassed by these half-power points. The bandwidth for the band specified by the half-power points should ideally be equivalent to that of the critical band for masking; the reference sound-pressure level for the band determined by the half-power points should be equivalent to that of a pure tone at the center frequency of the band. Commercially available audiometers do not generate NBN bandwidths as narrow as the critical bands; they employ wider NBN band-

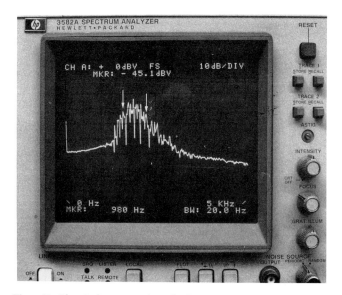

Figure 7 Electrical spectrum for a third-octave narrow-band noise signal having a center frequency of 2000 Hz routed from the GSI-10 audiometer through a real-time analyzer. The arrows represent the half-power points. The ordinate represents relative amplitude and the abscissa represents frequency Hz (5 KHz full scale).

widths based on, for example, third-octave bandwidths or BBN bandwidths.

As mentioned earlier, a pure-tone signal (maskee) at a given intensity and frequency will be masked by a masking noise (masker) whose energy in the frequency range corresponding to the critical band for the maskee is equivalent to the energy of the maskee. The intensity of the maskee can be referred to as the effective masking level (EML) of the masker. The difference between the intensity of the masker which just masks a given tone and the EML is the minimum effective masking (MEM) (see Chapter 2, Section VI,D). For example, if a pure tone is presented at 60 dB HL (hearing level) (the EML is 60 dB HL) and the intensity of an NBN centered at 2000 Hz which just masks the tone is 70 dB HL, the MEM is 10 dB HL (70 dB HL masker intensity − 60 dB HL EML).

With biologic calibration, MEM can be established for NBN and BBN maskers. With electroacoustic calibration, the masker levels corresponding to various EMLs can be established for NBN and BBN maskers. For biologic calibration, data from a group of at least 10 normal-hearing, otologically normal young adults should be obtained. In establishing the MEM of the NBN and BBN maskers, subjects should be randomly selected, and only one ear from each subject should be evaluated. The masker should be introduced at 50 dB HL (on continuously) and the intensity of the tone (maskee) presented in the same ear should be increased in 5-dB steps (pulsed tones) until the tone becomes barely audible. Then the maskee (test tone) is decreased in 5-dB steps until it just becomes inaudible. The decibel difference between the intensity of the masker and the intensity of the maskee when it just becomes inaudible (EML) is the MEM. The mean MEM should be calculated for the group, based on the mean of three trials for each person.

For clinical purposes, the MEM is the mean MEM calculated for the group plus a 10-dB safety factor to sufficiently account for intersubject variability. Table I shows the dB differences between the masker levels which just mask the test tone and the EML of the masker; the MEMs with the safety factor added are also shown. The values reported in Table I are based on a GSI-10 audiometer from a particular clinic. Each center must establish its own MEM values. The initial masking levels presented in Chapter 2 are based on the MEM values described here.

The electroacoustic method for establishing masker levels for various EMLs was described by Sanders (1972). For the electroacoustic method, the intensity level (energy) per cycle for the masker must be determined as described in Section 1,A. That is, the bandwidth of the masker is converted into decibels and the dB SPL of the masker is divided by the dB of the bandwidth. This resultant quantity is the intensity level (energy) per cycle of the masker. The critical

Table I Differences between the Masker Level (dB HL) Which Just Masks the Test Tone and the EML of the Masker (dB HL) with a Center Frequency at the Nominal Frequency of the Test Tone.

Frequency (Hz)	MEM		MEM + 10-dB Safety factor	
	Right channel	Left channel	Right channel	Left channel
250	0	0	+10	+10
500	+5	0	+15	+10
1000	+5	+5	+15	+15
2000	0	0	+10	+10
3000	0	+10	+10	+20
4000	+5	+5	+15	+15
6000	0	0	+10	+10
8000	0	0	+10	+10

[a] These decibel differences (MEMs) added to a safety factor as a function of test-tone frequency are also shown. These values, rounded off to the nearest 5-dB step, were obtained for a GSI-10 audiometer.

bandwidth is then converted into dB of bandwidth. In order to obtain the total energy of the critical band (in dB SPL), the level per cycle of the masker is multiplied by the dB of the critical bandwidth. The EML of the masker is determined by subtracting the audiometric zero level (expressed in dB SPL) from the total energy of the critical band. The EML should be derived for masker levels ranging 20 dB SPL to the maximum output of the audiometer. In pure-tone clinical masking situations, the intensity of the masker needed is based on an EML equivalent to the air-conduction threshold of the nontest ear at the test frequency. In speech clinical masking situations, the intensity of the masker needed is based on the average of the air-conduction thresholds at 500, 1000, and 2000 Hz in the nontest ear. To employ the electroacoustic approach to masking, equipment is needed to determine the overall SPL of the masker and the frequency response of the transducer (which affects the number of cycles of the masker).

IV. SHORT-DURATION STIMULI

A. CLICKS

A click is produced by rapidly switching on a voltage pulse of 100 μs duration and then rapidly switching off this pulse (see Figs. 2B and 3). A filtered click is obtained by passing a short-duration electrical pulse through a band-pass filter with and low-frequency cutoffs set to the nominal frequency of the click. For filtered clicks, the spectrum broadens as the nominal frequency of the filtered click increases, because of the inverse relation of signal bandwidth to signal duration. Because of this broadening, the use of filtered clicks during brainstem auditory evoked potentials testing (see Chapter 6) to achieve a frequency-specific signal has been abandoned by most investigators.

B. TONEBURSTS/TONE-PIPS, TONEBURST

For brainstem auditory evoked potentials testing, short-duration stimuli such as clicks are used. A limitation of using clicks, however, is the broadness of their spectra, which precludes frequency specificity. A compromise can be obtained between a signal with a broad spectrum (i.e., the click) that is effective in eliciting a brainstem auditory evoked potential and a signal with a narrow spectrum (i.e., the pure tone) that is ineffective in eliciting a brainstem auditory evoked potential. The toneburst/tone-pip represents this compromise.

We define tone of a very brief duration (only a few ms) as toneburst/tone-pip (Burkard, 1984). Beyond 10 ms short-

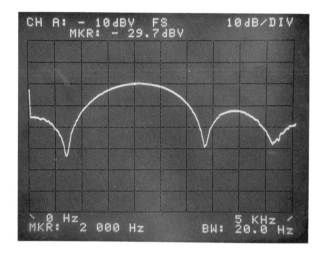

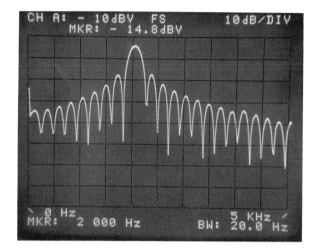

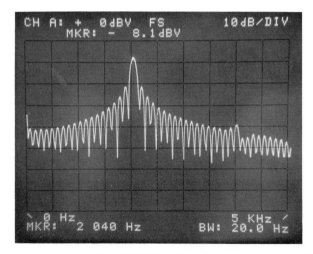

Figure 8 (A) The electrical spectrum for a 2000-Hz toneburst/tone-pip with a rise–fall time of 100 μs and a duration of 1 ms. (B) The electrical spectrum for a 2000-Hz toneburst/tone-pip signal with a rise–fall time of 100 μs and a duration of 5 ms. (C) The electrical spectrum for a 2000-Hz toneburst/tone-pip signal with a rise–fall time of 100 μs and duration of 10 ms. Note the narrowing to the center lobe as stimulus duration increases. Also note that the amplitude of the side lobes (reflecting spectral splatter) decreases as stimulus duration increases. The ordinate represents relative amplitude and the abscissa represents frequency Hz (5 KHz full scale).

duration tones are commonly referred to as tonebursts. When the duration reaches over several hundred milliseconds, the signal is a pure tone (although ideally a pure tone has infinite duration). The waveforms of tonebursts/tone-pips are trapezoidal in shape. The rise–fall time of a toneburst/tone-pip is commonly specified in milliseconds. Toneburst/tone-pip signals have short durations which are longer than those of clicks but shorter than those of pure tones. Because of the short duration of toneburst/tone-pip signals, there is always some spectral splatter resulting in energy being present at frequencies distant from the nominal frequency of the toneburst/tone-pip. There is an inverse relation between the duration of a toneburst/tone-pip and degree of spectral splatter. The longer the duration of a toneburst/tone-pip, the narrower the spectrum, and the less the spectral splatter. Figure 8 shows the effect of toneburst/tone-pip duration on the electrical spectra of toneburst/tone-pip signals. This figure reveals the inverse relation between toneburst/tone-pip duration and degree of spectral splatter.

The rise–fall time of a toneburst/tone-pip also affects its spectrum. Figure 9 shows the electrical spectrum for a toneburst/tone-pip signal that has the same duration as the signal in Figure 8B but with an increased rise–fall time. As can be seen from Figure 9, the center lobe is narrower and the degree of spectral splatter is decreased in comparison with Figure 8B. Thus, the toneburst/tone-pip in Figure 9 is a more frequency-specific signal than the one in Figure 8B. Spectral

splatter also occurs when the tone is turned on at phases other than 0 or 180°, even if the signal duration is long.

A logon is similar to a toneburst/tone-pip, except the envelope of the spectrum is Gaussian rather than trapezoidal in shape. The amplitude of the secondary side lobes of the logon is approximately 4–5 dB less than that of tonebursts/tone-pips. A typical logon, such as the one described by Davis, Hirsh, Popelka, and Formby (1984), is a 2-1-2 logon, which has 2 cycles rise time 1 cycle plateau, and 2 cycles fall time. For the 2-1-2 logon, for example, as its nominal frequency increases, the total duration decreases.

Very short rise–fall times will result in spectral splatter regardless of the duration; longer rise–fall times of at least 15 ms are sufficient to prevent spectral splatter (see Figure 2A).

V. SPEECH NOISE

Speech noise is BBN with a narrower frequency range extending from at least 250 Hz to 4000 Hz. The slope of the speech noise spectrum is +3 dB per octave from 250 Hz to 1000 Hz; the slope is −12 dB per octave from 1000 Hz to 4000 Hz. The acoustic spectrum of speech noise follows the configuration of the acoustic spectrum of a speech signal. Masking of speech signals can be done using either BBN shaped by the earphone or speech noise. Many audiometers calibrate speech noise in effective masking, that is, 50 dB HL of speech noise will mask a 50 dB HL speech signal. (BBN is generally not calibrated in effective masking; it is calibrated in dB SPL.) For NBN signals we recommend generating normative data on the MEMs using speech noise and BBN maskers; the MEM normative data for monosyllabic phonetically balanced (PB) words should be obtained separately from those for spondaic words. To obtain the normative data on masking of spondaic and monosyllabic PB words, the speech signals should be introduced at a level of 50 dB HL and the speech noise or BBN noise increased in the same ear until the subjects can no longer repeat 6 of 6 words.

ACKNOWLEDGMENT

George Bing and William Resnick photographed the figures in this chapter.

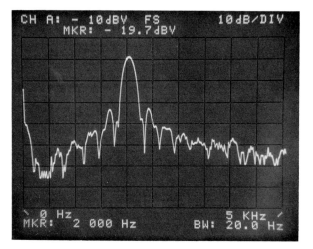

Figure 9 The electrical spectrum for a 2000-Hz toneburst/tone-pip with a rise–fall time of 2 ms and a plateau of 1 ms. Note that the duration of this signal is the same as that in Figure 8B. Compared with Figure 8B, the amplitudes of the side lobes are markedly decreased. This toneburst/tone-pip can also be classified as a logon. The ordinate represents relative amplitude and the abscissa represents frequency Hz (5 KHz full scale).

REFERENCES

Burkard, R. (1984). Sound pressure measurement and spectral analysis of brief acoustic transients. *Electroencephalogr. Clin. Neurophysiol., 57,*

83–91.

Davis, H., Hirsch, S. K., Popelka, G. R., & Formby, C. (1984). Frequency selectivity and thresholds of brief stimuli suitable for electric response audiometry. *Audiol. 23,* 59–74.

Egan, J. P., & Hake, H. W. (1950). On the masking pattern of a simple auditory stimulus. *J. Acoust. Soc. Am., 22,* 622–630.

Fletcher, H., & Munson, W. A. (1937). Relation between loudness and masking. *J. Acoust. Soc. Am., 9,* 1–10.

Hawkins, J. E., & Stevens, S. S. (1950). Masking of pure tones and of speech by white noise. *J. Acoust. Soc. Am., 22,* 6–13.

Sanders, J. W. (1972). Masking. In J. Katz (Ed.), *Handbook of clinical audiology,* pp. 111–142. Baltimore: Williams & Wilkins.

CHAPTER 2

BASIC AUDIOLOGIC TESTING

I. THE AUDITORY SYSTEM

The auditory system consists of the outer ear, middle ear, inner ear, eighth cranial nerve, and central auditory nervous system which includes the auditory brainstem and auditory cortex. The inner ear includes the vestibular system and the cochlea. The eighth cranial nerve includes the cochlear nerve branch and the vestibular nerve branch. The auditory brainstem begins with the cochlear nuclei and, proceeding rostrally in the brainstem, also includes the nuclei and projections of the superior olivary complex, lateral lemniscus, inferior colliculus, medial geniculate body, and auditory cortex. The auditory cortex is located in the temporal lobe, and the right and left auditory cortices are connected by the corpus callosum.

The conductive mechanism includes the outer and middle ears. The sensorineural mechanism includes the cochlea, eighth cranial nerve, and cochlear nuclei.

Conductive hearing impairment refers to hearing impairment from damage to the conductive mechanism. Sensorineural hearing impairment refers to hearing impairment from damage to the sensorineural mechanism. A central auditory disorder refers to disorder of the central auditory nervous system. Central auditory disorders affecting the brainstem can be classified as extra-axial brainstem or intra-axial brainstem disorders. Extra-axial brainstem disorders affect the cerebellopontine angle at the junction of the eighth cranial nerve and brainstem and the area of the brainstem caudal to the first major decussation. Thus, extra-axial brainstem disorders include disorders of the cochlear nuclei. Intra-axial brainstem disorders affect the brainstem at the first major decussation and in areas rostal to this decussation, including the superior olivary complex caudally and the medial geniculate body rostrally.

The term "retrocochlear" will be used to refer to disorders of the peripheral auditory nervous system including the eighth cranial nerve and extra-axial brainstem. Thus, the term "central auditory nervous system" will not include the retrocochlear sites. There is lack of agreement in the literature regarding the definitions of retrocochlear and central auditory disorders. Our terminology is consistent with that employed by Davis and Silverman (1970), Jerger (1973), Newby (1972), Noffsinger and Kurdziel (1979), and Pinsker (1972). Figure 1 shows the anatomical divisions of the auditory system as related to the anatomical terms used to describe hearing impairment.

II. AIR-CONDUCTION MEASUREMENT

Air-conduction measurement is the most fundamental aspect of audiologic assessment. Air-conduction measurement involves determination of the pure-tone thresholds at 250–8000 Hz. The pure-tone stimuli reach the cochlea through the air-conduction route: outer ear, middle ear, and inner ear. The total auditory system, including the conductive portion (outer ear and middle ear) and the sensorineural portion (cochlea and the eighth cranial nerve), are involved in air-conduction testing. The stimuli for this test are delivered through earphones or insert receivers or in soundfield through the speakers. Air-conduction testing represents the first test of the routine basic audiologic test battery.

Air-conduction testing is done (a) to determine the type of hearing loss present by comparison of the air- and bone-conduction thresholds, (b) to determine the magnitude of hearing loss, (c) to detect the presence of functional hearing loss by comparison of the pure-tone average with the speech-recognition threshold (see Chapter 4 on functional hearing loss), (d) to monitor the effectiveness of medical intervention by comparing pre- and post-treatment air-conduction thresholds, (e) to predict auditory handicap and phoneme-recognition ability, and (f) to assess the need for and the benefit from amplification. A discussion of the nondiagnostic aspects of air-conduction testing is beyond the scope of this book.

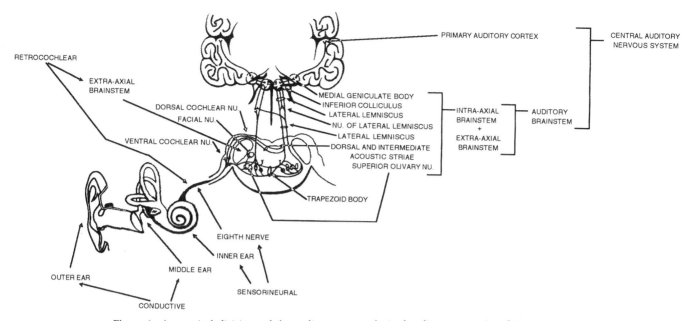

Figure 1 Anatomical divisions of the auditory system, loci of auditory system in relation to terms referring to type of hearing impairment, and anatomical terms relating to the auditory system. Partially adapted from Noback and Demarest (1981).

A. CONVENTIONAL PURE-TONE THRESHOLDS

According to the American National Standards Institute (ANSI, 1973), the threshold of hearing is the threshold of audibility. This threshold is defined as the "minimum effective sound pressure level of the signal that is capable of evoking an auditory sensation in a specified fraction of the trials" (ANSI S3.20-1973, p. 55). The procedure for obtaining audiometric thresholds is based on the psychophysical Method of Limits (or the Method of Minimal Change).

1. METHOD OF LIMITS

The Method of Limits (Fechner, 1860) is a classical psychophysical method for the measurement of threshold. Series of stimuli that are either ascending or descending in intensity are presented. The intensity increments are fixed and equal. Both ascending and descending trials are employed because the threshold varies as a function of the direction of the run or trial.

The subject's task is to indicate whether the sound is perceived. In an ascending run, the sound is first presented at a level known to be below threshold and then is increased in fixed, equal increments until the subject perceives the sound (positive response). In a descending run, the sound is first presented at a level known to be well above threshold and then is decreased in fixed, equal increments until the subject no longer perceives the sound (negative response). The ascending and descending runs are alternated. Each run is initiated and terminated at a different intensity in order to prevent the subject from standardizing the response by counting the number of stimuli given before changing the response. The absolute threshold is determined for each run by calculating the series transition (T) point, which is the midpoint between the last negative and first positive response in an ascending run or the last positive and first negative response in a descending run. The overall threshold is the average of the T values for at least 6 runs. Figure 2 shows threshold measurement using the Method of Limits for an individual.

A source of variation in the threshold as determined by the Method of Limits is a persistence effect. Errors of anticipation and errors of habituation constitute the persistence

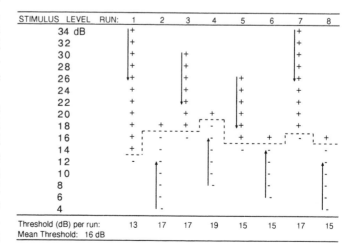

Figure 2 Method of Limits. Reprinted with permission from Gelfand (1990).

effect. In an error of anticipation, the subject changes the response before it is applicable. For example, in an ascending series, the subject may say "no" for the first few stimuli and then say "yes" before the stimulus is heard because the stimulus is anticipated. In an error of habituation, the subject continues to respond to the stimulus in the same manner, even when the response is no longer applicable. For example, in a descending series, the subject may say "yes" for the first few stimuli and continue to say "yes" out of habit even when the stimulus is no longer heard. The persistence effect is minimized by altering the direction of the runs and by using a large number of runs.

The threshold concept is predicated on the assumption that the subject's sensitivity fluctuates from moment to moment (Stevens, 1951). The subject's minimum response level at a specified moment is determined by his or her status at that moment. As a result, many runs must be given in order to statistically estimate the threshold, defined psychophysically as the stimulus value at which a positive response is obtained 50% of the time. The runs are presented according to one of the classical psychophysical methods of threshold measurement such as the Method of Limits.

2. Method for Clinical Determination of Pure-Tone Thresholds
Air- and bone-conduction thresholds are determined using the same method.

a. Hughson–Westlake (1944)
In the Hughson–Westlake (1944) method for determination of pure-tone thresholds, the stimulus presentations are always ascending from a level where the sound is inaudible to the lowest level where the sound is audible. The threshold is defined as the lowest level at which the sound is audible in more than half of the ascending trials. The Hughson–Westlake method represents an ascending version of the psychophysical Method of Limits.

b. Carhart–Jerger Modified Hughson–Westlake (1959)
Carhart and Jerger (1959) revised the Hughson–Westlake method. The procedure follows.

1. A tone is presented at a level well above threshold, that is, at 30–40 dB HL if the subject appears to have normal hearing sensitivity and at 70 dB HL if a moderate hearing loss appears to be present. If the initial level is insufficient, the intensity is increased in 15-dB steps until the subject responds.
2. The duration of the pure-tone stimuli is 1–2 s.
3. A convenient response involves finger-raising whenever the stimulus is heard.
4. After the first response, the intensity is decreased in 10–15 dB steps until no response is obtained.
5. When inaudibility is reached, the threshold search is initiated. The intensity is increased in an ascending series of 5-dB steps until a response is obtained. When

a response is obtained, the intensity is decreased 10–15 dB and another ascending trial (5-dB increments) is begun.
6. The criterion for threshold is the lowest intensity at which three responses are obtained on ascending runs.
7. The stimuli are separated by toneless intervals.

Carhart and Jerger (1959) employed 5-dB increments for ascending runs since moment-to-moment fluctuations in auditory sensitivity are generally less than this increment size. When 5-dB steps are employed, the threshold cannot be statistically defined. Therefore, the technique need not be one of the classical psychophysical techniques. The technique employed should be one that yields high reliability.

Carhart and Jerger (1959) recommended employing brief tonal durations in order to maximize the on-effect phenomenon, minimize adaptation, and enhance the reliability of the threshold. The on-effect refers to the fact that the auditory system responds most vigorously at the onset of the tone. When the stimulus is a sustained tone, the on-effect is followed by adaptation, that is, a reduction in responsiveness (decrease in loudness or change in tonality) even when the tone is not intense enough to yield fatigue. Full recovery from adaptation is generally regained during an interstimulus interval of 1–2 s. (See the SISI and Adaptation sections of Chapter 5 for further information regarding the on-effect and adaptation.)

c. ASHA (1978a) Guidelines for Manual Pure-Tone Threshold Audiometry
The ASHA (1978a) guidelines for manual pure-tone threshold audiometry is essentially based on the recommendations of Carhart and Jerger (1959) and Reger (1950). The guidelines indicate that variations in procedure may be necessary for difficult-to-test populations. The procedure follows.

1. The subject is instructed to respond whenever and as soon as the tone comes on, regardless of how faint it is and to stop responding as soon as the tone goes off. The subject is also instructed that first one ear and then the other ear is tested.
2. The mode of response can be any which is overt, for example, raising and lowering the finger, hand, or arm, or pressing and releasing a signal light switch.
3. A response should not be considered as one unless the latency of the response is consistent and the subject responds appropriately to the termination as well as the initiation of the tone. If the latency of the response to the first tone in an ascending run is delayed, the response to the tone that is 5-dB higher should be without hesitation.
4. Subjects should be reinstructed if false-positive responses (response in the absence of a tone) or false-negative (failure to respond when a tone is present and heard). False-positive responses can be

minimized by varying the interval between audible stimuli, employing pulsed or warbled tones, or by having the subject report the number of pulsed tones presented at a given level.

5. The subject is familiarized with the tone by one of two methods. In the first method, the attenuator is set at the lower limits and the intensity is slowly and continuously increased until a response occurs. In the second, the tone is presented at 30 dB HL, and at 50 dB HL if no response occurs at 30 dB HL; if there is no response at 50 dB HL, the tone is increased in 10-dB steps until a response occurs.
6. The duration of the tone is 1–2 s.
7. The interstimulus interval is varied but is never less than the duration of the stimulus.
8. After the first response, the tone is decreased by 10 dB whenever the subject responds and increased by 5 dB whenever the subject fails to respond.
9. The threshold is defined as the lowest intensity at which the subject responds at least half the time and at least three times on ascending runs.
10. Variations in technique should be recorded on the audiogram, for example, descending method, pulsed tones substituted, or warbled tones substituted.
11. The audiometer and earphones must meet the specifications in ANSI S3.6–1969.
12. The ambient noise levels in the test environment must meet the specifications in ANSI S3.1–1977.
13. The tester should check for cerumen blockage or collapsed canals with or without earphones. The tester should place the headphones so that the grid is directly over the entrance to the ear canal. Hair should be manipulated so that it is not trapped underneath the headphones and other obstacles such as earrings should be removed.
14. Diagnostic testing should be done at the following octave frequencies: 250, 500, 1000, 2000, 4000, and 8000 Hz. Testing is also done at 125 Hz when a low-frequency hearing loss is present. The interoctave frequency is tested whenever the difference in threshold between two adjacent octave frequencies is at least 20 dB.
15. If information concerning which ear is the better ear is available, the better ear should be tested first. The order of test frequencies employed should be (a) 1000, 2000, 4000, and 8000 Hz, retest at 1000, 500, and 250 Hz or (b) 1000, 500, and 250 Hz, retest at 1000, 2000, 4000, and 8000 Hz.

d. ANSI S3.21–1978 Method for Manual Pure-Tone Audiometry

The ANSI S3.21–1978 method for manual pure-tone audiometry is slightly different from the ASHA (1978a) guidelines. The ANSI standard recommends initial presentation of the tone at 30 dB HL for everyone; if no response

occurs, the intensity is increased by 20 dB and by 10 dB thereafter until a response occurs. An alternative approach recommended by ANSI (1978) involves setting the attenuator at the lowest intensity level and then slowly and continuously increasing the intensity until a response occurs. The tone is then turned off for at least two seconds and then presented again at the same intensity. If no response occurs when the tone is presented again, this familiarization procedure is repeated. According to Yantis (1985), the approach of starting at the minimum attenuator setting is preferred by many audiologists since this approach is less time consuming, the intensity range around threshold is decreased, and some of the behavioral characteristics associated with functional hearing loss and loudness recruitment may be detected more easily.

B. DISCRETE-FREQUENCY OR SWEEP-FREQUENCY TESTING BY AUTOMATIC AUDIOMETRY

Bekesy audiometry is based on a combination of the classical psychophysical Method of Limits and Method of Adjustment and on the adaptive procedure. In the Method of Adjustment (Fechner, 1860), the subject controls the stimulus levels, both ascending and descending trials are employed, and the stimulus level is varied in continuous rather than discrete steps. Similar to the Method of Limits, the Method of Adjustment is also biased by persistence effects.

In the adaptive procedure (Levitt, 1971; Zwislocki, Maire, Feldman, & Ruben, 1958), the level yielding a specified percentage response such as 50% can be obtained. The procedure is adaptive in the sense that the intensity level on any one trial is dependent on the responses and intensity levels used on the preceding trials. In the simple up–down procedure, the intensity level is reduced by a fixed increment if the subject responds and it is increased by the same fixed increment if the subject fails to respond. A run is considered a series of trials in one direction (e.g., a series of intensities at which the subject failed to respond or a series of intensities at which the subject responded). The average of all the midpoints between the positive and negative responses corresponds to the threshold.

1. Sweep Frequency

Bekesy (1947) developed an audiometer that enabled the subject to track his or her own threshold. Most Bekesy audiometers produce frequencies between 100 and 10,000 Hz. The subject holds a switch that is pressed as soon as the tone comes on and is released as soon as the tone goes off. When the button of the handswitch is pressed, the intensity decreases automatically. When the button of the handswitch is released, the intensity increases automatically. The motor-driven attenuator is connected to a recorder which plots the intensity as a function of frequency.

For the purpose of threshold measurement, pulsed-tone presentation is employed with an attenuation rate of 2.5 dB/s and a continuous frequency change from low to high frequency of 1 octave/min. The duty cycle is 50% with an on-time of 200 ms. The threshold is generally determined from the midpoints of the excursions (Price, 1963; Reger, 1970; Stream & McConnell, 1961).

Automatic audiometers are frequently used in mass-screening settings since they enable testing of several persons simultaneously.

2. FIXED FREQUENCY

In fixed-frequency automatic audiometry, the patient's threshold is sampled at a given frequency for a period of at least 0.5 min and not more than 4 min.

For a more complete discussion of automatic audiometry, see the Bekesy section of Chapter 5.

C. RATIONALE FOR FREQUENCY RANGE USED IN AUDIOMETRIC TESTING

As mentioned earlier, the range of frequencies for air-conduction testing is generally 250–8000 Hz. As will be discussed later, the range of frequencies for bone-conduction testing is 250–4000 Hz. The overall intensity level of conversational speech is approximately 65–70 dB SPL. Pascoe (1978) determined the sensation level re: minimum sound pressure level for audibility of the speech stimulus at the third-octave bands centered at 125, 250, 1000, 2000, 4000, and 8000 Hz. Real-ear measurements with a probe microphone were employed in order to account for head-shadow and ear-canal effects. Since the study was done on normal-hearing listeners, the sensation level can be considered equivalent to hearing level. Figure 3 shows the hearing level for speech at each frequency when the speech has an overall level of 65 dB SPL. As can be seen from Figure 3, the hearing level for long-term speech at 65 dB SPL is approximately 20 dB at 125 Hz, 40 dB at 250 Hz, 55 dB at 500 Hz, 52 dB at 1000 Hz, 55 dB at 2000 Hz, 50 dB at 4000 Hz, and 40 dB at 8000 Hz.

Audibility of the entire speech range is not essential for good speech-recognition ability in quiet. Hirsh, Reynolds, and Joseph (1954) found that the speech-recognition score for monosyllabic W-22 PB words decreased only slightly when frequencies above 1600 Hz were filtered. This led to the erroneous concept that high frequencies above 1500–2000 Hz do not contribute significantly to speech-recognition ability. The Hirsh *et al.* (1954) study, however, was done in quiet and on normal-hearing listeners who utilize high-frequency sensitivity in noisy situations when low-frequency hearing is masked by the noise. Persons with high-frequency hearing loss, on the other hand, cannot efficiently utilize their high-frequency hearing in noisy situations.

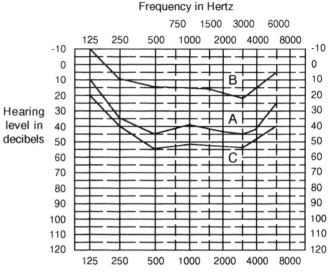

Figure 3 Speech spectrum on an audiogram format. A is the 50th percentile level, B is the 90th percentile level, and C is the 10th percentile level of speech having an overall spectrum level of 65 dB SPL. Adapted from Pascoe (1980). Reprinted with permission from Olsen *et al.* (1987).

Skinner and Miller (1983) investigated the speech-recognition score for speech presented in quiet and in noise for subjects with moderate sensorineural hearing losses. The bandwidth of a master hearing aid was varied to determine the bandwidth yielding the highest speech-recognition score in quiet and in noise. The highest speech-recognition score was obtained with the widest bandwidth (266–6000 Hz). Thus, frequencies above 4000 Hz are important for hearing-impaired listeners in quiet and noise as well as for normal-hearing listeners in noisy situations.

Another rationale for testing 250 and 500 Hz is for the detection of many conductive pathologies yielding a stiffness-loaded middle-ear or outer-ear system as in cases of otosclerosis and otitis media. In such cases, hearing impairment is revealed by air-conduction testing. As will be discussed later, such pathologies yield air–bone gaps at these frequencies. The threshold information at these frequencies may also yield information about the presence of early Meniere's disease, which is characterized by a low-frequency sensorineural hearing impairment.

Another rationale for testing 4000 and 8000 Hz is to assist in differentiating between noise-induced and other high-frequency sensorineural hearing losses. In noise-induced hearing loss, there is a notch usually at 3000–6000 Hz with recovery at 8000 Hz. In most other high-frequency hearing losses, the audiometric configuration is sloping; the hearing loss at 8000 Hz is greater than that at 4000 Hz. The threshold information at the high frequencies may also yield information about the presence of conductive pathologies yielding a mass-loaded outer- or middle-ear system, as in cases of ossicular discontinuity and impacted tympanic membrane. In such cases, a hearing impairment is detected by air-conduction testing at the high frequencies with air–bone gaps.

D. REFERENCE THRESHOLD LEVELS

The average sound-pressure level that makes a tone at a specified frequency just barely audible for a group of normal listeners, is called the zero hearing level or the standard audiometric threshold. The sound-pressure level is a measure of intensity in relation to a specified physical reference value. The standard physical reference value is 0.0002 dynes/cm^2 (2×10^{-4} d/cm^2) which is equivalent to 0.0002 μbar or 0.00002 Pascals (20 μPa or 2×10^{-5} Pa). The sound-pressure reference which is now used in acoustics is 20 μPa. The sound-pressure levels at audiometric zero for each frequency are incorporated in an audiometer. The reference levels for audiometric zero are based on ANSI S3.6–1989 in the United States and on ISO R389 (ISO, 1975) in Europe.

1. Earphones

ANSI S3.6–1989 specifies the dB SPL values equivalent to audiometric zero at the audiometric frequencies for various supra-aural earphones as measured in an NBS 9A 6-cc artificial ear. Supra-aural earphones fit over the ear so that the volume of air under the cushion is small, in contrast with circumaural earphones, which fit around the ear so that the volume of air under the cushion is large. These reference levels were based on large surveys of hearing levels. The TDH-39, TDH-49, and TDH-50 earphones, mounted in an MX-41AR cushion, are most commonly supplied with the audiometer. The ANSI S3.6–1981 refer-

ence equivalent threshold sound-pressure levels for the various earphones are shown in Table II of the Appendix.

The ANSI S3.6–1989 specifications replace the older American standard (ASA–1951) for audiometric zero based on the TDH-39 earphone. The reference levels specified in ANSI S3.6–1989 are, on average, approximately 10 dB lower than those specified in ASA–1951. The procedure for measurement of these output levels from the earphone and the equipment used in calibration of output levels are described in the Appendix.

The reference equivalent threshold sound-pressure levels specified in ISO R389 (1964, reaffirmed in 1975) are shown in Table I. The ISO values apply for all earphones calibrated with the IEC 318 coupler. Table I reveals that the ISO reference equivalent threshold sound-pressure levels are similar to the ANSI S3.6–1989 values. The IEC 318 coupler, however, is not yet commercially available in the United States.

2. Insert Earphones

Insert earphones are often substituted for traditional supra-aural earphones, particularly in cases of masking dilemma (see Section VI, Clinical Masking), in cases of collapsed ear canals, and when testing in a noisy environment. As will be mentioned later in this chapter in the masking section, insert earphones increase the interaural attenuation for air-conduction testing. Insert earphones are also used during brainstem auditory evoked potentials testing in conjunction with canal electrodes to remove the stimulus artifact, thereby enhancing wave I, and to increase the interaural attenuation.

Etymotic Research developed the ER-3A insert earphone, which is commercially available. Figure 4 illustrates the ER-3A insert earphones. The ANSI S3.6–1989 interim reference threshold sound-pressure levels for the ER-3A insert earphones are shown in Table III of the Appendix.

Wilber, Kruger, and Killion (1988) calculated the interim reference equivalent threshold sound-pressure levels reported in the ANSI S3.6–1989 standard (see Appendix) for

Table I Reference Threshold Levels for Audiometric Earphones[a]

Frequency (Hz)	Reference threshold levels, all earphones[b] (μPa)
125	45.0
250	27.0
500	13.5
750	—
1000	7.5
1500	7.5
2000	9.0
3000	11.5
4000	12.0
6000	16.0
8000	15.5

[a] ISO R389 (1964, R1975.)
[b] IEC 318 coupler.

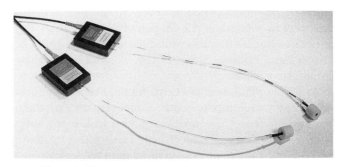

Figure 4 The Etymotic Research ER-3A insert earphones.

Page 15, first column, last paragraph, last line: 1981 should be 1989.

ER-3A insert earphones based on direct measurements reported in five studies. Wilber *et al.* (1988) obtained the mean output levels (across five studies) of the ER-3A at threshold (in dB SPL) using a 2-cc coupler. These mean values were then corrected for differences in coupler and eartip insertion. The values were corrected to apply to the HA-1 coupler and deep insertion (2–3 mm past the canal entrance, yielding a total insertion depth of approximately 16 mm as measured from the plane of the concha floor). These corrected values were compared with the mean output sound-pressure threshold levels (across the same five studies) under supra-aural earphones. The sound-pressure levels at threshold with the insert earphones, as measured in a 2-cc coupler, were subtracted from the threshold levels (dB HL) under earphones and rounded off to the nearest 0.5 dB to yield the reference equivalent threshold sound-pressure levels for the insert earphones as measured with an HA-1 coupler. The Appendix (Table III) shows these reference levels for an HA-1 coupler and shows the values to be added to the reference levels for an HA-1 coupler to yield the reference equivalent threshold sound-pressure levels in a Zwislocki coupler. For example, if the threshold under insert earphones is 60 dB HL at 1000 Hz for a patient, then the measured output sound-pressure level in the HA-1 2-cc coupler will be 63.5 dB SPL and the measured output sound-pressure level in a Zwislocki coupler will be 69.0 dB SPL.

E. SOUNDFIELD TESTING

Air-conduction testing using frequency-specific stimuli in soundfield may be necessary in situations where air-conduction thresholds cannot be obtained under earphones. Some pediatric patients and mentally retarded patients, for example, do not tolerate the earphones. Pure-tone stimuli cannot be employed in soundfield because of standing waves from interaction between the incident wave from the loudspeaker and the reflected wave from the walls of the audiometric booth. These standing waves cause variation in the sound-pressure level around the patient's head. Ideally, the test stimuli should not vary by more than ±2 dB in intensity around the patient's head (Skinner, 1988). When pure tones are delivered through speakers in an audiometric booth, the intensity levels around the patient's head vary by more than ±2 dB. Soundfield uniformity can be obtained using frequency-modulated (warble) tones or narrow-band noises. (For a further description of these stimuli, see Chapter 1.)

No ANSI or ISO standard exists for pure-tone soundfield testing in an audiometric booth. Moreover, since modulation rate and frequency deviation of the warble tones, spectrum of the narrow-band noises, loudspeaker azimuth (placement of the loudspeaker in relation to the patient's ear), and size and shape of the audiometric booth vary considerably from clinic to clinic, the reference equivalent threshold sound pressure levels for warble-tone or narrow-band noise soundfield testing should be obtained in each clinic on a group of normal-hearing listeners for a specified stimulus and loudspeaker azimuth. The potentiometer or the digital memory of the audiometer should be adjusted so that 0 dB HL in soundfield is equivalent to the reference equivalent threshold sound-pressure level (as determined on a group of normal-hearing persons) in soundfield. We recommend that, for warble-tone or narrow-band noise soundfield testing, the loudspeakers be located between 40° and 60° azimuth as suggested for speech soundfield testing in the ANSI S3.6–1989 standard (see Appendix), to maximize the correspondence between the pure-tone average and the speech-recognition threshold. (The ANSI S3.6–1989 standard provides guidelines for speech soundfield testing for informational purposes only.)

According to Staab (1971) and Staab and Rintelmann (1972), no significant differences were obtained between pure-tone thresholds measured in an anechoic chamber and the warble-tone thresholds measured in an audiometric booth when the frequency deviation did not exceed ±10% and the modulation rate did not exceed 32 Hz. Many of the existing audiometers have a modulation rate of 10 Hz for the warble tones. Although this modulation rate is adequate for normal-hearing listeners, it may be low for some patients with sensorineural hearing loss who have smaller-than-normal integration times (Skinner, 1988).

Since the bandwidth of narrow-band noises is considerably larger than that for warble tones, the threshold obtained in soundfield with narrow-band noises may be for a frequency within the narrow-band noise bandwidth other than the nominal center frequency.

Thresholds for stimuli presented in soundfield (through the loudspeakers) reflect the hearing sensitivity of the better ear.

F. PEDIATRIC TESTING

1. BEHAVIORAL OBSERVATION AUDIOMETRY

In behavioral observation audiometry (BOA), stimuli are presented in soundfield through the loudspeakers without reinforcement of responses and the clinician observes whether overt behavioral responses to the stimuli occurred. This procedure is used for testing neonates and older infants. Response behaviors for neonates and infants up to 4 months of age include eye widening, eyeblink, arousal from sleep, a shudder of the body, and observable definite movement of the arms, legs, or body (Northern & Downs, 1984). The best responses are obtained when the infant is in a light stage of sleep in which there is eye or body movement when the eyelid is flicked (Mencher, 1972). Speech signals are more effective signals than narrow-band noises which, in turn, are more efffective signals than warble tones (Eisenberg, 1976). Table II shows the expected levels required for responses in infants and young children from birth to 2 years of age. As can be seen from this table, the thresholds decrease as a function of age. Thompson and Weber (1974) reported that the spread between the 10th and 90th percentiles for BOA in infants and children is very wide. For example, for the 3–5 month-old child, the dispersion between the 10th and 90th percentiles, using band-pass filtered complex noise, is 65 dB. There is large intrasubject variability in thresholds measured with BOA in infants and young children because of habituation to repeated presentations of the test stimulus. According to Thompson and Weber (1974), BOA does underestimate the child's hearing sensitivity and therefore should be regarded as a screening technique.

2. Visual Reinforcement Audiometry

As can be seen from Table II, localization responses (head-turn to sound) occurs at 4–7 months of age. Suzuki and Ogiba (1960, 1961) developed conditioned orientation reflex (COR) audiometry. With COR, there was an initial conditioning procedure involving presentation of a warble tone through the loudspeaker in soundfield paired with illumination of a doll above the speaker. After a few conditioning trials, the sound was presented in isolation. Reinforcement by illumination of the doll occurred only if there was an appropriate localization (head-turn) response. Suzuki and Ogiba (1960, 1961) found that most children between 1 and 3 years of age could be tested successfully with COR audiometry.

The term visual reinforcement audiometry (VRA) applies to a modified COR technique in which any overt behavioral response is reinforced (Wilson & Thompson, 1984). Liden and Kankkunen (1969) developed the VRA procedure. Some investigators (Haug, Baccaro, & Guilford, 1967), including ourselves, have been able to employ this procedure in children as young as 5 months. Ear-specific information can be obtained if VRA is done under earphones. The visual reinforcer commonly used in VRA is an animated illuminated toy such as a clown playing the drums and percussion.

3. Play Audiometry

With play audiometry, the child is conditioned to respond to a sound by putting a block in a box, a peg in a pegboard, and so forth. The clinician and the child together make the responses during the conditioning trials. During the conditioning trials, the sound and the reinforcement, which may be social ("That's good, Johnny!") or visual (animated illuminated toy), are presented simultaneously. After the conditioning trials, the sound is presented and reinforcement is provided only when the child makes the appropriate motoric response. Play audiometry can be done in soundfield or under earphones.

When the reinforcement is tangible, for example, provision of candy or cereal, the procedure is called tangible reinforcement operant conditioning audiometry (TROCA). TROCA is commonly employed with mentally retarded children. We have modified the TROCA procedure so the child sucks a lollipop or eats a cereal piece in response to the sound so that the behavioral response is also the reinforcement. This modified technique appears to be easier for the mentally retarded and for young children because only two steps (hearing the sound and eating the candy) rather than three steps (hearing the sound, performing a motoric response such as putting a block in a box, and then receiving a tangible reinforcement) are involved.

Table II Auditory Behavior Index for Infants: Stimulus and Level of Response[a,b]

Age	Noisemakers (approx. dB SPL)	Warbled pure tones (dB HL)	Speech (dB HL)	Expected response	Startle to speech (dB HL)
0–6 wk	50–70	78	40–60	Eye widening, eye blink, stirring, or arousal from sleep, startle	65
6 wk–4 mo	50–60	70	47	Eye widening, eye shift, eye blinking, quieting, beginning rudimentary head turn by 4 mo	65
4–7 mo	40–50	51	21	Head-turn on lateral plane toward sound, listening attitude	65
7–9 mo	30–40	45	15	Direct localization of sounds to side, indirectly below ear level	65
9–13 mo	25–35	38	8	Direct localization of sounds to side, directly below ear level, indirectly above ear level	65
13–16 mos	25–30	32	5	Direct localization of sound on side, above, and below	65
16–21 mos	25	25	5	Direct localization of sound on side, above, and below	65
21–24 mos	25	26	3	Direct localization of sound on side, above, and below	65

[a] Reprinted with permission from Northern and Downs (1984).
[b] Testing done in a sound room.

Another modification of play audiometry that we have employed involves having the child slap the clinician's hands whenever a sound is presented. Again, the response also serves as a reinforcement. We have also paired tickle with the sound so that a response to the sound will be a laugh or giggle or movement away from the clinician. The tickle response habituates very quickly in a given test session so the tickle modification of play audiometry is employed as a last resort with the very difficult-to-test.

G. HIGH-FREQUENCY AUDIOMETRY

High-frequency air-conduction testing refers to air-conduction testing between 8000 and 20,000 Hz. There are commercially available audiometers for testing in this frequency range, such as the Monitor/Demlar Model 20K extended high-frequency audiometer.

Clinical applications of high-frequency audiometry include (a) differentiation between noise-induced hearing impairment and other high-frequency sensorineural hearing impairment such as presbycusis (Laukli & Mair, 1985), (b) early detection of ototoxicity (Dreschler, Van der Hulst, & Tange, 1984; Tange, Dreschler, & Van der Hulst, 1985; Tonndorf, & Kurman, 1984), and (c) measurement of speech-recognition ability in persons with significant hearing impairment at the routine audiometric frequencies with good speech intelligibility and articulation (Berlin, 1982).

Tonndorf and Kurman (1984) questioned the validity of doing extended high-frequency air-conduction audiometry. They found calibration of audiometers to be problematic. When one-fourth of the wavelength of the incident sound approximated the length of the ear canal, resonances and antiresonances developed at the tympanic membrane which resulted in large intersubject variability in sound-pressure level at the tympanic membrane. This problem could be remedied with the use of a probe microphone to measure the sound-pressure level of the eardrum. Nevertheless, even probe microphones cannot overcome the problem of transverse waves above 15000 Hz associated with half-wave resonance. Tonndorf and Kurman (1984) overcame the calibration problem by using a special electric transduction mode in which a 60-Hz carrier frequency is modulated by the desired audiofrequency. The carrier frequency and the desired frequency were applied to the skin through the electrodes placed on both mastoids or on one mastoid and the arm. According to J. Tonndorf (personal communication, 1987) and B. Kurman (personal communication, 1988), the procedure involving the special electric transduction mode has drawbacks when masking is introduced to the nontest ear; upon introduction of the masking, measurement errors occur. Therefore, further research is needed on masking using the special electric transduction mode before the clinical feasibility of high-frequency air-conduction audiometry can be evaluated.

III. BONE-CONDUCTION MEASUREMENT

Bone-conduction threshold measurement is an integral part of basic audiologic evaluation. In bone-conduction testing, an oscillator or vibrator is positioned on the mastoid process of the temporal bone or on the middle of the forehead. Electrical energy is delivered to the oscillator to drive it into vibration against the skull, thereby causing the skull bones to vibrate. The vibrational energy is transmitted directly to the cochlea, bypassing the outer and middle ears which make up the conductive portion of the auditory system. The bone-conduction threshold assesses the integrity of the cochlea and eighth cranial nerve. The inner ear and eighth cranial nerve represent the sensorineural portion of the auditory pathway. Thus, bone-conduction testing measures the sensorineural sensitivity or reserve. The bone-conduction test derives its name from the fact that the oscillator is placed against the bone. Bone-conduction hearing from airborne sound does not occur until the intensity of the sound exceeds the air-conduction threshold by at least 60 dB (Dirks, 1985). The high threshold for bone-conducted stimulation of the skull resulting from air-conducted sound is a consequence of the difference in impedance between the skull and air (Dirks, 1985).

Unlike air-conduction measurement, the purpose of bone-conduction testing is not to determine how intense a sound must be to attain audibility (Hodgson, 1980). Rather, the purpose of bone-conduction measurement is to determine the type of hearing loss present by comparison of the air- and bone-conduction thresholds. Recall from the previous section that air-conduction stimulation is mediated through the outer, middle, and inner ear, and beyond whereas bone-conduction stimulation is mediated through the inner ear and beyond. Information regarding the sensorineural sensitivity can be obtained directly from the bone-conduction thresholds and information about the conductive (outer and middle ear) status can be obtained from comparison of the air- and bone-conduction thresholds. If there is a problem in the conductive portion of the auditory system, the bone-conduction threshold will be normal, since the sound bypasses that part of the auditory system, but the air-conduction threshold will be affected since air-conducted sound travels through the entire auditory pathway including the outer and middle ears. In such cases, therefore, there will be a difference between the air- and bone-conduction thresholds; the latter will be better than the former, indicating the presence of a conductive hearing loss. If there is a problem in the sensorineural portion of the auditory system, the bone-conduction threshold will be affected since the bone-conduction transmission route includes the inner ear and eighth cranial nerve. The air-conduction threshold will also be affected equally since the air-conduction transmission route includes the outer, middle, and inner ear, and beyond. In such cases, therefore, the air-conduction thresholds will be as poor as the bone-conduction thresholds, indicating the presence of a sensori-neural hearing loss. The air- and bone-conduction thresholds are also equal (but normal) in the case of normal hearing since no problem interferes with either the air-conduction or the bone-conduction transmission route.

Bekesy (1932) was the first to show that air- and bone-conduction stimulation excite the sensory cells and move the basilar membrane in the cochlea in the same manner, as evidenced by the results of his experiment involving cancellation of an air-conducted signal with a bone-conducted signal out of phase by 180°. Similar findings were obtained by Lowy (1942), who observed cancellation of the cochlear microphonic when the Bekesy experiment was replicated. Thus, the cochlear activity is the same regardless of whether the sound enters the cochlea by air or bone conduction so the bone-conduction thresholds can validly be compared with the air-conduction thresholds to determine the type of hearing loss (Gelfand, 1990).

A. MECHANISM

The early investigators of the mechanism of bone conduction suggested that there were three modes involved: compressional bone conduction, ossicular inertial bone conduction, and the external-canal component involving radiation from the walls of the external auditory meatus (Barany, 1938; Bekesy, 1932; Groen, 1962; Herzog & Krainz, 1926; Huizing, 1960; Kirikae, 1959).

1. COMPRESSIONAL MODE

Herzog and Krainz (1926) hypothesized that the cochlear capsule was alternately expanded and compressed in phase with the applied alternating force. An implication of this theory was that the round-window membrane, which is more compliant than the oval-window membrane, would bulge upon compression of the cochlear capsule (since the cochlear fluids are incompressible) and the basilar membrane would be deformed, leading to excitation of the sensory cells of the cochlea. Figure 5 illustrates compression of the inner ear and displacement of the basilar membrane according to this theory. Figure 5A shows that no basilar movement will occur if the compliance at both the round and oval windows is equal. Figure 5B shows that downward deformation will occur (compression of the cochlear capsule during the positive phase of the wave) if the round window is more compliant than the oval window. Figure 5C shows that the presence of the semicircular canals and vestibule near the oval window will increase the deformation shown in Figure 5B because there is also compression of the semicircular canals and vestibule, which forces more fluid against the basilar membrane. It was postulated that the contribution of the compressional mode was greatest at frequencies above 1500 Hz.

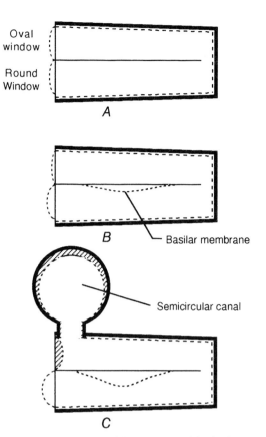

Figure 5 Compression of the inner ear and the displacement of the basilar membrane. The broken lines indicate the position of the various membranes during compression. (A) shows a hypothetical case of equal yielding at both windows, symmetrical compression, and no movement of the basilar membrane. The round window actually yields more than the oval window (B), and the compression is nonsymmetrical, leading to a downward displacement of the basilar membrane. Since semicircular canals are also compressed (C), more fluid is forced into the upper canal, and the basilar membrane is forced downward even more. Reprinted with permission from Bekesy and Rosenblith (1958).

2. INERTIAL–OSSICULAR MODE

Barany (1938) reported that, because the ossicles are loosely coupled to the skull, vibration of the temporal bone will not cause simultaneous vibration of the ossicles. The ossicles lag behind the movement of the temporal bone. During outward movement of the middle-ear walls, which are part of the skull, the ossicles will be essentially at rest, so force is exerted against the oval window, which has approached the stapes, leading to cochlear stimulation in the same manner as that produced by an air-conducted stimulus. Figure 6 illustrates the inertial component of bone conduction. The inertial component has its greatest contribution below 800 Hz.

3. EXTERNAL-CANAL MODE

Tonndorf (1968) provided the explanation for the external-canal component of bone conduction in order to

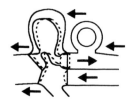

A. During lateral movement of
    the temporal bone, inertial lag
    of the ossicular chain results in
    a relative inward movement of
    the stapes footplate.

B. Medial movement of
    the temporal bone. Inertial lag
    of the ossicular chain
    result in an outward
    movement of the stapes,
    with respect to the temporal
    bone.

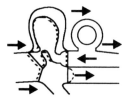

C. During air conduction the
    compressional wave results in
    a medial movement of the stapes
    footplate. The effect is the
    same as the inward movement
    produced by the inertial lag as in A.

D. A rarefaction wave results in
    lateral movement of the stapes
    footplate. The effect is the same
    as that produced by inertial lag,
    as in B.

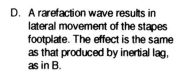
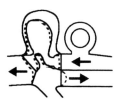

Figure 6 Bone conduction produced by inertial lag of the ossicular chain. Reprinted with permission from Zemlin (1988).

account for the occlusion effect, in which low-frequency bone-conducted signals are perceived as louder when the ear canal is occluded than when it is unoccluded. When a signal is introduced to a skull through an oscillator, the osseous and cartilaginous walls of the external auditory meatus vibrate with the skull. As a result, sound energy is radiated into the space within the external auditory meatus. Some of this energy is transmitted through the ear to the cochlea. If the ear canal is unoccluded, the ear canal acts as a high-pass filter. If the canal is occluded, the high-pass filter effect is eliminated so low-frequency transmission is improved.

4. Modern Theory

Tonndorf conducted a number of experimental animal studies on bone conduction between 1961 and 1964. Based on the results of these studies, Tonndorf (1966, 1968, 1972) introduced a new theory of the mechanism of bone conduction. Tonndorf questioned the validity of the compressional component since occlusion of both the round and oval windows did not significantly affect bone-conduction hearing. He proposed that the inner ear contributes to bone-conduction hearing

through a distortional rather than a compressional mechanism.

In the distortional mechanism, the shape of the cochlear capsule changes in synchrony with the applied alternating force. This theory does not require the presence of cochlear windows which differ in compliance. If the scala tympani and scala vestibuli are equal in volume, then the distortional vibrations cannot change the ratio of the scala vestibuli volume to the scala tympani volume and the basilar membrane will not be deformed. Since the scala vestibuli has a larger volume than the scala tympani, distortional vibrations will alter the volume ratio between the two scalae leading to deformation of the basilar membrane. Figure 7 illustrates the effect of distortional vibrations on the cochlear partition.

Tonndorf (1966, 1968, 1972) concluded that the outer ear, through the external-canal component, the middle ear, through the inertial-ossicular component, and the inner ear, through the distortional component, contribute together as a single unit for hearing by bone conduction. All operate throughout the frequency range although at a given frequency, one component may be predominant, as illustrated in Figure 8.

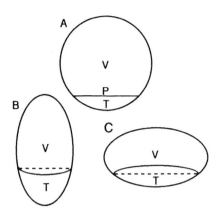

Figure 7 Distortional vibrations of the cochlear shell and their effect upon the instantaneous position of the basilar membrane (schematic). The shell undergoes periodic changes in shape. The three instances shown are 90° apart in phase, the sequence being A-B-A-C-A-B- . . . . If the cochlear partition (P) were dividing the entire space into two perilymphatic scalae of equal size, the ratio of their cross-sectional areas would remain unaltered at all times, and no displacement of the partition would ensue. However, when scala tympani (T) is smaller than scala vestibuli (V), the following is seen to happen. (The drawing overstates this case considerably.) At instant C, the area T becomes relatively smaller (it tends toward zero). At instant B it becomes relatively larger. Since the slice of fluid bounded within T cannot change its volume, the partition must be displaced in the manner indicated. Note the asymmetry of the positive and negative displacements (larger in C than in B). The resulting distortion (prominent 2nd harmonic) was actually observed in the model experiments in a correct phase relationship re the displacement of the partition. Reprinted with permission from Tonndorf (1964).

B. ARTIFICIAL MASTOID

In order to calibrate bone-conduction vibrators, the output of the bone vibrator should be measured in a device resembling the average human head with respect to its mechanical impedance characteristics. Under these conditions, it is assumed that the force developed at the output of such a mechanical device is equal to the force at the output of the

skull to the cochlea. Such devices are known as artificial mastoids.

The specification of the mechanical impedance of such devices was put forward by the International Electrotechnical Commission (Recommendation 373, 1971) and the American National Standards Institute (S3.13–1972). These specifications were based on the characteristics of the mechanical impedance of the human mastoid described by Dadson, Robinson, and Grieg (1954) and Corliss and Koidan (1955).

Until recently, two artificial mastoids—the Beltone Model 5A and the Bruel and Kjaer Model 4930—were commercially available in the United States and one artificial mastoid, which was developed in accordance with the British Standard 4009 (1966), was commercially available in Europe. The Beltone Model 5A was developed by Weiss (1960) and the Bruel and Kjaer Model 4930 was developed by Stisen and Dahm (1969). Currently only the Bruel and Kjaer Model 4930 artificial mastoid is commercially available and used for bond conduction calibration in the United States and Europe. According to Dirks, Lybarger, Olsen, and Billings (1979) and Dirks (1985), however, no available artificial mastoid meets the ANSI S3.13–1972 and IEC 373 (1971) specifications.

ficial mastoids have been put forward by the American National Standards Institute (S3.13–1987).

C. BONE VIBRATOR

The currently available bone-vibrator headband assemblies include the Radioear B-71 and B-72 developed in the United States and the Oticon A-20 and Pracitronic KH-70 developed in Europe. The Radioear B-71 is shown in Figure 9 and the Pracitronic KH-70 is shown in Figure 10. The Radioear B70A is no longer in use. The Radioear B-71 and Pracitronic KH-70 are used more frequently than Radioear B-72 and Oticon A-20. The Pracitronic KH-70 is used for high-frequency bone-conduction audiometry to 16,000 Hz. Both IEC 373 (1971) and ANSI S3.13-1972

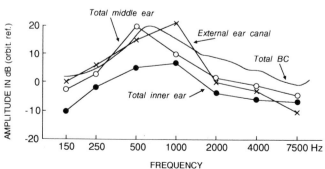

Figure 8 The frequency response curve of the three bone conduction (BC) components derived in the external canal, the middle ear, and the cochlea. The response of the whole ear is also shown. Data derived from experiments in cats. Reprinted with permission from Tonndorf (1968).

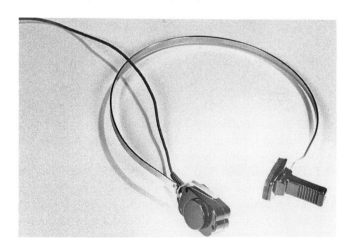

Figure 9 Radioear B-71 bone vibrator.

Page 21, second column, third paragraph should read in its entirety "New specifications of the mechanical impedance of artificial mastoids have been put forward by the American National Standards Institute (S3. 13-1987)."

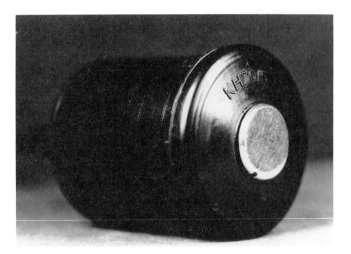

Figure 10 Pracitronic KH 70 bone vibrator. Courtesy of Thomas Frank.

Table III Mastoid RMS Force Levels

Frequency (Hz)	Beltone M5A artificial mastoid[b] (dB/1 dyne)	B & K 4930 artificial mastoid[c] (dB/1 dyne)
250	43	41.4
500	37.5	30.7
750	29	19.3
1000	23	16.9
1500	20.5	15.4
2000	20	8.1
3000	10.5	6.6
4000	15	11.2

[a] Reprinted with permission from Hodgson (1980).
[b] Lybarger (1966).
[c] Wilber (1972).

specify that bone vibrators must have a circular contact tip area of 1.75 cm² and are to be coupled to the head with a static force of 5.5 newtons (N) or ~550 gm/weight. The procedure for calibration of a bone vibrator with an artificial mastoid is discussed in the Appendix .

D. REFERENCE LEVELS

The Hearing Aid Industry Conference (HAIC) gathered data on the normal-hearing bone-conduction threshold levels (in force units). The data were obtained using the Beltone M5A artificial mastoid and were applicable for the Sonotone B-9 and Radioear B70A bone vibrators placed on the mastoid process. Lybarger (1966) published the mean data collected from eight laboratories. These values were known as the HAIC interim bone-conduction thresholds. The Lybarger (1966) norms were incorporated in the ANSI S3.13–1972 standard values for normal-hearing bone-conduction thresholds.

Since the Bruel and Kjaer Model 4930 (B & K 4930) artificial mastoid was developed in 1969, after the Lybarger norms were published in 1966, and has a lower mechanical impedance and different force response than the Beltone M5A artificial mastoid, the normal-hearing bone-conduction threshold values (in force units) for the B & K 4930 are slightly different from those for the Beltone M5A artificial mastoid. Table III shows the force values for the Beltone M5A (values reported by Lybarger, 1966, using the Sonotone B-9 and Radioear B70A bone vibrators) and B & K 4930 (values reported by Wilber, 1972, using the Radioear B70A bone vibrator) artificial mastoids.

Dirks, Lybarger, Olsen, and Billings (1979) specified the normal threshold sensitivity by bone conduction based on the results obtained on a group of 60 young, otologically normal listeners. The data were collected from three laboratories which used the (then) most recent version of the B &

K 4930 artificial mastoid and the B-71 bone vibrator. The newer version of the B & K 4930 had new pads which increased the uniformity of the mechanical impedances among the units. The B-71 bone vibrator was used since comparison of the 870A, B-71, and B-72 output levels revealed greater agreement among the three laboratories with the B-71 bone vibrator and since the B70A had a contact area larger than that recommended in the standards. Support for the use of the B-71 rather than the B-72 also comes from the study by Richards and Frank (1982), who found that the maximal output voltage variations of the artificial mastoid were smaller for the B-71 than B-72 bone vibrator. The mean values, rounded off to the nearest half-decibel, were incorporated in the ANSI S3.26–1981 standard specifying force values for normal threshold sensitivity by bone conduction using the B-71 bone vibrator. (See Table V in the Appendix for the ANSI S3.26–1981 specifications for reference equivalent threshold force levels for audiometric bone vibrators for mastoid placement.) Frank, Byrne, and Richards (1988) reported that, for their sample of 100 subjects, the reference equivalent threshold force levels differed among the B-71, B-72, and KH-70 bone vibrators. Therefore, Frank *et al.* (1988) recommended that the bone-vibrator type should be specified in bone-conduction studies.

Frank and Crandell (1986) found that the B-71 bone vibrator produced 4.3 dB of acoustic radiation (occluded bone-conduction threshold minus the unoccluded bone-conduction threshold) whereas the B-72 produced 8.3 dB of acoustic radiation, on average. They contended that ANSI S3.26–1981 did not take into account the effect of acoustic radiation when specifying the reference force levels at 4000 Hz for the B-71 bone vibrator. The newest standard, ISO DIS 7566 (1987), only partially considers the influence of acoustic radiation at 4000 Hz and the reference level is approximately 4 dB higher at 4000 Hz than the ANSI S3.26–1981 standard.

Table IV ISO DIS 7566 (1987) Specifications for the Reference Equivalent Threshold Force Levels (RETFLs) Referenced to 1 μN for Location of the Vibrator on the Mastoid Bone Based on a Combined Study Using the B-71 and KH 70 Bone Vibrators with the Mechanical Output Measured on a B & K 4930 Artificial Mastoid

	Frequency (Hz)							
	250	500	750[a]	1000	1500[a]	2000	3000	4000
RETFL[b]	67.0	58.0	48.5	42.5	36.5	31.0	30.0	35.5

[a] Values at these frequencies are derived from the results in one country only.
[b] Values rounded to the nearest 0.5 dB.

Table IV shows the ISO DIS 7566 (1987) specifications for normal-hearing threshold sensitivity by bone conduction based on data collected using the B-71 and KH-70 bone vibrators and calibrated with the B & K 4930 artificial mastoid. These specifications concur with ISO DIS 7566 (1987). Comparison of Table V in the Appendix and Table IV in this chapter reveals noticeable differences in the reference equivalent threshold force levels between the ANSI S3.26–1981 and ISO DIS 7566 (1987) specifications. Dirks and his colleagues are now completing the development of new ANSI specifications for normal-hearing threshold sensitivity by bone conduction based on the data collected in the United States and Europe after 1981 using the B & K 4930 artificial mastoid. D. D. Dirks (personal communication, 1991) stated that their findings concur with the ISO DIS 7566 (1987) specifications.

Even after the ANSI specifications now being developed by Dirks and his colleagues are published, new specifications for normal-hearing sensitivity by bone conduction have to be developed in accordance with the ANSI S3.13–1987 specifications for artificial mastoids. In the interim, D. D. Dirks (personal communication, 1991) suggests the use of the ANSI S3.26–1981 standard specifying force values for normal-hearing threshold sensitivity by bone conduction using the B-71 bone vibrator and the B & K 4930 artificial mastoid.

E. VIBRATOR PLACEMENT

Bone-conduction measurements are made with the bone vibrator at the mastoid process of the temporal bone or on the frontal bone. As noted by Dirk (1985), early investigators advocated the use of the frontal-bone placement for the following reasons.

1. Several investigators (Bekesy, 1932; Hart & Naunton, 1961; Studebaker, 1962a) reported that intrasubject variability is smaller with forehead than mastoid placement because the forehead has a more homogeneous surface and a lower degree of pneumatization than the mastoid process. More recent studies on bone vibrators with large contact areas have

failed to reveal significant intrasubject variability differences between forehead and mastoid placement (Dirks, 1964).

2. The intersubject variability is slightly smaller at the forehead than the mastoid because the forehead has a more homogeneous surface and a lower degree of pneumatization than the mastoid process (Dirks, 1964; Studebaker, 1962a).

3. The frontal-bone placement measurement excludes the contribution of the middle-ear inertial-ossicular component of bone conduction, in contrast with mastoid placement. In some cases of middle-ear pathology, such as otitis media and otosclerosis, the elevation of the bone-conduction thresholds (sensorineural component) will be less for mastoid than for forehead placement because of the loss of the inertial-ossicular component. Studebaker (1962a) and Dirks and Malmquist (1969) reported that the average threshold difference between the forehead and mastoid placements was approximately 5 dB. Dirks and Malmquist (1969), however, observed that the average threshold difference between the forehead and mastoid placement exceeded 10 dB in certain patients with middle-ear pathology.

The major disadvantage of frontal placement for bone-conduction testing is the reduced sensitivity at this site when compared with the mastoid site. More vibratory energy is required to reach threshold at the forehead than at the mastoid site. Therefore, the dynamic range is smaller at the frontal than at the mastoid site (Dirks, 1985; Naunton, 1963; Studebaker, 1962a).

Table VI in the Appendix shows the ANSI S3.26–1981 constants to be added to the mastoid reference equivalent threshold force levels (Table V in the Appendix) to yield the forehead reference equivalent threshold force levels for audiometric bone vibrators.

We recommend the use of mastoid placement over forehead placement because the reference levels in ANSI S3.26–1981 are based on mastoid placement and the dynamic range is larger for mastoid than forehead placement. Nevertheless, in some cases of middle-ear pathology, when bone-conduction thresholds measured using mastoid placement are elevated, the clinician may desire to obtain the forehead as well as the mastoid bone-conduction thresholds, in order to attempt to measure the size of the "artificial" sensorineural component.

F. ACOUSTIC RADIATION

Acoustic radiation is the sound energy leakage from the bone vibrator that is heard by air conduction. Significant acoustic radiation can result in a spuriously low bone-conduction threshold, leading to an artifactual air–bone gap, particularly at the high frequencies, in patients without middle-ear impairment or collapsing ear canals (Bell, Goodsell, & Thornton, 1980; Frank & Crandell, 1986;

Frank & Holmes, 1981; Shipton, John, & Robinson, 1980).

Several studies (Bell *et al.*, 1980; Frank & Holmes, 1981; Shipton *et al.*, 1980) reported that acoustic radiation was greatest at 4000 Hz. Acoustic radiation was measured by subtracting the unoccluded bone-conduction threshold from the occluded bone-conduction threshold. Bell *et al.* (1980), Frank & Holmes (1981), and Shipton *et al.* (1980) recommended eliminating the acoustic-radiation effect by occluding the ear canal with an earplug at frequencies above 2000 Hz during bone-conduction measurement.

As mentioned earlier, ANSI 3.26–1981 did not consider the effect of acoustic radiation in their specifications for the reference bone-conduction thresholds obtained with the B-71 bone vibrator. Similarly, the ISO DIS 7566 (1987) standard, which is based on three international studies using the B-71 and Pracitronic KH-70 bone vibrator, did not entirely eliminate the effect of acoustic radiation because one of the three studies was not done with the ear canal occluded (ipsilateral to the placement of the bone vibrator).

Frank and Crandell (1986) measured the acoustic radiation at 4000 Hz produced by B-71, B-72, and East German Pracitronic KH-70 bone vibrators. The acoustic radiation produced, on average, was 8.3 dB for the B-72, 4.3 dB for the B-71, and −0.3 dB for the KH-70. The range for the B-71 bone vibrator was −2.8 to +10.1 dB at the test and −3.7 to +10.2 at the retest. Greater than 5 dB of acoustic radiation was obtained for approximately 80% of the subjects with the B-72, for approximately 38% of the subjects with the B-71, and for approximately 8% of the subjects with the KH-70 bone vibrator. The differences in acoustic radiation among the bone vibrators was statistically significant. The results revealed that acoustic radiation was highest with the B-72 and negligible with the KH-70 bone vibrator, which is housed in cylindrical rubber.

In Appendix D of ANSI S3.26–1981, it is suggested (for informational purposes only) that occluded (with a small insert-type ear protector) as well as unoccluded bone-conduction thresholds be obtained to rule out the effect of acoustic radiation at 3000 and 4000 Hz. If occluded bone-conduction thresholds are obtained at 4000 Hz, then the ANSI S3.26–1981 reference levels underestimate the bone-conduction threshold measured with a B-71 bone vibrator by approximately 4 dB. Although the ISO DIS 7566 (1987) reference level is higher than the ANSI reference level at 4000 Hz by 4 dB, factors other than acoustic radiation accounted for this higher bone-conduction reference level. We support the recommendation of Frank and Crandell (1986) to occlude the better ear or both ears with an earplug during bone-conduction testing at frequencies above 2000 Hz if the air–bone gap exceeds 10 dB when the other

audiologic and acoustic-immittance data fail to reveal the presence of a middle-ear component.

G. EFFECT OF MIDDLE-EAR PATHOLOGY ON BONE-CONDUCTION THRESHOLDS

In some cases of middle-ear pathology, the bone-conduction thresholds may be either increased or decreased.

1. OSSICULAR FIXATION

The bone-conduction threshold is often elevated at frequencies around 2000 Hz in patients with ossicular fixation; this elevation is referred to as the Carhart notch (Carhart, 1950). The elevation occurs because of the loss of the middle-ear inertial-ossicular component of bone conduction. The Carhart notch occurs at approximately 2000 Hz since, in humans, the ossicular chain resonates at 2000 Hz. The classical Carhart notch usually shows a bone-conduction threshold of approximately 15 dB HL. Figure 11 shows an audiogram for a patient with early otosclerosis who demonstrates the classical Carhart notch.

Often, as otosclerosis advances, the air-conduction thresholds continue to increase whereas the bone-conduction thresholds remain essentially unchanged (with the classical Carhart notch) from the levels seen in early otosclerosis. This pattern is revealed in Figure 12, which shows an audiogram for a patient with advanced otosclerosis. Carhart (1962) reported that, in unusual cases of advanced otosclerosis, the bone-conduction threshold in the Carhart notch can be as great as 40 dB, as shown in Figure 13. Carhart (1962) contended that the sharply depressed bone-conduction threshold at 2000 Hz reflected the loss of

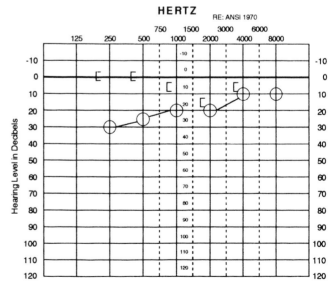

Figure 11 Audiogram for a patient with early otosclerosis who demonstrates the Carhart notch. Adapted from Carhart (1962).

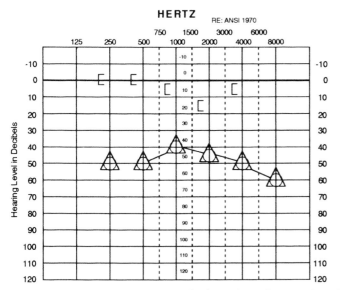

Figure 12 Audiogram for a patient with advanced otosclerosis. Adapted from Carhart (1962).

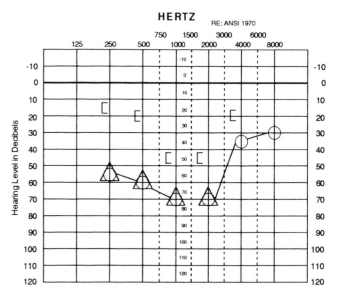

Figure 14 Audiogram for a patient with advanced otosclerosis in which the bone-conduction threshold elevation reveals a true sensorineural component. Adapted from Carhart (1962).

the middle-ear contribution in advanced otosclerosis if the air-conduction configuration was not parallel to the bone-conduction configuration, and reflected a true sensorineural component in advanced otosclerosis if the air-conduction configuration was parallel to the bone-conduction configuration. Figure 14 illustrates an audiogram for a patient with advanced otosclerosis in which the bone-conduction elevation reveals a true sensorineural component.

If the increased bone-conduction threshold around 2000 Hz is associated with the loss of the inertial-ossicular com-

ponent in bone conduction, then surgery may bring the bone-conduction threshold to within normal limits.

An increase in bone-conduction threshold, similar to that obtained in otosclerosis (Carhart notch), has been reported for some cases of radical mastoidectomy (Bekesy, 1939; Tonndorf, 1966).

2. OTITIS MEDIA

Several investigators observed that, in some cases of otitis media, the bone-conduction thresholds are decreased at the low frequencies and increased at the high frequencies (Huizing, 1964; Hulka, 1941; Naunton & Fernandez, 1961; Paparella, Morizono, Le, Mancini, Sipila, Choo, Liden, & Kim, 1984). According to Huizing (1964), Hulka (1941), and Naunton and Fernandez (1961), the alteration in bone-conduction threshold is related to resonance changes because of mass loading of the middle-ear system. This hypothesis is supported by the results of experimental studies involving the loading of the tympanic membrane in animals (Abu-Jaudeh, 1964; Allen & Fernandez, 1960; Barany, 1938; Brinkmann, Marres, & Tolk, 1965; Kirikae, 1959; Legouix & Tarab, 1959; Rytzner, 1954; Tonndorf, 1966) and humans (Huizing, 1960; Kirikae, 1959). Paparella *et al.* (1984) contended that, in cases of high-frequency conductive hearing loss in persons with acute purulent otitis media or chronic suppurative otitis media, the alteration in bone-conduction threshold resulted not only from mechanical factors associated with mass loading of the middle-ear system, but also from temporary or permanent threshold shifts associated with the passage of inflammatory agents through the round window.

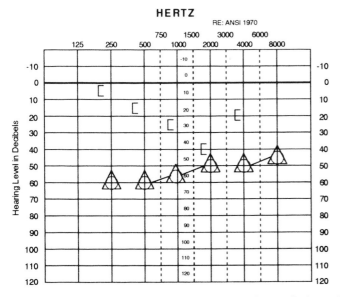

Figure 13 Audiogram for a patient with an unusual case of advanced otosclerosis. Note that the bone-conduction threshold at 2000 Hz (Carhart notch) is 40 dB HL. Adapted from Carhart (1962).

H. TACTILE BONE-CONDUCTION THRESHOLDS

Bone-conduction thresholds obtained at the upper limits of the audiometer at 250 and 500 Hz are occasionally tactile rather than auditory responses. Nober (1970) found that some patients with severe hearing loss feel the vibrations of the bone vibrator and respond to the vibrations rather than to the auditory sensation resulting in an artifactual bone-conduction threshold. Similar findings were obtained by Martin and Wittich (1966). When bone-conduction thresholds are present near the limits of the audiometer, the clinician must rule out the possibility of tactile responses by asking the patient directly whether the stimulus was heard or felt and by considering the other audiologic, acoustic-immittance, and otolaryngologic findings.

I. HIGH-FREQUENCY BONE-CONDUCTION THRESHOLDS

There is very little research on high-frequency bone-conduction hearing sensitivity. High-frequency bone-conduction thresholds have been obtained using mastoid placement of a specially constructed piezoelectric bone vibrator referenced in sound-pressure level (Corso, 1964) and referenced in acceleration levels (Bednin & Sagalovich, 1976) and using electrostimulation through an electrode-type transducer (Tonndorf & Kurman, 1984; Tonndorf, 1985).

Richter and Frank (1985) found stable mechanical impedance curves and force sensitivity curves for the B & K 4930 artificial mastoid up to 16000 Hz. They also measured the frequency response curves between 8000 and 16000 Hz for several electromagnetic-type bone vibrators calibrated with the B & K 4930 artificial mastoid. They found that all the bone vibrators, except the Atlas K and Pracitronic KH-70 bone vibrators, had poor test–retest reliability. Since the Pracitronic KH-70 had a higher output than the Atlas K for the same input voltage, Richter and Frank (1985) recommended the use of the Pracitronic KH-70 for high-frequency bone-conduction audiometry.

Frank and Ragland (1987) evaluated the test–retest reliability of high-frequency bone-conduction thresholds between 8000 and 16000 Hz using the Pracitronic KH-70 bone vibrator calibrated with a B & K 4930 artificial mastoid. The pure-tone stimuli were generated from an oscillator monitored by a frequency counter. The results, obtained on a group of 30 subjects with normal hearing thresholds between 250 and 8000 Hz, revealed that the initial bone-conduction thresholds were not significantly different from the retest bone-conduction thresholds, regardless of whether or not the bone vibrator was replaced at the re-peat session. Future research is needed to assess the relation between high-frequency air-conduction and bone-conduction thresholds within a given subject, to determine whether masking for high-frequency bone conduction is needed, and to develop a bone vibrator with a higher output level than the KH-70, particularly at 16000 Hz (Frank & Ragland, 1987). If such data are established and the clinical utility of high-frequency bone-conduction thresholds is demonstrated, commercially available clinical high-frequency audiometers are needed (Frank & Ragland, 1987).

J. PROCEDURE

The procedure for bone-conduction measurement is similar to that for air-conduction measurement described earlier in this chapter. Bone-conduction measurement is done after air-conduction measurement. The order of frequencies for bone-conduction testing is 1000, 2000, 4000, 500, and 250 Hz. Measurement of the bone-conduction thresholds at the interoctaves is not essential, even when more than a 15-dB difference exists between octaves, since bone-conduction thresholds are obtained for diagnostic purposes rather than for the purpose of evaluating hearing sensitivity by bone conduction. If the mastoid site is used, the clinician should make certain that the bone vibrator does not touch the pinna, thereby causing sound transmission into the ear canal.

K. TUNING-FORK TESTS

The two major tuning-fork tests that have the most relevance for audiologic testing are the Rinne test and the Weber test. These tests can be administered using a tuning fork or a bone vibrator.

1. RINNE TEST

The Rinne test is based on the concept that patients with a conductive hearing impairment will hear better by bone than by air conduction and patients with sensorineural hearing impairment will hear better by air than by bone conduction. A tone, usually at 500 Hz, is presented using a bone vibrator or tuning fork. The tone is alternated quickly between the mastoid and at the entrance to the ear canal. The patient's task is to indicate whether the tone is louder at the ear canal or mastoid. If the tone is louder at the ear canal (air conduction), the result is considered a positive Rinne. A positive Rinne indicates that the test ear is normal hearing or sensorineural hearing impaired, since air conduction transmits sound more efficiently than bone conduction. A negative Rinne indicates that the test ear has a conductive hearing impairment, since bone conduction transmits sound more efficiently than air conduction. A false-negative

Rinne may occur when the nontest instead of the test ear responds. A false-negative Rinne may occur when the bone-conduction threshold of the nontest ear is better than that of the test ear. Since physicians usually do not employ masking during the Rinne test, the audiologist should consider the possibility of a false-negative Rinne when a negative Rinne is obtained. In our experience, a false-positive Rinne may result from ears with mild conductive hearing impairment; this has also been reported in the literature (Gelfand, 1977).

2. WEBER TEST

The procedure for the Weber test involves placement of the tuning fork or bone vibrator on the center of the forehead, the midline of the skull, or on the midline of the nasal bones, chin, or upper teeth. The audiometric Weber is usually done at the center of the forehead. The subject's task is to indicate in which ear the sound is heard. If the tone is heard in the middle of the head, is equally loud at the two ears, or the patient cannot determine where the tone is heard, the result is considered to be consistent with normal hearing bilaterally or bilaterally symmetrical air- and bone-conduction thresholds (mixed, conductive, or sensorineural). Lateralization to the better ear (as evidenced by the air-conduction thresholds) indicates that there is a sensorineural hearing impairment in the poorer ear or that the poorer ear has a conductive hearing impairment with a bone-conduction threshold that is worse than the threshold of the better ear. Lateralization to the poorer ear (as evidenced by the air-conduction thresholds) indicates that there is a conductive hearing impairment in the poorer ear.

The mechanism for lateralization to the better ear when there is a sensorineural hearing impairment in the poorer ear reflects the Stenger phenomenon. The Stenger phenomenon states that when two tones of equal frequency are presented simultaneously to the two ears, the tone will be heard only in the ear which it is louder.

Several theories have been proposed to account for lateralization to the poorer ear when there is a conductive hearing impairment in the poorer ear. In cases of middle-ear effusion, the resonant frequency of the middle ear shifts downward because the middle ear is a mass-loaded system. Therefore, the sound will be louder in the ear with a resonant frequency that is shifted downward, that is, the ear with middle-ear effusion. According to Tonndorf (1964), cases of ossicular discontinuity and ossicular fixation are characterized by phase advances so the sound will be louder in the ear with the phase advance. We hypothesize that, in cases of ossicular discontinuity, the middle-ear system is mass loaded so there is a downward shift in resonant frequency. In cases with impacted ear canals, an occlusion effect may occur, causing the sound to be louder in the impacted ear.

IV. VARIABLES AFFECTING PURE-TONE AIR- AND BONE-CONDUCTION MEASUREMENT

A. PATIENT VARIABLES

1. COLLAPSED EAR CANALS

In some patients, particularly the elderly, when the earphones are placed on the head, the pressure from the earphones causes ear-canal collapse because of decreased skin elasticity in the cartilaginous part of the external auditory meatus. This results in a high-frequency conductive hearing loss and lack of test–retest reliability. The phenomenon of the collapsed ear canal was first reported by Ventry, Chaiklin, and Boyle (1961). There is a controversy regarding the prevalence of collapsed ear canals. On the one hand, Randolph and Schow (1983) reported that 36% of a group elderly listeners between 60 and 79 years old had collapsed canals and Schow and Goldbaum (1980) reported that the prevalence rate is higher in nursing homes. On the other hand, Marshall, Martinez, and Schlaman (1983) found that none of their elderly patients had collapsed canals. The problem of collapsed ear canals during audiometric testing can be alleviated by using insert earphones, canal-retaining earphones, soundfield testing, or pulling the pinna up and back prior to earphone placement (Maurer & Rupp, 1979). A screening procedure to detect the presence of collapsed canals involves getting the thresholds at 4000 Hz with the jaw closed and then with the jaw wide open (Reiter, Letzer, & Silman, 1984). If a discrepancy exists between these thresholds, one of the previously mentioned procedures to alleviate the collapsed ear-canal problem should be used. As mentioned earlier in this chapter, high-frequency air–bone gaps are also associated with ear pathology or technical factors such as acoustic radiation in bone-conduction measurement.

2. STANDING WAVES

The average length of the ear canal is approximately 1.5 inches. The wavelength of an 8000 Hz tone is also approximately 1.5 inches. When an 8000-Hz tone is delivered via the earphone into the ear canal, and the distance between the tympanic membrane and the earphone diaphragm is approximately 1.5 inches, the reflected wave from the tympanic membrane will be 180° out of phase with the incident wave and cancellation of the sound will result in persons in whom the distance between the tympanic membrane and the earphone diaphragm is 1.5 inches. We have observed that standing waves occur more frequently in children than in adults and may also occur at 6000 Hz. Whenever there is a disparity between the 4000 and 6000 or 8000 Hz thresholds, the presence of standing waves should be suspected and the clinician should readjust the earphones. If there is improvement in threshold at 8000 or 6000 Hz when the earphone is readjusted, the disparity resulted from standing waves. If no improvement occurs, the disparity is a true reflection of the person's hearing sensitivity.

3. FALSE RESPONSES

There are two types of false responses—false positives and false negatives. False positives (false alarms) occur when the patient signals that a tone is heard when in fact no tone was presented. False negatives occur when the patient indicates that no tone was heard when in fact, the tone was presented at a level that is audible to the patient. False positives occur in many patients with tinnitus and in patients who are anxious to respond. False-positive responses should be disregarded if they occur infrequently.

If the false-positive responses occur frequently, the following procedures can be employed to reduce the number of false alarms. (a) The clinician should reinstruct the patient and tell them they are responding when there is no sound. (b) The clinician should use the descending approach to threshold measurement. (c) The interstimulus interval should be varied more significantly. (d) The patient should count the number of pulses in a pulsed tone. (e) Warble tones should be employed.

If there are false-negative responses, the patient should be reinstructed and alerted to the signals. Alerting the patient to the signal is often necessary to increase attention to the task, especially in the case of distractible and very young children, elderly persons, and sick people. If reinstruction and alerting fail to eliminate the false-negative responses, the possibility of functional hearing loss (see Chapter 4) should be suspected. A descending approach can be used if the clinician suspects lack of attention as the cause of false-negative responses. An ascending approach can be employed when functional hearing loss is suspected to be the cause of the false-negative responses.

4. PATHOLOGY

Some patients with marked adaptation associated with retrocochlear pathology will display large intrasubject variability in thresholds. When the clinician suspects marked adaptation associated with retrocochlear pathology, the following modifications can be employed: (a) the use of short stimulus durations, (b) the use of lengthened interstimulus intervals, and (c) the use of an ascending approach to threshold measurement.

In some patients with mastoid abnormalities, good bone-vibrator placement may be difficult. In such cases, the clinician should place the vibrator on the better mastoid or move the bone vibrator around the mastoid process with the tone continuously on until a site is reached where the tone is loudest.

In some elderly patients, the mastoid process may be ossified, possibly leading to bone-conduction thresholds that are more than 15 dB poorer than the air-conduction thresholds at the low frequencies.

The effects of middle-ear pathology, such as ossicular fixation, otitis media, and radical mastoidectomy, on the bone-conduction thresholds have already been discussed.

B. INSTRUMENTATION AND ENVIRONMENTAL VARIABLES

1. EQUIPMENT OPERATION

Inaccurate thresholds can be obtained if the earphone plugs are not plugged into or are incompletely plugged into the correct jack, if there is excessive winding of the earphone leads, if the earphones are placed on the wrong ears, if the transducer and stimulus buttons on the audiometer are incorrect, and if the amplifiers have not been activated properly for soundfield testing. Clinicians should be especially suspicious of equipment problems in cases of asymmetrical or unilateral hearing, or when normal hearing thresholds are obtained despite the patient's report of a hearing loss.

Listening Check

In order to avoid inaccurate thresholds because of equipment problems, a listening check should be performed at the start of each testing day. A listening check is performed on a normal-hearing person by following this procedure.

1. The earphone cushions should be checked. They should not be hard and they should be free of cracks.
2. Check that the tension in the bone vibrator and earphone headband is adequate.
3. Check for loose dials on the audiometer.
4. Check for static or other noises on the earphone cords by flexing the earphone cords while a continuous tone is on at 1000 Hz at 40 dB HL. Do this first for one earphone and then the other. Then do this for the bone-vibrator cord.
5. Check for hum or other noises in the earphones by listening to the tone through one of the earphones at 1000 Hz at 90 dB. Also listen to the tone to check for distortions in tonal quality. Interrupt the signal and listen again for hum, clicks, or other noises. Do the same thing at 50 and then 0 dB HL. Repeat for the other earphone and then repeat for the bone vibrator using 70 dB HL as the highest intensity for the check.
6. Noise in the attenuator should be checked at 1000 Hz, for example, by setting the attenuator at the lowest level and then increasing slowly from minimum to maximum with the tone continuously on. The listener should check for noise or interruptions in the signal or decreases in loudness.
7. Check for gross linearity at 1000 Hz, for example, by setting the attenuator at 10 dB HL and then increasing in 10-dB steps up to 90 dB HL. The listener should determine whether the increases in

loudness are roughly equivalent from one 10 dB increment to the next. This should be done for both earphones and for the bone vibrator. (For the bone vibrator, the maximum intensity should be the output at the frequency tested.)

8. Check for crosstalk by disconnecting the earphone plug for the right earphone, applying a signal at 1000 Hz at 60 dB HL to the right earphone, and listening to the left earphone. The procedure should be repeated for the other earphone by disconnecting the plug for the left earphone, applying a signal at 1000 Hz at 50 dB HL to the left earphone, and listening to the right earphone. Although we recommend that all of these steps be done daily, the Professional Services Board of the American Speech–Language–Hearing Association (ASHA, 1978b) recommends that steps 5, 6, and 8 be done monthly.

2. TEMPERATURE AND VENTILATION

High temperatures exceeding 85°F and lack of ventilation in the booth can affect the accuracy of the pure-tone thresholds, especially in children (Wilber, 1979).

3. CALIBRATION

Lack of accuracy in the pure-tone thresholds can also stem from inadequate calibration. According to the Professional Services Board of the American Speech–Language–Hearing Association (ASHA, 1978b), electroacoustic calibration of sound-pressure levels for tones, masking noise, and speech under the earphones and in soundfield; attenuator linearity; and force levels for the bone vibrator should be done quarterly. The annual electroacoustic calibration should also include a frequency check with an electronic frequency counter, measurement of the rise and fall times, and measurement of the individual harmonics of each frequency with a distortion wave analyzer (ASHA, 1978b). (For a further discussion of the procedures for calibration, see the Appendix.)

4. AMBIENT NOISE

Ambient noise is another source of inaccuracy in audiometric measurement. The noise levels at each octave band should meet ANSI S3.1–1977 standards. Table V shows the maximum permissible noise levels at each octave band in the audiometric booth used for testing done to 0 dB HL in soundfield or by bone conduction (the criteria are stricter in soundfield or by bone conduction than they are under earphones).

C. CLINICIAN VARIABLES

Clinician variables that affect the accuracy of the pure-tone thresholds include the following.

1. *Earphone placement* The clinician should ensure that

Table V Maximum Permissible Sound-Pressure Levels for Ambient Noise during Audiometric Testing[a]

Frequency (Hz)	Ears uncovered		Ears covered	
	Octave band	1/3-octave band	Octave band	1/3-octave band
125	28.0	23.0	34.5	29.5
250	18.5	13.5	23.0	18.0
500	14.5	9.5	21.5	16.5
750	12.5	7.5	22.5	17.5
1000	14.0	9.0	29.5	24.5
1500	10.5	5.5	29.0	24.0
2000	8.5	3.5	34.5	29.5
3000	8.5	3.5	39.0	34.0
4000	9.0	4.0	42.0	37.0
6000	14.0	9.0	41.0	36.0
8000	20.5	15.5	45.0	40.0

[a] Values for ears not covered apply to bone-conduction and soundfield testing. Values for ears covered apply to air-conduction testing. Adapted from ANSI (1977).

the earphone diaphragm is against the entrance of the ear canal. The earphones must also fit snugly to reduce the problem of low-frequency leakage around the earphones.

2. *Bone-vibrator placement* As mentioned earlier, the bone vibrator must be placed on the mastoid process no closer than a thumb's width to prevent acoustic radiation.

3. *Visual clues* Visual clues, such as looking down or making certain body gestures everytime the tone is presented, relating to tonal presentation should not be given.

4. *Rapport with the patient* A friendly and understanding attitude increases the motivation of the patient.

5. *Instructions* Instructions should be clear and the clinician should check that the instructions are understood. The patient may need to listen to some tones or words before the test begins.

For further details on many of these variables, see the excellent discussion in Hannley (1986).

V. SPEECH-RECOGNITION THRESHOLD

The speech-recognition threshold (SRT) is the hearing threshold level for speech. It is an important tool serving many clinical purposes, such as (a) permitting the evaluation of the well-documented relation between speech and pure-tone sensitivity, thereby providing a check on the validity of the pure-tone thresholds essential for speech recognition (Carhart, 1952; Chaiklin & Ventry, 1964); (b) providing a reference intensity level for suprathreshold speech-recognition testing (ASHA, 1979; Wilson & Margolis, 1983); (c) providing an estimate of the hearing sensitivity in the speech-frequency range in difficult-to-test patients (e.g., mentally retarded and developmentally disabled) who cannot be conditioned to respond to pure-tone stimuli (ASHA, 1988; Wilson & Margolis, 1983); and (d) assessing amplification performance and monitoring progress in aural rehabilitation/habilitation (ASHA, 1979, 1988; Wilson & Margolis, 1983). The last purpose, unrelated to diagnostic audiology, is beyond the scope of this book.

A. TERMINOLOGY

1. SPEECH-RECOGNITION THRESHOLD

The SRT is the lowest hearing level at which a person correctly recognizes the speech stimuli 50% of the time. Usually, recognition is indicated by repetition of the speech-stimulus item. Terms other than "speech-recognition threshold" for reporting the speech threshold include spondee threshold and speech-reception threshold. The terms "speech-reception threshold" and "spondee threshold" have been used synonymously with "speech-recognition threshold." The term "spondee threshold" specifies the test material used and obviates the need for recording and reporting the type of test material used (ASHA, 1979). The term "speech-recognition threshold" rather than the terms "speech-reception threshold" and "spondee threshold" is recommended since the other terms do not specify the nature of the task—detection, recognition, or discrimination—performed by the listener (ASHA, 1988; Wilson & Margolis, 1983).

The most commonly employed and recommended speech stimuli for speech-recognition testing are spondaic words (ASHA, 1979, 1988; Wilson & Margolis, 1983). A spondaic word (spondee) is a bisyllabic word with equal stress on both syllables. If the test materials used are not spondaic words, the clinician should report the test material used (ASHA 1979, 1988).

2. SPEECH-DETECTION THRESHOLD

The speech-detection threshold (SDT) is the lowest hearing threshold level at which a person correctly detects the presence of a speech stimulus 50% of the time. The term "speech-awareness threshold" (SAT) has been used synonymously with SDT. SDT is preferred to SAT because the nature of the listener's task is more precisely specified with the former than the latter term.

B. HISTORY OF THE DEVELOPMENT OF THE SRT TEST MATERIALS

Fletcher and Steinberg (1929) and their colleagues at Bell Telephone Laboratories assessed the efficiency of speech transmission through communication systems such as the telephone. Fletcher and his colleagues referred to the speech-recognition score as the articulation score. They measured the articulation scores as a function of intensity level using consonant–vowel (CV) or consonant–vowel–consonant (CVC) monosyllables. The plot of these data was considered the articulation function.

Hudgins, Hawkins, Karlin, and Stevens (1947) developed phonographic recordings at the Harvard Psychoacoustic Laboratories of two spondaic-word lists, each list containing 42 spondees. These lists, the PAL Auditory Test No. 9, were used clinically for measuring the patient's speech threshold. The criteria employed to construct the spondaic-word lists developed by Hudgins et al. (1947) were (a) familiarity with respect to vocabulary; (b) phonetic dissimilarity, so one spondaic word would not be easily confused with another spondaic word; (c) normal sampling of English speech sounds, so the proportion of occurrence of the various speech sounds in everyday conversation is essentially the same as the proportion of occurrence of speech sounds in the spondaic-word list; and (d) homogeneity with respect to audibility, that is, the thresholds for the various spondaic words are obtained at essentially similar intensity levels and the articulation function for each spondaic word is steep.

Hirsh, Davis, Silverman, Reynolds, Eldert, and Benson (1952) improved the PAL test by restricting the vocabulary to include only the most familiar words and by increasing the homogeneity with respect to audibility. The most familiar of the PAL spondaic words were obtained from the ratings of the judges on a 3-point scale of familiarity. Homogeneity with respect to audibility was first improved by eliminating the "easy" words (words missed once or less by all listeners when the spondee lists were presented at +4, +2, 0, −2, −4, and −6 dB SL re: threshold for the PAL Test 9) and "hard" words (words missed five or more times by all listeners when the spondee lists were presented at +4, +2, 0, −2, −4, and −6 dB SL with respect to the threshold for the PAL Test 9). This process resulted in a list of 36 homogeneous spondaic words. A correspondence existed between the degree of difficulty of a spondaic word and the intensity reading of the word on a volume unit (VU) meter; the easier words were monitored at higher levels and the harder words were monitored at lower levels even though each word's intensity did not vary by more than ±2 dB from the average intensity. Therefore, the homogeneity was further improved by boosting the intensity of the hard words by 2 dB and decreasing the intensity of the easy words by 2 dB. Homogeneity is important because it improves the accuracy with which the SRT can be measured (Young, Dudley, & Gunter, 1982) and it reduces the number of test items needed to establish the SRT, thereby reducing test time (Olsen & Matkin, 1979). A final attempt at homogeneity by Hirsh et al. resulted in a list of 36 spondees and 6 scramblings (lists A–F) which comprised the C.I.D.

Table VI Alphabetical List of the Spondaic
Words Used in the Original CID W-1 and W-2
Tests[a]

1. airplane	19. iceberg
2. armchair	20. inkwell
3. baseball	21. mousetrap
4. birthday	22. mushroom
5. cowboy	23. northwest
6. daybreak	24. oatmeal
7. doormat	25. padlock
8. drawbridge	26. pancake
9. duckpond	27. playground
10. eardrum	28. railroad
11. farewell	29. schoolboy
12. grandson	30. sidewalk
13. greyhound	31. stairway
14. hardware	32. sunset
15. headlight	33. toothbrush
16. horseshoe	34. whitewash
17. hotdog	35. woodwork
18. hothouse	36. workshop

[a] Reprinted with permission from Hirsh *et al.* (1952).

Auditory Test W-1. Table VI shows the spondaic words in the C.I.D. Auditory Test W-1 list.

On the W-1 tape, a 1000-Hz calibration tone is recorded at the intensity level of the carrier phrase "Say the word . . .", which is 10 dB above the level of the test item. The calibration tone is calibrated to the carrier-phrase intensity rather than to the test-item intensity to prevent the indicator of the VU meter from pinning against the right side if the needle is monitored at zero during playback. "The talker monitored the carrier phrase 'Say the word . . .' carefully on a VU meter, and then spoke the following test word with 'equal effort' " (Hirsh *et al.*, 1952, p. 324). Egan (1948) felt that a carrier phrase was necessary to alert the patient to the fact that the test word would follow. Presenting the carrier phrase at an intensity 10 dB above that of the test item allows the patient to identify the space in which the test word occurs. The C.I.D. Auditory Test W-2 used the same words as the W-1 test but differed in intensity level. The intensity level of the taped W-2 words was attenuated by 3 dB after each group of three words, whereas the intensity of the taped W-1 words remained constant.

Bowling and Elpern (1961) obtained articulation functions for each of the spondaic words on the C.I.D. Auditory Test W-2 in 24 normal-hearing subjects. The results revealed a 10 dB range in thresholds (50% point on the psychometric function) for the individual spondaic words. Bowling and Elpern suggested that only the 22 spondaic words varying in threshold by only 3.5 dB be included in the spondaic-word list.

Curry and Cox (1966) also obtained articulation functions for the C.I.D. Auditory Test W-1 on a group of normal-hearing subjects. They found the range of thresh-

olds was 8 dB. The homogeneity was improved if a sub-sample of 27 of the 36 words was taken.

Beattie, Svihovec, and Edgerton (1975) identified a subsample of 18 spondaic words which had only a 1.5 dB range in thresholds. The slope of the 36-item list was 12% per decibel over the 20–80% range, compared with the 8% slope reported by Hirsh *et al.* (1952). Beattie *et al.* found a 7.6 dB difference between the mean SDT and the mean SRT based on the 36-item list.

According to Young *et al.* (1982), there is little agreement among the previous investigations on the homogeneity of the C.I.D. Auditory Test W-1 spondaic words. Agreement regarding homogeneity was obtained for only 4 of the 36 spondaic words. Young *et al.* (1982) contended that the previous studies were confounded by a learning effect, did not determine the rate at which the spondaic words became audible, and did not determine whether the SRT based on the subsample of homogeneous words was significantly different from that based on the entire 36-item list.

Young *et al.* (1982) overcame the methodologic limitations of the previous studies on homogeneity. They determined the sound-pressure level at which 50% intelligibility was obtained for each spondaic word and the percentage of listeners who correctly identified each spondaic word at each intensity level. Individual articulation functions were obtained for each spondaic word. The range of threshold levels was 6.4 dB. A spondaic word was considered homogeneous if its threshold was within one standard deviation of the mean SRT and had an equal rate of growth in intelligibility. Of the spondaic words, 15 met both criteria, and two randomizations of this homogeneous subgroup were developed. This subsample of homogeneous words is shown in Table VII. The test–retest reliability for the homogeneous subgroup was not significantly different from that derived from the full list ($r = 0.71$) and there was also no significant difference between the SRT obtained from the homogeneous group and that derived from the full list. Young *et al.* (1982) concluded that only 15 rather than 36 spondaic words need to be used to quickly and accurately measure the SRT. Moreover, "the use of these 15 spondaic words can be expected to minimize nonauditory factors such as memory, learning, and so on" (Young *et al.*, 1982, p. 592).

Table VII List of 15 Spondees That Are
Homogeneous in Terms of their Threshold
Intensities and the Slope of their Intelligibility
Function[a]

1. inkwell	6. grandson	11. playground
2. eardrum	7. sidewalk	12. toothbrush
3. railroad	8. northwest	13. woodwork
4. mousetrap	9. baseball	14. drawbridge
5. workshop	10. padlock	15. doormat

[a] Young *et al.* (1982).

C. RELATION BETWEEN THE SRT AND PURE-TONE AVERAGE

Fletcher (1929) reported that the average of the pure-tone thresholds at 512, 1024, and 2048 Hz could predict the speech sensitivity. Carhart (1946a) found a correlation of 0.69 between the Fletcher three-frequency pure-tone average (PTA) and the speech-recognition threshold. In another study on the relation between the SRT and three-frequency PTA, Carhart (1946b) reported that the correlation was 0.80 across all audiometric configurations, 0.79 for flat audiometric configurations, 0.75 for gradually sloping audiometric configurations, and 0.29 for markedly sloping audiograms. According to Fletcher (1950), the mean of the best two of the three thresholds at the speech frequencies (500, 1000, and 2000 Hz), correlated better with the SRT than the three-frequency PTA. Nevertheless, the three-frequency PTA adequately predicts the SRT in most cases, although it yields an exaggeratedly high estimate of the SRT in cases of high-frequency sloping audiometric configurations.

Harris, Haines, and Myers (1956) reported that the correlation between the predicted SRT for monosyllabic phonetically balanced (PB) words based on a multiple-regression formula involving the pure-tone thresholds and the actual SRT was 0.90; the standard error of measurement was 3.4 dB. Quiggle, Glorig, Delk, and Summerfield (1957) found the standard error of measurement, based on the use of a multiple-regression formula for the pure-tone audiogram, to be between 5.0 and 10.3 dB.

Carhart and Porter (1971) reported that the single frequency at which the pure-tone threshold best correlated with the SRT was 1000 Hz, except in cases with markedly sloping audiometric configurations. In our experience with the Veterans Administration population, the SRT may correlate best with 500 Hz in cases of precipitously sloping losses. Carhart (1971) recommended obtaining the average of the pure-tone thresholds at 500 and 1000 Hz and then subtracting 2 dB from this average to predict the SRT.

Graham (1960) found high correlations between the SRT and several measures of the pure-tone audiogram (three-frequency PTA, two-frequency PTA, Quiggle *et al.* multiple-regression formula, and the Zarcoff technique based on noise bands) and concluded that higher correlations were obtained with the two- or three-frequency PTA than the other methods. Siegenthaler and Strand (1964) evaluated the correlations between the SRT and the various audiogram-average methods. They found that the SRT correlated best with the two-frequency PTA overall. The method involving the multiplication of the mean of the pure-tone thresholds between 250 and 4000 Hz by 0.83, the two multiple-regression methods (Harris *et al.*, 1956, and Quiggle *et al.*, 1957), and the method involving the three-frequency PTA yielded correlations with the SRT that were nearly as high as that of the two-frequency PTA with the SRT. The audiogram-average methods yielding the poorest correlations with the SRT were the revised AMA method (AMA, 1947) and the Fowler (1942) method. Wilson, Morgan, and Dirks (1973) found small differences on the order of 0.3 to 3.1 dB between the various audiogram-average methods (three-frequency PTA, two-frequency PTA, and Carhart, 1971, mean based on 500 and 1000 Hz minus 2 dB) and the SRT. They also found high correlation coefficients (0.95 to 0.98) between the three audiogram-average methods and the SRT.

In summary, the three-frequency pure-tone average is a good predictor of the SRT except in cases of sharply sloping losses. In such cases of sharply sloping high-frequency hearing loss, the SRT is best predicted by the two-frequency average. In precipitously sloping audiometric configurations, the SRT may correlate best with the pure-tone threshold at 500 Hz.

Wilson and Margolis (1983) have noted that, because of the relation between the SRT and the PTA, many investigators refer to the frequencies on which the three-frequency pure-tone average is based as the "speech frequencies," leading many to the misconception that the frequencies above 2000 Hz and below 500 Hz are unimportant for speech recognition. Fletcher (1929) noted that frequencies above 3000 Hz are as important as frequencies below 1000 Hz for speech recognition. More recent research indicates that the frequencies between 4000 and 6000 Hz are important for consonant recognition (Bornstein and Randolph, 1983; Lawton & Cafarelli, 1978; Skinner & Miller, 1983; Skinner, Pascoe, Miller, & Popelka, 1982).

D. THE SRT–PTA AGREEMENT

According to Ventry and Chaiklin (1965), the SRT is compared with the three-frequency PTA when the speech-frequency thresholds do not differ by more than 5 dB. The SRT is compared with the two-frequency PTA when the thresholds at two of the speech frequencies differ by 10 dB or more. They considered the SRT to be in agreement with the PTA if there was less than a 12-dB difference between these measures; the SRT was considered to be in agreement with the PTA if there was not more than a 25-dB difference between these measures in cases of sharply sloping losses with at least a 25-dB drop in thresholds between 500 and 1000 Hz. (See Chapter 4 for further details concerning the SRT–PTA agreement.)

Reasons underlying an SRT–PTA discrepancy include (a) functional hearing loss (see Chapter 4 for further details), (b) audiologic instrumentation malfunction, (c) misunderstanding of the instructions by the patient, (d) pathology along the central auditory nervous system including the eighth cranial nerve, (e) developmental age, (f) irregular hearing sensitivity such as normal hearing at frequencies above 8000 Hz (Berlin, Wexler, Jerger, Halperin, & Smith, 1978) or significant hearing loss with an island of normal hearing (Roeser, 1982), (g) cognitive disorder, and (h) language disorder (ASHA, 1988). In cases of functional hearing loss or irregular hearing sensitivity, the SRT is better than would be predicted from the PTA. The other factors mentioned can yield an SRT which is substantially poorer than would be predicted from the PTA.

E. THE RELATION BETWEEN THE SRT AND SDT

Chaiklin (1959) and Thurlow, Silverman, Davis, and Walsh (1948) reported that the mean difference between the SRT and SDT is approximately 9 dB, with the SDT better than the SRT. Beattie, Svihovec, and Edgerton (1975) reported that the difference between the SRT and SDT was 7.6 dB for live-voice presentation of the speech stimuli. Thus, the SRT is approximately 8 to 9 dB higher than the SDT. According to Olsen and Matkin (1979), the SDT should be consistent with the best pure-tone threshold between 250 and 4000 Hz. The type of speech stimulus (e.g., running speech) employed is not as important a consideration for obtaining the SDT as it is for obtaining the SRT (ASHA, 1988). Nevertheless, the type of speech material used should be recorded on the audiogram form.

F. RECORDED VERSUS LIVE-VOICE PRESENTATION

The use of recorded speech standardizes the composition and presentation of the speech stimuli and controls for signal intensity. The disadvantages of recorded presentation include lack of flexibility, which may be important for the difficult-to-test population, and deterioration of phonographic and tape recordings resulting in signal distortion and the introduction of noise. The problems of signal distortion and the introduction of noise can be averted with digitized recordings (ASHA, 1979, 1988).

The advantage of live voice is the flexibility in presentation of the stimuli, especially with regard to the interstimulus interval. The disadvantages of live voice include lack of control of signal test intensity despite peaking each syllable at 0 on the VU meter and loss of standardization (ASHA, 1979, 1988).

Several investigators have reported that the SRTs obtained using monitored live voice are reliable (Beattie, Forrester, & Ruby, 1976; Carhart, 1946a; Creston, Gillespie, & Krahn, 1966).

Thus, recorded presentation is preferred to monitored live-voice presentation. Nevertheless, monitored live voice may be preferred with the difficult-to-test population, for example, children who may require restriction of test items and consideration of vocabulary and geriatric pa-

tients who may require lengthened interstimulus intervals. The type of presentation—recorded or monitored live voice—should be recorded and reported in the results.

G. CARRIER PHRASE

Egan (1948) felt that the carrier phrase "Say the word . . ." was necessary to alert the patient to the fact that the test word was to follow. Presenting the carrier phrase at a level 10 dB above that of the test word allows the patient to identify the interval in which the test item occurs. The Auditec of St. Louis recording of the CID W-1 spondees, for example, does not have a carrier phrase preceding the test item. Instead, the test item is presented at a constant interstimulus interval, for example, 5 s, which is sufficient to alert the patient that a test item is forthcoming. Regardless of whether a carrier phrase is used in a recording, the calibration tone preceding the SRT test is calibrated to the level of the test item and not to that of the carrier phrase. The SRT obtained with a carrier phrase is essentially the same as that obtained without a carrier phrase. Therefore, the carrier phrase is not a critical consideration when obtaining the SRT.

H. RESPONSE MODE

Alternative responses to oral repetition of the stimulus include (a) writing, provided a person is available to convey the responses to the clinician, (b) pointing to pictures or toy representations of the items, and (c) visual scanning of picture or toy representations of the items. The response mode for SDT testing can be any one of these employed in basic air- and bone-conduction testing. ASHA (1988) suggested that when the response mode was not oral repetition of the item, the response mode employed should be recorded and reported in the results.

I. FAMILIARIZATION AND PRACTICE

Tillman and Jerger (1959) found that the practice effect on the SRT is slight (1.1 dB, on average) whereas familiarization with the test list prior to the administration of the test improved the SRT by 4–5 dB on average. The finding regarding the familiarization effect was supported by the results of Conn, Dancer, and Ventry (1975). These findings suggest that practice has a negligible effect on the SRT and that familiarization is necessary to prevent intersubject differences in the SRT resulting from prior knowledge of the test vocabulary. Familiarization is provided by having the clinician say the words (or present the written list) and having the patient repeat the words. It ensures that the words are known to the patient, that the patient can give the appropriate response, and that the clinician can sufficiently understand the response in order to score properly.

J. PROCEDURE

The Committee on Audiometric Evaluation of the American Speech and Hearing Association recommended an SRT procedure in 1977 based on the ascending technique using 5-dB increments. The guidelines were approved in 1978 and published in 1979 (ASHA, 1979). Their recommended method was reached on the basis of consensus since there were no definitive research data supporting the superiority of one method over another. The ascending technique was recommended since it was the basis of the method recommended by ASHA for manual pure-tone threshold audiometry. ASHA recommended that the clinician familiarize the patient with the test items prior to the test by either reading aloud the items face-to-face or over the speech circuit of the audiometer, having the patient repeat the items, and eliminating spondees that are difficult for the patient to understand or repeat. ASHA also recommended that the patient be instructed regarding the nature of the test, the mode of response, the nature of the test material, the need to respond even when the stimuli are soft, the encouragement of guessing, and the importance of responding only with items from the test list.

The ASHA (1979) recommended technique for SRT determination follows.

1. Start at the lowest attenuation dial setting and present one spondee per level, ascending in 10-dB increments until a correct response is obtained.
2. Then decrease the intensity by 15 dB and begin the first descending sampling series by presenting four spondees at this level. The level is increased by 5-dB steps with four spondaic words presented at each level until a level is reached where at least three correct responses are obtained.
3. Additional ascending series are presented until the criterion for threshold is met. "Threshold is defined arbitrarily as the lowest level at which at least half of the spondaic words are repeated correctly with a minimum requirement of two ascending sampling series" (ASHA, 1979, p. 355).

The Chaiklin, Font, and Dixon (1967) ascending speech-recognition procedure involves starting at the lowest attenuator dial setting and then increasing the intensity in 10-dB steps while presenting one item per level until a correct response is obtained. The intensity is then decreased by 20 dB rather than by the 15 dB recommended by ASHA (1979). Three to six words rather than four words as recommended by ASHA (1979) are presented at this level. The intensity is increased by 5-dB increments with three to six words presented at each level until a level is reached at which at least three words are correctly repeated. This level is considered the SRT.

Tillman and Olsen (1973) proposed a descending method for SRT measurement that was based on the method proposed by Hirsh et al. (1952) that, in turn, was based on the method proposed by Hudgins et al. (1947). The Tillman and Olsen procedure follows.

1. After familiarization, a spondaic word is presented at 30 to 40 dB SL with respect to the estimated threshold. If the response is correct, the intensity is decreased in 10-dB increments with one spondaic word per level until an incorrect response is obtained.
2. A second spondaic word at this level is then presented. If this second response is correct, decrease the intensity in 10-dB steps, presenting two spondaic words per level until a level is reached at which two incorrect responses are obtained, and begin the test at 10 dB above this level. On the other hand, if this second response is incorrect, increase the intensity by 10 dB and begin the test at this level.
3. Two spondaic words are presented at this starting level of threshold testing. If both responses are correct, the level is decreased in 2-dB increments until at least five of the last six responses are incorrect. The starting level must be high enough to enable the patient to correctly repeat at least five of the first six spondaic words. If this criterion is not met, the starting level must be increased by 4 dB.
4. The SRT is equivalent to the starting level of threshold testing (described in step 3) minus the number of correct responses after threshold testing was begun at the starting level plus one (a correction factor added to take into account the extra word with a 1-dB value which was given at the starting level of threshold testing).

Wilson, Morgan, and Dirks (1973) reported that the calculation of threshold has a statistical basis derived from the Spearman–Karber method (Finney, 1952). The Spearman–Karber formula is

$$T_{50\%} = i + \tfrac{1}{2}(d) - [d(r)/n]$$

where $T_{50\%}$ is the threshold, i is the initial test intensity, d is the dB-increment size, r is the number of correct responses, and n is the number of words given at each intensity level. Thus, by inserting the desired values for d and n into the Spearman–Karber formula, the clinician can determine the SRT for any decrement size and any number of words per level. When d and n are equal, the formula is reduced to

$$T_{50\%} = i + \tfrac{1}{2}(d) - r$$

Wilson et al. (1973) showed that the threshold obtained when five spondaic words are presented at each level and 5-dB increments are used at the start of threshold testing is essentially the same as that obtained when two spondaic words are presented at each level and 2-dB increments are used when threshold testing is begun. Wilson et al. (1973)

suggested that, if the 5-dB variation is employed, threshold testing should continue until a level is reached at which all five responses are correct.

Huff and Nerbonne (1982) compared the Tillman–Olsen (1973) method as modified by Wilson *et al.* (1973) to permit the use of 5-dB increments with five spondaic words per level (after threshold testing is begun) with the ASHA (1979) method. They obtained test and retest (1 wk later) SRTs from 60 subjects. The SRTs were obtained using both methods. The results revealed that the mean SRT obtained with the revised Tillman–Olsen method was significantly different (about 2.7 dB lower) from that obtained using the ASHA (1979) method. The SRT–PTA agreement was similar and the test–retest correlation was high for both methods. The ASHA method took 63 sec longer, on average, than the revised Tillman–Olsen method. Huff and Nerbonne indicated that the saving in time with the revised method is underestimated since the starting level with the ASHA method was modified in their study. They suggested that, although one method was not conclusively shown to be superior to the other, the revised Tillman–Olsen method provided the more favorable outcome where differences between the two methods occurred and took less time to administer than the ASHA (1979) method. Therefore, Huff and Nerbonne (1982) recommended the revised Tillman–Olsen method with the 5-dB modification over the ASHA (1979) method for clinical practice.

An SRT method based on a descending technique other than the Tillman–Olsen method was proposed by Chaiklin and Ventry (1964). In this method, a spondaic word is presented at 25 dB SL with respect to the two-frequency PTA. The intensity is decreased in 5-dB steps, and one spondaic word per level is presented until an incorrect response is obtained. The intensity is then increased by 10 dB and three to six words are given at that level. If at least three correct responses are obtained at that level, the intensity is decreased in 5-dB steps until at least four incorrect responses are obtained at two consecutive levels. The threshold is the lowest level at which three correct responses are obtained. Chaiklin and Ventry (1964) suggested that 5-dB rather than 2-dB increments be employed for the following reasons. First, "if a variable is continuously distributed, a relatively small increase (2 or 3 dB) in size of measurement interval should have a negligible effect on precision, and no effect on reliability" (p. 47). Second, they contended that the intensity variations among spondaic words were larger than the 2-dB increment. Third, they questioned the obtaining of SRTs with increments smaller than those used on pure-tone threshold measurement.

Wall, Davis, and Meyers (1984) evaluated the ASHA (1979) ascending method, the Chaiklin *et al.* (1967) ascending method, the revised Tillman–Olsen (1973) descending method, and the Chaiklin and Ventry (1964) method for determination of the SRT in normal and sensorineural hearing-impaired adults with respect to (a) test–retest reliability, (b) SRT–PTA agreement, (c) test-administration time, and (d) number of words necessary to obtain the SRT. Their results revealed that no significant differences in the SRTs were obtained among the methods in both groups of subjects. The SRT–PTA agreement was poorer for the revised Tillman–Olsen procedure than for the other methods, and best for the ascending methods. Nonetheless, improved SRT–PTA agreement for the revised Tillman–Olsen method was obtained when the two-frequency PTA was employed in cases with steeply sloping configurations. Test–retest correlations exceeded 0.95 for all SRT methods. The ASHA (1979) method required approximately twice as many spondaic words as the other methods and took between 1.5 and 1.67 min longer than the other methods. Wall *et al.* (1984) suggested using the Chaiklin *et al.* (1967) method if an ascending method is desired and either the Chaiklin–Ventry (1964) or Tillman–Olsen (1973) method if a descending method is desired.

The ASHA Committee on Audiologic Evaluation presented new guidelines for SRT measurement which were approved in 1987 and published in 1988 (ASHA, 1988). The new guidelines were developed because the adequacy of the ASHA (1979) method for SRT measurement had been questioned. Ventry (1979) objected to the fact that ASHA (1979) endorsed an SRT method based on consensus rather than research evidence. Olsen and Matkin (1979) contended that the ASHA (1979) method had an excessively lengthy test-administration time. In the ASHA (1979) method, "a clear-cut 50% speech threshold criterion could not be found" and procedures for obtaining the SDT were not clearly specified (ASHA, 1988). ASHA (1988) recommended the use of the revised Tillman–Olsen method with either recorded or monitored live-voice presentation. A sample worksheet to be used for tallying the responses and calculating the SRT based on the revised Tillman–Olsen procedure is shown in Figure 15. ASHA (1988) recom-

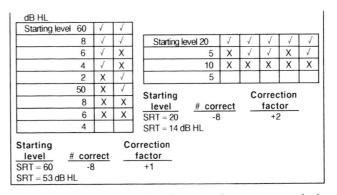

Figure 15 Sample worksheet for tallying test phase responses and calculating the speech recognition threshold, using the descending procedure in 2-dB steps (*left panel*) or 5-dB steps (*right panel*). Starting level has already been determined, as reflected on the panels. Reprinted with permission from ASHA (1988).

Table VIII Alphabetical Full Lists and Half Lists of Spondaic Words which are Revisions of the CID W-1 Auditory Test, Emphasizing the Criteria of Dissimilarity and Homogeneity of Audibility[a]

Alphabetical full list

airplane	drawbridge	hotdog	padlock
armchair	duck pond	icecream	pancake
backbone	eardrum	inkwell	playground
baseball	earthquake	mousetrap	railroad
birthday	eyebrow	mushroom	stairway
blackboard	greyhound	northwest	sunset
cookbook	hardware	nutmeg	toothbrush
cowboy	headlight	oatmeal	whitewash
doormat	horseshoe	outside	woodwork

Half lists

List A   List B

airplane	icecream	armchair	headlight
baseball	mousetrap	backbone	inkwell
blackboard	northwest	birthday	mushroom
cowboy	oatmeal	cookbook	nutmeg
drawbridge	pancake	doormat	outside
duck pond	playground	earthquake	padlock
eardrum	railroad	eyebrow	stairway
horseshoe	sunset	greyhound	toothbrush
hotdog	whitewash	hardware	woodwork

[a] Reprinted with permission from ASHA (1979).

mended that either a modified list of 36 spondaic words or the list of 15 words found to be homogeneous by Young *et al.* (1982) be used with adults. Table VIII shows the alphabetical and half lists of spondaic words recommended by ASHA (1979, 1988). For children aged 6–12 years, ASHA (1988) suggested the use of the list of 20 spondaic words recommended by Frank (1980). This pediatric list is shown in Table IX. ASHA (1988) suggested a standard procedure but did not intend to mandate this procedure as the only method for SRT measurement. For SDT measurement, ASHA (1988) recommended that the technique employed should follow that used for pure-tone threshold measurement. Familiarization was considered unessential.

K. CONSIDERATIONS FOR THE PEDIATRIC POPULATION

ASHA (1988) recommended the use of the pediatric lists of words for children between 6–12 years of age and possibly for younger children, depending upon their capability.

Table IX Spondaic Word List Recommended by Frank (1980) for Testing the Pediatric Population

airplane	cupcake	ice cream	seesaw
baseball	fire truck	mailman	shoelace
bathtub	flashlight	popcorn	snowman
bluebird	football	reindeer	toothbrush
cowboy	hotdog	sailboat	toothpast

Young children, children with restricted expressive language skills, multiply handicapped children, hyperactive children, mentally retarded children, developmentally delayed children, or emotionally disturbed children may require a modified SRT procedure. Keaster (1947) suggested using common nouns embedded in directives to obtain the SRT (e.g., put the "rabbit" on the floor, give the lady the "airplane"). Picture SRT cards are available which illustrate the appropriate spondaic words on cards. The picture SRT tests require the child to respond to the carrier phrase ("Point to . . ." or "Show me . . .") by pointing to or holding up the card. The pointing response can also be employed with small toys. ASHA (1988) recommended that if pointing responses are employed with picture cards or toy representations of the spondaic words, then between 6 and 12 items are appropriate. ASHA (1988) noted that an excessively high number of items "may be distracting and increase response time" and an excessively low number of items "increases the probability of chance performance." Social, visual, or tangible reinforcement of correct responses may be necessary to keep a highly distractible child involved with the task.

Another alternative SRT method to be used in selected situations involves directives concerning body parts such as "Show me your nose." The use of monosyllabic rather than spondaic words may inflate the SRT.

The techniques for SRT measurement in the pediatric population may also be appropriate for other difficult-to-test populations.

VI. CLINICAL MASKING

Clinical masking of the nontest ear during pure-tone and speech-recognition threshold testing, assessment of speech-recognition ability, and site-of-lesion testing (except for acoustic immittance) is often necessary to prevent the responses of the nontest ear from contaminating the responses of the test ear. In some cases, when testing the test ear by air-conduction or bone-conduction, the nontest rather than the test ear will respond to the stimulus. Masking is a noise which is presented to the nontest ear to elevate the threshold in that ear.

A. INTERAURAL ATTENUATION

1. BONE CONDUCTION

A signal presented through a bone-conduction oscillator or through an earphone can cross from the test ear to the nontest cochlea by bone conduction. That is, a signal presented to the test ear causes vibration of the skull so sound travels through the skull bones to the nontest cochlea. Consequently, the better cochlea responds to the stimulus regardless of which ear is being tested by bone conduction. The bone-conducted stimulus crosses from the test ear to the nontest cochlea without loss of intensity at the low frequencies and with a slight loss of intensity at the high frequencies. The loss of intensity as the sound travels from the test to the nontest ear is referred to as interaural attenuation (Chaiklin, 1967). The interaural attenuation for bone-conducted stimuli with mastoid placement of the bone oscillator ranges from approximately 0 dB at 250 Hz to approximately 15 dB at 4000 Hz (Studebaker, 1967). Our clinical experience shows that the interaural attenuation for bone-conduction at 2000 and 4000 Hz ranges from 0 to 15 dB. At the low frequencies, the skull vibrates as a whole so the signal crosses by bone conduction through the skull unattenuated. At the high frequencies, the temporal bone vibrates first; then the whole skull vibrates segmentally. The interaural attenuation for bone-conducted stimuli with forehead placement of the bone oscillator is approximately 0 dB (Studebaker, 1967).

The passage of sound from the test to the nontest ear is referred to as crossover. Crossover, however, is not synonymous with crosshearing (also described as transcranial hearing or shadow hearing). Crosshearing occurs only if the sound which arrived at the nontest cochlea by crossover from the test ear is heard by the nontest cochlea. For example, if a sound is presented by bone conduction at 50 dB HL at 250 Hz in the test ear, it will cross over to the nontest cochlea at 50 dB HL (that is, there is 0 dB interaural attenuation). If the nontest cochlea has a bone-conduction threshold of 70 dB HL at 250 Hz, that cochlea will not be sensitive to the sound that crossed over so crosshearing does not occur, that is, despite the crossover resulting in the presence of a 50-dB sound at the nontest cochlea, crosshearing does not occur. On the other hand, if the nontest cochlea has a bone-conduction threshold of 50 dB HL at 250 Hz, that cochlea will be sensitive to the sound that crossed over so crosshearing will occur at threshold (i.e., 0 dB SL), so the crossover resulting in the presence of a 50-dB sound at the nontest ear is accompanied by crosshearing. If the nontest cochlea has a bone-conduction threshold of 20 dB HL, that cochlea will be sensitive to the sound that crossed over, so crosshearing will occur at 30 dB SL re: bone-conduction threshold in the nontest ear (50 dB crossover level − 20 dB bone-conduction threshold in the nontest ear).

The following example illustrates the interaural attenuation for bone conduction at the high frequencies. Suppose that a 55 dB HL sound is presented by bone conduction to the right ear. The sound will cross over to the left cochlea at 40 dB HL, that is, there is 15 dB interaural attenuation. If the left cochlea has a bone-conduction threshold of 30 dB HL at 4000 Hz, it will be sensitive to the sound that crossed over, so crosshearing will occur at 10 dB SL re: bone-conduction threshold in the left ear (40 dB HL crossover level −30 dB HL bone-conduction threshold).

The 0 dB interaural attenuation for bone conduction at the low and mid frequencies has implications for the bone-conduction testing procedure. Only one ear need be tested by bone conduction in the unmasked condition since the better cochlea will respond regardless of which ear is being tested, so the unmasked bone-conduction threshold will be the same regardless of which ear is being tested by bone-conduction at the low and mid frequencies.

The interaural attenuation for bone conduction at the high frequencies can, in some cases, assist the clinician in determining when the unmasked bone-conduction thresholds for both the right and left ears should be obtained. If the bone oscillator is routinely placed on the ear with the better air-conduction threshold, time will often be wasted in obtaining the unmasked bone-conduction threshold of both ears as illustrated in Figure 16. As Figure 16 shows, if the better (left) ear has an air-conduction threshold of 30 dB HL at 4000 Hz, the poorer (right) ear has an air-conduction of 50 dB HL at that frequency, and the bone oscillator is placed on the better ear (yielding an unmasked bone-conduction threshold of 30 dB HL), a significant unmasked air–bone gap will be present for the poorer (right) ear. Therefore, the clinician will need to obtain the unmasked bone-conduction threshold for the right as well as the left ear to determine whether the masked bone-conduction threshold is needed for the right ear. Often in these cases the unmasked bone-conduction threshold with the bone vibrator on the poorer ear is similar to the air-conduction threshold of the poorer ear. Thus, if the bone oscillator is placed on the ear with the poorer air-conduction threshold, unnecessary measurement of the unmasked bone-conduction thresholds for both the right and left ears will be avoided. In the example just given, if the bone oscillator is placed on the poorer (right) ear rather than the better (left) ear, the unmasked bone-conduction threshold might be 45 dB HL instead of 30 dB HL, so the unmasked bone-conduction threshold would not have to be obtained for the left ear also (see Figure 16B). Nevertheless, if at 2000 or 4000 Hz the unmasked bone-conduction threshold (bone oscillator placed on the poorer ear) minus 15 dB (maximum interaural attenuation for bone conduction) results in a significant unmasked air–bone gap in the better ear, then the unmasked bone-conduction threshold should also be obtained with the bone oscillator placed on the ear with the better air-conduction threshold at these frequencies. It is otherwise unnecessary to obtain the unmasked bone-conduction threshold with the bone oscillator placed on the better ear. Thus, in some situations, when the bone oscillator is placed on the poorer ear, the unmasked bone-conduction threshold at 2000 or 4000 Hz may reflect the true bone-conduction threshold of the poorer rather than the better ear. When the bone oscillator is placed on the better ear at 2000 or 4000 Hz, the unmasked bone-conduction threshold will reflect the true bone-conduction

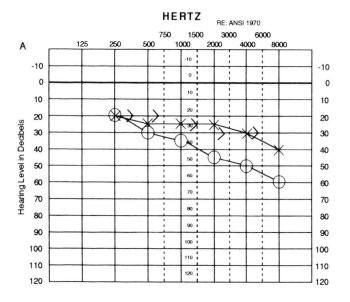

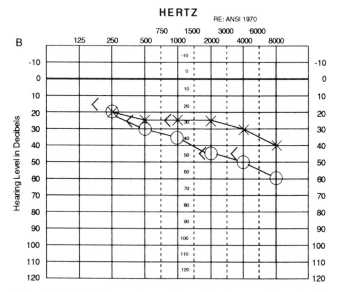

Figure 16 (A) Audiogram for a patient with a bone oscillator placed on the left, better ear. The unmasked bone-conduction thresholds and the air-conduction thresholds for both ears are shown. (B) Audiogram for the same patient with the bone oscillator placed on the right, poorer ear. The unmasked bone-conduction thresholds and air-conduction thresholds for both ears are shown.

threshold of the better ear. At the other test frequencies, regardless of whether the bone oscillator is placed on the poorer or the better ear, it can be assumed that the unmasked bone-conduction threshold reflects the true bone-conduction threshold of the better ear.

2. Air Conduction

According to Bekesy (1948), a signal presented at high intensities through the test earphone can leak from under the rubber cushions and cross over to the nontest earphone. That is, the mechanism for crossover during air-conduction

testing is by around-the-head (air conduction) leakage rather than through-the-head (bone conduction) transmission. Other investigators have contended that, for air-conduction testing, crossover occurs by means of the bone-conduction mechanism (Sparrevohn, 1946; Studebaker, 1962b; Wegel & Lane, 1924; Zwislocki, 1953). That is, when a sound is presented by air conduction to the test ear, it will be transmitted through the skull bones to the nontest cochlea. Chaiklin (1967) suggested that crossover from the test to the nontest ear for strong air-conducted stimuli occurs through the bone-conduction (through-the-head) as well as the air-conduction (around-the-head) mechanism. In the process, the sound will be attenuated by 40 dB because sound has to travel from the air into the skull. According to Chaiklin (1967), crossover by the bone-conduction mechanism occurs before crossover by the air-conduction mechanism at most frequencies. Thus, air-conducted stimuli presented to the test ear will cross over first by the bone-conduction mechanism and then by the around-the-head mechanism to the nontest ear regardless of the type or magnitude of hearing loss in the test ear. Thus, the intensity at the cochlea of the nontest ear depends only on the intensity at the external auditory meatus of the test ear and the interaural attenuation for air-conducted stimuli from the test to the nontest ear.

The interaural attenuation for air-conducted stimuli can be determined by obtaining the unmasked air-conduction thresholds bilaterally in patients with complete unilateral deafness and 0-10 dB HL air- and bone-conduction thresholds in the normal-hearing ear, and then subtracting the good-ear air-conduction thresholds from the poor-ear air-conduction thresholds. The intensities at which responses are obtained reflect crosshearing as well as crossover in the normal-hearing, nontest ear.

Table X shows the unmasked air-conduction threshold levels for both ears of subjects with unilateral deafness

Table X Mean Thresholds for Each Ear with Phones and Interaural Attenuation[a]

Frequency (Hz)	Mean thresholds (dB SPL)		Interaural attenuation		
	Deaf ear	Better ear	Mean	Maximum	Minimum
125	87	49	38	45	32
250	77	26	51	58	44
500	70	11	59	65	54
750	74	5	69	71	62
1000	66	5	61	66	57
1500	73	6	67	76	45
2000	69	8	61	72	55
3000	75	7	68	72	56
4000	73	3	70	85	61
6000	83	18	65	76	56
8000	76	19	57	69	51

[a] Modified from Chaiklin (1967).

presented by Chaiklin (1967). As can be seen from this table, a tone of 70 dB SPL at 500 Hz presented to the dead ear is heard in the nontest ear at 11 dB SPL. Thus, the interaural attenuation for air-conduction at 500 Hz is 59 dB on average, with a minimum value of 54 dB and a maximum value of 65 dB. The average, minimum, and maximum interaural values for air-conduction at each frequency are also shown in Table X. The minimum interaural attenuation at frequencies between 250 and 8000 Hz found by Chaiklin (1967) was 44 dB at 250 Hz. Note that the interaural attenuation for air-conducted stimuli increases directly with frequency. The maximum interaural attenuation for air-conduction stimuli reported by Chaiklin (1967) was 85 dB at 4000 Hz. Liden, Nilsson, and Anderson (1959b) reported minimum interaural attenuation values for air-conducted stimuli of 45–50 dB at 250–8000 Hz. Coles and Priede (1968) reported minimum interaural attenuation values for air-conducted stimuli of 40–50 dB at 250–4000 Hz. Thus, the smallest interaural attenuation value for air-conducted stimuli reported by any investigator is 40 dB. It is recommended that, for clinical purposes, the interaural attenuation value for air-conducted stimuli be considered as 40 dB to minimize the possibility of cross-hearing.

B. WHEN TO MASK

When masking is required, masking noise is introduced into the nontest ear while testing the test ear. The purpose of the masking noise is to shift the air- and bone-conduction threshold in the nontest ear so there will not be crosshearing in the nontest ear. The masking noise used during pure-tone air- and bone-conduction testing is narrow-band noise presented through the earphones. The masking noise used dur-

ing speech-recognition (suprathreshold and threshold) testing is speech noise presented through the earphones. (For further details about the masking noises, or maskers, see Chapter 1.)

1. BONE-CONDUCTION THRESHOLD MEASUREMENT

The masked bone-conduction threshold for the test ear should be obtained whenever the air–bone gap in the test ear exceeds 10 dB. Narrow-band noise is introduced into the nontest ear and the masked bone-conduction threshold is established for the test ear. Figure 17 shows an audiogram of the unmasked bone-conduction thresholds and air-conduction thresholds at 250, 500, and 1000 Hz. The masked bone-conduction thresholds need to be obtained for the left ear at 250 Hz, where there is a 15-dB air–bone gap, for the right ear at 500 Hz, where there is a 25-dB air–bone gap, and for both ears at 1000 Hz, where there is a 15-dB air–bone gap in the left ear and a 40-dB air–bone gap in the right ear. At 250 Hz, the masked bone-conduction threshold is established for the left ear and masking noise is introduced into the right ear. At 500 Hz, the masked bone-conduction threshold is established for the right ear and masking noise is introduced into the left ear. At 1000 Hz, the masked bone-conduction threshold is established for either the right or left ear first with masking noise in the opposite ear. If the masked bone-conduction threshold for the first ear tested (e.g., the right ear) shifts significantly (by more than 10 dB), it is not necessary to obtain the masked bone-conduction threshold for the other (left) ear; it is assumed, in such cases, that the unmasked bone-conduction threshold reflects the true bone-

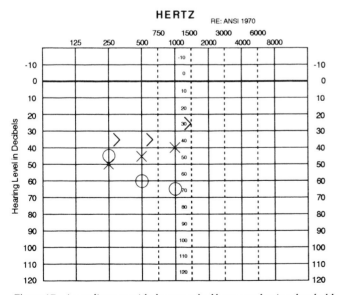

Figure 17 An audiogram with the unmasked bone-conduction thresholds and air-conduction thresholds at 250, 500, and 100 Hz.

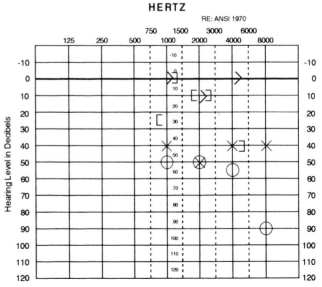

Figure 18 An audiogram with the unmasked and masked bone-conduction thresholds and the unmasked air-conduction thresholds at 1000–8000 Hz.

conduction threshold of the other (left) ear. If there is no shift in the masked bone-conduction threshold of the initial (right) ear, then the masked bone-conduction threshold must also be obtained for the other (left) ear.

2. AIR-CONDUCTION THRESHOLD MEASUREMENT

The masked air-conduction threshold is needed for the test ear if the air-conduction threshold for the test ear exceeds the true bone-conduction threshold (or air-conduction threshold, whichever is lower) of the nontest ear by at least 40 dB. If the masked air-conduction threshold is needed, masking noise is introduced into the nontest ear and the masked air-conduction threshold is established for the test ear. Because the decision to obtain the masked air-conduction threshold depends on knowledge of the true bone-conduction thresholds, masking for bone conduction should be done before masking for air conduction. Figure 18 shows an audiogram with the masked and unmasked bone-conduction thresholds and unmasked air-conduction thresholds at 1000, 2000, 4000, and 8000 Hz.

The masked air-conduction threshold is needed at 1000 Hz, where there is a 50-dB difference between the right air-conduction threshold and the left masked bone-conduction threshold, at 2000 Hz, where there is a 40-dB difference between both air-conduction thresholds and both masked bone-conduction thresholds, at 4000 Hz, where there is a 40-dB difference between the left air-conduction threshold and the left unmasked bone-conduction threshold (reflecting right-ear response), and at 8000 Hz, where there is a 50-dB difference between the left and right air-conduction thresholds. At 1000 Hz, the masked air-conduction threshold is established for the right ear while masking noise is introduced into the left ear. At 2000 Hz, the masked air-conduction threshold is established for the left ear while masking noise is introduced into the right ear and for the right ear while masking noise is introduced to the left ear. At 4000 Hz, the masked air-conduction threshold is established for the left ear while masking noise is introduced into the right ear. At 8000 Hz, the masked air-conduction threshold is established for the right ear with masking noise in the left ear.

At 4000 Hz, if the decision to obtain the masked air-conduction threshold had been based on the unmasked rather than masked bone-conduction threshold, the masked air-conduction threshold would have been obtained unnecessarily for both ears. Note that the masked left bone-conduction threshold of 40 dB HL made it unnecessary to obtain the right masked air-conduction threshold. At 1000 Hz, if the decision to obtain the masked air-conduction threshold had been based on the unmasked rather than the masked bone-conduction threshold, the masked air-conduction threshold would have been obtained unnecessarily for both ears. Note that the masked

right bone-conduction threshold of 25 dB HL made it unnecessary to obtain the left masked air-conduction threshold.

3. SPEECH-RECOGNITION THRESHOLD

The masked speech-recognition threshold (SRT) is needed if the SRT of the test ear exceeds the bone-conduction threshold of the nontest ear by at least 40 dB at any frequency. Martin (1986), based on the research by Martin and Blythe (1977) and the recommendations made by ASHA (1979), recommended that the SRT of the test ear be compared with the bone-conduction thresholds only at 500, 1000, and 2000 Hz. Goldstein and Newman (1985) recommend that the SRT of the test ear be compared with the bone-conduction or air-conduction pure-tone average or SRT of the nontest ear. It is our experience that, although the 500, 1000, and 2000 Hz are the most important for hearing spondaic words, the other frequencies can also be responsible for the recognition of spondaic words, so the SRT should be compared with the bone-conduction and air-conduction thresholds at each frequency. Our experience with the Veterans Administration population (the majority of whom have sharply sloping sensorineural hearing loss) shows that, in a considerable number of cases, the SRT is in agreement with the hearing threshold level at any single frequency between 250 and 8000 Hz; there was good intratest and intertest reliability for these findings over the years. Although many investigators (Goldstein & Newman, 1985; Konkle & Berry, 1983) employ 45 dB as the interaural attenuation for speech, we confirm Martin's (1986) recommendation for setting the interaural attenuation for speech presented by air conduction at 40 dB.

C. OCCLUSION EFFECT

The occlusion effect is the improvement in the bone-conduction threshold when the external ear is covered by an earphone (as is the case when obtaining the masked bone-conduction threshold) or when the ear canal is occluded by a finger, ear insert, earmold, or ear protector over the bone-conduction threshold when the ear canal is unoccluded (during unmasked bone-conduction testing) (Studebaker, 1979). The occlusion effect occurs primarily at the low frequencies and is, on average, approximately 2 dB at 250 Hz, 15 dB at 500 Hz, 5 dB at 1000 Hz, and 0 dB at 2000 Hz and above (Goldstein & Hayes, 1965; Martin, Butler, & Burns, 1974).

Under the unmasked bone-conduction testing condition, some of the sound generated in the ear canal by vibration of the bony part of the external auditory meatus leaves the ear through the external auditory meatus. When the external auditory meatus is occluded, the sound generated in the external auditory meatus is prevented from leaving the ear canal, so the sound-pressure level rises at the tympanic membrane. The occlusion effect does not reflect an improved hearing sensitivity by bone conduction. Rather it reflects an increase in the total energy delivered to the cochlea. (For further details on the occlusion effect, see Section III,A,3.) The occlusion effect is present in normal-hearing and sensorineural-hearing-impaired ears but not in conductive-hearing-impaired ears.

Several investigators (Goldstein & Newman, 1985; Studebaker, 1979) employ a fixed number for the occlusion effect based on the average occlusion-effect values reported in the literature. Following Martin (1986), we recommend calculating the patient's individual occlusion effect by subtracting the bone-conduction threshold just prior to masking for bone conduction (with the earphone covering the nontest ear) from the bone-conduction threshold when the ear canal is not covered by an earphone.

D. EFFECTIVE MASKING

The effective masking level (EML) is the intensity in dB HL of a signal or threshold (maskee) that a masker will just mask and the minimum effective masking (MEM) is the amount of masking noise in dB beyond the effective masking level. For example, if the hearing threshold level at 500 Hz is 50 dB, and this threshold is just masked (i.e., the air-conduction and bone-conduction thresholds are shifted by 5 dB) by a masker of 65 dB HL, the EML is 50 dB HL and the MEM is 15 dB (65 dB HL − 50 dB HL).

Although most audiometers are calibrated in MEM, we recommend that each clinic establish its own MEM on a group of 10 normal-hearing young adults. The MEM should include a 10–15 dB safety factor. Recall from Chapter 1 that the manufacturers calibrate the audiometer masking noises in MEM based on computation with the critical band data. The behavioral procedure for establishing MEM is also described in Chapter 1.

E. INITIAL MASKING

The minimum amount of noise in dB HL required to shift the air-conduction and bone-conduction threshold by 5 dB in the nontest ear is the initial masking (Martin, 1986). Initial masking is equivalent to EML plus MEM (which has a built-in safety factor).

1. BONE CONDUCTION

Several formulas have been suggested for deriving the initial masking (IM) when obtaining the masked bone-conduction threshold. For example, Liden, Nilsson, and Anderson (1959b) proposed this formula for IM:

$$IM = Bt + (Am - Bm)$$

where Bt is the bone-conduction threshold in the test ear, Am is the air-conduction threshold in the masked ear, and

Bm is the bone-conduction threshold in the masked ear (assuming the dial is calibrated in effective masking). Goldstein and Newman (1985), based on Beedle's (1971) finding, employed the following formula for IM:

$$IM = Ant + OE + 15 \text{ dB MEM}$$

where Ant is the air-conduction threshold of the nontest ear, OE is the occlusion effect, and MEM is minimum effective masking. Martin (1986) recommends this formula for obtaining IM:

$$IM = Ant + MEM + OE$$

where Ant is the air-conduction threshold of the nontest ear, MEM is minimum effective masking for bone conduction, and OE is the occlusion effect. The MEM is established based on the calibration of narrow-band noise in units of effective masking on a group of normal-hearing subjects.

The formula used by Liden et al. (1959b) involves subtraction so it involves lengthy computation at each frequency. The formula used by Goldstein and Newman is essentially the same as the one used by Martin (1986) except that the former assigned a fixed number for MEM whereas the latter derived the MEM based on calibration of the narrow-band noise from the particular audiometer on a group of normal-hearing persons. We recommend the formula for IM described by Martin (1986).

2. AIR CONDUCTION

We recommend the following formula for deriving IM when obtaining the masked air-conduction threshold based on Martin (1986):

$$IM = Ant + MEM$$

where Ant is the air-conduction threshold of the nontest (masked) ear and MEM is the minimum effective masking for air-conduction testing. The introduction of IM to the masked ear will shift the air-conduction and bone-conduction thresholds in that ear by 5 dB.

3. SPEECH-RECOGNITION THRESHOLD

Following Martin (1986), the IM when obtaining the masked SRT can be derived from the following formula:

$$IM = SRTnt + MEM$$

where SRTnt is the speech-recognition threshold of the nontest (masked) ear and MEM is the minimum effective masking for speech-recognition threshold testing.

F. OVERMASKING

Overmasking occurs when the masking noise crosses from the nontest to the test ear and shifts the air-conduction and bone-conduction threshold in the test ear by at least 5 dB. Similar to the mechanism for crossover of the test signal from the test ear to the nontest ear in air conduction, the crossover of the masking noise from the nontest ear to the test ear during overmasking occurs by bone conduction. That is, the masking noise, presented by air conduction, has an interaural attenuation of approximately 40 dB during crossover from the nontest to the test ear. Crosshearing of the masking noise does not necessarily result in overmasking unless the masker is sufficient in intensity to shift the air-conduction and bone-conduction threshold in the test ear by at least 5 dB.

According to Martin (1986), overmasking (OM) during bone-conduction, air-conduction, and speech-recognition threshold testing may occur when the masker intensity in the nontest ear is greater than or equal to the bone-conduction threshold of the test ear plus the interaural attenuation for air conduction (40 dB). That is, OM may occur if $MLnt \geq Bt + IA$, where Bt is the bone-conduction threshold of the test ear, IA is the interaural attenuation for air conduction, and $MLnt$ is the intensity of the masking noise in the nontest ear in dB HL. Overmasking actually does not occur until the masker intensity in the nontest ear is greater than or equal to the bone-conduction threshold of the test ear plus 40 dB plus MEM. It is accepted clinical practice, however, not to consider the MEM when determining whether overmasking is occurring because it is desirable to be conservative when determining whether overmasking is occurring.

G. MAXIMUM MASKING

The maximum amount of masking noise that one can introduce into the nontest ear without resulting in overmasking of the test ear is called maximum masking (MM). Maximum masking is the amount of masking noise in dB HL which is just insufficient to result in overmasking of the test ear. The formula for determining maximum masking during bone-conduction, air-conduction, and speech-recognition testing is:

$$MM = Bt + IA - 5 \text{ dB}$$

where Bt is the bone-conduction threshold of the test ear and IA is the interaural attenuation for air conduction (40 dB).

H. CENTRAL MASKING

The introduction of a masker into the nontest ear can result in a threshold shift even when the masker intensity is insufficient to result in overmasking. Central masking occurs because the two ears are not completely independent neurologically. The most rostral, shared neural pathways usually available to the test ear are occupied by the masker (Ward, 1963). Liden, Nilsson, and Anderson (1959b) suggested that the central-masking effect is probably mediated by the efferent pathways. Although Zwislocki (1953) reported that the central-masking effect did not exceed 5 dB, Liden et al. (1959b) found that the central-masking effect was as large as 15 dB. Several investigators (Dirks, 1964; Dirks & Malmquist, 1964; Martin & DiGiovanni, 1979; Studebaker, 1962b) have observed that the central-masking effect increases as the intensity of the masker increases. We have observed that, when the masking noise in the test ear is interrupted and the patient is reinstructed to ignore the masking and respond to the test signal, the threshold shift seen when the masking noise is initially introduced to the nontest ear is often eliminated, especially in elderly persons. Since this phenomenon occurs only in some patients, it may not be related to the central-masking effect. Nevertheless, this finding on the elimination of the threshold shift by interrupting the masking noise and reinstructing the patient suggests that further research is necessary on the nature of the central-masking effect.

I. TECHNIQUE FOR CLINICAL MASKING

Whenever masking is needed for bone conduction, the bone-conduction threshold should be re-established with the earphone on the nontest ear in order to determine the magnitude of the occlusion effect. Then the IM using narrow-band noise should be introduced into the nontest ear. With the masker in the nontest ear, the bone-conduction threshold should again be established. If there is no shift in the bone-conduction threshold in comparison with the bone-conduction threshold in the uncovered-ear condition (unmasked), the masking procedure is terminated and this threshold is considered the masked bone-conduction threshold for the test ear. If there is an increase in the bone-conduction threshold with the introduction of IM to the nontest ear (in comparison with the bone-conduction threshold in the uncovered-ear condition), the following plateau procedure should be employed.

After re-establishing the bone-conduction threshold upon introduction of IM in the nontest ear, increase the masker intensity by 5 dB and determine if the patient still hears the test signal. Suppose, for example, that a patient has an unmasked bone-conduction threshold of 25 dB HL, a masker of 30 dB HL is presented to the nontest ear, and the bone-conduction threshold with the IM in the nontest ear is 35 dB HL (threshold shift). The masker intensity is then increased to 35 dB HL and the clinician determines whether the patient hears the bone-conducted signal of 35 dB HL. If the patient still hears the bone-conducted signal at 35 dB HL, the masker is again increased by 5 dB to 40 dB HL and the clinician again determines whether the patient hears the bone-conducted signal of 35 dB HL. If the patient still hears the bone-conducted signal at 35 DB HL, the masker is again increased by 5 dB to 45 dB HL and the clinician once again determines whether the patient hears the bone-conducted signal of 35 dB HL. If the patient hears the bone-conducted signal at 35 dB HL, the plateau procedure is terminated and the masked bone-conduction threshold is 35 dB HL for this patient. Thus, the plateau procedure involves the introduction of IM to the nontest ear and re-establishment of the bone-conduction threshold with the IM in the nontest ear. If there is an increase in the bone-conduction threshold, the masking noise is increased by 5 dB. If the patient continues to hear the bone-conducted signal at the same intensity, the noise is again increased by 5 dB. If the patient continues to hear the bone-conducted signal at the same intensity, the noise is again increased by 5 dB and if the patient continues to hear the bone-conducted signal at the same intensity, that intensity is taken as the masked bone-conduction threshold.

If, at any time, the patient fails to hear the test signal when the masking noise is increased by 5 dB, the intensity of the test signal must be increased in 5-dB steps until the patient responds. Then the plateau procedure is once again employed, until three or four 5-dB masking increments do not change the threshold of the test signal.

The plateau principle developed by Hood (1960) actually involved increasing the masker intensity and test intensity in 10-dB steps. A common clinical practice in masking is to use a plateau procedure involving 10-dB increments in the masking noise but only 5-dB increments in the test signal. This practice may be theoretically feasible when broadband rather than narrow-band noise close to the critical band is used. Since most audiometers are calibrated in effective masking, it is advisable to use the same increment size for both the test signal and masker level. We recommend that the increment size be 5 dB since the clinical procedure for threshold determination involves intensity increases in 5-dB steps. Martin (1980) contended that, although the use of 10-dB increments increases the speed of the masking procedure, it decreases the accuracy slightly.

This technique can also be applied directly to obtaining the masked air-conduction threshold, except that the test signal is an air-conducted one. This technique can be applied to speech-recognition threshold testing but with a slight modification. In this case, the test signal is speech presented by air conduction and the masker is speech noise. Also, the patient responds by repeating the word rather than by indicating (by raising the hand) that the word is heard. Whenever masking is done, the patient should be instructed to ignore the noise and to respond only to the test signal.

J. MASKING DILEMMA

Situations can occur in which introduction of initial masking results in overmasking. Suppose, for example, a patient has the unmasked air- and bone-conduction thresholds

shown in Figure 19. Assume MEM is 15 dB at 1000 Hz and the occlusion effect is 0 dB. The IM is 65 dB HL (50 dB HL + 15 dB + 0 dB). Overmasking can occur when the masker intensity in the nontest ear is greater than or equal to 40 dB HL (0 dB for the bone-conduction threshold of the test ear + 40 dB IA). Thus, in this case, the IM of 65 dB HL can result in overmasking. Therefore a threshold shift that occurs upon the introduction of IM to the nontest ear may reflect OM if the IM level is sufficient to result in OM. If no threshold shift occurs with the introduction of 65 dB HL IM into the test ear, OM did not occur and it can be assumed that, for this patient, the IA was greater than 40 dB. If the introduction of 65 dB HL of IM resulted in a threshold shift but a plateau was obtained, OM did not occur even though the masking intensity exceeded the level which may result in OM. When OM occurs, no plateau will be obtained. That is, for every increment in the masker in the nontest ear, there will be an equal shift in the threshold for the signal in the test ear. This situation is referred to as a masking dilemma because it is unknown whether the threshold shift and lack of plateau in the test ear did or did not result from OM. That is, either the masking noise crossed over and caused a shift in the threshold of the test ear or a plateau could not be reached because the maximum output level for the masking noise was reached before establishing the plateau. Masking dilemmas are commonly encountered in patients whose unmasked air- and bone-conduction thresholds reveal 40-60 dB air–bone gaps, bilaterally. If OM occurs (i.e., threshold shift in the test ear upon introduction of the masker to the nontest ear, masker intensity exceeds maximum masking level, and lack of plateau), the clinician should mark on the audiogram "CNT-masking dilemma" at that test frequency.

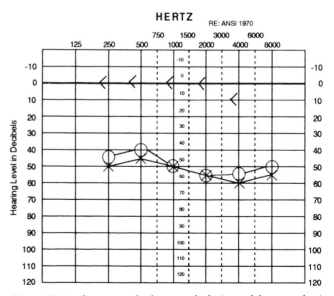

Figure 19 Audiogram with the unmasked air- and bone-conduction thresholds. Masking dilemma is illustrated.

Sometimes a plateau is not reached when the masking noise reaches the maximum output level of the audiometer, and the initial masker intensity level is insufficient to possibly cause OM. In such cases, the clinician should use the audiometric symbol indicating that the masked threshold is greater than the test signal intensity level when the masking noise reached the limits of the audiometer.

In some situations, a plateau will not be reached because the threshold of the test signal is beyond the output limits of the audiometer. If OM is not a possibility, the clinician should put the symbol representing a masked threshold beyond the audiometer output limits on the audiogram. For example, suppose 40 dB IM is introduced into the nontest ear of a patient and the bone-conduction threshold with the masker in the nontest ear increases to beyond 65 dB HL (the limits of the audiometer). If the possibility of OM does not occur until the masker intensity reaches 60 dB HL (for example) for this patient, the clinician should indicate that the masked bone-conduction threshold in the test ear for this patient was greater than 65 dB HL.

K. INSERT EARPHONES

Insert earphones have been used to increase the interaural attenuation for air conduction, thereby reducing the frequency of clinical situations in which the masked bone-conduction or air-conduction threshold is needed. Furthermore, the use of insert earphones reduces the frequency of occurrence of masking dilemmas since the increased interaural attenuation for the masker means OM is less likely to occur.

Table XI Mean Interaural Attenuation Values in dB and Ranges for the Deeply Inserted ER-3A,[a] Supra-Aural TDH-39 Earphones,[b] and Supra-Aural TDH-49P Earphones[c]

Transducer	.25	.50	.75	1.0	1.5	2.0	3.0	4.0	6.0	Speech
ER-3A										
Mean	—	94+	89	81	74	71	69	77	75+	75
Minimum	75+	85	80	75	65	55	50	60	60+	68
Maximum	100+	105	100	90	85	90	80	85	95	84
TDH-39										
Mean	50	60	60	60	55	60	60	62		
Minimum	45	52	53	52	47	50	50	52		
Maximum	65	65	65	65	65	68	68	74		
TDH-49										
Mean	54	59	63	62	59	58	57	65	65	58
Minimum	45	45	55	60	50	45	45	60	50	54
Maximum	60	75	75	65	65	70	70	75	80	68

[a] Sklare & Denenberg (1987).
[b] Killion, Wilber, & Gudmundsen (1985).
[c] Sklare & Denenberg (1987).

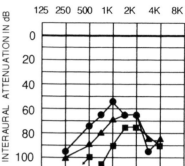

Figure 20 Interaural attenuation obtained on subject ER with deep earplug insertion in both ears (■), with shallow insertion in dead ear only (▲), and with shallow insertion in both ears (●). Reprinted with permission from Killion, Wilber, and Gudmundsen (1985).

According to Zwislocki (1953), the IA for air-conducted signals is inversely proportional to the surface area exposed to acoustic or mechanical force. With insert earphones, the surface area vibrated is reduced, resulting in decrease in the intensity of the air-conducted signal transmitted through the skull bones to the other cochlea (crossover involves the bone conduction route). As a result, the interaural attenuation for air conduction is increased.

The most commonly used insert earphone is the ER-3A manufactured by Etymotic Research. With deep insert earphone insertion (back surface flush with the orifice), the IA values were increased significantly over those for the TDH-39 and TDH-49 earphones, especially at the low and mid frequencies. Table XI shows the means and ranges for the IA values obtained with the ER-3A insert earphones (Sklare & Denenberg, 1987), the TDH-39 earphones (Killion, Wilber, & Gudmundsen, 1985), and TDH-49 earphones (Sklare & Denenberg, 1987). As can be seen from this table, the IA for the insert earphones is as much as or greater than 100 dB below 1000 Hz. The IA values obtained with shallow insert earphone placement (back surface of the plug is slightly lateral to the orifice of the ear canal) is less than those for deep-insert earphone insertion. Figure 20 shows the IA values obtained in a patient with deep earphone insertion in both ears, shallow insertion in the hearing-loss ear only, and shallow insertion bilaterally.

VII. AUDIOMETRIC INTERPRETATION

A. HYPOTHETICAL CASES FOR MASKING BY AIR- AND BONE-CONDUCTION

The pure-tone unmasked and masked air- and bone-conduction thresholds are plotted in graphic form on an audiogram or in tabular form. Figure 21 shows an audiogram and the audiometric symbols. The audiometric sym-

FREQUENCY IN HERTZ (Hz)

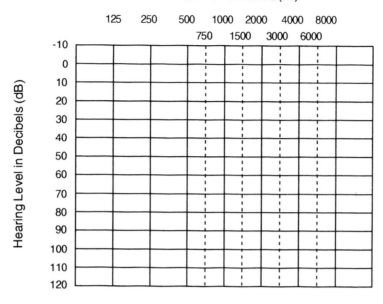

EFFECTIVE MASKING LEVELS

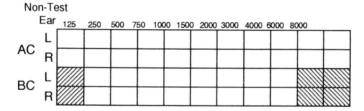

Response

MODALITY	EAR		
	LEFT	UNSPECIFIED	RIGHT
AIR CONDUCTION-EARPHONES			
UNMASKED	✗		○
MASKED	◻		△
BONE CONDUCTION-MASTOID			
UNMASKED	>	⊓	<
MASKED	⌋		⌊
BONE CONDUCTION-FOREHEAD			
UNMASKED		⋁	
MASKED	⌐		⌐
AIR CONDUCTION-SOUND FIELD	⋇	$	∅
ACOUSTIC-REFLEX THRESHOLD			
CONTRALATERAL	>—		—<
IPSILATERAL	⊢		⊣

No Response

MODALITY	EAR		
	LEFT	UNSPECIFIED	RIGHT
AIR CONDUCTION-EARPHONES			
UNMASKED	✗		○
MASKED	◻		△
BONE CONDUCTION-MASTOID			
UNMASKED	>	⊓	<
MASKED	⌋		⌊
BONE CONDUCTION-FOREHEAD			
UNMASKED		⋁	
MASKED	⌐		⌐
AIR CONDUCTION-SOUND FIELD	⋇	$	∅
ACOUSTIC-REFLEX THRESHOLD			
CONTRALATERAL	>—		—<
IPSILATERAL	⊢		⊣

Figure 21 Audiogram and key for audiogram symbols as recommended by ASHA (1990).

bols used are those recommended by ASHA (1988b). In Figure 21, frequency, in Hz, is represented along the abscissa and intensity, in dB HL, is represented along the ordinate.

Figure 22 shows the air-conduction thresholds only for a hypothetical patient. These results were plotted during air-conduction testing. Figure 23 shows the air- and bone-conduction thresholds for the same patient as in Figure 22. Note that the mastoid bone-conduction thresholds for the left ear have been added to the audiogram. Figure 23 reveals the presence of significant air–bone gaps for the left ear of approximately 45 dB. Recall from the section on masking that the masked bone-conduction thresholds are obtained whenever there are air–bone gaps of 15 dB or more.

Figures 24, 25, 26, and 27 show four possibilities (there are more than four) for the masked left bone-conduction thresholds after masking for bone conduction. The masked left bone-conduction thresholds are obtained by routing masking noise through the earphone to the right ear while obtaining the bone-conduction thresholds with the bone vibrator on the left ear. In Figures 24–27, the left masked bone conduction thresholds have been added to the unmasked air- and bone-conduction thresholds in Figure 23. In Figure 24, the masked left bone-conduction thresholds are the same as the unmasked bone-conduction thresholds shown in Figure 23. In Figures 25, 26, and 27, the masked

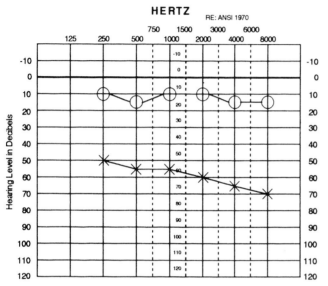

Figure 22 Audiogram shows the unmasked air-conduction thresholds.

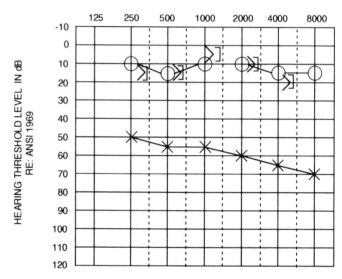

Figure 24 Audiogram shows the unmasked air- and bone-conduction thresholds for the patient in Figures 22 and 23 and one possibility for the masked, left bone-conduction thresholds.

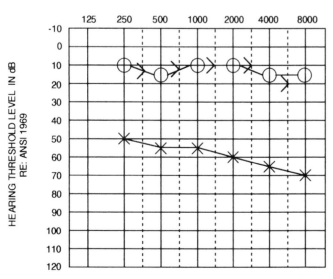

Figure 23 Audiogram shows the unmasked air- and bone-conduction thresholds for the patient in Figure 22.

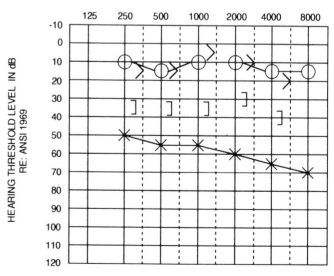

Figure 25 Audiogram shows the unmasked air- and bone-conduction thresholds for the patient in Figures 22 and 23 and a second possibility for the masked, left bone-conduction thresholds.

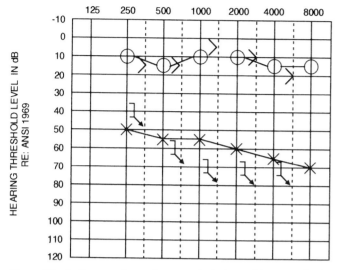

Figure 26 Audiogram shows the unmasked air- and bone-conduction thresholds for the patient in Figures 22 and 23 and a third possibility for the masked, left bone-conduction thresholds.

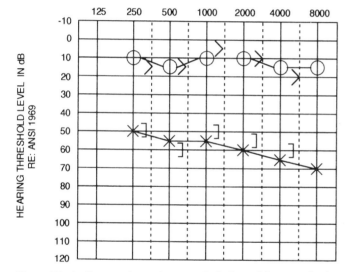

Figure 27 Audiogram shows the unmasked air- and bone-conduction thresholds for the patient in Figures 22 and 23 and a fourth possibility for the masked, left bone-conduction thresholds.

left bone-conduction thresholds are worse than the unmasked bone-conduction thresholds shown in Figure 23.

Now the clinician must determine whether the masked air-conduction thresholds are needed after obtaining the masked bone-conduction thresholds. Figures 24–27 must be examined to determine whether there is a 40-dB or greater difference between the bone-conduction threshold of one ear and the air-conduction threshold of the other ear. (Recall the rules for masking for air conduction in the section on air-conduction masking.) Inspection of Figures 24–27 reveals that the masked air-conduction thresholds need to be obtained for the left ear in all of these situations

since the left unmasked air-conduction thresholds are at least 40 dB worse than the right bone-conduction thresholds.

Figures 28, 29, 30, and 31 show two possibilities (there are more) for the masked left air-conduction thresholds, after masking for air conduction, based on the masked bone-conduction thresholds shown in Figures 24, 25, 26, and 27, respectively. The masked left air-conduction thresholds are obtained by routing narrow-band noise through the earphone to the right ear while obtaining the left air-conduction thresholds. In Figure 28, the first possi-

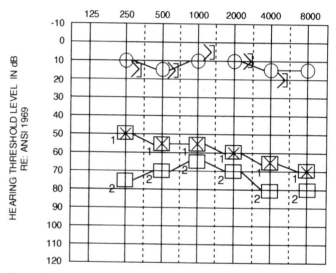

Figure 28 Audiogram shows the unmasked air-conduction thresholds, masked and unmasked bone-conduction thresholds, and two possibilities for the left, masked air-conduction thresholds for the patient in Figure 24.

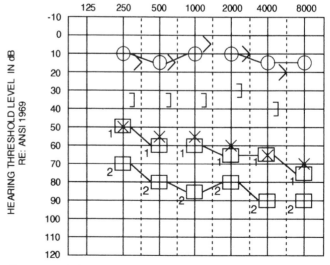

Figure 29 Audiogram shows the unmasked air-conduction thresholds, masked and unmasked bone-conduction thresholds, and two possibilities for the left, masked air-conduction thresholds for the patient in Figure 25.

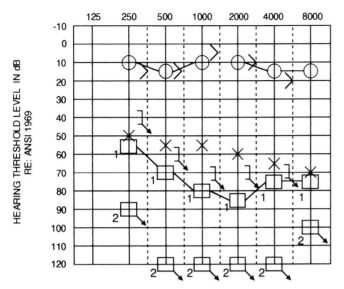

Figure 30 Audiogram shows the unmasked air-conduction thresholds, masked and unmasked bone-conduction thresholds, and two possibilities for the left, masked air-conduction thresholds for the patient in Figure 26.

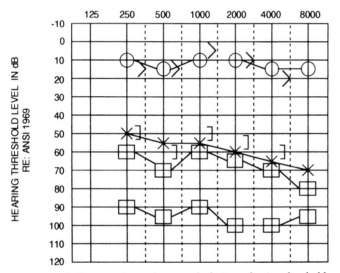

Figure 31 Audiogram shows the unmasked air-conduction thresholds, masked and unmasked bone-conduction thresholds, and two possibilities for the left, masked air-conduction thresholds for the patient in Figure 27.

bilities for the masked left air-conduction thresholds are the same as the unmasked left air-conduction thresholds; the second possibilities for the masked left air-conduction thresholds are worse than the unmasked left air-conduction thresholds. In Figure 29, the first possibilities for the masked left air-conduction thresholds are essentially the same as the unmasked left air-conduction thresholds; the second possibilities for the left masked air-conduction thresholds are worse than the left unmasked air-conduction thresholds. In Figure 30, both possibilities for the masked left air-conduction thresholds are worse than the unmasked

left air-conduction thresholds. In Figure 31, the first possibilities for the masked left air-conduction thresholds are slightly worse than or similar to the unmasked left air-conduction thresholds; the second possibilities for the masked left air-conduction thresholds are worse than the unmasked left air-conduction thresholds. Observe that the masked air–bone gaps (based on both possibilities for the masked left air-conduction thresholds) for the left ear after air- and bone-conduction masking in Figure 28 are approximately 35–60 dB and do not exceed the 60 dB maximum air–bone gap limits mentioned earlier in the masking section.

B. TYPE OF HEARING LOSS

The etiologies and loci of conductive, sensorineural, mixed, and central hearing loss were discussed at the beginning of this chapter. Determination of the type of hearing loss is made by comparing the bone-conduction thresholds to the air-conduction thresholds (masked thresholds, if masked thresholds are needed).

The three major classifications of hearing impairment are conductive, sensorineural, and mixed. A conductive hearing loss is present if the bone-conduction thresholds are within normal limits, air–bone gaps of 15 dB or more are present, and the air-conduction thresholds are outside the normal limits, that is, are more than 25 dB HL. Some clinicians consider the bone-conduction thresholds to be within normal limits if they are 25 dB HL or less. We consider bone-conduction thresholds to be within normal limits only if they are 15 dB HL or better. Thus, a conductive hearing impairment is characterized by good bone-conduction thresholds, signaling the absence of a problem in the sensorineural mechanism, significant air–bone gaps, signaling better hearing sensitivity by bone conduction than by air conduction, and poor air-conduction thresholds, signaling a problem in the outer and/or middle ear (inner-ear problem ruled out by the good bone-conduction thresholds).

A sensorineural hearing impairment is present if the bone-conduction thresholds are outside of the normal limits, that is, greater than 15 dB HL, no significant air–bone gaps are present (i.e., air–bone gaps do not exceed 10 dB), and the air-conduction thresholds are outside of the normal limits, that is, are greater than 25 dB HL. Thus, a sensorineural hearing impairment is characterized by poor bone-conduction thresholds, signaling a problem in the sensorineural mechanism, and essentially equally poor air-conduction thresholds.

A mixed hearing impairment is present if the bone-conduction thresholds are outside of the normal limits, that is, greater than 15 dB HL, significant air–bone gaps exceeding 10 dB are present, and the air-conduction thresholds are outside of the normal limits, that is, are greater than 25 dB HL. Thus, a mixed loss is characterized by poor bone-conduction thresholds, signaling a problem in the sensori-neural mechanism, significant air–bone gaps exceeding 10 dB, signaling better hearing sensitivity by bone conduction than by air conduction, and air-conduction thresholds worse than the bone-conduction thresholds, signaling a problem in the outer and/or middle ear (conductive mechanism) in addition to the problem in the sensorineural mechanism indicated by the poor bone-conduction thresholds.

If a patient has a 0 dB HL bone-conduction (BC) threshold and 40 dB HL air-conduction (AC) threshold at 1000 Hz, a conductive impairment is present because the BC threshold is within normal limits, a significant air–bone gap (ABG) is present (40 dB), and the AC threshold is outside of the normal limits. If, on the other hand, the patient has a 25 dB HL BC threshold and 40 dB HL AC threshold, we would consider this a mixed hearing impairment whereas some other clinicians would consider this a conductive hearing impairment. We would consider this a mixed hearing impairment because the BC threshold is depressed, a significant ABG is present (15 dB), and the AC threshold is outside of the normal limits. We consider the BC threshold depressed in this case because if the AC and BC threshold are improved by the amount of the BC depression, 25 dB, there is clearly a shift in diagnostic category, in this case from mixed to normal hearing with air–bone gaps. Other clinicians would consider a BC threshold of 25 dB to be within normal limits, making this a conductive rather than a mixed hearing impairment. If a patient has a 20 dB HL BC threshold and a 25 dB HL AC threshold, we would consider this to be normal hearing because of the absence of a significant air-bone gap and an AC threshold within normal limits despite the elevated BC threshold.

Classification of type of hearing impairment is done for each ear. Both possibilities shown in Figure 28 represent a case with a conductive hearing impairment in the left ear and normal hearing sensitivity in the right ear. Conductive hearing impairment, as mentioned earlier in this chapter, may be caused by ossicular fixation, ossicular discontinuity, middle-ear effusion, Eustachian-tube dysfunction without middle-ear effusion, middle-ear tumor, or other lesions. Acoustic-immittance testing may enable distinction among these conductive pathologies, as will be shown in the chapter on acoustic immittance testing. Both possibilities in Figure 29 represent a case with a mixed hearing impairment in the left ear and normal hearing sensitivity in the right ear. A mixed hearing impairment results from a combined conductive and sensorineural hearing impairment at a given frequency or frequencies. For example, a person with congenital sensorineural hearing impairment may develop a conductive component from middle-ear disease such as middle-ear effusion, resulting in a mixed hearing impairment. Figure 30 represents a case with normal hearing sensitivity in the right ear and a sensorineural hearing impairment in the left ear, based on the first possibilities for the masked left air-conduction thresholds; based on the second

possibilities for the masked left air-conduction thresholds, Figure 30 shows a sensorineural or mixed hearing impairment in the left ear. (Differentiation between sensorineural and mixed hearing impairment based on just the audiogram cannot be done since the air–bone gap sizes remain unknown.) A sensorineural hearing impairment, as mentioned earlier, can be caused by damage to the cochlea, eighth cranial nerve, and/or cochlear nuclei. Traditional site-of-lesion testing, acoustic immittance testing, and brainstem auditory evoked potentials testing may distinguish between peripheral (cochlear) and retrocochlear (eighth cranial nerve and cochlear nuclei) sites of sensorineural hearing impairment. Figure 31 represents a case with normal hearing sensitivity in the right ear and sensorineural hearing impairment in the left ear, based on the first possibilities for the masked air-conduction thresholds; based on the second possibilities for the masked left air-conduction thresholds, Figure 31 shows a case with mixed hearing impairment in the left ear.

C. AUDIOMETRIC CONFIGURATION

The audiometric configuration with respect to the positive or negative slope of the air-conduction thresholds is classified as flat, gradually sloping, sharply sloping, precipitously sloping, rising, trough, or saucer. Table XII shows the criteria for the classification of audiometric configuration modified from Carhart (1945) and Lloyd and Kaplan (1978). A trough (also called saddle, dipper, or U-shaped) has an essentially equivalent loss (within 10 dB) for two or more mid frequencies, with recovery at the extreme frequencies. A notch has a dip at a single frequency with recovery at the immediately adjacent frequencies. A notch at a high frequency is usually associated with noise exposure or head trauma. A trough audiometric configuration occurs in some children with rubella, for example. A rising conductive loss reflects a stiffness tilt such as that associated with otosclerosis and middle-ear effusion. A sloping conductive loss reflects a mass tilt such as that associated with

Table XII Criteria for Classifying Audiometric Configurations[a]

Term	Description
Flat	<5 dB Rise or fall per octave
Gradually sloping	5–12 dB Threshold increase per octave
Sharply sloping	15–20 dB Threshold increase per octave
Precipitously sloping	Flat or gradually sloping, then threshold increasing at rate of 25+ dB per octave
Rising	5 dB or More threshold decrease per octave
Trough	20 dB or Greater loss at the mid frequencies than at the extreme frequencies
Notch	Sharp dip at a single frequency with recovery at the immediately adjacent frequencies
Saucer	20 dB or Greater loss at the extreme frequencies than at the mid frequencies

[a] Adapted from Carhart (1945) and Lloyd and Kaplan (1978).

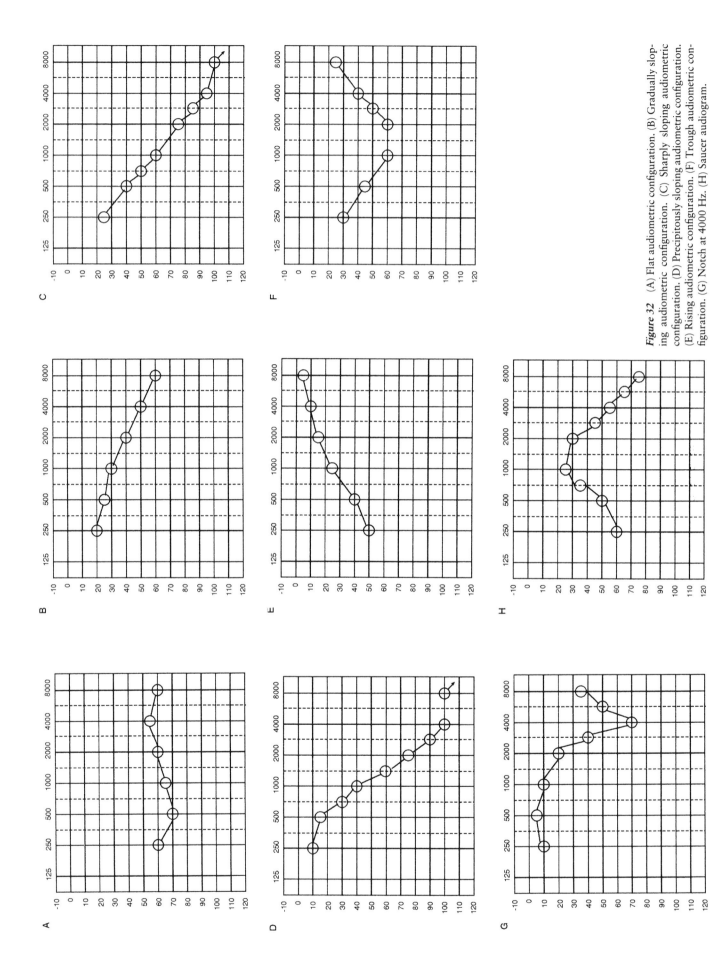

Figure 32 (A) Flat audiometric configuration. (B) Gradually sloping audiometric configuration. (C) Sharply sloping audiometric configuration. (D) Precipitously sloping audiometric configuration. (E) Rising audiometric configuration. (F) Trough audiometric configuration. (G) Notch at 4000 Hz. (H) Saucer audiogram.

ossicular discontinuity, middle-ear tumor, thickened tympanic membrane, and impacted ear canal. A saucer audiogram has poorer air-conduction thresholds at the high and low frequencies than at the mid frequencies. Figure 32 illustrates eight audiometric configurations.

D. MAGNITUDE OF HEARING IMPAIRMENT

The degree of magnitude of hearing impairment, as well as the type and configuration of hearing impairment, should be classified. Most magnitude-of-hearing-impairment classification systems are based on the pure-tone average for the air-conduction thresholds at 500, 1000, and 2000 Hz. Table XIII shows a commonly employed classification system for describing the severity of hearing impairment in adults. A similar classification system is used for describing the severity of hearing impairment in children, except that a pure-tone average less than or equal to 15 dB HL is considered normal hearing, a pure-tone average between 16 and 25 dB HL is considered a slight hearing loss, and a pure-tone average between 26 and 40 dB HL is considered a mild hearing loss.

As mentioned earlier in Sections II,C and V,C of this chapter, high-frequency hearing sensitivity affects the hearing in noise in normal-hearing and hearing-impaired persons and the hearing in quiet in hearing-impaired persons. Therefore, classification of the magnitude of hearing loss should be based on the hearing sensitivity at high as well as low frequencies.

Another shortcoming of the traditional classification system for magnitude of hearing loss is that a pure-tone average based on the best two of the three speech frequencies (Fletcher, 1950; Martin, 1975; Newby, 1972; Siegenthaler & Strand, 1964), or a three-frequency pure-tone average in cases of significantly rising or sloping audiometric configurations, often underestimates the hearing handicap. For example, a patient with 0 dB HL at 500 Hz, 10 dB HL at 1000 Hz, and 50 dB HL at 2000 Hz would have normal hearing using either the two- or three-frequency pure-tone average. Clinical experience shows that persons with such hearing threshold levels will have difficulty hearing in noisy situations.

A modified system for classification of magnitude of

hearing impairment is proposed which is based on the hearing sensitivity at high as well as low frequencies and which, at least partially, overcomes the problem of underestimation of the hearing handicap in significantly sloping and rising audiometric configurations. We recommend that magnitude of hearing impairment be determined for the low–mid frequencies (500, 1000, and 2000 Hz) and for the high frequencies (3000 and 4000 Hz). Table XIV shows the proposed classification system. Table XV shows the air- and bone-conduction thresholds, audiometric configuration, low–mid frequency average, high frequency average, low–mid frequency magnitude of hearing impairment, high frequency magnitude of hearing impairment, low–mid frequency type of hearing impairment, and high frequency type of hearing impairment for five cases.

We also propose that the type of hearing impairment be classified along similar lines as the magnitude of hearing impairment is classified. Classifying the type of hearing impairment for a given ear varies enormously from clinic to clinic and even from audiologist to audiologist. We propose that, if 500, 1000, and 2000 Hz show the same type of impairment, the low–mid frequencies should be classfied as having that type of impairment. If all of these frequencies do not show the same type of hearing impairment, then the

Table XIII Classification of Magnitude of Hearing Impairment[a]

dB HL Range	Term
<26	Normal hearing
26–40	Mild hearing impairment
41–55	Moderate hearing impairment
56–70	Moderately severe hearing impairment
71–90	Severe hearing impairment
>90	Profound hearing impairment

[a] Modified from Lloyd and Kaplan (1978).

Table XIV Proposed System for Classifying Magnitude of Hearing Impairment in the Low–Mid Frequencies (500, 1000, and 2000 Hz) and High Frequencies (3000–4000 Hz)

Criterion	Procedure for determining average based on one, two, or three frequencies
Low–mid frequency magnitude	
1. If the 500 Hz threshold is within 20 dB of the 2000 Hz threshold	Traditional three-frequency pure-tone average
2. If the 500 Hz threshold is not within 20 dB of the 2000 Hz threshold and there is not more than a 20-dB difference between the two worst speech frequencies (500, 1000, or 2000 Hz)	Two-frequency pure-tone average based on the two worst speech frequencies
3. If the 500 Hz threshold is not within 20 dB of the 2000 Hz threshold and there is more than a 20-dB difference between the two worst speech frequencies	Two-frequency pure-tone average based on the worst speech frequency and the interoctave between the two worst speech frequencies
High frequency magnitude	
1. If the 2000 Hz threshold is within 20 dB of the 4000 Hz threshold	Threshold at 4000 Hz
2. If the 2000 Hz threshold is not within 20dB of the 4000 Hz threshold	Two-frequency pure-tone average based on 3000 Hz and 4000 Hz

Table XV The Air- and Bone-Conduction Threshold Levels, Audiometric Configuration, and Magnitude and Type of Hearing Impairment for the Low–Mid Frequencies and High Frequencies for Five Cases Using the Proposed Classification System

Case	Conduction	Frequency (Hz) 250	500	750	1000	1500	2000	3000	4000	6000	8000	Audiometric configuration	Average (dB HL) Low–mid1[a]	Low–mid2[b]	Low–mid3[c]	High1[d]	High2[e]	Magnitude Low–mid	High	Type of hearing impairment Low–mid frequencies	High frequencies
1	Air	5	10	—	10	—	5	5	10	—	15	Flat	8	—	—	10	—	normal	normal	normal hearing	normal hearing
	Bone	5	5	—	15	—	15	—	10	—	—										
2	Air	15	25	40	55	—	65	75	90	100	>100	Sloping	—	60	—	—	83	moderate–severe	severe	essentially sensorineural	sensorineural
	Bone	15	15	—	45	—	70	—	>75	—	—										
3	Air	15	20	—	25	35	50	50	55	—	>50	Sloping	—	—	43	55	—	moderate	moderate	essentially normal hearing with significant air-bone gaps	conductive
	Bone	0	5	—	5	—	10	—	15	—	—										
4	Air	30	40	55	65	—	65	85	90	95	>100	Sloping	—	65	—	—	88	moderate–severe	severe	mixed	sensorineural
	Bone	15	25	—	30	—	35	—	>75	—	—										
5	Air	75	70	60	45	—	40	50	40	—	45	Rising	—	—	65	40	—	moderate–severe	mild	essentially mixed	mixed
	Bone	15	15	—	30	—	25	—	20	—	—										

[a] Based on low–mid frequency criterion 1 in Table XIV.
[b] Based on low–mid frequency criterion 2 in Table XIV.
[c] Based on low–mid frequency criterion 3 in Table XIV.
[d] Based on high frequency criterion 1 in Table XIV.
[e] Based on high frequency criterion 2 in Table XIV.

word "essentially" should modify the type of hearing impairment shared by the majority of the frequencies (500, 1000, and 2000 Hz). The type of hearing impairment at the high frequencies should be based on the type of hearing impairment at 4000 Hz.

VIII. MAJOR ETIOLOGIES OF AUDITORY DISORDERS

A. CONDUCTIVE HEARING IMPAIRMENT

Conductive hearing impairment resulting from disorders of the outer and/or middle ear usually can be treated surgically or medically. Conductive hearing impairment, therefore, is generally reversible.

1. EXTERNAL EAR
a. Atresia
The absence of the external auditory meatus because of failure in embryologic development is called atresia. If a partial opening is present, the condition is called stenosis rather than atresia. Atresia is often accompanied by microtia, the total or partial absence of the auricle, because the auricle and external auditory meatus develop embryologically at the same time. Atresia can be hereditary (as an isolated genetic disorder or part of a cranio-facial syndrome such Treacher–Collins Syndrome), associated with interruptions during embryologic development (e.g., rubella, thalidomide), or associated with chromosomal abnormalities. Atresia is usually unilateral and associated with a maximum conductive hearing impairment (60 dB HL).

b. Cerumen Impaction
Cerumen, or ear wax produced by glands underneath the skin of the external auditory meatus, lubricates the skin, prevents foreign bodies from entering the ear canal, and protects against maceration. The cerumen usually migrates laterally and falls out of the ear canal. In some persons, however, the anatomy of the ear canal prevents cereumen from falling out so the wax becomes impacted and causes occlusion of the ear canal. Impacted cerumen also occurs when cotton-tipped applicators are used to clean the ear; the use of these swabs actually pushes the cerumen more deeply into the ear canal. Cerumen impaction often occurs in persons who wear hearing aids since the earmolds prevent outward migration of the cerumen. Sometimes diving causes wax to be pushed deep into the ear canal. Cerumen accumulates gradually and a conductive hearing loss occurs only when the meatus is completely occluded. As long as there is a tiny opening in the meatus, sound will travel through the ear canal. The loss associated with impacted cerumen is of sudden onset. It may be mild to moderate.

c. Foreign Bodies in the External Auditory Meatus
Foreign bodies such as beans, cotton, roaches, buttons, paper, or pens may be present in the ear canal. The foreign bodies are often present in the ear canals of children. They can cause occlusion of the ear canal with concomitant conductive hearing loss and can irritate the skin of the ear

canal, resulting in external otitis. Tympanic membrane perforation can sometimes result from foreign objects in the ear canal.

d. Bony Growths

Exostoses are multiple, hard, bony growths of the ear canal covered with skin. A contributing factor in the development of exostoses may be frequent swimming in cold salt water. Exostoses are often bilateral. Osteomas are spongy bony growths of the ear canal covered with skin. They occur singly rather than as multiple growths. Unlike exostoses, osteomas usually continue to grow. Neither osteomas nor exostoses are associated with conductive hearing loss unless they cause cerumen impaction or occlude the meatus.

e. External Otitis

External otitis, an infection of the skin of the external auditory meatus, is also known as "swimmer's ear." It is a very commonly occurring condition. Signs and symptoms of external otitis include itching and severe pain, especially upon manipulation of the affected area. Sometimes aural discharge occurs. Fever is occasionally present. The ear canal is swollen and tender. Conductive hearing loss occurs only if the canal is completely closed. External otitis may result from trauma to the ear canal such as that caused by foreign bodies, fungi (molds), bacteria, chemicals, and sparks. External otitis is most common during the summer months because of water maceration or trauma from swimming.

2. MIDDLE EAR

a. Tympanic Membrane Perforations

Tympanic membrane perforations are caused by direct trauma to the tympanic membrane (for example, from bobby pins), indirect trauma, (for example, from pressure from a slap on the head or explosion near the ear), hot slag (metal) burns commonly occurring in welders, or middle-ear infection resulting in necrosis and perforation of the tympanic membrane. Accompanying signs and symptoms include pain, bleeding, a hollow sensation in the ear, and conductive hearing impairment, the degree of which depends on the size and site of the perforation.

b. Tympanosclerosis

Tympanosclerosis is a condition characterized by the formation of white plaques on the tympanic membrane, causing thickening and scarring of the tympanic membrane. The white plaques reflect degeneration of the hyaline cartilage within the middle layer of the tympanic membrane, and calcium deposition. Tympanosclerosis usually results from repeated middle-ear infections. Tympanosclerosis may be present in some elderly persons with a history of chronic rheumatism or arthritis (Calavita, 1978).

c. Otitis Media

Otitis media is an inflammation of the middle ear. When there is bacterial infection of the associated middle-ear effusion and pus is present, the condition is termed acute purulent otitis media. Acute purulent otitis media often follows or occurs simultaneously with an upper respiratory infection. Eustachian-tube dysfunction is present. There are four progressive stages of inflammation. (a) Hyperemia is a reddening and thickening of the tympanic membrane accompanied by discomfort. The hearing sensitivity may be within normal limits. (b) Exudation is the development of serous (nonpurulent) liquid in the middle-ear space accompanied by pain, fever, and fluctuating conductive hearing impairment. (c) In suppuration, the liquid becomes purulent and the tympanic membrane may rupture. (With rupture, the pain and fever decrease.) (d) In uncomplicated cases, resolution occurs: the perforation heals spontaneously, the liquid becomes serous and thin before diminishing, and the hyperemia decreases. Acute purulent otitis media occurs most frequently during the cold winter season, particularly in children less than 6 years of age. Repeated occurrences of acute purulent otitis media are referred to as acute otitis media.

Acute purulent otitis media present for 12 weeks or more is called chronic otitis media with effusion (Pashley, 1984). According to Pashley (1984), chronic otitis media with effusion may have three progressive stages: (a) initiation, which is the twelfth week of constant effusion; (b) full expression, which is the constant presence of effusion beyond twelve weeks; and (c) degeneration, in which tympanosclerosis and/or tympanic membrane retraction may be present. Rare complications of chronic otitis media with effusion include labyrinthitis, coalescent mastoiditis, petrositis, meningitis, lateral sinus thrombophlebitis, otic hydrocephalus, and intracranial abscesses (Pappas, 1985). Sequelae of chronic otitis media with effusion include structural damage to the middle ear, such as atrophy of the tympanic membrane and epithelial layers of the middle-ear mucosa, osteitis with erosion of the ossicular chain, tympanosclerosis, formation of granulation tissue, cholesteatoma, and cholesterol granuloma (Pappas, 1985). Perforation of the tympanic membrane and a pus discharge from the ear may also occur.

Serous otitis media is an inflammation of the middle ear accompanied by nonpurulent, thin, watery effusion. It results from Eustachian-tube dysfunction or blockage which leads to failure to ventilate the middle ear. Eustachian-tube dysfunction is often present in children with cleft palate who have decreased function of the palate muscles, children with Down's syndrome who have alterations in Eustachian-tube anatomy or musculature, and persons with other cranio-facial abnormalities. Other causes of Eustachian-tube dysfunction or blockage include infection, allergies, adenoid hypertrophy, tumors of the nasopharynx, barotrauma from rapidly changing air pressure (such as that encountered during airplane descent or scuba diving), radiotherapy of the nasopharynx, nasal obstruction from a deviated nasal septum, and recurrent nasopharyngitis (Pashley, 1984). Eustachian-tube dysfunction first results in absorption of air by the middle-ear tissues followed by negative middle-ear pressure followed by secretion of liquid from the middle-ear tissues into the middle-ear space. Serous otitis media is often accompanied by fluctuating conductive hearing impairment.

Prolonged and/or recurrent serous otitis media may result in adhesive otitis media, sometimes referred to as "glue ear," which is characterized by very thick and viscous liquid in the middle ear that adheres to the ossicles, thickening of the tympanic membrane, and retraction of the tympanic membrane. Adhesive otitis media is accompanied by conductive hearing impairment.

d. Otosclerosis

Otosclerosis, also known as otospongiosis, is a disease of the labyrinthine capsule and stapedial footplate. It most frequently affects the site just anterior to the oval window (Derlacki, 1984). Initially, otosclerosis is characterized by the active growth of soft, spongy, vascular bone. The phase of active growth is followed by an inactive phase in which the growth hardens and becomes dense and sclerotic. Involvement of the stapes, particularly the stapedial footplate, results in impairment of stapedial movement (stapedial fixation), leading to progressive conductive hearing impairment. There is controversy concerning the existence of cochlear otosclerosis associated with pure sensorineural hearing impairment, in which there is otosclerotic involvement of the cochlear capsule (medial rather than lateral growth of new bone).

The etiology of otosclerosis has not yet been established. There appears to be a genetic factor with an autosomal dominant mode of inheritance with a penetrance of 25–40% (Shambaugh, 1967; Schuknecht, 1971). Otosclerosis is prevalent in approximately 10% of Caucasians and 1% of Blacks. It occurs rarely in Orientals. It occurs in twice as many females as males. The onset of otosclerosis in women is often associated with pregnancy. Otosclerosis usually begins between 20 and 30 years of age. It is bilateral in approximately 85–90% of the cases.

Signs and symptoms of otosclerosis include gradually progressive conductive hearing impairment (which may stabilize), tinnitus, and sometimes vertigo and nausea. In approximately 10% of the cases, otoscopic examination reveals a positive Schwartze sign, which is a reddish glow of the posterior–inferior promontory visible through the tympanic membranes (Derlacki, 1984).

Early otosclerosis is characterized by a low-frequency conductive hearing loss. As the disease progresses, the air-conduction audiometric configuration flattens because a mass component as well as a stiffness component is added to the middle-ear system. When a resistive component is added to the middle-ear system, the magnitude of the hearing impairment is increased. The Carhart notch (Carhart, 1950), which is an elevation of the bone-conduction threshold (but not air-conduction threshold) at that frequency, is often present at 2000 Hz.

Ossicular fixations other than otosclerosis are sometimes present at birth and are termed congenital ossicular fixations.

e. Cholesteatoma

Cholesteatoma, also known as keratoma, is a cyst which usually occurs in the middle-ear cavity but may occur in the temporal bone. Cholesteatomas are often associated with tympanic-membrane perforation or retraction. A cholesteatoma is more likely to be associated with perforation in the posterior superior pars tensa margin or on the pars flaccida involving the attic than with a perforation in the central tympanic membrane. Cholesteatomas may develop following chronic or recurrent otitis media, are occasionally idiopathic, and are rarely congenital. As the disease progresses, it may cause necrosis of the ossicular chain, labyrinthine fistula, paralysis of the facial nerve, and may invade the mastoid, internal auditory canal, or cerebellopontine angle. The disease usually progresses slowly but may progress rapidly if an active infection is also present.

Signs and symptoms of cholesteatoma include earache, tinnitus, conductive hearing loss, and a foul-smelling aural discharge. Symptoms may be absent in cases with a small cholesteatoma which develops in the attic. A sensorineural component may be present in cases in which the cholesteatoma involves the bony labyrinth, the internal auditory canal, or the cerebellopontine angle.

f. Glomus Jugulare and Glomus Tympanicum Tumors

Glomera jugularae are very small, neural bodies that are normally present in the body (Jerger & Jerger, 1981). In the temporal bone, they may be present superior to the jugular bulb (which is inferior to the floor of the middle ear), on the glossopharyngeal and vagus nerves, or in the mucosa and tympanic plexus of the cochlear promontory (Jerger & Jerger, 1981).

Neoplasms of the glomus jugular usually originate in the middle-ear cavity or the jugular bulb region. When a neoplasm develops in the jugular bulb region, it may invade the floor of the middle ear and spread into the middle-ear space (Jerger & Jerger, 1981). Neoplasms which originate in and are contained in the middle-ear space are often called glomus tympanicum tumors, whereas neoplasms which originate in the jugular bulb region and spread into the middle ear are termed glomus jugulare tumors. Glomus jugulare tumors, commonly occurring neoplasms of the middle ear, are almost always unilateral. Of 209 temporal bone lesions investigated by Greer, Cody, & Weiland (1976), approximately 39% were glomus jugulare tumors and approximately 9% were glomus tympanicum tumors. Approximately 80% of the cases with glomus tumors are females; the age of diagnosis is usually between 40 and 60 years of age (Jerger & Jerger, 1981). The onset of the symptoms precedes diagnosis by approximately 4–6 years (Alford & Guilford, 1962; Greer, Cody, & Weiland, 1976). Although glomus tumors are slow-growing, they can metastasize and be fatal (Cole, 1977).

Signs and symptoms of glomus tumors generally include pulsatile tinnitus, hearing loss, aural fullness, and ear pain. Facial-nerve paralysis may be present in cases with glomus tympanicum, and cranial nerves 8–12 may be affected in cases with glomus jugulare tumors (Jerger & Jerger, 1981). The hearing impairment may be progressive conductive, mixed, or sensorineural.

g. Ossicular Discontinuity

Ossicular discontinuity, or a break anywhere along the ossicular chain, often occurs in cases of head trauma or may be a congenital malformation of the middle ear. Congenital ossicular discontinuity may be associated with other craniofacial abnormalities such as Pierre–Robin and Treacher–Collins syndromes and atresia with microtia, or may be associated with musculoskeletal diseases such as osteogenesis imperfecta. Ossicular discontinuity may occur in some cases of chronic or recurrent otitis media and cholesteatoma. Incudostapedial joint separation is the most common site of ossicular disruption. Signs and symptoms of ossicular discontinuity include conductive hearing impairment. When associated with head trauma, skull fracture and facial-nerve impairment may be present.

B. SENSORINEURAL HEARING IMPAIRMENT

Sensorineural hearing impairment results from disorders of the cochlea, eighth cranial nerve, or cochlear nuclei. Generally, sensorineural hearing impairment is irreversible. Usually, in contrast to conductive hearing impairment, sensorineural hearing impairment cannot be alleviated surgically or by medical intervention except in some cases of Meniere's disease, sudden hearing impairment associated with interruption of the cochlear blood supply, or perilymphatic fistula. Generally, sensorineural hearing impairment is managed through aural rehabilitation or habilitation including amplification.

1. Congenital

Some genetic forms of hearing impairment are associated with other anomalies, although most are not. Those associated with other genetic anomalies are usually called syndromes (Konigsmark, 1971). Etiologies of nongenetic congenital hearing impairment may be maternal infection, birth complications such as asphyxia or anoxia, accident during pregnancy, malformation during embryologic development, drugs, or metabolic disorders.

a. Nongenetic

Most perinatal infections resulting in sensorineural hearing impairment in the offspring are nonbacterial. These perinatal infections may cross the placental barrier and result in a sensorineural hearing impairment in the fetus. The acronym TORCHS stands for toxoplasmosis, other infections such as bacterial meningitis, rubella, cytomegalovirus, herpes simplex, and syphilis.

Toxoplasmosis is a protozoal infection which causes a slowly progressive sensorineural hearing impairment which may be associated with hydrocephalus, seizures, mental retardation, visual impairment, and neuromuscular impairment. Transmission from the mother to the fetus is transplacental. Approximately 17% of infants with toxoplasmosis have hearing impairment (Abrams, 1977).

Maternal rubella (German measles) acquired during the first trimester of pregnancy may result in congenital cataracts or glaucoma, congenital heart disease, microcephaly, mental retardation, and/or sensorineural hearing impairment. The sensorineural hearing impairment is usually a bilateral severe-to-profound sensorineural hearing impairment with a trough audiometric configuration. The loss may be progressive. After the first trimester, visual and cardiac impairments are less common although hearing and neurologic impairment may still result. In general, the later in pregnancy maternal rubella is acquired, the less severe the malformations. The fetus may be affected by maternal rubella even if the infection appears in a subclinical form and is asymptomatic in the mother.

Cytomegalovirus (CMV) is the most commonly occurring infection in the TORCHS group. Approximately 0.5–2.5% of all infants are born with CMV infection. Approximately 90% of the infants evidence no symptoms at birth; ther other 10% manifest symptoms of CMV. Unilateral or bilateral sensorineural hearing impairment is present in approximately 7–17% of those who are asymptomatic at birth but excrete this virus in the urine (Stagno, 1984). The symptomatic infants who survive—approximately 29% die—manifest microcephaly, mental retardation, chorioretinitis (inflammation of the choroid and retina), neuromuscular disorders, hepatosplenomegaly, (enlargement of the spleen and liver), hyperbilirubinemia, thrombocytopenia (decrease in the number of blood platelets) with skin discolorations from blood escape (petechiae or purpura), and cerebral calcifications. Unilateral or bilateral sensorineural hearing impairment is present in 30% of infants with CMV (Pass, Stagno, Meyers, & Alford, 1980). The hearing impairment associated with CMV is generally progressive and may be associated with cochlear and retrocochlear pathology and with central auditory disorders.

Herpes simplex virus is a sexually transmitted disease which is usually transmitted during passage through the birth canal rather than through the placenta during pregnancy. More than half of the infants born with herpes simplex virus die. The infection in the surviving infants is generalized and severe. According to Northern and Downs (1984) and Gerkin (1984), there are no reported cases of hearing impairment associated with herpes simplex virus, although studies reveal that the sensory cells of the labyrinth are affected.

Maternal syphilis (lues) may be transmitted through the placental barrier to the fetus and result in congenital syphilis. Syphilis is a protozoal infection and is the least common of the TORCHS infections. Congenital syphilis is asymptomatic in approximately 50% of infants. Signs and symptoms of congenital syphilis include saddle nose, frontal projections, corneal scars (interstitial keratitis), dental abnormalities such as mulberry molars and Hutchinson's teeth, sensorineural hearing impairment, and vestibular signs. The sensorineural hearing impairment is usually bilateral, of sudden onset, and can occur any time between birth and 60 years of age. The loss is of cochlear and/or neural origin. When onset of the loss occurs in adulthood, it begins as a low-frequency sensorineural hearing impairment and develops into a flat, asymmetrical sensorineural hearing impairment which may also fluctuate. Vestibular involvement may be present as indicated by falling and walking difficulties. Congenital syphilis can be fatal, particularly when it is untreated.

b. Genetic

Most forms of genetic congenital sensorineural hearing impairment is autosomal recessive. Genetic congenital sensorineural hearing impairment may occur in isolation or in a syndrome.

Waardenburg's syndrome is an autosomal dominant disorder having variable penetrance. Signs and symptoms of the syndrome include white forelock, heterochromia iridis (multicolored eyes or one eye differently colored than the other), wide displacement of the medial canthi, flattening of the bridge of the nose, cupid's bow of the lips, hyperplasia of the medial portion of the eyebrows, prominent mandible, congenital unilateral or bilateral sensorineural hearing impairment which may be progressive, and sometimes cleft or high-arched palate.

Albinism, absence of coloring pigmentation, may be associated with congenital sensorineural hearing impairment. It is a dominant disorder. Signs and symptoms of albinism include white fine hair, very fair skin, severe congenital sensorineural hearing impairment, and sometimes heterochromia iridis.

The mode of inheritance of Klippel–Feil syndrome, an otocervical disorder, has not been established. Signs and symptoms of this syndrome include short or absent neck, reduced head movement, clubfoot, cleft palate, neurologic disturbances, and hearing impairment. There may be malformations of the middle ear (e.g., atresia, malformed ossicles) and/or inner ear (e.g., a malformed cochlea or vestibular labyrinth) and/or auditory nerve absence. The hearing impairment is usually sensorineural, but may also be conductive or mixed. A central auditory disorder may also be present.

Usher's syndrome involves retinitis pigmentosa and sensorineural hearing impairment. Retinitis pigmentosa is a degenerative, bilateral visual condition initially characterized by loss of night vision and later by loss of the peripheral field vision (tunnel vision). As the disease progresses, it leads to central visual dysfunction and eventually blindness. Retinitis pigmentosa represents a group of diseases. Approximately 0.3–0.5% of persons in the general population are carriers of an Usher's syndrome gene. Usher's syndrome is the most frequent cause of deaf–blindness. The mode of inheritance of Usher's syndrome is autosomal recessive. The onset of the sensorineural hearing impairment apparently occurs at the same time as that of the visual problems (Karp & Santore, 1983). The onset of the hearing impairment is variable from childhood to adulthood. According to Merin, Abraham, and Auerbach (1974), there may be two forms of Usher's syndrome; Type I involves retinitis pigmentosa, profound sensorineural hearing impairment, and vestibular abnormalities and Type II involves slowly progressive sensorineural hearing impairment, no vestibular abnormalities, and less severe visual dysfunction.

Mucopolysaccharidosis, an autosomal recessive disorder, is characterized by excessive excretion of mucopolysaccharides in the urine. The two most common forms of mucopolysaccharidosis associated with hearing impairment are Hunter's syndrome and Hurler's syndrome. Hunter's syndrome is not as severe as Hurler's syndrome and the former affects only males where as the latter can affect both males and females. Signs and symptoms of mucopolysaccharidosis include mental impairment, reduced stature, malformations of the bones and joints, large head, widely spaced eyes, flattening of the bridge of the nose, coarse facial features, hepatosplenomegaly, corneal clouding, hirsutism, joint stiffness, cardiac deformities, humpback, blindness, prominent eyebrows, wide lips, protruding abdomen, and sensorineural or conductive hearing impairment. The prevalence of hearing impairment is 5.2% in Hurler's syndrome and 43% in Hunter's syndrome (Northern & Downs, 1978).

Down syndrome is an autosomal aberration syndrome. It is also referred to as mongolism and Trisomy 21 syndrome. The disorder usually results from an extra chromosome (21). Down syndrome occurs in approximately 0.12–0.16% of live births (Northern & Downs, 1978). Signs and symptoms of Down syndrome include stenosis of the external auditory canal (which normalizes in later childhood), increased incidence of serous otitis media and cholesteatoma with associated conductive hearing impairment, mild–moderate hearing impairment in approximately 17% (Balkany, Downs, Jafek, & Krajicek, 1979), mental retardation, stubby fingers (particularly the fifth), simian creases in the palms, flattened facial expression, and upward slant of the lateral canthi of the eyes.

Crouzon's disease is an autosomal dominant disorder with variable expression. Signs and symptoms of Crouzon's disease may include exophthalmos (bulging of the eyes), hypertelorism (great width between the eyes), strabismus (deviation of the eye), beaklike nose, malformed head with a protruding forehead, bifid uvula, cleft palate, low-set ears, middle-ear malformations such as ossicular fixation, atresia of the external auditory meatus, and nonprogressive hearing impairment which may be conductive or sensorineural. When malformed (lobster-claw) hands or feet are also present, the disorder is known as Apert's syndrome.

Treacher–Collins syndrome has an autosomal dominant mode of inheritance with high penetrance and variable expression. Characteristic features of Treacher–Collins syndrome include microtia, atresia, eyes that slope downward at the lateral canthi, receding chin, fishlike mouth, dental abnormalities, coloboma (notch of the lower lid), middle-ear abnormalities such as absence or fixation of the ossicular chain, inner-ear abnormalities, and hearing impairment. The hearing impairment may be conductive, sensorineural, or mixed.

2. ADVENTITIOUS

Adventitious hearing impairment is postnatally acquired hearing impairment. Causes of adventitious hearing impairment include drugs, noise, age, systemic disease, degenerative disorders, infections, trauma, and tumors. Some cases of adventitious hearing impairment are idiopathic (of unknown cause).

a. Idiopathic

Meniere's disease affects the membranous labyrinth and is characterized by hydropic distention of the endolymphatic system (Hallpike & Cairns, 1938). The three types of Meniere's disease are classic Meniere's disease, cochlear Meniere's disease, and vestibular Meniere's disease (Pulec, 1984). Features of classic Meniere's disease include fluctuating and progressive sensorineural hearing impairment (of cochlear origin), aural fullness and pressure, roaring tinnitus, and vertigo. Cochlear Meniere's disease is classic Meniere's disease without vertigo. Vestibular Meniere's disease is classic Meniere's disease without hearing impairment. Cochlear and vestibular Meniere's disease may later develop into classic Meniere's disease. Initially, the hearing loss affects the low frequencies and, later on, also affects the high frequencies. The attacks of vertigo are episodic and are often accompanied by nausea and vomiting along with tinnitus, aural pressure and fullness, and hearing loss (in classic Meniere's disease). Early in the classic form of the disease, the hearing impairment and vestibular functioning recover but later on in the disease the hearing impairment becomes permanent (and increases during attacks), tinnitus may be permanent (and worsen during attacks), and there may be instability between spells. Syphilis is considered to be the great imitator of Meniere's disease. Meniere's disease is unilateral in more than 85% of cases, occurs more frequently in males than females, and is rare in Blacks (Gerber & Mencher, 1980). The onset of this disease occurs usually before 50 years of age (Gerber & Mencher, 1980).

The disease is idiopathic in 45% of those affected (Pulec, 1984). Known causes of Meniere's disease include allergy, particularly to foods, insufficiency of the pituitary and adrenal glands, hypothyroidism, stenosis of the internal auditory canal causing compression inside the canal, head or acoustic trauma, vascular disease, estrogen insufficiency, viral disease, or a combination of these causes (Pulec, 1984).

Sudden idiopathic sensorineural impairment refers to sensorineural hearing impairment of sudden onset. Sudden idiopathic sensorineural hearing impairment can be established only when known etiologies are ruled out. Etiologies which must be excluded include known infections, trauma, definitive vascular disease, known otologic disease, and others. Postulated etiologies for this disorder include viruses and vascular disturbances (Alford, Shaver, Rosenberg, & Guilford, 1965).

The hearing impairment may be of cochlear and/or eighth-cranial-nerve origin and may be accompanied by tinnitus or vertigo. It is usually unilateral. Recovery to normal or improvement in the degree of hearing impairment occurs in approximately two-thirds of patients (Snow, 1973). Simmons (1978) has reported that spontaneous recovery occurs in 92% of the cases of sudden idiopathic sensorineural hearing loss with rising audiometric configurations and 28% of the cases with sloping sensorineural audiometric configurations.

b. Trauma

Perilymphatic fistula is rupture of the round or oval window resulting from abrupt increase in fluid pressure through the cochlear aqueduct (Pappas, 1985). Etiologies of perilymphatic fistula include head trauma, congenital conditions, diving, physical exertion (e.g., heavy lifting, sneezing), acoustic trauma, and idiopathic causes. Estimates of the percentage of fistula cases with idiopathic causes range from 12 to 33% (Wofford, 1981). Signs and symptoms of perilymphatic fistula include vertigo and sudden or progressive sensorineural hearing impairment of cochlear origin. Hearing impairment is not necessarily present. A negative fistula test does not rule out perilymphatic fistula, although a positive fistula test is a strong indicator of perilymphatic fistula.

Head injury can result in hearing impairment. Longitudinal fracture of the temporal bone, transverse fracture of the temporal bone, and labyrinthine concussion without fracture of the temporal bone may be associated with hearing impairment (Pappas, 1985). Longitudinal fractures are often associated with blows to the side of the head and typically affect the outer and middle ear; the facial nerve is also affected in approximately 25% of the cases. The hearing impairment associated with longitudinal fractures is usually sudden conductive hearing impairment (Pappas, 1985). Transverse fractures are usually associated with strong blows to the head which may result in unconsciousness and typically affect the inner ear and audiovestibular nerve; the facial nerve is also affected in approximately 50% of the cases. Vertigo and sudden sensorineural hearing impairment (often total) is often present in transverse fractures (Pappas, 1985). Signs and symptoms of labyrinthine concussion without temporal-bone fracture include vertigo, tinnitus, and sudden sensorineural hearing impairment. The hearing impairment in labyrinthine-concussion cases (without temporal-bone fracture) may be characterized by a notched, sloping, flat, or parabolic audiometric configuration (Wofford, 1981). The hearing impairment in head injuries may be unilateral or bilateral.

c. Drugs

Certain drugs can result in hearing impairment and/or vestibular dysfunction (ototoxicity). Drugs that primarily affect the cochlea, resulting in hearing impairment, are cochleotoxic whereas drugs that affect the vestibular system, resulting in vestibular dysfunction, are vestibulotoxic. Some drugs are both cochleotoxic and vestibulotoxic. The severity of the ototoxicity depends on the concentration of the drug in the blood (as indicated by the serum level in blood tests), the period of time the drug has been used, individual susceptibility (probably determined primarily by heredity), whether other ototoxic drugs are also being used, whether renal function is unimpaired, and whether there is concurrent noise exposure. Ototoxicity can occur any time in childhood or adulthood and may also be congenital, because an ototoxic drug administered to a pregnant woman can cross the placental barrier to the fetus. A common precursor of ototoxicity is tinnitus. Halting administration or reducing the dosage of an ototoxic drug when tinnitus occurs may prevent hearing impairment due to drug use.

Ototoxic drugs enter the inner ear through the bloodstream (Bergstrom & Thompson, 1984). The mechanism of hearing impairment from cochleotoxic drugs is damage to the sensory hair cells (outer and then inner) and stria vascularis of the cochlea (Boettcher, Henderson, Gratton, Danielson, & Byrne, 1987). Monitoring the serum level of the drug to prevent ototoxicity may not necessarily prevent ototoxicity since the drug persists longer in the inner-ear fluids than in the blood (Gerber 7 & Mencher, 1980). Since the kidney filters drugs from the bloodstream and excretes them from the body, renal insufficiency can lead to overaccumulation of ototoxic drugs and increase their ototoxic effect. Some ototoxic drugs also affect the kidney, at least temporarily (Bergstrom & Thompson, 1984). When ototoxic drugs are used in combination, they may have an ototoxic effect at lower serum levels than when the drugs are used singly. Recent studies show that hearing impairment from continuous noise can be increased by ototoxic drugs (this effect is enhanced when the noise occurs in combination with vibration) and the interaction may be synergistic (Boettcher et al., 1987).

Aminoglycoside antibiotics, antibacterial agents, are one class of ototoxic drug which may be administered to adults in cases of life-threatening infections and to neonates with sepsis (Boettcher et al., 1987). Aminoglycoside antibiotics include streptomycin, dihydrostreptomycin, kanamycin, gentamycin, nentilmycin, neomycin, tobramycin, and amikacin. Not all "mycin" drugs are ototoxic. For example, terramycin and aureomycin are not ototoxic.

Certain potent diuretics, used to treat refractory edema, are ototoxic. Ototoxic diuretics include furosemide (Lasix®), ethacrynic acid (Edecrin®), and bumetanide (Bumex®).

Salicylates are salicylic acids which are antipyretic (relieve fever), antiseptic (inhibit the growth of microorganisms), and antirheumatic agents. They represent another class of ototoxic drug. Salicylates include aspirin, Alka Seltzer®, Anacin®, and Bufferin®. Unlike the effects of other ototoxic drugs, the effects of these drugs are temporary so the hearing impairment (preceded by tinnitus) may be reversible upon cessation of drug use. These drugs are generally ototoxic at the high dosage levels common to arthritics, for example.

Other ototoxic drugs include cisplatinum (used to treat cancer), quinine (used to treat malaria and as an abortifacient), chloroquinine phosphate (used to treat malaria and some collagen diseases), thalidomide (a drug now removed from the market that was used to relieve discomfort in pregnancy), nitrogen mustard (used to treat cancer), tetanus antitoxin (innoculation against tetanus), and others.

Cochleotoxic drugs are associated with sensorineural hearing impairment of cochlear origin, generally bilateral and symmetrical, although some cases of unilateral or asymmetrical losses have been reported. It is usually of abrupt onset but may be of gradual onset. Tinnitus usually precedes or occurs in conjunction with the hearing impairment, which is permanent except in the case of salicylates. Vestibulotoxic drugs may cause disequilibrium, ataxia, unsteadiness, and/or vertigo. The vestibular damage associated with vestibulotoxic drugs is generally bilateral and permanent.

d. Noise

Exposure to hazardous levels of noise can result in what is known as noise-induced hearing impairment. The term "noise-induced hearing impairment" generally refers to hearing impairment from long-term, repeated exposure to noise (e.g., noise encountered in certain occupational and military settings or in recreational activities such as snowmobiling) whereas the term "acoustic trauma" generally refers to hearing impairment from a single exposure to a short-term noise (e.g., gunshot, explosion, or firecracker).

Excessive noise levels can cause damage, primarily in the cochlea, leading to sensorineural hearing impairment of cochlear origin. With exposure to very intense but not necessarily long-duration noise, the physical and mechanical stress properties of the structures within the cochlea may be surpassed, resulting in morphologic and circulatory changes in the cochlea and, in severe cases, degeneration of the eighth-cranial-nerve fibers (Melnick, 1984). With chronic exposure to moderate levels of noise, there may be metabolic and physiological/mechanical exhaustion (Melnick, 1984). Metabolic exhaustion is evidenced by decreases in oxygen and energy supply to the cochlea and swelling of the hair cells—first the outer and then the inner. Continued prolonged exposure to noise may lead to further auditory degeneration involving the eighth cranial nerve.

Auditory damage from exposure to high-frequency noise is typically associated with damage to the basal coil of the cochlea, resulting in high-frequency hearing impairment. Auditory damage from exposure to low-frequency noise is typically associated with damage to the apical coil of the cochlea, resulting in low-frequency hearing impairment. With continued, prolonged exposure, the damage spreads basally. The region of the cochlea showing maximal damage from broad-band noise, which is commonly found in industrial settings, is usually the basal coil because the resonance of the outer- and middle-ears is between 1000 and 4000 Hz and experimental observation shows that the frequency most affected by an intense signal of a particular frequency is one-half to one octave above the signal frequency.

Initially, exposure to hazardous noise levels results in a temporary threshold shift [threshold elevation that usually recovers after a short time (several hours or a few days) unless the sound is very intense] that is often accompanied by tinnitus, a sensation that speech is muffled, and aural fullness. With continued exposure to noise, the threshold shift becomes permanent. The development of permanent threshold shift is usually gradual.

Factors which affect the magnitude of permanent threshold shift from noise exposure include the acoustic characteristics of the noise (its intensity, duration, spectrum, and temporal pattern) and individual susceptibility. Continuous noises have a more adverse effect on hearing than intermittent noise. As mentioned previously in the section on drugs, the hearing impairment from noise exposure is enhanced by drugs and exposure to vibration. The hearing impairment associated with noise exposure is also increased in conditions that affect the acoustic reflex such as cases with congenital absence of the middle-ear muscles, stapedectomy, and Bell's palsy causing paralysis of the stapedius muscle.

The hearing impairment from noise exposure is sensorineural of primarily cochlear origin and the audiometric configuration characteristically reveals a notch at 3000–6000 Hz. Noise-induced hearing impairment is typically a bilateral hearing impairment and is usually symmetrical. It may be asymmetrical if there is "handedness" in the source of the sound, as evidenced by the audiograms of truck drivers and ambulance paramedics (Dufresne, Alleyne, & Reesai, 1988; Johnson, Hammond, & Sherman, 1980). Hearing impairment from acoustic trauma may be bilateral or unilateral. The prevalence of hearing impairment from noise exposure is greater in males than in females. Noise is the most common cause other than aging of sensorineural hearing impairment.

e. Aging

Presbycusis refers to hearing impairment associated with aging. Aging results in anatomic and physiologic degeneration at all levels of the auditory system. Age-related alterations of the auditory system include loss of elasticity in the pinna and external auditory meatus, freckling of the auricle, excessive coarse hair growth in the pinna, increased pinna size, a stiffened and more translucent tympanic membrane, stiffening of the ossicular chain, degeneration of the middle-ear muscles and ossicles, degeneration of the sensory hair and support cells and stria vascularis, decrease in the number of functional spiral ganglia and eighth-cranial-nerve fibers, loss of elasticity of the basilar membrane, reduced cochlear blood supply, reduction in the number of functional neurons in the central auditory system, and cortical atrophy (Belal & Stewart, 1974; Calavita, 1978; Crowe, Guild, & Palvogt, 1934; Hansen & Reske-Nielsen, 1965; Kirikae, Sato, & Shitara, 1964; Krmpotic-Nemanic, 1971; Nadol, 1981; Nerbonne, 1988; Rasmussen, 1940).

Schuknecht (1955, 1964, 1974) categorized four forms of presbycusis. In sensory presbycusis, the auditory damage is in the form of epithelial atrophy and degeneration of the hair and supporting cells of the cochlea, particularly in the basal coil. Sensory presbycusis is slowly progressive. In neural presbycusis, the auditory damage is in the form of slow reduction in the number of functional eighth-cranial-nerve fibers and other nerve fibers in the central auditory nervous system. Neural presbycusis is manifested by impairment in speech recognition that is greater than expected based on hearing sensitivity, which is not affected until the population of neuronal units is significantly decreased. Neural presbycusis is also referred to as central presbycusis (Johnson & Hawkins, 1972) since the brainstem and cortical auditory system as well as the peripheral auditory pathway are affected. In strial (metabolic) presbycusis, the auditory damage is characterized by atrophy of the stria vascularis, particularly in the middle and apical coils of the cochlea. The cochlear bioelectric capability is affected by stria vascularis atrophy. In cochlear conductive (mechanical) presbycusis, the auditory damage is characterized by degeneration of the mechanical properties of the cochlear duct (particularly the spiral ligament) and middle ear as evidenced by atrophy of the spiral ligament and stiffening of the basilar membrane and middle-ear structures. These forms occur either singly or in any combination.

The mechanism by which damage to the auditory system relating to aging occurs may be through vascular changes, genetic makeup affecting the time of onset and rate of aging, and cellular aging (Hansen & Reske-Nielsen, 1965; Nadol, 1981; Schuknecht, 1974). Environmental factors which accumulate through one's lifetime and which contribute to the aging process and affect the hearing impairment associated with aging include high-fat diet, occupational/environmental/recreational noise exposure, and ototoxic drugs (Corso, 1963a,b; Schow, Christensen, Hutchinson, & Nerbonne, 1978; Spencer, 1975).

The hearing impairment associated with presbyscuis is usually bilateral and sensorineural of cochlear and/or neural origin. A central auditory disorder may also be present. The hearing impairment is usually a slowly progressive one, affecting first the high frequencies and then the low frequencies (sloping configuration). Several investigators (Corso, 1963a; Lebo & Reddell, 1972) have reported that the onset of presbycusis occurs earlier in males than in females. Several studies also suggest that the magnitude of hearing impairment is greater in males than in females (Corso, 1963a,b; Moller, 1981; Moscicki, Elkins, Baum, & McNamara, 1985). There is evidence that the audiometric configuration associated with presbycusis slopes more abruptly for men than women (Corso, 1963a,b; Moscicki et al., 1985). Sensory presbycusis is associated with an abruptly sloping, slowly progressive, high-frequency hearing impairment (Schuknecht, 1974). Neural presbycusis generally shows substantial reduction in speech-recognition ability with onset of hearing impairment in relatively late adulthood (Schuknecht, 1974). Cochlear conductive presbycusis is associated with a steeply sloping hearing impairment affecting the low as well the high frequencies (Schuknecht, 1974). Strial presbycusis is generally associated with a flat, slowly progressive hearing impairment (Schuknecht, 1974). The results of a survey based on questionnaire data, done in 1977 and reported in 1982 (NCHS, 1982), reveal that approximately 24% of persons between 65 and 74 years of age and 38.5% of persons 75 years of age and older have hearing impairment. The prevalence of hearing impairment is markedly higher in the nursing-home population.

f. Systemic Disease

Disorders which affect the general metabolic system and/or chemical hemeostasis can cause hearing impairment (Gerber & Mencher, 1980). Hypothyroidism can result in conductive, sensorineural, or mixed hearing impairment that sometimes improves after medical treatment (Schuknecht, 1974). There is controversy in the literature regarding the effect of renal disease on hearing impairment. On the one hand, several studies show that sensorineural hearing impairment occurs in some patients with chronic renal failure because of the ototoxic drugs administered to treat the disease; the effect of the ototoxic drugs is enhanced by the renal dysfunction. On the other hand, a report by Laitakari (1977) showed that hearing impairment occurred more commonly in patients with chronic renal insufficiency than in a control group of nonrenal patients taking the same medication, indicating that ototoxicity is not the primary cause of the hearing impairment in patients with renal failure. Diabetes mellitus may be associated with sensorineural hearing impairment of cochlear and/or eighth-cranial-nerve origin. The prevalence of hearing impairment in diabetics ranges from 10 to 55% (Jerger & Jerger, 1981). The loss is progressive and bilateral and may be accompanied by dizziness. The primary mechanism of damage from diabetes is through vascular changes, including those in the cochlea.

g. Infections

Labyrinthitis is a disorder of the ear accompanied by sensorineural hearing impairment and vertigo. Serous labyrinthitis reflects an irritative process which may occur as a complication of otitis media or ear surgery. The damage may be transient or progress to destruction of the inner ear. Suppurative labyrinthitis reflects an irreversible, destructive process in the inner ear and may occur as a complication of bacterial infection such as bacterial meningitis. Labyrinthitis may also be caused by viral diseases such as measles, mumps, and rubella. Labyrinthitis is often misdiagnosed as vestibular neuronitis. The latter disorder is not, however, accompanied by hearing impairment.

Bacterial meningitis is an inflammation of the meninges (coverings) of the brain and the cerebrospinal fluid. Bacterial meningitis was discussed previously in the section on congenital nongenetic sensorineural hearing impairment. Bacterial meningitis is the most common cause of adventitious sensorineural hearing impairment in children. The mechanism of hearing impairment from bacterial meningitis is inflammation of the cochlea by transmission of the infection through the cochlear aqueduct or internal auditory canal. The infection may be accompanied by bilateral vestibular dysfunction and progressive sensorineural hearing impairment, which is also fluctuant in some cases. The sensorineural hearing impairment associated with bacterial meningitis may be of cochlear or eighth-cranial-nerve origin and is usually bilateral.

Sensorineural hearing impairment from acquired syphilis occurs far less frequently than from congenital syphilis. As mentioned earlier, congenital syphilis may result in sensorineural hearing impairment which is initially unilateral and then progresses quickly to a bilateral, symmetrical, and profound hearing impairment.

Other infections which can result in sensorineural hearing impairment through invasion of the inner ear include rubella, scarlet fever, herpes zoster, influenza, and other viral diseases of childhood. Mumps are the most common cause of unilateral sensorineural hearing impairment in children; it rarely causes bilateral impairment.

Some genetic forms of sensorineural hearing impairment related to recessive or dominant forms of inheritance do not appear at birth and may begin in childhood or early adulthood. Degenerative disorders associated with sensorineural hearing impairment are progressive.

h. Acoustic Schwannomas

Acoustic schwannoma is a neoplasm arising within the internal auditory canal, usually from the vestibular branch of the auditory nerve. Other terms used to refer to this neoplasm include acoustic neuroma, vestibular schwannoma, acoustic neurinoma, acoustic neurilemmoma, and acoustic neurofibroma. Since tumors of the auditory nerve affect the Schwann cells, they are more properly termed schwannomas. The overwhelming majority of acoustic schwannomas arise from the vestibular branch of the auditory nerve; slightly more than half originate from the inferior vestibular nerve and slightly less than half originate from the superior vestibular nerve (Linthicum, 1983).

The growth of acoustic schwannomas is extremely slow and insidious. Very fast tumor growth usually results from hemorrhage within the tumor. Malignant degeneration occurs very rarely. Sometimes the tumor growth is self-limited and asymptomatic. Most tumors, however, continue to enlarge and initially stretch and thin out the nerve fibers of the branch of origin over the surface of the tumor and later affect, by pressure and/or infiltration, the other nerves in the internal auditory canal.

There are three stages in the growth of acoustic schwannomas. The canal phase is associated with vestibular and auditory signs and symptoms caused by destruction and displacement of the sensory nerve branches. The cochlear phase is characterized by indirect involvement of the cochlear vascular system or direct invasion of the cochlea. The angle phase is characterized by growth into the cerebellopontine angle with signs and symptoms depending upon its size, position, and the degree to which the tumor interferes with the circulation of cerebrospinal fluid. Although the canal phase is always the first phase, the other phases do not necessarily occur and the cochlear phase does not necessarily precede the angle phase. Some tumors, for example, have predominantly cochlear expansion whereas other tumors have predominantly angle expansion.

There is no direct relation between tumor size and the signs and symptoms. Early symptoms do not necessarily indicate that the tumor is in an early stage of development. Conversely, total hearing impairment can result from a small, strategically situated canal tumor. The strong propensity for origination of the tumor from the vestibular branch is hypothesized to result from an embryologic over-accumulation of neuroglial cells supporting the vestibular nerves.

Acoustic schwannomas represent 8–10% of all brain tumors and 75–80% of all cerebellopontine angle tumors. Other commonly occurring cerebellopontine angle tumors include meningiomas and cholesteatomas. The cerebellopontine angle tumors usually demonstrate angle symptoms.

The age of onset is variable, occurring usually before age 70 with a medial age of onset of 30–40 years. In 50% of the cases, the initial symptom is hearing impairment, usually of gradual onset but of sudden onset in approximately 5–10% of the cases. Unilateral tinnitus is the initial symptom in approximately 12% of the cases. Tinnitus and hearing impairment occur together as initial symptoms in approximately 75% of the cases.

Dizziness is the initial symptom in only 7% of the cases. Nevertheless, as the tumor progresses, eventually 80% of those affected develop dizziness and unsteadiness, with balance problems that are chronic rather than episodic. Vertigo occurs rarely. In some unusual cases, there is an attack of vertigo which then subsides over time.

In 7% of cases, the initial symptom reflects involvement of the trigeminal (fifth) nerve (e.g., loss of pain, touch, and temperature sensibility of the face, or corneal anesthesia). As the tumor progresses, eventually 72% of the cases develop fifth-cranial-nerve symptoms. The fifth cranial nerve is the second most frequently involved cranial nerve in acoustic schwannomas.

Signs and symptoms of facial-nerve involvement occur initially in only 1% of those affected. As the tumor progresses, facial weakness develops eventually in less than 10% of the cases.

Signs and symptoms of angle involvement (e.g., headache, ataxia, and vomiting) occur initially in 8% of the patients. As the tumor progresses, angle symptoms eventually develop in 50–75% of cases and ultimately 100% of cases which go untreated. Large tumors which grow posteroinferiorly may occasionally affect the ninth and tenth cranial nerves, resulting in a jugular foramen syndrome (hoarseness, swallowing difficulty, aspiration of food). Ultimately, tumors which go untreated may interrupt circulation of cerebrospinal fluid, causing internal hydrocephalus, headaches, papilledema, diplopia, vomiting, and death from respiratory failure. In very rare cases, there is lateral rectus palsy reflecting involvement of the third, fourth, and sixth cranial nerves. The presence of oculomotor paralysis is generally suggestive of cerebellopontine angle tumors other than acoustic schwannomas.

The hearing impairment associated with acoustic schwannomas is of eighth-cranial-nerve origin with possible secondary sites of the cochlea or brainstem. The hearing impairment is generally a progressive, unilateral one but the onset is abrupt in a small percentage of cases. The complaint of difficulty understanding speech may precede a hearing impairment.

Bilateral acoustic schwannomas occur commonly in Von

Recklinghausen's disease (neurofibromatosis), a hereditary disorder characterized by schwannomas of myelinated and unmyelinated nerves, racemose angiomas (groupings of small tumors with blood or lymph vessels), skin abnormalities, and intracranial tumors. The mode of inheritance of the disease is autosomal dominant.

A report on audiologic manifestations of bilateral acoustic tumors (Bess, Josey, Glasscock, & Wilson, 1984) revealed that approximately 41% of 44 ears of 22 patients with bilateral acoustic schwannomas were normal hearing. When hearing impairment was present, it was usually bilateral. Of those with normal hearing or mild hearing impairment, approximately 61% had lesions exceeding 1.5 cm and approximately 26% had lesions of at least 4 cm. Thus, the occurrence of normal hearing or mild hearing impairment in cases with large bilateral acoustic schwannomas is more common than in cases with large unilateral acoustic schwannomas. To account for this, it has been hypothesized that, in unilateral cases, the uninvolved neurons are squeezed between the tumor and the wall of the internal auditory meatus because the tumor expands against the nerve (Bess *et al.*, 1984). In bilateral cases, the uninvolved neurons are not compressed to one side since the tumor expands within and through the nerve (Bess *et al.*, 1984).

C. CENTRAL AUDITORY DISORDERS

Central auditory disorders result from lesions of the auditory brainstem pathway or auditory cortex. It is controversial whether some children and adults who manifest auditory difficulties and yield central auditory test results similar to patients with organic central auditory disorders, but who are without apparent organic lesions of the central auditory nervous system have a central auditory disorder. Central auditory disorders may be characterized by auditory difficulties even in those with normal hearing sensitivity. Musiek (1985), for example, reported that auditory signs and symptoms of patients with organic lesions of the central auditory system and normal hearing sensitivity include tinnitus, auditory hallucinations, difficulty understanding speech in noisy or reverberant situations, difficulty understanding complex auditory directions or commands, difficulty attending auditorily with marked distractibility, difficulty localizing, and loss of appreciation of music. Although medical and surgical treatment may remove the organic lesion in some cases of organic cerebral lesions causing central auditory disorders, the central auditory disorder itself often is not alleviated by this treatment. Speech–language therapy may also be required. Treatment of children with central auditory disorders may consist of medication, educational management, and speech–language therapy. Central auditory disorders may be congenital or acquired.

1. CONGENITAL

Congenital central auditory disorders can result from toxoplasmosis acquired during pregnancy, hyperbilirubinemia, birth trauma, asphyxia, or erythroblastosis fetalis. Many of the factors producing congenital sensorineural hearing impairment can also cause central auditory disorders (Gerber & Mencher, 1980).

2. ACQUIRED

Intracranial tumors may be benign or malignant. Those intracranial tumors growing on the meninges (coverings of the brain and spinal cord) are called meningiomas. Intracranial tumors growing in the brain tissue include astrocytomas, glioblastomas, ependymomas, medulloblastomas, and pinealomas. The rate of growth of intracranial tumors is variable; some grow very slowly and others grow very rapidly. Children usually demonstrate fewer symptoms than adults because their brains are more elastic and can compensate for deficits, children are also less able to verbalize their difficulties. The signs and symptoms of temporal-lobe lesions are hemiparesis, seizures, memory impairment, emotional blunting or instability, gustatory/olfactory/auditory hallucinations, visual-field defects, deja vu phenomena, personality changes, and central auditory disorder (Gerber & Mencher, 1980; Jerger & Jerger, 1981). Approximately 10% of the cases demonstrate vertigo and/or tinnitus (Jerger & Jerger, 1981). Many cases with temporal-lobe pathology in the dominant hemisphere demonstrate aphasia. The signs and symptoms of brainstem tumors are hemiparesis, sensory loss, visual abnormalities, ocular–motor weakness, involuntary movement or tremors, abnormal corneal reflex, hydrocephalus, nystagmus, dizziness, facial paralysis, ataxia, vomiting, inadequate gag and cough reflexes, defective swallowing, hoarseness of the voice, and central auditory disorder (Jerger & Jerger, 1981). Intra-axial brainstem and temporal-lobe tumors are usually associated with normal hearing sensitivity or a mild, bilaterally symmetrical, high-frequency sensorineural hearing impairment.

As one gets older, the brain tends to fall caudally and arteriosclerosis and deterioration of vascular collagen result in distended or tortuous arteries (Moller & Moller, 1985). This vascular collagen in the brainstem exerts stress on the nerves of the cerebellopontine angle, for example, the audiovestibular nerve, leading to hyperactive syndromes and modified or progressive loss of nerve function (Moller & Moller, 1985). Signs and symptoms of vascular brainstem compression affecting the audiovestibular nerve include tinnitus, sensorineural hearing impairment, disequilibrium, and vertigo. Vascular compression of the brainstem affecting the audiovestibular nerve may result from elongation of one of the loops of the anterior inferior cerebellar artery between, under, or above the seventh and eighth cranial nerves (Moller & Moller, 1985). Cryptogenic (of obscure origin) hemifacial spasm results from cross-compression of the root entry zone of the facial nerve, leading to hyperactive facial-nerve dysfunction usually characterized by unilateral facial spasm. The cross-compression at the facial-nerve root entry zone may also affect the eighth cranial nerve and/or brainstem auditory pathway (Moller & Moller, 1985). Vascular compression of the brainstem can also result from elongation of arteries, usually a loop of the superior cerebellar artery, in the posterior fossa, leading to trigeminal neuralgia, a hyperactive dysfunction of the trigeminal nerve characterized by severe pain (more often on the right than on the left side). This type of vascular compression may exert pressure on the eighth cranial nerve and/or auditory brainstem pathways (Moller & Moller, 1985).

Multiple sclerosis is a degenerative disease affecting the central nervous system through demyelination (destruction of the myelin sheath of the nerves) while sparing the nerve axons. Plaque-like scars form at the sites of myelination (Cohn, 1981). The disease, ultimately progressive, is characterized by remissions and exacerbations (Keith & Jacobson, 1985). Although plaques may form anywhere in the brain and spinal cord, the brainstem, visual system, cerebellum, and/or pyramidal motor system are the sites most commonly affected (Cohn, 1981). The etiology is unknown.

Early signs and symptoms of multiple sclerosis include paresthesia (abnormal sensation such as burning or prickling), sensation of heaviness or numbness in one or more of the extremities, diplopia and blurring, mild ataxia, or vertigo (Jerger & Jerger, 1981). Classic signs and symptoms of multiple sclerosis may include visual difficulties, nystagmus, dysarthria, ataxia, bladder problems, paraplegia, muscle weakness or spasticity in the extremities, and mood changes such as euphoria, depression, or lability (Jerger & Jerger, 1981). Up to 75% of patients experience vertigo (Cohn, 1981). Temporal-lobe involvement may be manifested by apathy and lack of judgment, seizures, speech abnormalities (e.g., scanning speech, dysarthria, and slow speech rate) and sometimes word-retrieval difficulties (Gerber & Mencher, 1980). Complaints of auditory difficulties including tinnitus occur infrequently. Multiple sclerosis can cause sensorineural hearing impairment of eighth-cranial-nerve origin which may be bilateral or unilateral. When the cortical or brainstem auditory pathways are involved, a central auditory disorder may be present.

Multiple sclerosis is more prevalent in higher than in lower latitudes, in Caucasians than in Blacks, and in females than in males (Keith & Jacobson, 1985). The onset of symptoms is usually between 20 and 40 years of age. In approximately 10% of patients, there is a positive family history of the disease (Noffsinger, Olsen, Carhart, Hart, & Sahgal, 1972).

IX. CASE HISTORY

Prior to performing audiologic testing, the audiologist should obtain a complete history from the patient and then examine the ears to rule out the presence of cerumen. The case history enables the audiologist to understand the patient's difficulties and to develop strategies for testing. For example, knowledge of the better ear can guide the audiologist in terms of which ear to start testing and the presence of speech or language difficulties can guide the audiologist in terms of how speech-recognition testing should be done. The presence of tinnitus may suggest the need for using interrupted rather than continuous tones. Observation of patient difficulties in hearing the interview questions may guide the audiologist in terms of starting intensity in pure-tone testing. The absence of hearing difficulties during the interview together with the presence of a significant hearing impairment may alert the audiologist regarding testing for functional hearing impairment.

The case history can help establish the audiologic diagnosis. For example, the complaint of running ears helps establish the audiologic diagnosis of conductive hearing impairment as indicated by audiologic and acoustic-immittance testing. Difficulty hearing in noisy situations or on the telephone can confirm the audiologic diagnosis of sensorineural hearing impairment. Difficulty understanding speech in the presence of normal hearing sensitivity may confirm the audiologic diagnosis of retrocochlear disorder or central auditory disorder. Better hearing in noisy situations may confirm the audiologic diagnosis of conductive hearing impairment. The complaint that people are mumbling may confirm the audiologic diagnosis of high-frequency sensorineural hearing impairment. The complaint of difficulty hearing children's or women's voices may confirm the audiologic diagnosis of high-frequency sensorineural hearing impairment.

The degree of correspondence between the case history and the audiologic test results may alert the audiologist to measurement error associated with calibration, instrumentation, earphone placement, and so forth. For example, if a patient complains of a very mild problem but yields a severe hearing impairment upon audiologic testing, the audiologist should suspect a measurement error such as improper earphone placement.

The case history may also guide the audiologist in terms of patient management such as medical referral, referral for speech–language testing, hearing-aid evaluation, site-of-lesion testing, counseling, and so forth. The presence of medical complaints such as ear pain, tinnitus, ear discharge, and so forth should guide the audiologist to make a medical referral. The presence of vertigo should alert the audiologist to do site-of-lesion testing. The presence of communication difficulties in the absence of hearing impairment as evidenced by audiometric testing should alert the audiologist to do site-of-lesion testing and to make a medical referral. The presence of unilateral tinnitus should indicate the need for site-of-lesion testing and medical referral.

The case history may help the audiologist understand the etiology of the hearing impairment and thereby develop testing and management strategies. For example, a history of noise exposure together with a sensorineural notch at 3000–6000 Hz may indicate the need for audiologic monitoring and counseling. A history of perinatal infections should alert the audiologist to monitor the child's hearing. A case history of familial hearing impairment should alert the audiologist to the need for monitoring and genetic counseling. The use of ototoxic drugs should alert the audiologist to monitor the patient's hearing.

In the case of the adult, identifying information, purpose of referral, communication history, audiologic history, otologic history, and medical history should be obtained. In the case of the child, in addition to this information, the educational history, developmental history, prenatal history, and perinatal history should be obtained.

The following is an outline for obtaining a history.

1. Identifying information
   a. Name, address, telephone number
   b. Sex, age
   c. Occupation
   d. Referral source
2. Purpose of referral and presenting complaint
3. Audiologic history
   a. Onset: date, sudden or gradual, to what onset was related
   b. Better ear
   c. Unilateral or bilateral
   d. Stable, progressive, or fluctuating
   e. Family history of hearing impairment
   f. Exposure to noise: military, industrial, recreational, environmental
   g. Drugs: prescription and nonprescription
   h. Previous hearing tests
   i. Head trauma or accidents
4. Communication history
   a. Situations in which hearing difficulty is detected: telephone, noise, television, movie, theater, parties, temple, in quiet, conferences, classroom
   b. Difficulty hearing men's, women's, children's voices
   c. Difficulty localizing
   d. Use of amplification
   e. Speech–language therapy or evaluation

   f. Communication needs: retired, live alone, recreational interests
5. Otologic history
   a. Previous ear, nose, or throat surgery
   b. Ear pain
   c. Ear discharge
   d. Tinnitus: unilateral or bilateral, continuous or fluctuating, onset, character (buzzing, hissing, thumping, ringing, rushing, steam, high-pitched, low-pitched, roaring), frequency, degree of severity
   e. Dizziness: character (lightheadedness, faintness, giddiness, unsteadiness, spinning—room or within oneself), date of onset, gradual or sudden onset, episodic or constant, frequency, duration, associated symptoms (nausea, vomiting, sweating, hearing impairment, tinnitus, ear fullness, ear pain, ear drainage, gait disturbances, imbalance, visual problems), exacerbating and remitting factors (head turn, lying down, sitting down, standing up, walking in the dark), precipitating factors, alleviating factors, dysarthria, blackouts
   f. Ear infections
6. Medical history
   a. General health
   b. Kidney disease
   c. Cancer
   d. Diabetes
   e. Hypertension
   f. Other vascular or cardiac problems
   g. Other diseases: measles, mumps, chicken pox, meningitis, syphilis, tuberculosis, malaria, scarlet fever, AIDS, thyroid disease
   h. History of smoking
   i. History of alcohol
   j. Allergies
   k. Visual problems: nightblindness, tunnel vision, diplopia, blurring, corrective lenses
   l. Sinus problems
   m. Seizures
   n. Neurologic or neuromuscular problems
   o. Bone diseases
   p. Native language
   q. Head and neck defects
   r. Psychologic or psychiatric therapy or counseling
   s. Financial information (Medicaid, unemployed, receiving disability)

The outline of the case history for children should include the following information in addition to the previously mentioned information for adults.

1. Prenatal history
   a. Ototoxic medications
   b. Maternal diseases

c. Rubella immunization
d. Spontaneous abortions or miscarriages
2. Perinatal history
   a. Congenital infections
   b. Low birth weight
   c. Hyperbilirubinemia
   d. Asphyxia
   e. Congenital cranio-facial abnormalities
3. Developmental history
   a. Speech–language milestones
   b. Motoric milestones
   c. Auditory milestones
4. Educational history
   a. Special education
   b. Special educational assistance
   c. Repeated grades
   d. School performance
   e. Learning disability
   f. Psychoeducational evaluations
   g. Mental retardation

REFERENCES

Abrams, I. F. (1977). Nongenetic hearing loss. In B. F. Jaffe (Ed.), *Hearing loss in children*, pp. 367–375. Baltimore: University Park Press.

Abu-Jaudeh, C. N. (1964). The effect of simultaneous loading of the tympanic membrane of the external auditory canal on the bone conduction sensitivity of the normal ear. *Ann. Ontol., 73,* 934–947.

Alford, B., & Guilford, F. (1962). A comprehensive study of tumors of the glomus jugulare. *Laryngoscope, 72,* 765.

Alford, B., Shaver, E., Rosenberg, J., & Guilford, F. (1965). Physiologic and histopathologic effects of microembolism of the internal auditory artery. *Ann. Otol. Rhinol. Laryngol., 74,* 728.

Allen, G. W., & Fernandez, C. (1960). The mechanism of bone conduction. *Ann. Otol., 69,* 5–29.

American Medical Association (1947). Tentative standard procedure for evaluating the percentage loss of hearing in medico-legal cases. *J. Am. Med. Assoc., 133,* 396–397.

American National Standards Institute (1972). American national standard for an artificial headbone for the calibration of audiometer bone vibrators. *ANSI* S3.13–1972. New York: American National Standards Institute.

American National Standards Institute (1973). American national standard psychoacoustical terminology. *ANSI* S3.20–1973. New York: American National Standards Institute.

American National Standards Institute (1977). Criteria for permissible ambient noise during audiometric testing. *ANSI* S3.1–1977. New York: American National Standards Institute.

American National Standards Institute (1978). Methods for manual pure-tone threshold audiometry. *ANSI* S3.21–1978. New York: American National Standards Institute.

American National Standards Institute (1981). American national standard for reference equivalent threshold force levels for audiometric bone vibrators. *ANSI* S3.26–1981. New York: American National Standards Institute.

American National Standards Institute (1987). American national standards for mechanical coupler for measurement of bone vibrators. *ANSI* S3.13–1987. New York: American National Standards Institute.

American National Standards Institute (1989). American national standard specification for audiometers. ANSI S3.6–1989. New York: American National Standards Institute.

American Speech and Hearing Association (1974). Guidelines for audiometric symbols. *Asha, 16,* 260–264.

American Speech and Hearing Association (1979). Guidelines for determining the threshold level for speech. *Asha 21,* 353–356.

American Speech and Hearing Association, Committee on Audiometric Evaluation (1978a). Guidelines for manual pure-tone threshold audiometry. *Asha, 20,* 297–301.

American Speech and Hearing Association, Professional Services Board (1978b). *PSB accreditation manual.* Rockville, Maryland: American Speech and Hearing Association.

American Speech–Language–Hearing Association (1988). Guidelines for determining threshold level for speech. *Asha, 30,* 85–89.

American Speech–Language–Hearing Association (1990). Guidelines for audiometric symbols. *Asha Suppl., 32,* 25–30.

American Standards Association (1951). American standard specification for audiometers for general diagnostic purposes. *Asa* Z24.5–151. New York, American National Standards Institute.

Balkany, T. J., Downs, M. P., Jafek, B. W., & Krajicek, M. J. (1979). Hearing loss in Down's syndrome. *Clin. Pediatr., 18,* 116–118.

Barany, E. (1938). A contribution to the physiology of bone conduction. *Acta Otolaryngol. Suppl., 26,* 1–223.

Beattie, R. C., Svihovec, D. V., & Edgerton, B. J. (1975). Relative intelligibility of the CID spondees as presented via monitored live voice. *J. Speech Hear. Dis., 40,* 84–91.

Beattie, R. C., Forrester, P. W., & Ruby, B. K. (1976). Reliability of the Tillman–Olsen procedure for determination of spondee threshold using recorded and live voice presentations. *J. Am. Audiol. Soc., 2,* 159–162.

Bednin, F. V., & Sagalovich, B. M. (1976). Human equivalent bone-conduction thresholds measured by an artificial mastoid with an expanded frequency range. *Sov. Phys. Acoust., 21,* 417–420.

Beedle, R. K. (1971). Unpublished manuscript.

Bekesy, G. v. (1932). Zur Theorie des Hörens bei der Schallaufnahme durch Knochenleitung. *Ann. Physik, 13,* 111–136.

Bekesy, G. v. (1939). Über die piezoelektrische Messung der absoluten Hörschwelle bei Knochenleitung. *Akust. Z., 4,* 113–125.

Bekesy, G. v. (1947). A new audiometer. *Acta Otolaryngol., 35,* 411–422.

Bekesy, G. v. (1948). Vibration of the head in a sound field and its role in hearing by bone conduction. *J. Acoust. Soc. Am., 20,* 749–760.

Bekesy, G. v., & Rosenblith, W. A. (1958). The mechanical properties of the ear. In S. S. Stevens (Ed.), *Handbook of experimental psychology,* pp. 1075–1115. New York: John Wiley & Sons.

Belal, A., & Stewart, T. J. (1974). Pathologic changes in the middle ear joints. *Ann. Otol. Rhinol. Laryngol., 83,* 159–167.

Bell, J., Goodsell, S., & Thornton, A. R. D. (1980). A brief communication on bone conduction artifacts. *Br. J. Audiol., 14,* 73–75.

Bergstrom, L., & Thompson, P. (1984). Ototoxicity. In J. L. Northern (Ed.), *Hearing disorders,* 2d ed., pp. 119–134. Boston: Little, Brown.

Berlin, C. I. (1982). Ultra-audiometric hearing in the hearing impaired and the use of upward-shifting translating hearing aids. *Volta Rev., 84,* 352–363.

Berlin, C. I., Wexler, K. F., Jerger, J. F., Halperin, H. R., & Smith, S. (1978). Superior ultra-audiometric hearing: A new type of hearing loss which correlates highly with unusually good speech in the "profoundly deaf." *Otolaryngol., 86,* 111–116.

Bess, F. H., Josey, A. F., Glasscock, M. E., & Wilson, L. K. (1984). Audiologic manifestations in bilateral acoustic tumors (von Recklinghausen's disease). *J. Speech Hear. Dis., 49,* 177–182.

Boettcher, F. A., Henderson, D., Gratton, M. A., Danielson, R. W., & Byrne, C. D. (1987). Synergistic interactions of noise and other oto-traumatic agents. *Ear Hear., 8,* 192–212.

Bornstein, S., & Randolph, K. (1983). Research on smooth, wideband frequency responses: Current status and unresolved issues. *Hear. Instruments, 34,* 12–16.

Bowling, L. S., & Elpern, B. S. (1961). Relative intelligibility of items of CID Auditory Test W-1. *J. Aud. Res., 1,* 152–157.

Brinkmann, W. F. B., Marres, E. H. A. M., & Tolk, J. (1965). The mechanism of bone conduction. *Acta Otolaryngol., 59,* 109–115.

British Standard Institute (1966). An artificial mastoid for the calibration of bone vibrators. British Standard 4009. London: British Standards House.

Calavita, F. B. (1978). Sensory changes in the elderly. Springfield Illinois: Thomas.

Carhart, R. (1945). Classifying audiograms: An improved method for classifying audiograms. *Laryngoscope, 55,* 640–662.

Carhart, R. (1946a). Monitored live voice as a test of auditory acuity. *J. Acoust. Soc. Am., 17,* 339–349.

Carhart, R. (1946b). Speech reception in relation to pattern of pure tone loss. *J. Speech Dis., 11,* 97–108.

Carhart, R. (1950). Clinical application of bone conduction. *Arch. Otolaryngol., 51,* 798–807.

Carhart, R. (1952). Speech audiometry in clinical evaluation. *Acta Otolaryngol., 41,* 18–42.

Carhart, R. (1962). Effects of stapes fixation on bone-conduction response. In H. F. Schuknecht (Ed.), *International symposium on otosclerosis,* pp. 175–197. Boston: Little, Brown.

Carhart, R. (1971). Observations on relations between thresholds for pure tones and for speech. *J. Speech Hear. Dis., 36,* 476–483.

Carhart, R., & Jerger, J. F. (1959). Preferred method for clinical determination of pure-tone thresholds. *J. Speech Hear. Dis., 24,* 330–345.

Carhart, R., & Porter, L. S. (1971). Audiometric configuration and prediction of threshold for spondees. *J. Speech Hear. Res., 14,* 486–495.

Chaiklin, J. B. (1959). The relation among three selected auditory speech thresholds. *J. Speech Hear. Res., 2,* 237–243.

Chaiklin, J. B. (1967). Interaural attenuation and cross-hearing in air-conduction audiometry. *J. Aud. Res., 7,* 413–424.

Chaiklin, J. B., & Ventry, I. M. (1964). Spondee threshold measurement: A comparison of 2- and 5-dB methods. *J. Speech Hear. Dis., 29,* 47–59.

Chaiklin, J. B., Font, J., & Dixon, R. F. (1967). Spondee thresholds measured in ascending 5-dB steps. *J. Speech Hear. Res., 10,* 141–145.

Cohn, A. (1981). Etiology and pathology of disorders affecting hearing. In F. N. Martin (Ed.), *Medical audiology: Disorders of hearing,* pp. 403–410. Englewood Cliffs, New Jersey: Prentice-Hall.

Cole, J. (1977). Glomus jugulare tumor. *Laryngoscope, 87,* 1244–1258.

Coles, R. R. A., & Priede, V. M. (1968). Problems in crosshearing and masking. *Annual Report, 26.* South Hampton, England: Institute of Sound and Vibration Research.

Conn, M., Dancer, J., & Ventry, I. M. (1975). A spondee list for determining speech reception threshold without prior familiarization. *J. Speech Hear. Dis., 40,* 388–396.

Corliss, E., & Koidan, D. (1955). Mechanical impedance of the forehead and mastoid. *J. Acoust. Soc. Am., 27,* 1164–1172.

Corso, J. F. (1963a). Aging and auditory thresholds in men and women. *Arch. Environmen. Health, 6,* 350–356.

Corso, J. F. (1963b). Age and sex differences in pure-tone thresholds. *Arch. Otolaryngol., 77,* 53–73.

Corso, J. F. (1964). Bone-conduction thresholds for sonic and ultrasonic frequencies. *J. Acoust. Soc. Am., 35,* 1738–1743.

Creston, J. E., Gillespie, M., & Krahn, C. (1966). Speech audiometry: Taped vs. live voice. *Arch. Otolaryngol., 83,* 14–17.

Crowe, S., Guild, S., & Palvogt, L. (1934). Observations on pathology of high-tone deafness. *Bull. Johns Hopkins Hospital, 54,* 315.

Curry, E. T., & Cox, B. P. (1966). The relative intelligibility of spondees. *J. Aud. Res., 6,* 419–424.

Dadson, R. S., Robinson, D. W., & Grieg, R. G. P. (1954). The mechanical impedance of the human mastoid process. *Br. J. Applied Physics, 5,* 435–442.

Davis, H., & Silverman, S. R. (1970). *Hearing and deafness.* New York, Holt, Rinehart, and Winston.

Derlacki, E. L. (1984). Otosclerosis. In J. L. Northern (Ed.), *Hearing disorders,* 2d ed., pp. 111–118. Boston: Little, Brown.

Dirks, D. (1964). Factors related to bone conduction reliability. *Arch. Otolaryngol., 79,* 551–558.

Dirks, D. (1985). Bone-conduction testing. In J. Katz (Ed.), *Handbook of clinical audiology,* 3d ed., pp. 202–223. Baltimore: Williams & Wilkins.

Dirks, D. D., & Malmquist, C. W. (1964). Changes in bone-conduction thresholds produced by masking in the non-test ear. *J. Speech Hear. Res., 7,* 271–278.

Dirks, D., & Malmquist, C. W. (1969). Comparison of frontal and mastoid bone conduction thresholds in various conduction lesions. *J. Speech Hear. Res., 12,* 725–746.

Dirks, D. D., Lybarger, S. F., Olsen, W. O., & Billings, B. L. (1979). Bone conduction calibration: Current status. *J. Speech Hear. Dis., 44,* 143–155.

Dreschler, W. A., Van der Hulst, R. J. A. M., & Tange, R. A. (1984). Ototoxicity and the role of high-frequency audiometry. *J. Acoust. Soc. Am. Suppl., 76,* 74.

Dufresne, R. M., Alleyne, B. C., & Reesai, M. R. (1988). Asymmetric hearing loss in truck drivers. *Ear Hear., 9,* 41–42.

Egan, J. (1948). Articulation testing methods. *Laryngoscope, 58,* 955–991.

Eisenberg, R. B. (1976). *Auditory competence in early life.* Baltimore: University Park Press.

Fechner, G. T. (1860). *Element der Psychophysik.* Leipzig: Breitkopf & Harterl.

Finney, D. J. (1952). *Statistical method in biological assay.* London: Griffen.

Fletcher, H. (1929). *Speech and hearing.* Princeton, New Jersey: Van Nostrand Reinhold.

Fletcher, H. (1950). A method of calculating hearing loss for speech from an audiogram. *J. Acoust. Soc. Am., 22,* 1–5.

Fletcher, H., & Steinberg, J. C. (1929). Articulation testing methods. *Bell Tel. Syst. Tech. Public., 8,* 806–854.

Fowler, E. P. (1942). A simple method of measuring percentage of capacity to hear speech. *Arch. Otolaryngol., 36,* 874–890.

Frank, T. (1980). Clinical significance of the relative intelligibility of pictorially represented spondee words. *Ear Hear., 1,* 46–49.

Frank, T., & Crandell, C. C. (1986). Acoustic radiation produced by B-71, B-72, and KH-70 bone vibrators. *Ear Hear., 7,* 344–347.

Frank, T., & Holmes, A. (1981). Acoustic radiation from bone vibrators. *Ear Hear., 2,* 59–63.

Frank, T., & Ragland, A. E. (1987). Repeatability of high-frequency bone conduction thresholds. *Ear Hear., 8,* 343–346.

Frank, T., Byrne, D. C., & Richards, L. A. (1988). Bone conduction threshold levels for different bone vibrator types. *J. Speech Hear. Dis., 53,* 295–301.

Gelfand, S. A. (1977). Clinical precision of the Rinne test. *Acta Otolaryngol., 83,* 480–487.

Gelfand, S. A. (1990). *Hearing: An introduction to psychological and physiological acoustics,* 2nd ed. New York: Dekker.

Gerber, S. E., & Mencher, G. T. (1980). *Auditory dysfunction: A text by and for audiologists.* Houston, College-Hill Press.

Gerkin, K. P. (1984). The high risk register for deafness. *Asha, 26,* 17–23.

Goldstein, B. A., & Newman, C. W. (1985). Clinical masking: A decision-making process. In J. Katz (Ed.), *Handbook of clinical audiology,* 3d ed., pp. 170–201. Baltimore: Williams & Wilkins.

Goldstein, D. P., & Haynes, C. S. (1965). The occlusion effect in bone-conduction hearing. *J. Speech Hear. Res., 8,* 137–148.

Goodman, A. (1965). Reference zero levels for pure-tone audiometer. *Asha, 7,* 262–263.

Graham, J. T. (1960). Evaluation of methods for predicting speech reception threshold. *Arch. Otolaryngol., 72,* 347–350.

Greer, J., Cody, T., & Weiland, L. (1976). Neoplasms of the temporal bone. *J. Otolaryngol., 5,* 17–22.

Groen, J. J. (1962). The value of the Weber test. In H. F. Schuknecht (Ed.), *International symposium on otosclerosis,* pp. 220–228. Boston: Little, Brown.

Hallpike, C. S., & Cairns, H. (1938). Observation on the pathology of Meniere's syndrome. *J. Laryngol. Otol., 53,* 625.

Hannley, M. (1986). *Basic principles of auditory assessment.* San Diego: College-Hill Press.

Hansen, C. C., & Reske-Nielsen, E. (1965). Pathological studies in presbycusis. *Arch. Otolaryngol., 82,* 115–132.

Harris, J. D., Haines, L., & Myers, C. K. (1956). A new formula for using the audiogram to predict speech hearing loss. *Arch. Otolaryngol., 63,* 158–176.

Hart, C., & Naunton, R. (1961). Frontal bone conduction tests in clinical audiometry. *Laryngoscope, 71,* 24–29.

Haug, O., Baccaro, P., & Guilford, F. R. (1967). A pure-tone audiogram on the infant: The PIWI technique. *Arch. Otolaryngol., 86,* 435–440.

Herzog, H., & Krainz, W. (1926). Das Knochenleitungsproblem. *Z. Hals Ohr Nasen Heilk., 15,* 300–306. Cited by Tonndorf, J. (1968). A new concept of bone conduction. *Arch. Otolaryngol., 87,* 595–600.

Hirsh, L., Davis, H., Silverman, S., Reynolds, E., Eldert, E., & Benson, R. (1952). Development of materials for speech audiometry. *J. Speech Hear. Dis., 17,* 321–337.

Hirsh, I., Reynolds, E., & Joseph, M. (1954). Intelligibility of different speech materials. *J. Acoust. Soc. Am., 26,* 530–538.

Hodgson, W. R. (1980). *Basic audiologic evaluation.* Baltimore: Williams & Wilkins.

Hood, J. D. (1960). The principles and practice of bone-conduction audiometry. *Laryngoscope, 70,* 1211–1228.

Hudgins, C., Hawkins, J., Karlin, J., & Stevens, S. (1947). The development of recorded auditory tests for measuring hearing loss for speech. *Laryngoscope, 57,* 57–89.

Huff, S. J., & Nerbonne, M. S. (1982). Comparison of the American Speech–Language–Hearing Association and revised Tillman–Olsen methods for speech threshold measurement. *Ear Hear., 3,* 335–339.

Hughson, W., & Westlake, H. (1944). Manual for program outline for rehabilitation of aural casualties both military and civilian. *Trans. Am. Acad. Ophthalmol. Otolaryngol. Suppl., 48,* 1–15.

Huizing, E. H. (1960). Bone conduction—The influence of the middle ear. *Acta Otolaryngol. Suppl., 155,* 1–99.

Huizing, E. H. (1964). Bone conduction loss due to middle ear pathology pseudoperceptive deafness. *Int. Audiol., 3,* 89–98.

Hulka, J. (1941). Bone conduction changes in acute otitis media. *Arch. Otolaryngol., 33,* 333–346.

International Electrotechnical Commission (1971). An IEC mechanical coupler for the calibration of bone vibrators having a specified contact area and being applied with a specific static force, IEC-373 1971. Geneva: International Electrotechnical Commission.

International Standards Organization (1975). Acoustics—Standard reference zero for the calibration of pure-tone audiometers. ISO R389, Geneva, Switzerland. Addendum 1-ISO DAD-1, 1981. Geneva: International Standards Organization.

International Standards Organization (1987). Acoustics—Standard reference zero for the calibration of pure-tone bone-conduction audiometers and guidelines for its practical application. ISO/DIS 7566. Geneva: International Standards Organization.

Jerger, J. (1973). Diagnostic audiology. In J. Jerger (Ed.), *Modern developments in audiology,* 3d ed., pp. 75–115. New York: Academic Press.

Jerger, S., & Jerger, J. (1981). *Auditory disorders: A manual for clinical evaluation.* Boston: Little, Brown.

Johnson, D. W., Hammond, R. J., & Sherman, R. E. (1980). Hearing in an ambulance paramedic population. *Ann. Emerg. Med., 9,* 557–561.

Johnson, L. G., & Hawkins, J. E. (1972). Sensory and neural degeneration with aging, as seen in microsections of the human inner ear. *Ann. Otolaryngol., 81,* 179–183.

Karp, A., & Santore, F. (1983). Retinitis pigmentosa and progressive hearing loss. *J. Speech Hear. Dis., 48,* 308–314.

Keaster, J. (1947). A quantitative method of testing the hearing of young children. *J. Speech Hear. Dis., 12,* 159–160.

Keith, R. W., & Jacobson, J. T. (1985). Physiological responses in multiple sclerosis and other demyelinating diseases. In J. T. Jacobson (Ed.), *The auditory brainstem response,* pp. 219–235. San Diego: College-Hill Press.

Killion, M. C. (1978). Revised estimate of minimum audible pressure: Where is the "missing 6 dB"? *J. Acoust. Soc. Am., 63,* 1501–1508.

Killion, M. C., & Revitt, L. J. (1987). Insertion gain repeatability versus loudspeaker location: You want me to put my loudspeaker WHERE? *Ear Hear. Suppl., 8,* 68S–73S.

Killion, M. C., Wilber, L. A., & Gudmundsen, G. I. (1985). Insert earphones for more interaural attenuation. *Hear. Instrum., 36,* 34–36.

Kirikae, I. (1959). An experimental study on the fundamental mechanism of bone conduction. *Acta Otolaryngol. Suppl., 145,* 1–111.

Kirikae, I., Sato, T., & Shitara, T. (1964). A study of hearing in advanced age. *Laryngoscope, 74,* 205–220.

Konigsmark, B. W. (1971). Hereditary and Congenital factors affecting newborn sensorineural hearing. In G. C. Cunningham (Ed.), *Conference on newborn hearing screening,* pp. 37–52. Berkeley: California Department of Health.

Konkle, D. F., & Berry, G. A. (1983). Masking in speech audiometry. In D. F. Konkle & W. F. Rintelmann (Eds.), *Principles of speech audiometry,* pp. 285–319. Baltimore: University Park Press.

Krmpotic-Nemanic, J. (1971). A new concept of the pathogenesis of presbycusis. *AMA Arch. Otolaryngol., 93,* 161–166.

Laitakari, K. (1977). Vestibular disorders in medically managed chronic renal insufficiency. *Acta Otolaryngol. Suppl., 349,* 1–30.

Laukli, E., & Mair, I. W. S. (1985). High-frequency audiometry: Normative studies and preliminary experiences. *Scand. Audiol., 14,* 151–158.

Lawton, R., & Cafarelli, D. (1978). The effects of hearing aid frequency response modification upon speech reception. *Instit. Sound Vibr. Res. Mem. No. 588.*

Lebo, C. P., & Reddell, R. C. (1972). The presbycusis component in occupational hearing loss. *Laryngoscope, 82,* 1339–1409.

Legouix, J. P., & Tarab, S. (1959). Experimental study of bone conduction in ears with mechanical impairment of the ossicles. *J. Acoust. Soc. Am., 31,* 1453–1457.

Levitt, H. (1971). Transformed up–down methods in psychoacoustics. *J. Acoust. Soc. Am., 49,* 467–477.

Liden, G., & Kankkunen, A. (1969). Visual reinforcement audiometry. *Acta Otolaryngol., 67,* 281–292.

Liden, G., Nilsson, G., & Anderson, H. (1959a). Narrow band masking with white noise. *Acta Otolaryngol., 50,* 116–124.

Liden, G., Nilsson, G., & Anderson, H. (1959b). Masking in clinical audiometry. *Acta Otolaryngol., 50,* 125–136.

Linthicum, F. H. (1983). Electronystagmography findings in patients with acoustic tumors. *Sem. Hear., 4,* 47–54.

Lloyd, L. L., & Kaplan, H. (1978). *Audiometric interpretation: A manual of basic audiometry.* Baltimore: University Park Press.

Lowy, K. (1942). Cancellation of the electrical cochlear response with air-conducted and bone-conducted sound. *J. Acoust. Soc. Am., 14,* 156–158.

Lybarger, S. F. (1966). Interim bone conduction thresholds for audiometry. *J. Speech Hear. Res., 9,* 483–487.

Marshall, L., Martinez, S., & Schlaman, M. (1983). Reassessment of high-frequency air-bone gaps in older adults. *Arch. Otolaryngol., 109,* 601–606.

Martin, F. N. (1975). *Introduction to audiology.* Englewood Cliffs, New Jersey: Prentice-Hall.

Martin, F. N. (1980). The masking plateau revisited. *Ear. Hear., 1,* 112–116.

Martin, F. N. (1986). *Introduction to audiology,* 3d ed. Englewood Cliffs, New Jersey: Prentice-Hall.

Martin, F. N., & Blythe, M. (1977). On the cross-hearing of spondaic words. *J. Aud. Res., 17,* 221–224.

Martin, F. N., & DiGiovanni, D. (1979). Central masking effects on spondee threshold as a function of masker sensation level and masker sound pressure level. *J. Am. Aud. Soc., 4,* 141–146.

Martin, F. N., & Wittich, W. W. (1966). A comparison of forehead and mastoid tactile bone conduction thresholds. *Ear Nose Throat Month., 45,* 72–74.

Martin, F. N., Butler, E. C., & Burns, P. (1974). Audiometric Bing test for determination of minimum masking levels for bone-conduction tests. *J. Speech. Hear. Dis., 39,* 148–152.

Maurer, F. J., & Rupp, R. R. (1979). *Hearing and aging: Tactics for intervention.* New York: Grune & Stratton.

McConnell, F., & Ward, P. H. (1967). *Deafness in childhood.* Nashville: Vanderbilt University Press.

Melnick, W. (1984). Auditory effects of noise exposure. In M. H. Miller & C. A. Silverman (Eds.), *Occupational hearing conservation,* pp. 100–132. Englewood Cliffs, New Jersey: Prentice-Hall.

Mencher, G. T. (1972). Screening infants for auditory deficits: University of Nebraska Neonatal Hearing Project. *Audiol. Suppl., 11,* 69.

Merin, S., Abraham, F., & Auerbach, E. (1974). Usher's and Hallgren's syndromes. *Acta Genet. Med. Gemelol., 23,* 49–55.

Moller, M. B. (1981). Hearing in 70- and 74-year-old people: Results from a cross-sectional and longitudinal population study. *Am. J. Otolaryngol., 2,* 22–29.

Moller, M. B., & Moller, A. R. (1985). Auditory brainstem-evoked responses (ABR) in diagnosis of eighth nerve and brainstem lesions. In M. L. Pinheiro & F. E. Musiek (Eds.), *Assessment of central auditory dysfunction: Foundations and clinical correlates,* pp. 43–66. Baltimore: Williams & Wilkins.

Moscicki, E. K., Elkins, E. F., Baum, H. M., & McNamara, P. M. (1985). Hearing loss in the elderly: An epidemiologic study of the Framingham Heart Study Cohort. *Ear Hear., 6,* 184–190.

Musiek, F. E. (1985). Application of central auditory tests: An overview. In J. Katz (Ed.), *Handbook of clinical audiology,* 3d ed., pp. 321–336. Baltimore: Williams & Wilkins.

Nadol, J. B. (1981). The aging peripheral hearing mechanism. In D. S. Beasley & G. A. Davis (Eds.), *Aging: Communication processes and disorders,* pp. 67–81. New York: Grune & Stratton.

Naunton, R. F. (1963). The measurement of hearing by bone conduction. In J. Jerger (Ed.), *Modern developments in audiology,* pp. 1–29. New York: Academic Press.

Naunton, R. F., & Fernandez, C. (1961). Prolonged bone conduction observations on man and animals. *Laryngoscope, 71,* 306–318.

Nerbonne, M. A. (1988). The effects of aging on auditory structures and functions. In B. B. Shadden (Ed.), *Communication behavior and aging: A sourcebook for clinicians,* pp. 137–161. Baltimore: Williams & Wilkins.

Newby, H. (1972). *Audiology.* New York: Appleton-Century-Crofts.

Noback, C. R., & Demarest, R. J. (1981). *The human nervous system,* 3d ed. New York: McGraw-Hill.

Nober, E. H. (1970). Cutile air and bone conduction thresholds of the deaf. *Except. Child., 36,* 571–579.

Noffsinger, P. D., & Kurdziel, S. A. (1979). Assessment of central auditory lesions. In W. F. Rintelmann (Ed.), *Hearing assessment,* pp. 351–377. Baltimore: University Park Press.

Noffsinger, D., Olsen, W., Carhart, R., Hart, C., & Sahgal, V. (1972). Auditory and vestibular aberrations in multiple sclerosis. *Acta Otolaryngol. Suppl., 303,* 5–63.

Northern, J. L., & Downs, M. P. (1978). *Hearing in children,* 2d ed. Baltimore: Williams & Wilkins.

Northern, J. L., & Downs, M. P. (1984). *Hearing in children,* 3d ed. Baltimore: Williams & Wilkins.

Olsen, W. O., & Matkin, N. D. (1979). Speech audiometry. In W. F. Rintelmann (Ed.), *Hearing assessment,* pp. 132–206. Baltimore: University Park Press.

Olsen, W. O., Hawkins, D. B., & Van Tasell, D. J. (1987). Representations of the long-term spectra of speech. *Ear Hear. Suppl., 8,* 100S–108S.

Paparella, M. P., Morizono, T., Le, C. T., Mancini, F., Sipila, P., Choo, Y.B., Liden, G., & Kim, C. S. (1984). Sensorineural hearing loss in otitis media. *Ann. Otol. Rhinol. Laryngol., 93,* 623–629.

Pappas, D. G. (1985). *Diagnosis and treatment of hearing impairment in children: A clinical manual.* San Diego: College-Hill Press.

Pascoe, D. (1978). An approach to hearing aid selection. *Hear. Instruments, 29,* 12–16.

Pascoe, D. (1980). Clinical implications of nonverbal methods of hearing aid selection and fitting. *Sem. Speech Lang. Hear., 1,* 217–229.

Pashley, N. R. T. (1984). Otitis media. In J. L. Northern (Ed.), *Hearing disorders,* pp. 103–110. Boston: Little, Brown.

Pass, R. F., Stagno, S., Meyers, G. J., & Alford, C. A., Jr. (1980). Outcome of symptomatic congenital CMV infection: Results of long-term longitudinal follow-up. *Pediatrics, 66,* 758–762.

Pinsker, O. T. (1972). Otological correlates of audiology. In J. Katz (Ed.), *Handbook of clinical audiology,* pp. 36–59. Baltimore: Williams & Wilkins.

Price, L. L. (1963). Threshold testing with Bekesy audiometer. *J. Speech Hear. Res., 6,* 64–69.

Pulec, J. L. (1984). Meniere's disease. In J. L. Northern (Ed.), *Hearing disorders,* 2d., pp. 135–142. Boston: Little, Brown.

Quiggle, R. R., Glorig, A., Delk, J. H., & Summerfield, A. B. (1957). Predicting hearing loss for speech from pure tone audiograms. *Laryngoscope, 67,* 1–15.

Randolph, L., & Schow, R. (1983). Threshold inaccuracies in an elderly clinical population: Ear canal collapse as a possible cause. *J. Speech Hear. Res., 26,* 54–58.

Rasmussen, A. (1940). Studies of the VIIIth cranial nerve of man. *Laryngoscope, 50,* 67–83.

Reger, S. N. (1950). Standardization of pure-tone audiometer testing technique. *Laryngoscope, 60,* 161–185.

Reger, S. N. (1970). Bekesy audiometry and the method of limits. *Int. Audiol., 9,* 24–29.

Reiter, L., Letzer, C. B., & Silman, S. (1984). A quick screening test and a solution for meatal collapse. Paper presented at the Annual Convention of the New York State Speech–Language–Hearing Association, Kiamesha Lake, New York.

Richards, W. D., & Frank, T. (1982). Frequency response and output variations of Radioear B-71 and B-72 bone vibrators. *Ear Hear., 3,* 37–38.

Richter, U., & Frank, T. (1985). Calibration of bone vibrators at high frequencies. *Audio. Acous., 24,* 52–62.

Ries, P. W. (1982). Hearing ability of persons by sociodemographic and health characteristics: United States. *Vital and Health Statistics, Series 10, No. 140.* [DHHS Publ. No. (PHS) 82-1568] Washington, D.C.: U.S. Govt. Printing Office.

Roeser, R. (1982). Moderate-to-severe hearing loss with an island of normal hearing. *Ear Hear., 3,* 284–286.

Rytzner, C. (1954). Sound transmission in clinical otosclerosis. *Acta Otolaryngol. Suppl., 117,* 1–137.

Schow, R. L., & Goldbaum, D. (1980). Collapsed ear canals in the elderly nursing home population. *J. Speech Hear. Dis., 45,* 259–267.

Schow, R. L., Christenson, J. M., Hutchinson, J. M., & Nerbonne, M. A. (1978). *Communication disorders of the aged.* Baltimore: University Park Press.

Schuknecht, H. F. (1955). Presbycusis. *Laryngoscope, 65,* 402–419.

Schuknecht, H. F. (1964). Further observation on the pathology of presbycusis. *Arch. Otolaryngol., 80,* 369–382.

Schuknecht, H. F. (1971). *Stapedectomy.* Boston: Little, Brown.

Schuknecht, H. F. (1974). *Pathology of the ear.* Cambridge: Harvard University Press.

Shambaugh, G. E., Jr. (1967). *Surgery of the ear,* 2d ed. Philadelphia: Saunders.

Shipton, M. S., John, A. J., & Robinson, D. W. (1980). Air radiated sounds from bone vibrator transducers and its implications for bone conduction audiometry. *Br. J. Audiol., 14,* 86–99.

Siegenthaler, B. M., & Strand, R. (1964). Audiogram-average methods and SRT scores. *J. Acoust. Soc. Am., 36,* 589–595.

Simmons, F. (1978). Fluid dynamics in sudden sensorineural loss. *Otolaryngol. Clin. North Am., 11,* 55.

Skinner, M. W. (1988). *Hearing aid evaluation.* Englewood Cliffs, New Jersey: Prentice-Hall.

Skinner, M., & Miller, J. (1983). Amplification bandwidth and intelligibility of speech in quiet and noise for listeners with sensorineural hearing loss. *Audiol., 22,* 253–279.

Skinner, M., Pascoe, D., Miller, J., & Popelka, G. (1982). Measurements to determine the optimal placement of speech energy within the listener's auditory area: A basis for selecting amplification characteristics. In G. Studebaker & F. Bess (Eds.), *The Vanderbilt hearing aid report: State of the art—Research Needs,* pp. 161–169. Upper Darby, Pennsylvania: Monographs in Contemporary Audiology.

Sklare, D. A., & Denenberg, L. J. (1987). Technical note: Interaural attenuation for Tubephone insert earphones. *Ear Hear., 8,* 298–300.

Snow, J. B. (1973). Sudden deafness. In M. M. Paparella & D. A. Shumrick (Ed.), *Otolaryngology,* Vol. 2, pp. 357–364. Philadelphia: Saunders.

Sparrevohn, U. R. (1946). Some audiometric investigations of monaurally deaf persons. *Acta Otolaryngol., 34,* 1–10.

Spencer, I. T. (1975). Hyperlipoproteinemia in inner ear disease. *Otolaryngol. Clin. North Am., 8,* 483–492.

Staab, W. J. (1971). *Comparison of pure-tone and warble-tone thresholds.* Ph.D. Thesis. East Lansing: Michigan State University.

Staab, W. J., & Rintelmann, W. F. (1972). Status of warble-tone in audiometers. *J. Aud. Comm., 11,* 244–255.

Stagno, S. (1984). Cited by D. G. Pappas. *Diagnosis and treatment of hearing impairment in children: A clinical manual.* San Diego: College-Hill Press.

Stevens, S. S. (1951). Mathematics, measurement, and psychophysics. In S. Stevens (Ed.), *Handbook of experimental psychology.* pp. 1–49. New York: John Wiley & Sons.

Stisen, B., & Dahm, M. (1969). *Sensitivity and mechanical impedance of artificial mastoid type 4930.* Bruel & Kjaer Technical Information.

Stream, R. W., & McConnell, F. (1961). A comparison of two methods of administration in Bekesy-type audiometry. *J. Aud. Res., 1,* 263–271.

Studebaker, G. A. (1962a). Placement of vibrator in bone conduction testing. *J. Speech Hear. Res., 5,* 321–331.

Studebaker, G. A. (1962b). On masking in bone-conduction testing. *J. Speech Hear. Res.,* 215–227.

Studebaker, G. A. (1967). Clinical masking of the non-test ear. *J. Speech Hear. Dis., 32,* 360–371.

Studebaker, G. A. (1979). Clinical masking. In W. F. Rintelmann (Ed.), *Hearing assessment,* pp. 51–100. Baltimore: University Park Press.

Suzuki, T., & Ogiba, Y. (1960). A technique of pure-tone audiometry for children under three years of age: Conditioned orientation reflex (COR) audiometry. Rev. *Laryngol. Otol. Rhinol., 81,* 33–45.

Suzuki, T., & Ogiba, Y. (1961). Conditioned orientation reflex audiometry. *Arch. Otolaryngol., 74,* 192–198.

Tange, R. A., Dreschler, W. A., & Van der Hulst, R. J. A. M. (1985). The importance of high-tone audiometry in monitoring for ototoxicity. *Arch. Otorhinolaryngol., 242,* 77–81.

Thompson, G., & Weber, B. A. (1974). Responses of infants and young children to behavior observation audiometry (BOA). *J. Speech Hear. Dis., 39,* 140–147.

Thurlow, W. R., Silverman, S. R., Davis, H., & Walsh, T. E. (1948). A statistical study of auditory tests in relation to the fenestration operation. *Laryngoscope, 58,* 43–66.

Tillman, T. J., & Jerger, J. F. (1959). Some factors affecting the spondee threshold in normal-hearing subjects. *J. Speech Hear. Res., 2,* 141–146.

Tillman, T. W., & Olsen, W. O. (1973). Speech audiometry. In J. Jerger (Ed.), *Modern developments in audiology,* pp. 37–74. New York: Academic Press.

Tonndorf, J. (1964). Animal experiments in bone conduction: Clinical conclusions. *Ann. Otol. Rhinol. Laryngol., 73,* 659–678.

Tonndorf, J. (1966). Bone conduction: Studies in experimental animals. *Acta Otolaryngol. Suppl., 213,* 1–132.

Tonndorf, J. (1968). A new concept of bone conduction. *Arch. Otolaryngol., 87,* 595–600.

Tonndorf, J. (1972). Bone conduction. In J. V. Tobias (Ed.), *Foundations of modern auditory theory,* pp. 84–99. New York: Academic Press.

Tonndorf, J. (1985). Electro-stimulation. *Seminars in Hear., 6,* 359–367.

Tonndorf, J., & Kurman, B. (1984). High frequency audiometry. *Ann. Otolaryngol., 93,* 576–582.

Ventry, I. M. (1979). Communication guidelines. (Letter to Editor.) *Asha, 21,* 639.

Ventry, I. M., & Chaiklin, J. B. (Eds.) (1965). Multidiscipline study of functional hearing loss. *J. Aud. Res., 3,* 175–272.

Ventry, I. M., Chaiklin, J. B., & Boyle, W. F. (1961). Collapse of the ear canal during audiometry. *Arch. Otolaryngol., 73,* 727–731.

Wall, L. G., Davis, L. A., & Myers, D. K. (1984). Four spondee threshold procedures: A comparison. *Ear Hear., 5,* 171–174.

Ward, W. D. (1963). Auditory fatigue and masking. In J. Jerger (Ed.), *Modern developments in audiology,* pp. 240–286. New York: Academic Press.

Wegel, R. L., & Lane, C. E. (1924). The auditory masking on one pure tone by another and its probable relation to the dynamics of the inner ear. *Phys. Rev., 23,* 266–285.

Weiss, E. (1960). An air damped artificial mastoid. *J. Acoust. Soc. Am., 32,* 1582–1588.

Wilber, L. (1972). Comparability of two commercially available artificial mastoids. *J. Acoust. Soc. Am., 52,* 1265–1266.

Wilber, L. A. (1979). Pure tone audiometry: Air and bone conduction. In W. F. Rintelmann (Ed.), *Hearing assessment,* pp. 29–49. Baltimore: University Park Press.

Wilber, L. A. (1985). Calibration: Puretone, speech, and noise signals. In J. Katz (Ed.), *Handbook of clinical audiology,* 3d ed., pp. 115–150. Baltimore: Williams & Wilkins.

Wilber, L. A., Kruger, B., & Killion, M. C. (1988). Reference thresholds for the ER-3A insert earphone. *J. Acoust. Soc. Am., 83,* 669–676.

Wilson, R. H., & Margolis, R. H. (1983). Measurements of auditory thresholds for speech stimuli. In D. F. Konkle & W. F. Rintelmann (Eds.), *Principles of speech audiometry.* pp. 52–76. Baltimore: University Park Press.

Wilson, R., Morgan, D., & Dirks, D. (1973). A proposed SRT procedure and its statistical precedent. *J. Speech Hear. Dis., 38,* 184–191.

Wilson, W. R., & Thompson, G. (1984). Behavioral audiometry. In J.

Jerger (Ed.), *Pediatric audiology: Current trends*, pp. 1–44. San Diego: College-Hill Press.

Wofford, M. (1981). Audiological evaluation and management of hearing disorders. In F. N. Martin (Ed.), *Medical audiology: Disorders of hearing*, pp. 257–326. Englewood Cliffs, New Jersey: Prentice-Hall.

Yantis, P. A. (1985). Puretone air-conduction testing. In J. Katz (Ed.), *Handbook of clinical audiology*, pp. 153–169. Baltimore: Williams & Wilkins.

Young, L. L., Dudley, B., & Gunter, M. B. (1982). Thresholds and psychometric functions of the individual spondaic words. *J. Speech Hear. Res.*, 25, 586–593.

Zemlin, W. R. (1988). *Speech and hearing science: Anatomy and physiology*, 3d ed. Englewood Cliffs, New Jersey: Prentice-Hall.

Zwislocki, J. (1953). Acoustic attenuation between the ears. *J. Acoust. Soc. Am.*, 25, 752–759.

Zwislocki, J., Maire, R., Feldman, A., & Ruben, A. (1958). On the effect of practice and motivation on the threshold of audibility. *J. Acoust. Soc. Am.*, 30, 254–262.

CHAPTER 3

ACOUSTIC-IMMITTANCE ASSESSMENT

In Chapter 2, the procedure for air- and bone-conduction testing to measure hearing sensitivity and classify the hearing impairment (conductive or sensorineural) was discussed. A limitation of air- and bone-conduction testing is its inability to differentiate between cochlear and retro-cochlear pathology. Another limitation is that air- and bone-conduction test results do not yield information concerning the nature of a conductive disorder. Also, air- and bone-conduction testing is often insensitive to mild conductive problems. Finally, the testing requires patient cooperation which is often difficult to obtain, particularly in neonates, the mentally retarded, the developmentally disabled, and the multiply handicapped.

In Chapters 5 and 9, the traditional site-of-lesion tests such as Bekesy, ABLB, and tone-decay will be discussed. As will be mentioned in those chapters, these tests are characterized by relatively low sensitivity rates ranging from approximately 50% to 75% (Turner, Shepard, & Frazer, 1984), the tests are relatively time-consuming, and the task involved may be difficult for the patient to understand or perform.

Acoustic-immittance testing represents a powerful tool in the clinician's armamentarium. It provides information regarding the nature of the conductive problem, for example, whether it is a stiffening or a loosening pathology, whether effusion is present, whether there is Eustachian-tube dysfunction, and so forth. Acoustic-immittance testing is sensitive to the presence of even a mild conductive pathology that does not result in an air–bone gap.

Since acoustic-immittance testing is not a behavioral test, is not time-consuming, is noninvasive, and is relatively easy to administer, it can be used to detect the presence of conductive pathology in the difficult-to-test. Furthermore, predictive statements concerning hearing sensitivity from the acoustic reflex thresholds can be made in the difficult-to-test population on whom traditional audiometric tests cannot be done.

As will be shown in Chapter 9, the sensitivity of acoustic-reflex testing to retrocochlear pathology (the hit rate) is substantially higher than the sensitivity of the traditional

site-of-lesion tests although it is not quite as high as that of brainstem auditory-evoked potentials testing. Nevertheless, since acoustic-reflex testing is used routinely for clinical assessment of middle-ear functioning, it is clinically feasible and convenient to do acoustic-reflex testing to detect retrocochlear as well as conductive pathology. Unlike brainstem auditory-evoked potentials testing, acoustic-reflex testing can be employed as a relatively low-cost screening device to identify persons who are otherwise at low risk for retrocochlear pathology.

Acoustic-reflex testing can also be used to help identify nonorganic hearing impairment, as will be described in Chapter 4.

The American National Standard Institute (1987) proposed the replacement of traditional acoustic-immittance measurement units with those now used in Europe. Since these proposed units are cumbersome, with the exception of the use of daPa for m H_2O, these units will not be discussed in this chapter.

I. CONCEPT OF IMMITTANCE

A. IMPEDANCE
1. Mechanical Impedance

a. CONSTANT FORCE

The concept of mechanical impedance will be discussed first in order to make the concept of acoustic impedance easier to understand. This discussion is based, in part, on the excellent work by Margolis (1981). The concept of mechanical impedance will be illustrated by examining the interaction between a constant force applied to an object, in this case, a block, and the resultant velocity of the object.

In Figure 1A, a block is being pushed by a constant force, that is, a force having an amplitude which does not change over time (unlike an alternating force). This force of 1 dyne pushes the block (which has a weight of 1 gm) over a smooth surface. As a result, the block moves with a velocity of 1 cm/s. Since a force of 1 dyne is required to move the 1-gm block a distance of 1 cm in 1 s, the block has an opposition to the force or mechanical impedance, Z, of

1A. F = 1 dyne⟶ ☐ $\underline{1\ cm/s}$ $Z = \dfrac{F}{v} = 1$ ohm

1B. F = 50 dynes⟶ ☐ $\underline{1\ cm/s}$ $Z = \dfrac{F}{v} = 50$ ohms

Z = 50 ohms Z = ? ohms

1C. F = 150 dynes⟶ ☐—☐ $\underline{1\ cm/s}$ $Z = \dfrac{F}{v}$

Figure 1 The relation between impedance (Z), force (F), and velocity (V).

1 ohm. In order to calculate the mechanical impedance, the force applied to the object, in this case, a block, is divided by the velocity of the object.

In Figure 1B, a greater force is applied to push a heavier block. In this case, a force of 50 dynes is needed to move this heavier block with a velocity of 1 cm/s. The mechanical impedance, Z, can be calculated by dividing the force of 50 dynes by the velocity of 1 cm/s. Thus, the mechanical impedance is equal to 50 dynes/cm/s or 50 ohms (Ω). More force is needed to move the block with a velocity of 1 cm/s in Figure 1B than in Figure 1A because the block in Figure 1B has more mechanical impedance than the one in Figure 1A.

In Figure 1C, another block is added in series to the block in Figure 1B. The force moves the blocks in series with a velocity of 1 cm/s. More force is needed to move the two blocks than was needed to move the block in Figure 1B since another block needs to be pushed, thereby increasing the opposition to the force. Let us suppose that a force of 150 dynes is needed to move the two blocks with a velocity of 1 cm/s. What is the total mechanical impedance of this two-block system? Also, what is the mechanical impedance of the second block alone? Using the formula

$$Z = F/V \qquad (1)$$

the total impedance of the two-block system can be calculated by dividing 150 dynes by 1 cm/s which yields 150 ohms. In order to determine the impedance of the second block, we subtract the impedance of the first block, 50 ohms, from the total impedance, 150 ohms, which yields 100 ohms. Thus, 150 dynes was needed to move the two blocks with a velocity of 1 cm/s compared with 50 dynes to move the block in Figure 1B with the same velocity. Thus, an additional 100 dynes of force was needed to move the second block in Figure 1C.

In Figure 1C, the mechanical impedance of one block was subtracted from the total mechanical impedance of the two-block system to yield the mechanical impedance of the second block. This was possible since both blocks had the same type of impedance, that is, they were both masses, and since the velocities were equal (they were attached in series).

b. Alternating Force
When an alternating force (a force having an amplitude

which changes over time) is applied to a system which has an object with mass, a spring fixed at one end, and a rough surface, the total mechanical impedance of the system cannot be obtained by simply adding the component impedances.

In Figure 2, a mechanical force (in this case, a human hand) is alternately pushing and pulling on a spring fixed at one end, that is, attached at one end to a wall. In Figure 2A, a mechanical force has just been applied to push a spring. The force, therefore, is at a minimum and the velocity of the spring is at a maximum since it has not yet been compressed. In Figure 2B, the mechanical force has pushed maximally on the spring. Although the force is at a maximum, the velocity of the spring is at a minimum since the spring is completely compressed. In Figure 2C, the mechanical force decreases until it reaches a minimum. The velocity of the spring increases until it reaches a maximum at the point at which the spring is completely uncompressed (the starting or resting position). In Figure 2D, the mechanical force is applied maximally in the opposite direction since it is now pulling rather than pushing on the spring. The velocity is at a minimum since the spring is maximally expanded. In Figure 2E, the mechanical force decreases until it reaches a minimum. The velocity increases until it reaches a maximum at the point at which the spring is no longer expanded.

The relation just discussed between a force applied to a

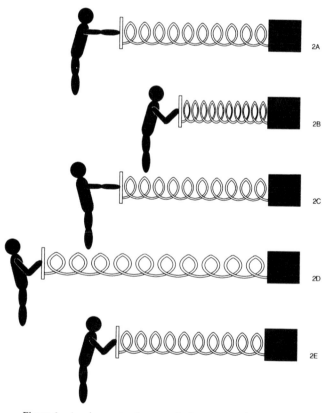

Figure 2 An alternating force applied to a spring fixed at one end.

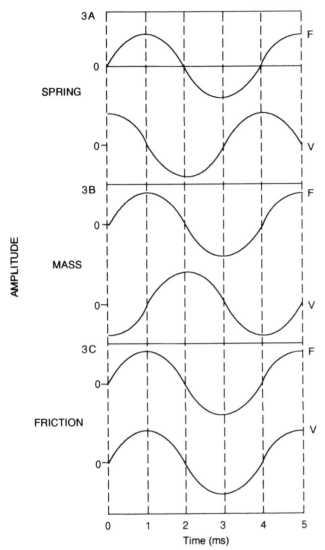

Figure 3 The relations among a sinusoidal force (F), velocity (V), and time for a spring (A), mass (B), and friction (C).

force is minimal and the velocity of the spring is maximal (in the positive direction), analogous to the situation in Figure 2E. Clearly, the velocity of the spring reaches a maximum 1 ms (90°) before the force applied to the spring reaches a maximum. Thus, velocity leads force by 90°.

In Figure 4, the relation between an alternating force applied to an object having mass and the resultant velocity of the mass is described. In this figure, a person is pushing and pulling on a heavy block. In Figure 4A, the maximum push on the block has been exerted. The block starts moving only after the maximum push is given because the block initially rejects the push as a result of its inertia. (Inertia is the tendency for a mass to oppose a change in position.) Thus, force is at a maximum and velocity is at a minimum. The mathematical analog of this situation is shown in Figure 3B at $t = 1$ ms. Between Figures 4A and B, the block moves faster (the velocity increases) and less pushing occurs (the force decreases). In Figure 4B, the block is moving at its fastest speed (velocity is maximal) and no more pushing is occurring (force is minimal). The mathematical analog of this situation is shown in Figure 3B at t = 2 ms. Between Figures 4B and C, the person starts to pull rather than push

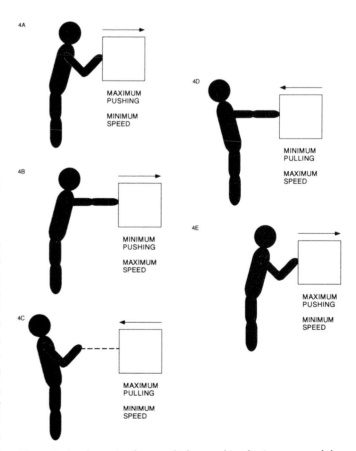

Figure 4 An alternating force applied to an object having mass, and the resultant velocity of the mass. The arrows represent the direction of the applied force.

spring and the resultant velocity of the spring can also be understood in mathematical terms, as illustrated in Figure 3. Figure 3A shows a sinusoidal force being applied to a spring which alternates at a rate of 250 times per second (250 Hz). In this example, it takes 4 ms for the amplitude of the force to undergo one cycle. At time (t) of 0 ms, the force is minimal (zero amplitude) and the velocity of the spring is maximal (in the positive direction), analogous to the situation in Figure 2A. At $t = 1$ ms, the force is maximal (in the positive direction) and the velocity of the spring is minimal, analogous to the situation in Figure 2B. At $t = 2$ ms, the force is minimal and the velocity of the spring is maximal (in the negative direction, analogous to the situation in Figure 2C). At $t = 3$ ms, the force is maximal (in the negative direction) and the velocity of the spring is minimal, analogous to the situation in Figure 2D. At $t = 4$ ms, the

the block in order to decrease the velocity of the block so it can be brought to a halt. Thus, the force increases, but in a different direction than shown in Figure 4A. In Figure 4C, the maximal pull has been exerted (force is maximal) and the block has been brought to a complete halt (velocity is minimal). The mathematical analog of this situation is shown in Figure 3B at $t = 3$ ms. Between Figures 4C and D, the amount of pulling on the block decreases (the force decreases). As a result, the block begins moving faster in the opposite direction, that is, toward the person rather than away from the person (the velocity increases). In Figure 4D, there is no more pulling on the block (force is minimal) and the block is moving at its fastest speed (velocity is maximal). The mathematical analog of this situation is shown in Figure 3B at $t = 4$ ms. Between Figures 4D and E, the person is now pushing rather than pulling on the block in order to slow down its speed and bring it to a halt. Thus, the force is increasing whereas the velocity is decreasing. In Figure 4E, the person exerts the maximal push, thereby bringing the block to a complete halt. Thus, the force is maximal and the velocity is minimal. The mathematical analog of this situation is shown in Figure 3B at $t = 5$ ms. In Figure 4, illustrated in Figure 3, velocity of the mass reaches a maximum 1 ms (90°) after the force applied to the mass reaches a maximum.

The relation between an alternating force and velocity of an object in a frictional system which contains negligible mass or stiffness components is illustrated in Figure 3C. If an alternating force is applied to a springless object having negligible mass over a rough, frictional surface, the velocity of the object will attain maximum and minimum values at the same time that the force attains maximum and minimum values, respectively. Thus, the velocity of the object moving over a frictional surface is in phase with the applied force. (Since the object is springless and has a negligible mass, it can be assumed that neither mass nor spring components modify this relation between force and velocity of the object over a frictional surface.)

As stated earlier, impedance (Z) = force/velocity (Eq. 1) and there are three impedance components. The impedance offered by mass is termed the mass reactance ($+ X_M$). The $+$ sign indicates that force attains a maximum value before the velocity attains a maximum value when an alternating force is applied to an object having mass. That is, the force leads velocity by 90°. The impedance offered by a spring is stiffness reactance ($- X_S$). The $-$ sign indicates that the force attains a maximum value after the velocity attains a maximum value when an alternating force is applied to a spring or an object having stiffness. Thus, the force lags velocity by 90°. The impedance resulting from friction is termed the resistance (R). For each impedance component, $+X_M$, $-X_S$, or R, the impedance is equal to the force divided by the velocity.

If a system consists of an alternating force applied to

several masses in series, then the total impedance of the system is simply the sum of the mass reactances offered by each mass component, since the relation between force and velocity is the same for each of the mass reactance components, that is, force leads velocity by 90°. If a system consists of an alternating force applied to several springs in series, the total impedance of the system is simply the sum of the stiffness reactances offered by each spring, since the relation between force and velocity is the same for each of the stiffness reactance components, that is, velocity leads force by 90°. If a system consists of an alternating force applied to several frictional surfaces in series, the total impedance of this system is simply the sum of the resistances offered by each frictional surface, since the relation between force and velocity is the same for each of the resistance components, that is, velocity is in phase with the force. It is rare to find a system which consists of only one type of impedance component. If the three types of impedance components exist in a system (mass reactance offered by a mass, stiffness reactance offered by a spring or an object having stiffness, and resistance offered by friction), then the total impedance is not simply the sum of the impedance components, since the relation between force and velocity is different for each of the impedance components.

Figure 5A shows a mechanical system containing a mass, spring, and friction. Thus, it contains all three types of impedance components—mass reactance, stiffness reactance, and resistance. Figure 5B shows the changes in veloc-

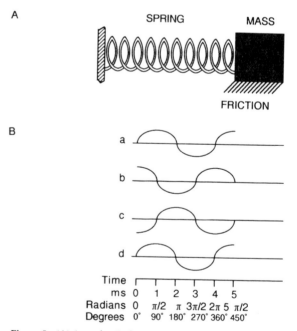

Figure 5 (A) A mechanical system containing mass, spring, and frictional components. (B) (a) the applied, alternating force as a function of time, (b) the velocity of a spring as a function of time, (c) the velocity of a mass as a function of time, and (d) the velocity of a frictional component as a function of time.

ity over time for each of the three components as related to the changes in the applied alternating force over time. Note that, in this system, the velocity values reach a maximum at different times during the force cycle. That is, the maximum velocity occurs at $t = 0$ ms in the force cycle for the stiffness reactance, at $t = 1$ ms for the resistance component, and at $t = 2$ ms for the mass reactance. Since the velocity maxima for the mass reactance, stiffness reactance, and resistance occur at different points along the force cycle, the maxima of the impedance occur at different points along the force cycle. Therefore, a vector system is required to obtain the sum of the impedance components (see Figure 6).

In Figure 6, the placement of the resistance (R) component of impedance on the abscissa represents the fact that, for this component, the velocity is in phase with the force. The placement of the stiffness-reactance component ($-X_S$) along the negative ordinate represents the fact that in the case of this component, the velocity leads the force by 90°. The placement of the mass-reactance component ($+X_M$) along the positive ordinate represents the fact that in the case of this component, the velocity lags the force by 90°. Note that the mass reactance ($+X_M$) and the stiffness reactance ($-X_S$) are out of phase by 180°. Therefore, to obtain the net reactance (X_T), the stiffness reactance is added to the mass reactance. If the system has more stiffness than mass reactance, the net reactance, X_T, will be negative. If the system has more mass than stiffness reactance, the net reactance, X_T, is positive.

Figure 7 shows the vectors for impedance, resistance, and the net reactance. The resultant impedance is the vector sum of the resistance and net reactance. The magnitude of the impedance vector (the diagonal line in Figure 7) can be calculated using the Pythagorean theorem which states that the hypotenuse squared equals the sum of the squares of the other two sides of a right triangle. Thus,

$$Z^2 = R^2 + X_T^2 \qquad (2)$$

and

$$Z = \sqrt{R^2 + X_T^2}$$

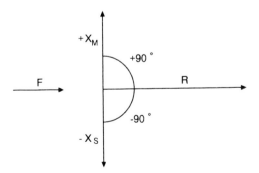

Figure 6 A vectorial representation of the impedance components. $+X_M$ is the mass reactance, $-X_S$ is the stiffness reactance, R is the resistance, and F is the applied alternating force.

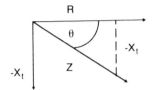

Figure 7 The vectors for the total impedance (Z), resistance (R), and the net reactance ($-X_T$). The phase angle (θ) is also shown in the figure. The formula for calculating the total impedance from the resistance and the net reactance is shown at the top of the figure.
reactance is shown at the top of the figure.

The phase angle of the impedance vector is calculated using the formula

$$\cos \theta = R/Z \qquad (3)$$

or

$$\sin \theta = X_T/Z \qquad (4)$$

Let us calculate the mechanical impedance of a system consisting only of stiffness reactance and resistance in which the velocity and force are known. The velocity of the spring is 5 cm/s and the force required to produce this velocity is 50 dynes. The velocity of the friction is 10 cm/s and the force required to produce this velocity is 50 dynes. The impedance offered by the spring ($-X_S$) is force divided by velocity (50/5) or 10 ohms. This stiffness reactance is the net reactance (X_T) since there is no mass reactance. The impedance offered by the friction (R) is force divided by velocity (50/10) or 5 ohms. To obtain the complex impedance of the system the Pythagorean theorem is employed, so $Z^2 = 5^2 + 10^2$ so $Z = \sqrt{25 + 100}$ and $Z = 5\sqrt{5}$, which means $Z = (5 \times 2.29)$ ohms, or 11.45 ohms.

In all the previous examples, the alternating force driving the mechanical system was a 250-Hz force. The mechanical impedance of a system also varies as the frequency of the applied force varies. The relation between mechanical stiffness reactance, stiffness, and frequency is illustrated by the formula

$$-X_S = S/(2 \pi f) \qquad (5)$$

where S is stiffness and f is frequency. According to this formula, the stiffer the spring, the larger the mechanical stiffness reactance; the higher the frequency, the smaller the stiffness reactance. Thus, the stiffness reactance can be increased by increasing the stiffness or by decreasing the frequency; it can be decreased by decreasing the stiffness or increasing the frequency. If there is no stiffness reactance at one frequency, one cannot conclude that there is no stiffness reactance in the system; it may be present at other frequencies.

The mass reactance also changes with frequency. The relation among mechanical mass reactance, mass, and frequency is illustrated in the formula

$$+X_M = 2\pi fM \qquad (6)$$

According to this formula, the mass reactance increases as the mass or frequency increases; it decreases as the mass or frequency decreases. Since mechanical mass reactance decreases whereas mechanical stiffness reactance increases as frequency decreases, and vice-versa, there is a frequency at which the stiffness and mass reactances are equal. At this frequency, there is no mass or stiffness reactance. This frequency is known as the resonance frequency, which can be calculated with the formula

$$f_0 = (1/2\pi)(S/M) \qquad (7)$$

where f_0 is the resonant frequency, S is stiffness, and M is mass. If there is no mass reactance at one frequency, one cannot conclude there is no mass reactance in the system; it may be present at other frequencies.

Resistance, unlike mass or stiffness reactance, does not change with frequency. That is, resistance is independent of frequency.

Since $-X_S = S/(2\pi f)$ (Eq. 5), the total impedance of a system which has a net reactance that is stiffness reactance can also be written as

$$Z^2 = R^2 + [S/(2\pi f)]^2 \qquad (8)$$

Since $+X_M = 2\pi fM$ (Eq. 6), the total impedance of a system which has a net reactance that is mass reactance can be written as

$$Z^2 = R^2 + (2\pi fM)^2 \qquad (9)$$

2. Acoustic Impedance

In acoustics, the analog of a mechanical mass is the air volume in a tube open at both ends. Similarly, the analog of a spring is the air volume in a tube closed at both ends. When the air volume in a tube is compressed, it will behave like a spring. The analog of friction is the collision of the air molecules.

According to Van Camp, Margolis, Wilson, Creten, and Shanks (1986), the ear is an "acoustico-mechanical" system that contains acoustical as well as mechanical impedance components. The tympanic membrane can be considered a mechanical spring. The air volume enclosed in the middle ear can be considered an acoustic spring. The ossicular chain can be considered a mechanical mass. The air molecules in the mastoid air cells can be considered an acoustic mass. The friction in the tympanic membrane, middle-ear tendons, and ligaments can be considered the mechanical friction. The air viscosity can be considered the acoustic friction. Figure 8 illustrates the mechanoacoustic model of the middle ear. The mechanoacoustic impedance of the middle ear is referred to in the literature as the acoustic impedance (Z_a) of the middle ear. The total acoustic impedance (Z_a) consists of acoustic mass reactance ($+X_a$),

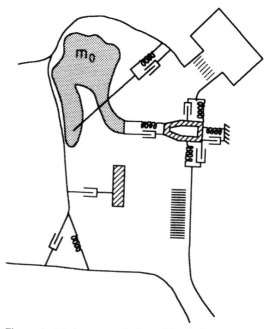

Figure 8 Mechanoacoustical model of the ear, containing masses, springs, and friction elements as mechanical elements, together with open and closed air-filled volumes as acoustical elements. Reprinted with permission from Marquet, Van Camp, Creten, Decraemer, Wolff, and Schepens (1973).

which is the acoustico-mechanical mass, acoustic stiffness reactance ($-X_a$), which is the acoustico-mechanical stiffness reactance, and acoustic resistance (R_a) which is the acoustico-mechanical resistance.

In the previous section, when the impedance of a mechanical system was measured, a force was applied and the resultant velocity was measured. In an acoustic system, sound pressure expressed in dynes/cm^2 is applied and the resultant volume velocity (expressed in cm^3) is measured. Volume velocity is defined as the volume (cm^3) of the sound-conducting medium which flows in a given area in a given amount of time (in s). The total acoustic impedance, therefore, can be expressed as

$$Z_a = P/U \qquad (10)$$

where P is the sound pressure (in dynes/cm^2), U is the volume velocity (in cm^3), and Z_a is acoustic impedance (in acoustic ohms). One acoustic ohm of acoustic impedance is equivalent to 10^5 Pa $\times$ s/m^3.

The formula for acoustic impedance having a net acoustic reactance that is acoustic stiffness reactance is

$$Z_a^2 = (-X_a)^2 + R_a^2 \qquad (11)$$

or

$$Z_a^2 = [S/(2\pi f)]^2 + R_a^2 \qquad (12)$$

The formula for acoustic impedance having a net acoustic reactance that is acoustic mass reactance is

$$Z_a^2 = (+X_a)^2 + R_a^2 \qquad (13)$$

or

$$Z_a^2 = (2\pi fM)^2 + R_a^2 \qquad (14)$$

B. ADMITTANCE

1. MECHANICAL ADMITTANCE

The ability of the system to transfer energy can also be expressed in terms of its acceptance rather than rejection of energy. If the force applied to System A is the same as that applied to System B and if the resultant velocity of System A is greater than that of system B, then System A has more admittance (less impedance) than System B. Since mechanical admittance is the reciprocal of mechanical impedance, it can be calculated using the formula

$$Y = V/F \qquad (15)$$

where Y is mechanical admittance, V is velocity, and F is force. The unit of admittance is mho (the reciprocal of ohms). Note that the relation between velocity and force for admittance is the reverse of that for impedance since admittance is the reciprocal of impedance. The ease with which energy flows into a mass is called mass susceptance ($-B_M$). The ease with which energy flows into a spring or an object having stiffness is called stiffness susceptance ($+B_S$). The ease with which energy flows into friction is called conductance (G). The relation among the admittance vectors is shown in Figure 9. Note that the stiffness susceptance is on the positive ordinate rather than the negative ordinate and the mass susceptance is on the negative ordinate rather than the positive ordinate. In this graph, the net reactance, (B_T), obtained by adding the negative mass susceptance to the positive stiffness susceptance, happens to be stiffness susceptance. The admittance vector is calculated using the Pythagorean theorem.

Admittance is calculated from the formula

$$Y^2 = B_t^2 + G^2 \qquad (16)$$

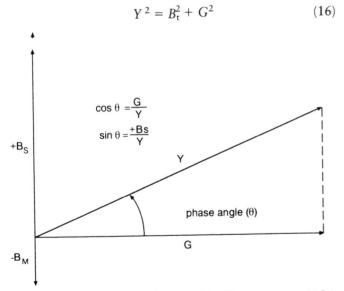

Figure 9 Relations among conductance (G), stiffness susceptance ($+B_S$), and mass susceptance ($-B_M$).

The unit of admittance, mass susceptance, stiffness susceptance, and resistance is mho (1000 mmhos). The relations among stiffness susceptance, stiffness, and frequency, and among mass susceptance, mass, and frequency are given by the formulas

$$+ B_S = (2\pi f/S) \qquad (17)$$

and

$$- B_M = 1/(2\pi fM) \qquad (18)$$

According to Eq. 17, the stiffness susceptance increases as the frequency increases or as the stiffness decreases; it decreases as the frequency decreases or as the stiffness increases. According to Eq. 18, the mass susceptance increases as the frequency or mass decreases; it decreases as the frequency or mass increases. If there is no mass or stiffness susceptance at one frequency it cannot be concluded that there is no mass or stiffness susceptance at other frequencies.

2. ACOUSTIC ADMITTANCE

The principles underlying mechanical admittance can be applied to acoustic admittance. Acoustic admittance is defined as the ease with which acoustic energy passes through a system. It is mathematically expressed as the ratio of volume velocity to sound pressure ($Y_a = U/P$). The unit of acoustic admittance is mho. One mmho equals $m^3/(10^8 Pa \times s)$. The admittance components include acoustic stiffness susceptance ($+B_a$), acoustic mass susceptance ($-B_a$), and acoustic conductance (G_a). The total acoustic admittance can be calculated from the formula

$$Y_a^2 = B_{ta}^2 + G_a^2 \qquad (19)$$

The acoustic admittance or impedance is expressed using rectangular or polar notation. In rectangular notation, one value is given to the acoustic conductance or resistance component and one value is given to the net acoustic susceptance or reactance component. For example, acoustic impedance can be written, using rectangular notation, as $Z_a = 1500 - j3000$, where j is the square root of -1. Since j represents an imaginary number, it cannot be added to real numbers such as the value 1500 in the given example.

In polar notation, one number is given to the magnitude of the acoustic impedance or admittance and one number represents the phase angle of the acoustic impedance or admittance vector. For example, $Y_a = 0.6 < + 30°$.

The term "immittance" is used to refer to either impedance or admittance.

C. ACOUSTIC-IMMITTANCE INSTRUMENTATION

Recall from Section I,A,2 that acoustic impedance is the ratio of sound pressure to volume velocity, that is, $Z_a = P/U$. Also recall from Section I,B,2 that acoustic admittance is the ratio of volume velocity to sound pressure, that is, $Y_a = U/P$. In the impedance equation, if U is kept constant, then P is directly proportional to Z_a. This concept can be illustrated by considering water flow from a hose directly into a container. If the water flow is kept constant, the pressure of the water in the container is inversely proportional to the size of the container. The water flow is the analog to the volume velocity, the pressure in the container is the analog to sound pressure, and the size of the cavity is the analog to the impedance of the ear. If the volume of the container decreases, the impedance increases; therefore, water pressure (sound pressure) will be directly related to the impedance of the container (ear impedance) if the water flow (volume velocity) is kept constant.

Modern commercially available acoustic-immittance devices are essentially constructed on the basis of the acoustic-impedance or acoustic-admittance formula. Devices constructed on the basis of the acoustic-impedance formula are called acoustic-impedance meters. Devices constructed on the basis of the acoustic-admittance formula are called acoustic-admittance meters.

The acoustic-impedance meter has a probe assembly which is inserted into the external auditory meatus. The probe assembly contains a loudspeaker (usually called the driver) which introduces a constant volume velocity in the ear canal by applying voltage from a source in the acoustic-impedance meter to the diaphragm of the driver. When the voltage is applied to the diaphragm, the air molecules in the ear canal are set in motion (the volume velocity). The probe assembly also contains a microphone that tranduces the sound pressure resulting from the volume velocity into electrical voltage; the electrical voltage is read in acoustic-impedance units (acoustic ohms). Figure 10, adapted from Van Camp *et al.* (1986), illustrates the components of an acoustic-impedance meter.

One of the disadvantages of the acoustic-impedance meter shown in Figure 10 is that acoustic impedance at the probe tip is affected by the ear-canal volume, since sound pressure and volume are inversely related. Therefore, in order to avoid the effect of ear-canal volume on sound pressure and consequently on the acoustic impedance at the probe, acoustic-immittance devices which measure acoustic impedance usually apply additional steps for keeping sound pressure constant at the probe. A balance meter in the acoustic-impedance device functions to maintain sound pressure at a predetermined level. That is, when the sound pressure level at the probe tip reaches a predetermined level such as 85 dB SPL, the balance meter will read 0 (arbitrary units). At the 0 unit balance-meter reading, the voltage at the microphone reaches a value equivalent to a reference voltage which produces 85 dB SPL in a cavity having a specified volume. Adjustment of the balance meter causes the driver voltage to change, leading to changes in volume velocity so the pressure can be adjusted to 85 dB SPL in a given ear canal.

Another disadvantage (which cannot be offset) of the acoustic-impedance meter shown in Figure 10 is that the amplitude of tympanograms produced by such a device cannot be expressed in physical units such as acoustic ohms because of nonlinearity in the impedance change during the ear-canal pressure change. These acoustic-impedance meters express the amplitude of the tympanogram in arbitrary units, often erroneously referred to as compliance units. Because arbitrary units are employed, such devices are called relative acoustic-impedance meters.

In acoustic-admittance meters, the acoustic admittance is derived from the volume velocity rather than from the sound pressure as is done for acoustic-impedance meters. In acoustic-immitance meters, P is kept constant so Y_a is directly proportional to U. With acoustic-admittance meters, an alternating voltage is applied to the loudspeaker. The alternating voltage is also applied to a rectifier filter which rectifies the voltage (changes it from an AC to a DC voltage), which is displayed as Y_a at the probe tip.

This admittance concept can be illustrated with the water hose analogy. The driver voltage can be considered the source of the water flow. The admittance can be likened to the size of the container; the larger the container, the larger the admittance. Using the water hose analogy, to maintain a constant water (sound) pressure, the flow of the water (volume velocity) has to be adjusted. The larger the container (admittance), the greater the water flow (volume velocity) to maintain the pressure.

The effect of ear-canal volume on sound-pressure level in the ear canal is offset by the AGC circuit. That is, sound-pressure level is continuously kept constant by a circuit which continuously adjusts the driver voltage depending on the voltage at the microphone. Since the acoustic admittance is calculated from the volume velocity rather than from the sound pressure, acoustic-admittance meters do not have the disadvantage of nonlinearity in acoustic-admittance changes with changes in ear-canal air pressure during tympanometry. Thus, the admittance changes can be

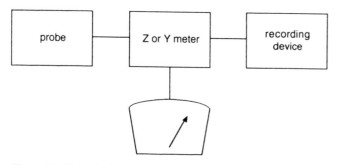

Figure 10 General scheme for an acoustic-immittance meter. Reprinted with permission from Van Camp, Margolis, Wilson, Creten, and Shanks (1986).

quantified in absolute admittance units, that is, mmho. Admittance devices which measure the admittance change in absolute units are called absolute acoustic-admittance meters.

Description of an acoustic-admittance meter that measures two components of admittance simultaneously, as reported by Van Camp et al. (1986), may provide us with information on the principle operation of admittance meters. In such devices the driver voltage consists of in-phase and out-of-phase components relative to the phase of the microphone voltage. The in-phase component represents the volume velocity of the acoustic conductance (G_a) and the out-of-phase component represents the volume velocity of the acoustic susceptance (B_a). If the voltage from the microphone and the voltage from the driver are fed to a multiplier,[1] the output voltage from the multiplier will be proportional to G_a and could be read out directly from the meter. If the driver voltage or microphone voltage is fed to a 90° phase shifter (in this case the driver voltage),[2] the output of which is fed to a multiplier, then the voltage output of the multiplier will be proportional to B_a and could be read out from the meter. Figure 11 illustrates a schematic of an acoustic-admittance meter that measures acoustic susceptance and conductance. When Y_a is calculated, the rectified driver voltage is measured before being routed to the phase shifter and multiplier.

The early acoustic-immittance meters used only a single low-frequency probe tone. The use of a low-frequency probe tone was based on the results of early studies showing that the normal middle ear is stiffness dominated at all probe-tone frequencies. The results of recent research, however, illustrate that the normal middle ear is stiffness

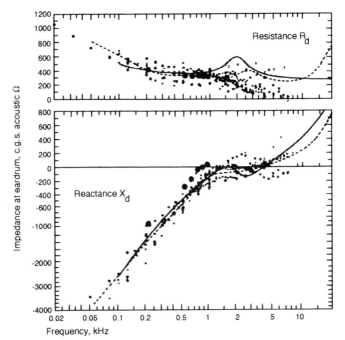

Figure 12 Acoustic resistance and acoustic reactance at the eardrum from 20 previous studies (from Shaw, 1980). Closed circles, current investigation; dashes, curves fitted to data; solid lines, middle-ear network with compound eardrum. Reprinted with permission from Margolis, Van Camp, Wilson, and Creten (1985).

dominated below 800 Hz; at probe-tone frequencies between 800 and 1200 Hz, the middle ear resonates (stiffness and mass reactance are cancelled out) and at probe-tone frequencies above 1200 Hz, the middle ear is mass loaded (Margolis, Van Camp, Wilson, & Creten, 1985). Figure 12 illustrates the middle-ear impedance (reactance and resistance) as a function of probe-tone frequency. As will be shown in Section II,D,1, high probe-tone frequencies are essential in detection of ear pathologies that alter the mass of the middle ear. Many commercially available acoustic-immittance devices incorporate a high-frequency probe tone such as 660 Hz or 1000 Hz in addition to a low-frequency probe tone.

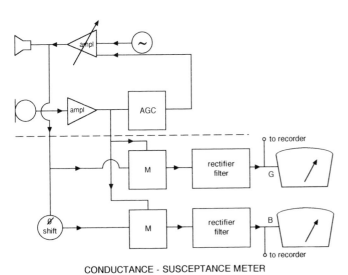

CONDUCTANCE - SUSCEPTANCE METER

Figure 11 Block diagram of a susceptance–conductance meter. Reprinted with permission from Van Camp, Margolis, Wilson, Creten, and Shanks (1986).

II. CLINICAL APPLICATIONS OF ACOUSTIC IMMITTANCE

Having discussed the principles and instrumentation used for measuring the acoustic immittance of the ear, we shall now explain how these principles and instrumentation can be used to measure the integrity of the auditory system up to the level of the lower brainstem. There are three major techniques which are routinely employed clinically: (a) static acoustic immittance of the middle ear, (b) tympanometry, and (c) acoustic-reflex testing.

1. A multiplier is a phase sensitive voltage amplifier that passes only in-phase components and cancel out-of-phase components.
2. Alters the phase of the incoming components from the speaker so that only the B_a component will be passed by the multiplier.

A. STATIC ACOUSTIC IMMITTANCE

The static acoustic immittance of the middle ear is the immittance of the middle ear under a predetermined value of air pressure in the external auditory canal.

1. PROCEDURE

a. Different Approaches

There are two approaches for measuring the static acoustic immittance of the middle ear. In the first approach, the static acoustic immittance of the outer ear (obtained with an ear-canal pressure of +200 or −400 daPa) is subtracted from the static acoustic immittance of the combined middle and outer ears at 0 daPa (atmospheric pressure). At +200 or −400 daPa, the tympanic membrane is very stiff so the middle ear is essentially excluded from the acoustic-immittance measurement. For exclusion of the middle ear from the static acoustic immittance measurement, Ter-kildsen and Scott-Nielsen (1960) recommended an ear-canal pressure of +200 daPa whereas Shanks and Lilly (1981) recommended an ear-canal pressure of −400 daPa. At 0 daPa, no pressure is applied against the tympanic membrane so the acoustic immittance consists of the immittance of both the outer and middle ears. This approach was advocated by Feldman (1975, 1976) and Zwislocki and Feldman (1970). With this approach, the test–retest reliability appears to be very poor Porter & Winston, 1973). Margolis and Popelka (1975) reported that the static acoustic immittance of the middle ear obtained with this approach is characterized by large intrasubject variability. Margolis (1981) attributed the large intrasubject variability to the day-to-day fluctuation in middle-ear pressure resulting from the ongoing absorption of air by the middle-ear tissues and replacement of the absorbed air.

In the second approach, the static acoustic immittance of the outer ear at +200 or −400 daPa is subtracted from the combined outer- and middle-ear static immittance at the peak pressure. The peak-pressure point is the pressure point which yields the peak amplitude in the tympanogram. This approach was advocated by Brooks (1968, 1971), Jerger (1970), Jerger, Jerger, and Mauldin (1972), Jerger, Anthony, Jerger, and Mauldin (1974a), and Margolis and Popelka (1975). In this approach the static acoustic middle-ear immittance appears to be stable since pressure against the tympanic membrane on one side is equivalent to pressure against the tympanic membrane on the other side, regardless of the middle-ear pressure. Therefore we recommend this second approach for determining the static acoustic middle-ear immittance.

b. Concepts Underlying the Static-Acoustic Middle-Ear Admittance

The middle ear and outer ear are considered, in the literature, analogous to parallel electric impedance components.

The input impedance of a parallel system shown in Figure 13 can be calculated using the formula

$$1/Z_T = 1/Z_1 + 1/Z_2 \qquad (20)$$

here Z_T is the total impedance of the system and Z_1 and Z_2 are the parallel impedance components. If the total impedance of the system and the impedance of one of the two parallel components are known, the formula, derived from the formula for the total impedance, used to determine the impedance of the second component is

$$Z_2 = (Z_1 \times Z_T)/(Z_1 - Z_T) \qquad (21)$$

where Z_2 is the impedance of the unknown component, Z_1 is the impedance of the known component, and Z_T is the total impedance. Equation 21 can be modified to obtain the middle-ear impedance as

$$Z_{me} = (Z_{oe} \times Z_{te})/(Z_{oe} - Z_{te}) \qquad (22)$$

where Z_{me} is the middle-ear impedance, Z_{oe} is the outer-ear impedance, and Z_{te} is the total impedance of the ear.

The relation between the impedance of the middle ear and the total impedance (combined middle and outer ears) is nonlinear (Margolis, 1981). The relation between the middle-ear admittance and the total admittance, however, is linear (Margolis, 1981), so admittance rather than impedance measurements are desirable for determining the middle-ear immittance. Since the total acoustic impedance in a parallel system is determined by Eq. 20, and since admittance (Y) is the reciprocal of impedance, the formula for calculating the total admittance in a parallel system is

$$Y_T = Y_1 + Y_2 \qquad (23)$$

where Y_T is the total admittance and Y_1 and Y_2 are the parallel admittance components. The admittance of the unknown component (Y_2) can be derived from the formula

$$Y_2 = Y_T - Y_1 \qquad (24)$$

Equation 24 can be modified to determine the static-acoustic admittance of the middle ear as

$$Y_{me} = Y_{te} - Y_{oe} \qquad (25)$$

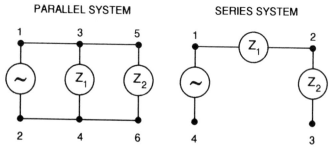

Figure 13 The left graph shows the impedance components in parallel to the applied force. The right graph shows the impedance components in series with the applied force.

where Y_{me} is the static-acoustic admittance of the middle ear, Y_{te} is the total static-acoustic admittance of the ear (combined middle and outer ears) and Y_{oe} is the static-acoustic admittance of the outer ear.

In some acoustic-immittance devices, the vector for acoustic admittance can be derived directly by subtracting the static-acoustic admittance of the outer ear from the static-acoustic admittance of the total ear. The clinician should be aware that errors may occur with such devices, in the calculation of the magnitude of the admittance vector, since the subtraction process involves admittance vectors which may differ in phase angle. With low-frequency probe tones, for example, 220 Hz, the conductance component is very small so the phase angle of the admittance vector approaches 90°. Thus, the magnitude of the admittance vector approaches that of the susceptance vector. Therefore, the error in calculation of the magnitude of the acoustic admittance vector by subtracting the static-acoustic admittance of the outer ear from the static-acoustic admittance of the total ear is nonsignificant— approximately 2% (Bennett, 1984). The error in calculation of the magnitude of the admittance vector using this subtractive process is large for high-frequency probe tones, for example, 660 Hz. With high-frequency probe tones, the conductance vector is large in magnitude compared with the magnitude of the susceptance vector so the phase angle is small. The magnitude of the admittance vector is dissimilar from that of the susceptance vector. Therefore, the error in calculating the static-acoustic admittance of the middle ear by subtracting the static-acoustic admittance of the outer ear from the static-acoustic admittance of the total ear may be as large as 50% (Wiley & Block, 1979). Thus, when high probe-tone frequencies are used, the clinician should not derive the middle-ear acoustic admittance by subtracting the acoustic admittance of the outer ear from that of the total ear. Instead, the acoustic susceptance of the middle ear should be directly calculated by subtracting the acoustic susceptance of the outer ear from that of the total ear. Similarly, the acoustic conductance of the middle ear can be derived. Then, the acoustic admittance of the middle ear, Y_{me}, can be obtained from the formula

$$Y_{me}^2 = G_{me}^2 + B_{me}^2 \qquad (26)$$

based on Eq. 19, where Y_{me} is the static-acoustic admittance of the middle ear, G_{me} is the acoustic conductance of the middle ear, and B_{me} is the acoustic susceptance of the middle ear.

c. Calculating the Static-Acoustic Middle-Ear Admittance

As mentioned previously, two measurements are needed to calculate the static-acoustic middle-ear admittance. The first measurement is made to obtain the admittance of the external auditory meatus. When relative immittance de-

vices are used, the external ear canal is subjected to a pressure of +200 or −400 daPa. (One daPa is equivalent to 1.02 mm water pressure.) The outer-ear static-acoustic admittance is obtained by balancing the admittance meter to 0 and reading the admittance value in cm³. (When the probe-tone frequency is approximately 220 Hz, 1 cm³ = 1 ml = 1 mmho.) For this reason, many acoustic-immittance devices use the 226-Hz rather than the 220-Hz probe tone and the 678-Hz rather than 660-Hz probe tone. When absolute admittance devices are used, the external ear canal is subjected to a pressure of +200 daPa. Then the pressure in the ear canal is gradually decreased to −400 daPa. The outer-ear static-acoustic admittance is obtained by reading from the tympanogram the difference between 0 mmhos and the number of mmhos at +200 or −400 daPa.

Figure 14A illustrates the static-acoustic admittance of the outer ear obtained using an absolute immittance device. Note that the static-acoustic admittance of the outer ear, measured at −400 daPa, is less than that measured at +200 daPa. This difference was attributed by Shanks and Lilly (1981) to the fact that the external ear canal is not completely excluded from the immittance measurement until a pressure of −400 daPa is reached. The second measurement is made to obtain the total static-acoustic admittance (combined admittance of the middle and outer ears). When relative immittance devices are used, the pressure in the external auditory meatus is reduced gradually from +200 daPa to −400 daPa (or increased from −400 to +200 daPa). The static-acoustic admittance of the total ear can be obtained by balancing the admittance meter at zero (the ear canal is subjected to the pressure that yields the greatest admittance—also called the tympanometric peak pressure) and reading the admittance value in cm³. Now, in

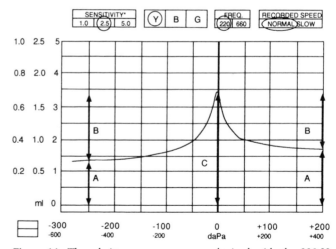

Figure 14 The admittance tympanogram obtained with the 220-Hz probe tone and recorded on the GS 1723 otoadmittance meter (absolute admittance device) from a normal middle ear. (A) The outer-ear static-acoustic admittance; (B) the middle-ear static-acoustic admittance; (C) the total (combined outer and middle) ear static-acoustic admittance.

order to calculate the static-acoustic admittance of the middle ear, Eq. 25 is employed.

When using absolute immittance devices, the static-acoustic admittance of the total ear can be obtained by reading from the tympanogram the difference between 0 mmhos and the number of mmhos at the peak pressure. Figure 14B is the static-acoustic admittance of the middle ear derived by subtracting the static-acoustic admittance of the outer ear (Figure 14A) from the static-acoustic admittance of the total ear (Figure 14C), according to Eq. 25.

In an otoadmittance meter, the acoustic admittance vector (Y_a) and its components, acoustic susceptance (B_a) and acoustic conductance (G_a) are obtained directly. The acoustic impedance vector (Z_a) and its components, acoustic net reactance (X_a) and acoustic resistance (R_a) can be calculated by obtaining the reciprocals of B_a, G_a, and Y_a.

$$X_a = B_a/(B_a^2 + G_a^2) \tag{27}$$

$$R_a = G_a/(G_a^2 + B_a^2) \tag{28}$$

$$Z_a = \sqrt{(X_a^2 + R_a^2)} \tag{29}$$

2. Normative Data

The normative data on the static-acoustic middle-ear admittance and impedance for the 220-Hz probe tone, when the ear-canal static-acoustic admittance and impedance were calculated at +200 daPa, are shown in Table I. The data by Brooks (1971) in Table I were obtained from school children, whereas the data by Jerger (1970) and Jerger *et al.* (1972) were obtained from older children and adults.

In Table II, the normative data on the static-acoustic middle-ear admittance and impedance for the 226-Hz probe tone, when the acoustic admittance and impedance of the ear canal were calculated at −400 daPa, are shown for children and adults at low pump speeds (≤50 daPa/s) and high pump speeds (200 daPa/s). Table II reveals that the static-acoustic middle-ear admittance of children differs from that of adults and that the static-acoustic middle-ear admittance in a given age group varies with pump speed.

It is reasonable to consider the normal static-acoustic middle-ear admittance and impedance ranges for 80% of

Table I The 10th and 90th Percentile Values for Y_A and Z_A Acoustic Immittance for Normal Middle Ear[a]

	Z_A (ohms)			Y_A (mmhos)	
	10%	90%		10%	90%
Jerger (1970)	769	2564	Jerger *et al.* (1972)	0.39	1.30
Brooks (1971)	952	2381	Brooks (1971)	0.35	1.05

[a] Measured using the 220-Hz probe tone and the +200 daPa pressure point to determine the ear-canal volume.

Table II Recommended Admittance and Impedance Norm[a,b]

		Pump speed			
		≤50 daPa/s		200 daPa/s	
		|Y|	|Z|	|Y|	|Z|
Children (3–5 yrs)	Lower limit	0.35	1100	0.40	970
	Median	0.53	1900	0.63	1600
	Upper limit	0.90	2900	1.03	2500
Adults	Lower limit	0.50	570	0.57	500
	Median	0.91	1100	1.08	925
	Upper limit	1.75	2000	2.00	1750

[a] Reprinted with permission from Van Camp, Margolis, Wilson, Creten, and Shanks (1986).
[b] Normative values are presented for a 226-Hz probe frequency for the admittance magnitude |Y| and the impedance magnitude |Z|. Under standard barometric conditions, the admittance magnitude units are equivalent to volume units (cm³) and the impedance units are equivalent to cgs acoustic ohms. The norms for children were obtained from 3- to 6-year-old audiometrically and otoscopically normal children (Koebsell & Margolis, 1986). The adult norms for the slow pump speed (≤ 50 daPa/s) were obtained from adult subjects (mean age = 25.6 years) with a pump speed of 25 daPa/s (Wilson *et al.*, 1984). The fast pump speed values for adults were calculated from the slow speed data, assuming that the effect of pump speed is proportionately the same for children and adults.

the school-age population (between the 10th and 90th percentiles) to be between 0.35 and 1.05 acoustic mmhos and between 952 and 2381 acoustic ohms, respectively, for the 220-Hz probe tone when the ear-canal static-acoustic immittance is calculated at +200 daPa. Similarly, it is reasonable to consider the normal static-acoustic middle-ear admittance and impedance ranges for 80% of the population of older children and adults (between the 10th and 90th percentiles) to be between 0.39 and 1.30 acoustic mmhos and between 769 and 2564 acoustic ohms, respectively, for the 220-Hz probe tone when the ear-canal static-acoustic immittance is calculated at +200 daPa.

It is also reasonable to consider the normal static-acoustic middle-ear admittance and impedance ranges for 90% of the school-age population (between the 5th and 95th percentiles) to be between 0.35 and 0.90 acoustic mmho and between 1100 and 2900 acoustic ohms, respectively, for the 226-Hz probe tone when the ear-canal static-acoustic immittance is calculated at −400 daPa with a low pump speed. Similarly, it is reasonable to consider the normal static-acoustic middle-ear admittance and impedance ranges for 90% of the school-age population to be between 0.40 and 1.03 acoustic mmhos and between 970 and 2500 acoustic ohms, respectively, for the 226-Hz probe tone when the ear-canal static-acoustic immittance is calculated at −400 daPa with a high pump speed.

The normal static-acoustic middle-ear admittance and impedance ranges for 90% of the adult population (between the 5th and 95th percentiles) can be considered, based on Table II, to be between 0.50 and 1.75 acoustic mmhos and between 570 and 2000 acoustic ohms, respectively, when the ear-canal static-acoustic immittance is calculated at −400 daPa with a low pump speed. Similarly, the normal static-acoustic middle-ear admittance and impedance ranges for 90% of the adult population (between the 5th and 95th percentiles) can be considered, based on Table II, to be between 0.57 and 2.00 acoustic mmhos and between 500 and 1750 acoustic ohms, respectively, for the 226-Hz probe tone when the ear-canal static-acoustic immittance is calculated at −400 daPa with a high pump speed.

3. Pathologic Data

a. Ranges for the Various Pathologic Groups

Most studies on the pathologic and normative ranges for the static-acoustic middle-ear admittance and impedance were based on the 220-Hz probe tone, the use of +200 daPa for the determination of the static-acoustic immittance or impedance of the outer ear, and the direct derivation of the admittance vector. Therefore, the following discussion is based on the middle-ear static-acoustic admittance findings with the use of the 220-Hz probe tone and +200 daPa for the determination of the ear-canal volume.

Based on the normative ranges in Table I for the static-acoustic middle-ear admittance and impedance, it would be expected that ears with stiffening pathology such as otosclerosis, congenital ossicular fixation, otitis media, and cholesteatoma would have impedance values above approximately 2600 acoustic ohms and admittance values below 0.35 acoustic mmho. Similarly, it would be expected that ears with loosening pathology such as partial erosion of the ossicular chain and complete ossicular disarticulation would have impedance values below approximately 800 acoustic ohms and admittance values greater than 1.3 acoustic mmhos. Nevertheless, these expectations are not completely fulfilled since many pathologic ears have admittance and impedance values within the normative range, as shown in Table III. Also, there is overlap in the static-acoustic middle-ear immittance values among the various pathologic middle-ear groups.

Approximately 30% of middle ears with otosclerosis have static-acoustic middle-ear immittance values within normal limits (Feldman, 1976; Jerger, 1970). Many ears with ossicular discontinuity have normal static-acoustic middle-ear immittance values (Jerger, 1970). Furthermore, ears with healed tympanic membrane perforation or tympanosclerosis due to aging otherwise normal middle ears lacking air–bone gaps) have abnormal static-acoustic middle-ear immittance values consistent with ossicular discontinuity in the former case and a stiffening pathology in the latter case. Such overlapping among the pathologic ears and between the normal and pathologic ears led Jerger

Table III The 10th and 90th Percentile Values for Y_A and Z_A Acoustic Immittance for Ears with Middle-Ear Pathology[a]

	Z_A (ohms)		Y_A (mmhos)	
	10%	90%	10%	90%
Ossicular discontinuity				
Jerger et al. (1974a)	374	977	0.76	>3.66
Otosclerosis				
Jerger et al. (1974a)	2345	6002	0.10	1.01
Otitis media				
Jerger et al. (1974a)			0.06	0.81
Cholesteatoma				
Jerger et al. (1974a)			0.04	0.44

[a] Measured with the 220-Hz probe tone and pressure point of +200 for determination of the ear-canal volume.

(1970) and Dempsey (1975) to question the clinical value of static-acoustic middle-ear immittance.

The ranges of the static-acoustic middle-ear admittance using the 220-Hz probe tone and −400 daPa for the determination of the ear-canal volume were determined by us for a group of adult ears with otosclerosis and a group of adult ears with ossicular discontinuity. The data are presented in Table IV. The ranges of the static-acoustic middle-ear admittance using the 220-Hz probe tone and +200 daPa for the determination of the ear-canal volume for the same ears are also shown in Table IV for comparative purposes. As can be seen from this table, only 50% of the ears with ossicular discontinuity had static-acoustic middle-ear admittance values (based on −400 daPa) which exceeded the adult normative range reported by Van Camp et al. (1986) in Table II. When the data on the ears with ossicular discontinuity in Table IV were compared with the normative data reported by Jerger et al. (1972) in Table I, 66% had static-acoustic middle-ear admittance values (based on +200 daPa) which exceeded the normative ranges.

As can be seen from Table II, 50% of the ears with otosclerosis in Table IV had static-acoustic middle-ear admittance values (based on −400 daPa) which fell below the adult normative range reported by Van Camp et al. (1986). When the data on the ears with otosclerosis were compared with the normative data reported by Jerger et al. (1972), 70% had static-acoustic middle-ear admittance values below the normative range reported by Jerger et al. (1974a). Furthermore, 30% of the otosclerotic ears in Table IV had static-acoustic middle-ear admittance (calculated using either method) which exceeded the upper limits for normal middle ears as reported by Van Camp et al. (1986) in Table II and Jerger et al. (1972) in Table I. This finding of large static-acoustic middle-ear admittance values in 30% of otosclerotic ears is similar to that expected for ears with ossicu-

Table IV Static-Acoustic Middle-Ear Admittance $(Y_A)^a$

Group	Method based on −400 daPa	Method based on +200 daPa
Ossicular discontinuity		
Case 1	1.7	2.0
Case 2	2.8	2.8
Case 3	3.0	2.5
Case 4	0.9	0.8
Case 5	1.9	1.6
Case 6	1.4	1.0
Ostosclerosis		
Case 1	0.8	0.4
Case 2	2.2	1.9
Case 3	0.4	0.3
Case 4	0.4	0.2
Case 5	0.2	0.2
Case 6	1.9	1.9
Case 7	0.3	0.1
Case 8	2.0	2.6
Case 9	0.2	0.3
Case 10	0.6	0.3

^{a}Based on the 220-Hz probe tone in ears with otosclerosis and ossicular discontinuity calculated with the method involving the use of −400 daPa for determining the ear-canal volume and with the method involving the use of +200 daPa for determining the ear-canal volume.

lar discontinuity. Further research using a large sample size is needed before the two methods for obtaining static-acoustic middle-ear admittance on pathologic ears can be compared. This preliminary analysis shows that either method cannot, by itself, differentiate accurately among the various pathologic groups. As shall be shown later in the chapter, tympanometry can be used in conjunction with static-acoustic middle-ear admittance to help differentiate among the various pathologic groups.

b. Perforated Tympanic Membrane

Although, as stated earlier, a static-acoustic middle-ear admittance value of less than 0.35 acoustic mmho is indicative of a stiffening pathology, this value can also be obtained in ears with a perforated tympanic membrane. That is, static-acoustic ear-canal admittance obtained at +200 daPa (or at −400 daPa) and the static-acoustic total-ear admittance at the tympanometric peak pressure may be the same or nearly so in ears with a perforated tympanic membrane. Thus, the difference between the static-acoustic total-ear admittance and the static-acoustic ear-canal admittance (that is, the static-acoustic middle-ear admittance) will be 0 acoustic mmho or close to 0 acoustic mmho. Small static-acoustic middle-ear admittance values, even as small as 0 acoustic mmho, can also be obtained in ears with a patent or clogged ventilation tube or a probe tip pressing against the canal and in ears with an extremely stiffening

pathology such as advanced otosclerosis, middle-ear effusion, cholesteatoma or other middle-ear tumor, or cerumen occluding the external canal. The presence of cerumen can be ruled out by otoscopic inspection of the ear canal and the possibility of a probe tip pressing against the canal wall can be ruled out by repositioning the probe tip.

At +200 daPa or −400 daPa with the 220-Hz probe tone, the static-acoustic ear-canal admittance (the first measurement taken to obtain the static-acoustic middle-ear admittance) should not exceed 2.5 acoustic mmhos in adults or 2.0 acoustic mmhos in children. If the static-acoustic middle-ear admittance is less than approximately 0.15 acoustic mmho and the static-acoustic ear-canal admittance is greater than 2.5 acoustic mmhos in adults or 2.0 acoustic mmhos in children, the presence of a perforated tympanic membrane or a patent ventilation tube is suspected. (If the static-acoustic middle-ear admittance value is small and there is known to be a ventilation tube in the ear, the ventilation tube is clogged.) A normal static-acoustic middle-ear admittance value with an abnormally large static-acoustic ear-canal admittance value usually reflects the presence of a larger than average ear canal. Our clinical experience suggests, however, that this finding is occasionally obtained in cases with small tympanic membrane perforations.

B. PRESSURE

The measurement of middle-ear pressure represents an important audiologic diagnostic tool for identifying some middle-ear disorders such as Eustachian-tube dysfunction and middle-ear effusion. The measurement of middle-ear pressure is part of tympanometric assessment.

1. BASIC CONCEPTS

The tympanic membrane best transmits sound energy when the air pressure on both sides of the membrane is equal. Under this condition, the tympanic membrane approximates a vertical position (with respect to the ear canal). If there is negative pressure on one side of the membrane, for example, in the middle ear, the tympanic membrane will be sucked in toward the side with the negative pressure, that is, the middle ear. The negative pressure has two results:

1. The tympanic membrane is stretched and is thereby stiffened.
2. The tympanic membrane is bent so energy is not transmitted equally across all parts of the surface.

Recall that acoustic impedance is the reciprocal of air volume under standard conditions for the 220-Hz probe tone. Therefore, the bending of the tympanic membrane inward results in a decrease in the air volume of the site where negative pressure exists. As a consequence of the decreased air volume in the middle ear, the acoustic impedance of the middle ear increases. As a result of the tympanic membrane's increased stiffness and unequal transmission of sound energy across all parts of its surface and the increased impedance of the middle ear, there is rejection of energy transmitted from the side of the positive pressure to the side of the negative pressure. Nevertheless, the capacity of the tympanic membrane to transmit energy can be completely restored if the air pressure on the positive side of the tympanic membrane is decreased until it equals that on the negative side.

The equalization of air pressure across both surfaces of the tympanic membrane is accomplished by air flow through the Eustachian tube into the middle ear in persons with normal middle ears. Whenever there is negative middle-ear pressure (relative to the atmospheric pressure), which results from absorption of the air in the middle-ear cavity by the wall tissues of the middle ear (an on-going process), the air pressure across both surfaces can be equalized by swallowing, which opens the Eustachian tube.

The middle-ear pressure can be grossly estimated by determining the tympanometric peak pressure, that is, the pressure in the external auditory meatus at which the tympanic membrane best transmits energy. The tympanometric peak pressure can be measured using tympanometry. In tympanometry, +200 daPa of air pressure (referenced to atmospheric pressure) is introduced into the outer ear canal. Using a relative acoustic-immittance device in which the volume velocity is kept constant and the sound-pressure level is measured as a function of air pressure in the external auditory meatus, the balance meter is set so the needle is at the rightmost setting (that is, the highest impedance setting in arbitrary units). Using an absolute acoustic-immittance device in which the sound-pressure level is kept constant and the volume velocity is measured as a function of the air pressure in the external auditory meatus, the selection of the +200 daPa pressure automatically yields the maximum absolute impedance value. The air pressure in the external ear canal is then reduced gradually to approximately −200, −300, or −400 daPa. The tympanometric peak pressure can be determined by inspection of the tympanogram. Figure 15 illustrates a tympanogram. The tympanometric peak pressure in this figure, the pressure at which the highest amplitude on the tympanogram is obtained, is −5 daPa. Thus, in Figure 15, the transfer of energy is greatest at the peak-pressure point of −5 daPa. Therefore, at −5 daPa, the air pressure across both surfaces of the tympanic membrane is equal.

2. THE RELATION BETWEEN THE TYMPANOMETRIC PEAK PRESSURE AND THE MIDDLE-EAR PRESSURE

It is often assumed that the tympanometric peak pressure is equivalent to the middle-ear pressure. The results of re-

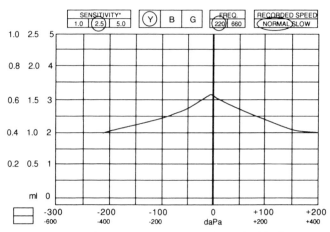

Figure 15 The admittance tympanogram obtained with the 220-Hz probe tone using the GS 1723 otoadmittance meter (absolute admittance device) from a normal middle ear. The tympanometric peak pressure is at −5 daPa.

cent studies, however, indicate that the tympanometric peak pressure can significantly differ from the actual middle-ear pressure (Porter & Winston, 1973; Renvall & Holmquist, 1976; Renvall & Liden, 1978). This disparity between the actual middle-ear pressure and the tympanometric peak pressure is attributed to several factors.

1. The movement of the tympanic membrane from the retracted toward the middle position during the introduction of negative-pressure changes (from a positive to negative direction) results in an artifactual increase in the middle-ear volume and a tympanometric peak pressure which underestimates the actual middle-ear pressure. This effect is very slight in persons with normal middle-ear pressure but can be substantial in persons with negative middle-ear pressure such as children, who commonly have transient negative middle-ear pressure (Renvall & Liden, 1978).

2. The presence of a flaccid tympanic membrane can affect the measurement of the middle-ear pressure by causing the tympanic membrane to be stretched to a degree beyond that seen in nonflaccid tympanic membranes during air-pressure variation in the ear canals, resulting in sizable changes in the middle-ear cavity and a tympanometric peak pressure which deviates even further from the actual middle-ear pressure (Margolis & Shanks, 1985).

3. The presence of a flaccid tympanometric membrane can affect the measurement of the middle-ear pressure in another manner in absolute electroacoustic immittance devices with automatic volume controls which maintain 85 dB SPL in the ear canal during tympanometry. In such devices, when measuring the tympanometric peak

pressure in persons with flaccid tympanic membranes that have a large impedance change at the tympanometric peak pressure, the automatic volume-control circuitry will be unable to track the impedance changes quickly. Therefore, the tympanometric peak pressure will significantly underestimate the middle-ear pressure if the pressure change is from positive to negative and will significantly overestimate the middle-ear pressure if the pressure change is in the negative to positive direction (Margolis & Shanks, 1985).

The aforementioned three factors, which at least partially account for the disparity between the actual middle-ear pressure and the tympanometric peak pressure, can be additive, present individually, or absent in a given person.

When the tympanometric peak pressure is very negative, the pressure-change direction is from positive to negative, and the rate of pressure change is 50 daPa/s (which is the recommended rate for clinical purposes), another tympanometric peak pressure should be obtained using the negative-to-positive pressure-change direction at the same pressure-change rate. The average of the two tympanometric peak pressures represents a better estimate of the middle-ear pressure than either tympanometric peak pressure by itself (Elner, Ingelstedt, & Ivarsson, 1971).

Clinicians are reminded not to equate middle-ear pressure with the tympanometric peak pressure. Nevertheless, the presence of a tympanometric peak pressure around atmospheric pressure (the range to be defined later) should be consistent with normal middle-ear pressure in children and adults. The presence of a significantly negative tympanometric peak pressure is consistent with significantly negative middle-ear pressure in adults but not necessarily in children. A significantly negative tympanometric peak pressure in children should be evaluated cautiously and its clinical significance should be considered in conjunction with other acoustic-immittance factors (to be discussed later).

3. Normal Middle-Ear Pressure

Whereas researchers are in accord regarding the range of tympanometric peak pressures consistent with normal middle-ear pressure in adults, they disagree about the range of tympanometric peak pressures consistent with normal middle-ear pressure in children. For example, Brooks (1980), Holmquist & Miller (1972), Peterson and Liden (1972), and Porter (1974) reported tympanometric peak pressures between -50 and $+50$ daPa in adults with normal middle ears. Holmquist and Miller's (1972) criterion for normal middle ears was based on otomicroscopically-normal tympanic membranes.

The lower limit of the range of tympanometric peak pressures considered to be consistent with normal middle ears in children varies considerably from study to study and

has been reported to be as high as -30 daPa and as low as -170 daPa (Brooks, 1968, 1969; Feldman, 1975; Jerger, 1970; Liden & Renvall, 1978; Renvall, Liden, Jungert, & Nilsson, 1975). Very few of these studies based the criterion of middle-ear normalcy on the presence of normal otoscopic findings. Instead, the majority of these studies employed nonmedical criteria for middle-ear normalcy. For example, Brooks (1968, 1969), who used -170 daPa as the lower limit of the normal range of tympanometric peak pressures, considered middle ears to be normal if the ART did not exceed 95 dB HL at 2000 Hz, bilaterally. Renvall et al. (1975) found that 90% of their sample of school children who were presumed to have normal middle ears had tympanometric peak pressures exceeding -150 daPa. Therefore, they considered -150 DaPa to be the lower limit for normal middle ears. The presence of lower tympanometric peak pressures in children than in adults is attributed to the ability of some children to maintain relatively lower middle-ear pressures than adults (Brooks, 1980).

Figure 16 from Renvall and Liden (1978) shows the tympanometric peak pressures in ears with (16B) and without (16A) surgically confirmed middle-ear effusion (in children). As can be seen from Figure 16B, 18.5% of the ears with middle-ear effusion are missed if -150 or -170 daPa is used as the lower limit of the normal range of tympanometric peak pressures as proposed by Renvall et al.

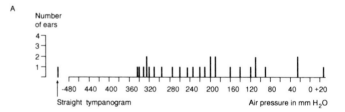

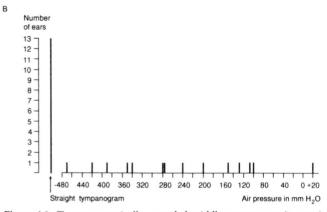

Figure 16 Tympanometrically recorded middle-ear pressure in ears in which myringotomy was performed within one hour of the tympanometric recording. (A) No effusion present at myringotomy. (B) Effusion present at myringotomy. Reprinted with permission from Renvall and Liden (1978).

(1975) and Brooks (1968, 1969). The false-negative rate is reduced from 18.5% to 7.4% (see Figure 16B) but the false-positive rate is increased to 17.8% (see Figure 16A) if −100 daPa is used as the lower limit of the normal range of tympanometric peak pressures as proposed by Jerger (1970). It is clear that screening for the presence of middle-ear effusion based on the tympanometric peak pressure is inefficient in children, resulting in either a high false-positive or false-negative rate depending upon the cutoff tympanometric peak pressure employed.

In children, since there is no cutoff tympanometric peak pressure which yields low false-positive and false-negative rates with respect to middle-ear effusion as illustrated in Figure 16, and since the correlation between otoscopic findings and tympanometric peak pressure is small (as will be discussed later), the presence of a pathologically negative middle-ear pressure cannot be determined solely from the tympanometric peak pressure. As mentioned earlier, the determination of the presence of a pathologically negative middle-ear pressure must be based on additional factors beyond the tympanometric peak pressure. It can be concluded with confidence in adults that the normal range of tympanometric peak pressures consistent with normal middle-ear pressure is between −50 daPa and +50 daPa.

4. ABNORMAL MIDDLE-EAR PRESSURE

A negative tympanometric peak pressure less than −50 daPa in adults is consistent with Eustachian-tube dysfunction by itself or in conjunction with middle-ear effusion. Since a valid normal range for tympanometric peak-pressure points could not be established for children, as discussed in the preceding section, the range of tympanometric peak pressures consistent with Eustachian-tube dysfunction also cannot be established in young children. The lack of relation between the tympanometric peak pressure and middle-ear pathology in young children is illustrated by the following findings in children.

1. There is essentially no relation between the tympanometric peak pressure and the presence or absence of middle-ear effusion (Beery, Bluestone, Andrus, & Cantekin, 1975; Fiellau-Nikolajsen, 1983; Renvall & Liden, 1978; Renvall et al., 1975). This finding is illustrated in Figure 15.
2. There is essentially no relation between the quality of the middle-ear effusion (graded as mucous, sero-mucous, or serous fluid) and the tympanometric peak pressure (Fiellau-Nikolajsen, 1983).
3. There is essentially no relation between the quantity of middle-ear effusion (graded as impaction, moderate, or minimal) and the tympanometric peak pressure Fiellau-Nikolajsen, 1983). Nevertheless, if middle-ear effusion is present with an abnormally negative tympanometric peak pressure, the middle-ear

space is not completely filled with fluid, that is, some air is present in the middle-ear space (Fiellau-Nikolajsen, 1983).
4. There is essentially no relation between the tympanometric peak pressure and the otoscopic findings (Cantekin, Bluestone, Fria, Stool, Beery, & Sabo, 1980; McCandless & Thomas, 1974; Roberts, 1976; Roeser, Soh, Dunckel, & Adams, 1978).

Absence of a peak-pressure point at −200 daPa does not necessarily indicate the absence of a tympanometric peak pressure altogether; a tympanometric peak pressure may be present at more extreme negative pressures (Feldman, 1976; Roeser et al., 1978). Feldman (1976) and Roeser et al. (1978) recommended that the pressure range be extended down to −400 daPa. It is important that the lower limit of the pressure range be extended downward to −400 daPa since the majority of cases with negative tympanometric peak pressures as low as −400 daPa resolve spontaneously (Fiellau-Nikolajsen, 1983; Renvall et al., 1975; Thomsen, Tos, Hancke, & Melchiors, 1982). Tos, Stangerup, Holm-Jensen, & Sorensen (1984) reported that persistent negative tympanometric peak pressures beyond −200 daPa are directly related to irreversible eardrum abnormalities such as attic retractions of varying degrees, atrophy, and/or tympanosclerosis of the pars tensa. These eardrum abnormalities have medical significance since atrophy and retraction of Shrapnell's membrane may lead to attic cholesteatoma and retraction of the pars tensa may lead to sinus or tensa cholesteatoma, adhesive otitis, and perforations of the eardrum. Therefore, the presence of negative middle-ear pressure beyond −200 daPa over an extended period of time should be considered significant, despite the possibility that the tympanometric peak pressure may not reflect the presence of a pathological middle ear.

Audiologists should be aware that the absence of a peak pressure (as well as increased static-acoustic middle-ear impedance) can also occur under the following conditions: (a) impacted external auditory meatus, (b) perforated tympanic membrane, (c) advanced otosclerosis, (d) clogged acoustic-immittance probe assembly, and (e) a large middle-ear tumor.

In the case of an impacted ear canal or perforated tympanic membrane, the sound pressure emitted through the probe assembly will be reflected by the hard wall of wax in the former case and the bony promontory of the cochlea in the latter case. In both cases, the impedance is so high that the pressure change will not be able to move the wax or promontory. The case of the clogged probe assembly is similar to that of the impacted ear canal or perforated tympanic membrane. That is, when the probe assembly is clogged, the sound pressure will be prevented from going into the middle ear so all of the sound will be reflected back into the microphone. Generally, tympanometric peak pressures are absent in ears with perforated tympanic membranes. In our experience, however, tympanometric peak pressures are sometimes observed in ears with perforated tympanic membrane if the perforation or pressure-equalization (p.e.) tube is inferiorly located; in such cases, the presence of perforation or patency of the p.e. tube should be judged on the basis of the physical volume test (ear-canal volume at +200 daPa) (see Section II,A,3,b). In cases of advanced otosclerosis and large middle-ear tumors, the impedance of the middle ear is so high, the pressure change at the tympanic membrane will not be able to elicit any movement of the tympanic membrane.

5. INTERPRETATION OF A POSITIVE PEAK PRESSURE

A positive tympanometric peak pressure refers to peak pressures occurring at greater than +50 daPa. Positive peak pressures can be obtained in patients who just blew their noses, went up quickly in an elevator, or were crying (Harford, 1980). Bluestone, Beery, and Paradise (1973) reported that effusion was usually present in ears with high positive peak pressures exceeding +200 daPa. Feldman (1976) reported that positive tympanometric peak pressures can occur in cases of resolving acute otitis media. In our combined experiences, positive tympanometric peak pressures lack diagnostic significance. Further research is needed to determine whether a positive tympanometric peak pressure has any diagnostic significance.

C. AMPLITUDE AND SHAPE

Earlier in this chapter, it was stated that when absolute acoustic-immittance devices are used, the static acoustic admittance of the middle ear can be obtained by calculating directly from the tympanogram the difference between the number of mmhos at +200 or −400 daPa and the number of mmhos at the peak-pressure point. This difference, which yields the static-acoustic immittance of the middle ear, is also the peak height or amplitude of the tympanogram. Using relative acoustic-immittance devices, however, the static-acoustic admittance of the middle ear cannot be derived directly from the peak amplitude of the tympanogram (height from the point at peak pressure to the baseline). Therefore, amplitude and shape of the tympanogram for relative acoustic-immittance devices will be discussed separately from those for absolute acoustic-immittance devices.

1. RELATIVE ACOUSTIC-IMMITTANCE DEVICES: NORMAL AMPLITUDE AND SHAPE

Alberti and Jerger (1974) described tympanometric peak amplitudes and shapes observed using various probe tones in normal middle ears. Figure 17 illustrates the relations

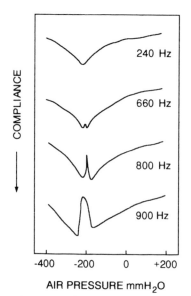

Figure 17 Effect of probe frequency on tympanogram in a patient with a grossly abnormal tympanic membrane. Note that a "W" shape is obvious at 800 and 900 Hz, but only barely discernible at 600 Hz. This tympanogram reflects the Scandinavian rather than American convention of recording since the acoustic-immittance changes are plotted downward rather than upward. Reprinted with permission from Alberti and Jerger (1974).

among peak amplitude, shape, and probe tone in persons with normal middle ears, as reported by Alberti and Jerger (1974) using a relative acoustic-immittance device. This figure shows that, as the probe-tone frequency increases, the amplitude also increases. When the probe-tone frequency approaches 660-Hz, notching of the tympanogram begins to occur. This notching becomes more prevalent as the probe-tone frequency increases beyond 660 Hz up to 900 Hz. Alberti and Jerger (1974) referred to the notching shape as "W-shaped." Figure 17 also shows a tympanogram recorded using the Scandinavian convention, in which increases in admittance are plotted downward rather than upward. (If the American convention of recording tympanograms is employed, the notching no longer appears W-shaped; rather, it appears "M-shaped.") The notching occurs in a small proportion of normal middle ears for probe-tone frequencies below 800 Hz. The majority of normal middle ears have W-shaped tympanograms for probe-tone frequencies above 900 Hz. Liden, Harford, and Hallen (1974) stated that since high-frequency probe tones around 800 Hz were near the resonance frequency of the middle ear and since ear-canal pressure changes cause changes in the resonance characteristics of the middle ear, the W-shaped tympanogram reflects increased interaction among the probe-tone frequency, resonance characteristics of the middle ear, and external ear-canal pressure.

Most clinicians obtain the tympanometric peak amplitude and shape using relative acoustic-immittance devices and the 220-Hz probe tone. The lower normal limit of peak amplitude using relative acoustic-immittance devices varies from one manufacturer to another. Figure 18A shows that, with the American Electromedics 83 impedance meter for example, a normal peak amplitude is defined as one which has a height of 5–10 arbitrary acoustic-immittance units. Figure 18B shows that, with the Madsen Z0-73 impedance meter, a normal peak amplitude is defined as one which has a height of 3–10 arbitrary acoustic-immittance units. Recall that, in relative acoustic-immittance devices, the amplitude at the tympanometric peak pressure is influenced by the ear-canal volume so the height of these tympanograms from relative acoustic-immittance devices must be cautiously interpreted.

2. ABSOLUTE ACOUSTIC-IMMITTANCE DEVICES: NORMAL AMPLITUDE AND SHAPE

Margolis, Van Camp, Wilson, and Creten (1985) described the amplitude and shape of susceptance, conductance, and admittance tympanograms obtained from young adults with normal middle ears using probe-tone frequencies varying between 220 and 910 Hz and an absolute acoustic-immittance device. Figure 19, from Margolis et al. (1985), shows the amplitude and shape of susceptance, conductance, and admittance tympanograms using probe tones which varied in frequency from 220 to 910 Hz using an absolute acoustic-immittance device. As can be seen from this figure, the peak amplitude on the susceptance tympanogram is greater than that on the conductance tympanogram and the peak amplitude on the admittance tympanogram is only slightly greater than that on the susceptance tympanogram for the 220-Hz probe tone. This relation among the peak amplitudes of the admittance, susceptance, and conductance tympanograms occurs since, at 220 Hz, the resistance component of the middle ear is very small so the admittance vector has an angle approaching 90°. Note also from Figure 19, that, as the probe-tone frequency increases (using an absolute acoustic-immittance device), normal middle-ears start to demonstrate notching in the susceptance, conductance, and admittance tympanograms obtained with absolute acoustic-immittance devices similar to the notching described by Alberti and Jerger (1974) using relative acoustic-immittance devices.

When the direction of pressure change is from positive to negative (+/−), the tympanometric pattern changes from the 1B–1G pattern (one peak on the susceptance tympanogram and one peak on the conductance tympanogram) to the 3B–1G pattern (3 peaks on the susceptance tympanogram and one peak on the conductance tympanogram) as the probe-tone frequency increases from 220 to 910 Hz. When the direction of the pressure change is in the negative to positive direction (−/+), the change in the tympanometric pattern from 1B–1G to 3B–3G occurs at a lower frequency, that is, 510 Hz; at 710 Hz, the 3B–3G

pattern develops, and above 710 Hz, the 5B-3G pattern occurs. Margolis et al. (1985) also reported that the susceptance and conductance tympanograms from most, but not all, of their 10 subjects with normal middle ears progressed through 1B–1G to 3B–1G to 3B–3G to 5B–3G as the probe-tone frequency increased.

Regardless of the direction of pressure change, the admittance tympanometric pattern changes from 1Y (one peak on the admittance tympanogram) at 220 Hz to 3Y at 610 Hz when the pressure-change direction is −/+ and at 810 Hz when the pressure-change direction is +/−.

Margolis et al. (1985) attributed the changes in the susceptance and conductance tympanometric patterns with probe-frequency changes to the shift in acoustic reactance from large negative values to small positive values as shown in Figure 12. These changes in the admittance, susceptance, and conductance tympanometric patterns as a function of probe-tone frequency were predicted by the model developed by Vanhuyse, Creten, and Van Camp (1975) and later described mathematically by Van Camp, Vanhuyse, Creten, and Vanpeperstraete (1978). The theoretical basis for these changes was given by Vanhuyse et al. (1975), Margolis (1978), and Shanks (1984).

According to Vanhuyse et al. (1975), Margolis (1978), and Shanks (1984), the 1B–1G tympanometric pattern with a single susceptance maximum and a single conductance maximum is obtained when the middle ear is a stiffness-dominated system and when the resistance of the middle ear is less than the absolute value of the stiffness reactance of the middle ear at all pressures. This tympanometric pattern is illustrated in Figure 20A.

In the 3B–1G tympanometric pattern, the maximum on the G tympanogram (which lies above the baseline) falls between the two maxima on the B tympanogram (which also lies above the baseline). The 3B–1G tympanometric pattern is illustrated in Figure 20B. According to Vanhuyse et al. (1975), Margolis (1978), and Shanks (1984), this tympanometric pattern is obtained when the resistance of the middle ear is larger than the absolute value of the stiffness reactance around 0 daPa and when the resistance of the middle ear is smaller than the absolute value of the stiffness reactance at the pressure extremes. The B minimum sits above the baseline (positive location), indicating that the middle ear is stiffness controlled.

In the 3B–3G pattern, there is a maximum on each side of the central minimum in both the conductance and susceptance tympanograms. The pressure interval between the conductance maxima is smaller than that between the susceptance maxima. The central minimum for susceptance occurs at nearly the same pressure as that for conductance. The 3B–3G pattern is illustrated in Figure 20C. According to Vanhuyse et al. (1975), Margolis (1978), and Shanks (1984), the 3B–3G tympanometric pattern occurs when the middle ear is mass controlled around 0 daPa but is stiffness

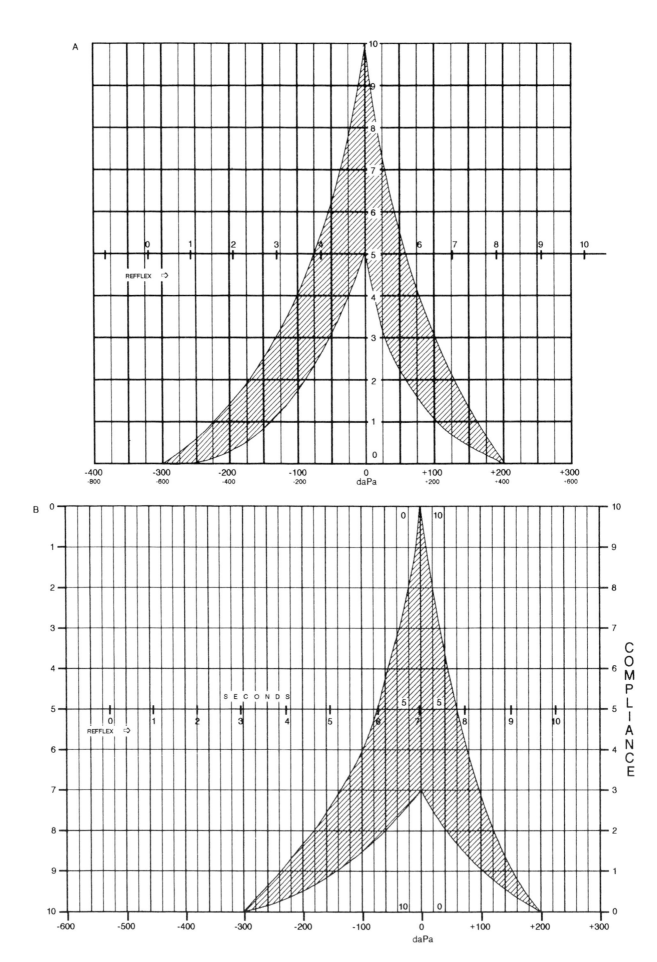

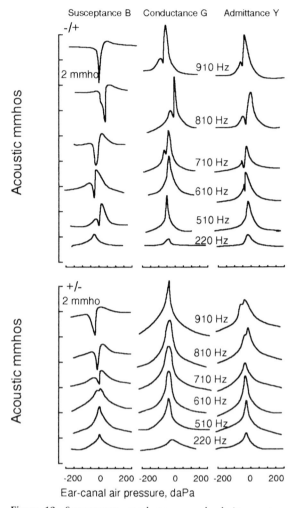

Figure 19 Susceptance, conductance, and admittance tympanograms from one normal subject at six probe frequencies and two pressure directions (negative to positive: −/+; positive to negative: +/−). Reprinted with permission from Margolis, Van Camp, Wilson, and Creten (1985).

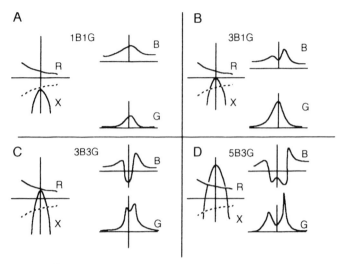

Figure 20 Four normal high-frequency tympanometric patterns modeled in acoustic impedance [resistance (R) and reactance (X)] and acoustic admittance [conductance (G) and susceptance (B)]. After Vanhuyse, Creten, and Van Camp (1975). Reprinted with permission from Shanks (1984).

reactance is larger than that for the middle-ear resistance at the pressure extremes.

Van Camp, Creten, Van de Heyning, Decraemer, and Vanpeperstraete (1983) reported the percentage occurrences of the four tympanometric patterns (1B–1G, 3B–1G, 3B–3G, 5B–3G) for a group of 132 normal middle ears using the 660-Hz probe tone. Of the sample, 56.8% displayed the 1B–1G pattern, 28.0% displayed the 3B–1G pattern, 6.1% displayed the 3B–3G pattern, and 9.1% displayed the 5B–3G pattern.

Wiley, Oviatt, and Block (1987) obtained similar findings to those reported by Van Camp et al. (1983). Wiley et al. (1983) reported that 75.8% of their group of 132 normal middle ears had the 1B–1G tympanometric pattern for the 660-Hz probe tone, 17.4% had the 3B–1G tympanometric pattern, 5.5% had the 3B–3G tympanometric pattern, and 1.2% had the 5B–3G tympanometric pattern.

Several investigators (Creten, Van Camp, Maes, & Vanpeperstraete, 1981; Van Camp et al., 1978, 1983; Van de Heyning, Van Camp, Creten, & Vanpeperstraete, 1982) described another characteristic feature of the 3B–3G and 5B–3G tympanograms at 660 Hz, relating to the pressure. The pressure difference between the first and last susceptance maxima is less than 75 daPa for the 3B–3G tympanograms and less than 100 daPa for the 5B–3G tympanograms.

controlled at the pressure extremes. At 0 daPa, the absolute value of the middle-ear resistance is larger than that of the mass reactance; at the pressure extremes, the absolute value of the stiffness reactance is larger than that of the middle-ear resistance.

The 5B–3G pattern is shown in Figure 20D. According to Vanhuyse et al. (1975), Margolis (1978), and Shanks (1984), the 5B–3G pattern occurs when the middle ear is mass dominated around 0 daPa but stiffness controlled at the pressure extremes. The mass reactance is larger than the resistance at 0 daPa; the absolute value of the stiffness

Figure 18 (A) Tympanogram form for American Electromedics impedance meter (relative immittance device). Reprinted with permission of American Electromedics Corp. (B) Tympanogram form for the Madsen

Electronics impedance meter (relative immittance device). Reprinted with permission of Madsen North America, Inc.

In summary, when low probe-tone frequencies are employed during tympanometry, the tympanometric amplitude but not shape is the salient feature, regardless of whether relative or absolute acoustic-immittance devices are used. In such cases, the peak amplitude is considered normal with relative acoustic-immittance devices when it has a height within normal limits (as specified by the manufacturer of the device); the peak amplitude is considered normal with absolute acoustic-immittance devices when the static acoustic immittance of the middle ear is within normal limits. When high probe-tone frequencies are employed during tympanometry, the shape but not the amplitude of the tympanogram is the salient feature, regardless of whether relative or absolute acoustic-immittance devices are employed. When absolute acoustic-immittance devices are employed with high-frequency probe tones, the shape of the admittance, susceptance, and conductance tympanograms should be described. Most relative acoustic-immittance devices do not enable measurement of the susceptance and conductance tympanograms as well as the admittance tympanogram. Therefore, when high-frequency probe tones from relative acoustic-immittance devices are used, only the shape and not the peak amplitude, should be interpreted.

> In the Vanhuyse *et al.* (1975) classification system, a normally notched tympanogram must meet the following criteria: (1) the number of extrema must not exceed five for the susceptance (B) and three for the conductance (G) tympanograms, (2) the distance (in decapascal) between the outermost conductance maxima must be smaller than the distance between the susceptance maxima, and (3) the distance between the outermost maxima must not exceed 75 daPa for tympanograms with three extrema (e.g., 3B3G), and must not exceed 100 daPa for tympanograms with five extrema (e.g., 5B3G). (Shanks, 1984, p. 274)

Margolis *et al.* (1985) and Shanks and Wilson (1986) reported that notching of tympanograms occurs more frequently and is more complex when the pressure-change direction is from negative to positive than from positive to negative when high-frequency probe tones are employed. Therefore, the criteria for normalcy developed by Vanhuyse *et al.* (1975) and described by Shanks (1984) apply only when the pressure-change direction is from positive to negative. According to Shanks and Wilson (1986), the rate of ear-canal pressure change has only a small effect on the tympanometric data at 226 and 678 Hz. They concluded that the most efficient clinical procedure involved the use of the pressure-change rate of 50.0 daPa/sec.

3. GRADIENT

Figure 21 shows the parameters of a tympanometric gradient.

The tympanometric gradient is defined as the ratio of *hp* to *ht*, where *hp* is the distance from the tympanometric peak to the horizontal line intersecting the tympanogram such that the distance between the points of intersection (*a* and *b*) is 100 daPa, and *ht* is the peak height of the tympanogram (see Figure 21). The smaller the gradient, the flatter the tympanogram, since the magnitude of the gradient is inversely related to the degree of flatness of the tympanogram. According to Brooks (1969) and Paradise, Smith, and Bluestone (1976), a gradient is small if it is less than or equal to 0.15. According to Fiellau-Nikolajsen (1983), a gradient is small if it is less than or equal to 0.1. Small gradients occur when the middle-ear space is completely or nearly completely filled with middle-ear effusion, in children as well as in adults.

Most of the studies on the tympanometric gradient have employed relative electroacoustic-immittance devices. The validity of using relative electroacoustic-immittance devices was challenged by Margolis and Shanks (1985). Margolis and Shanks (1985) stated that "the mean gradient value, calculated on undefined units, is not a meaningful expression of central tendency" (p. 470). They recommended the use of absolute electroacoustic-immittance devices for the measurement of tympanometric gradient. On the other hand, Fiellau-Nikolajsen (1983) contended that it is of little significance whether relative or absolute electroacoustic-immittance devices are employed, despite the fact that the type of device affects the tympanometric shape, since the gradient is a ratio. According to Fiellau-Nikolajsen (1983), who employed a relative electroacoustic-immittance device on 44 three-year-old children with bilateral myringotomies, a small gradient has a false-negative rate of 17% and a false-positive rate of 0% with respect to the presence of middle-ear effusion.

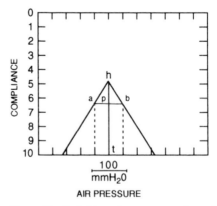

Figure 21 Definition of tympanometric gradient. Gradient is defined as the ratio *hp/ht* where *ht* equals the overall height of the tympanogram, and *hp* equals the vertical distance from the peak of the tympanogram to a horizontal line intersecting the tympanogram so that its width between the points of intersection (*a,b*) is 100 mm H₂O. The higher the ratio *hp/ht*, the steeper the gradient. Adapted from Brooks (1969). Reprinted with permission from Paradise, Smith, and Bluestone (1976).

Margolis and Heller (1987) and the American Speech–Language–Hearing Association (1989) suggested the measurement of the tympanometric gradient by calculating the pressure interval corresponding to 50% reduction in the static acoustic middle-ear admittance. For the measurement of static acoustic outer-ear admittance, +200 daPa was recommended by the American Speech–Language–Hearing Association (1989) and Margolis and Heller (1987). The American Speech–Language–Hearing Association (1989) and Margolis and Heller (1987) recommended the use of an absolute acoustic-immittance device for the measurement of tympanometric gradient.

The American Speech–Language–Hearing Association (1989) stated that the use of the 50% reduction in the static acoustic middle-ear admittance to define the tympanometric gradient was superior to other measures of tympanometric gradient because of "(a) normative distribution width in relation to the range of possible values, (b) invariance with pump speed, and (c) low correlation with (and, therefore, supplemental to) static admittance" (p. 73). Little clinical data were available until recently (Silman & Silverman, 1990) to support the use of the tympanometric gradient as defined by the American Speech–Language–Hearing Association (1989).

According to the American Speech–Language–Hearing Association (1989), the 90% ranges for tympanometric width (gradient) of normal persons are 60–150 daPa in children and 50–110 daPa in adults (regardless of pump speed). If the tympanometric gradient has a pressure interval wider than these values, middle-ear effusion is suspected.

In conclusion, negative tympanometric peak pressure, small static-acoustic middle-ear admittance, flat tympanogram, and the small tympanometric gradient, singly, do not have low false-negative and false-positive rates with respect to detection of middle-ear effusion. As will be discussed later, false-positive and false-negative rates are substantially reduced when all of the acoustic-immittance findings including the acoustic-reflex results are integrated.

4. Pathologic Ears

Figure 22 illustrates the various admittance tympanometric patterns observed in normal and pathologic ears when relative acoustic-immittance devices are employed with the 220-Hz probe tone. Figure 23 illustrates the various admittance tympanometric patterns observed in normal and pathologic ears using absolute acoustic-immittance devices with the 220-Hz probe tone. Several investigators observed these patterns (Beery, Andrus, Bluestone, & Cantekin, 1973; Bluestone, Beery, & Paradise, 1973; Feldman, 1976; Jerger, 1970; Jerger, Jerger, & Mauldin, 1972; Jerger, Anthony, Jerger, & Mauldin, 1974a; Jerger S., Jerger, Mauldin, & Segal, 1974). Table V shows the middle-ear conditions associated with

the admittance tympanometric patterns shown in Figures 22 and 23. This table can be applied to the general population since the clinical data on which the table is based are from the general population. As can be seen from Figures 22 and 23 and Table V, there is no one-to-one relation between the middle-ear condition and the tympanometric pattern for the 220-Hz probe tone. For example, the tympanometric pattern labeled "1" is associated with normal middle ears, otosclerosis, and ossicular discontinuity.

The findings of recent studies show that the lack of a one-to-one correspondence between the tympanometric pattern and the middle-ear condition can be resolved at least partially with the use of high-frequency probe tones for tympanometry (Alberti & Jerger, 1974; Beery et al., 1975; Colletti, 1975a, 1977; Margolis & Popelka, 1977; Margolis, Osguthorpe, & Popelka, 1978; Van Camp et al., 1983; Van de Heyning et al., 1982). The best probe-tone frequency for detecting a mass-loaded middle ear in an adult, as is found, for example, in ears with ossicular discontinuity, is around 660 Hz (Van Camp et al., 1983; Van Camp et al., 1986; Van de Heyning et al., 1982). Recall from Section I,C that the probe-tone frequency of 660 Hz is close to the resonant frequency of the human middle ear (approximately 800 to 1200 Hz). Thus, it will be sensitive to changes in the mass component of acoustic middle-ear impedance.

The tympanometric patterns that are consistent with the presence of ossicular discontinuity are (a) tympanograms containing more peaks than those specified by Vanhuyse et al. (1975) (see Section II,C.), (b) a distance between the outermost maxima exceeding 75 daPa in tympanograms with 3 extrema, (c) a distance between the outermost maxima exceeding 100 daPa in tympanograms with 5 extrema, and (d) a distance between the conductance outermost maxima which is larger than that between the susceptance outermost maxima. This association between the presence of ossicular discontinuity and tympanometric pattern for the 660-Hz probe tone has been confirmed by several experimental and clinical investigations (Margolis & Popelka, 1977; Van Camp, Creten, Vanpeperstraete, & Van de Heyning, 1980; Van de Heyning et al., 1982). Although it is recommended that the conductance and susceptance tympanograms at 660 Hz be recorded simultaneously, our clinical experience shows that separate recordings of susceptance and conductance tympanograms have high diagnostic value. Nevertheless, simultaneous recordings are preferred if the equipment allows.

Figure 24 shows the tympanometric susceptance and conductance patterns obtained using the 220-Hz and 660-Hz probe tones from a normal middle ear in a cadaver, prestapedectomy and poststapedectomy. The stapedectomy resulted in a mass-loaded ear since the stapes was removed without any prosthetic replacement. Note that the susceptance and conductance tympanograms obtained with the

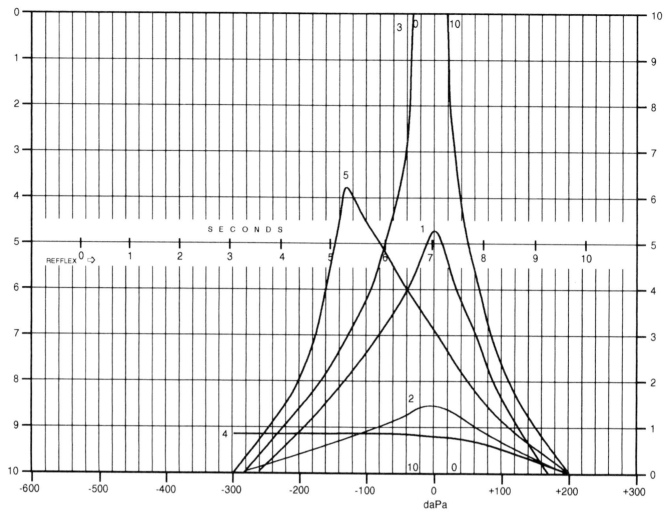

Figure 22 The various admittance tympanometric patterns observed in normal and pathologic ears when a relative acoustic-immittance device is employed with the 220-Hz probe tone.

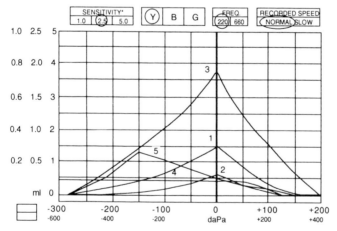

Figure 23 The various admittance tympanometric patterns observed in normal and pathologic ears when an absolute acoustic-immittance device is employed with the 220-Hz probe tone.

220-Hz probe tone prestapedectomy are similar to those obtained with the 220-Hz probe tone poststapedectomy. For the 660-Hz probe tone, the susceptance and conductance prestapedectomy tympanograms differed from the susceptance and conductance poststapedectomy tympanograms. That is, the prestapedectomy pattern at 660-Hz fit the 3B–3G pattern consistent with normal middle ears but the poststapedectomy tympanogram had more than 5 peaks for the susceptance and more than 3 peaks for the conductance, consistent with the presence of ossicular discontinuity.

Figure 25 shows the susceptance tympanograms obtained with the 660-Hz probe tone from a middle ear with myringostapediopexia and necrosis of the lenticular process of the incus that produced ossicular discontinuity. As can be seen in this figure, there are more than 5 susceptance peaks and more than 3 conductance peaks, consistent with the

Table V Description of Five Tympanometric Patterns with Respect to Amplitude and the Most Common Middle-Ear Conditions Associated with These Patterns

Tympanogram type	Peak amplitude[a]	Amplitude[b] (mmho)	Commonly occurring middle-ear conditions
#1	3–10 units	0.35–1.30	Normal middle ears Ossicular fixation Some cases of ossicular discontinuity
#2	<3 units	<0.35	Ossicular fixation Some cases of external otitis Tympanosclerosis
#3	Right and left slopes do not meet	>1.30	Ossicular fixation with flaccid tympanic membrane Ossicular discontinuity Normal middle ear with a flaccid tympanic membrane
#4	Absence of peak-pressure point	Absence of peak-pressure point	Middle-ear effusion Extreme cases of ossicular fixation Some large middle-ear tumors Impacted cerumen Perforated tympanic membrane
#5	3–10 units	0.35–1.30	Eustachian-tube dysfunction with or without ossicular fixation Eustachian-tube dysfunction with or without ossicular discontinuity

[a] Relative acoustic-immittance device (Madsen); for other relative acoustic-immittance devices, see manufacturer's specifications.
[b] Absolute acoustic-immittance device in which amplitude is the middle-ear admittance and the outer-ear static-acoustic admittance is calculated at +200 daPa.

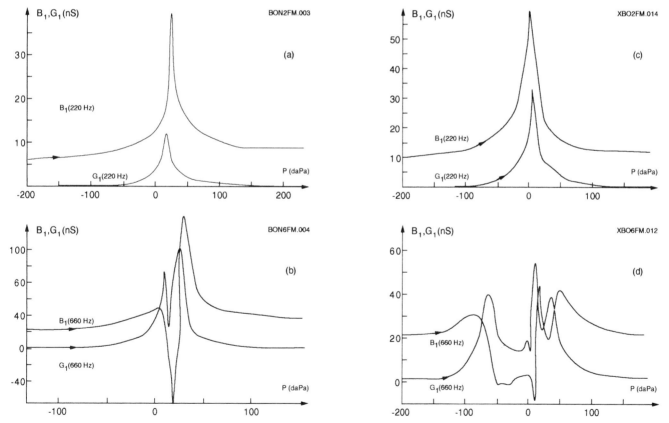

Figure 24 Comparison of simultaneously recorded tympanograms of the susceptance and conductance at the tip of the probe on an intact temporal bone (a,b) versus the same recordings on the same temporal bone after stapedectomy (c,d). Note: 1 daPa = 1 mm H_2O. Rate of pressure change: +28 daPa/s. Reprinted with permission from Van de Heyning, Van Camp, Creten, and Vanpeperstraete (1982).

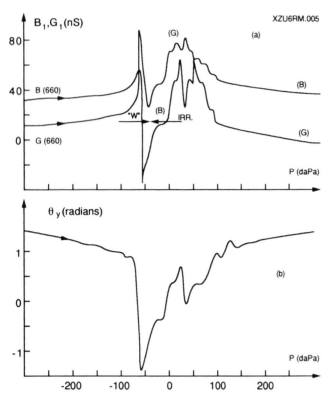

Figure 25 Tympanograms of the susceptance B1 and the conductance G1 at the tip of the probe and of the phase angle θ y at the drum, obtained with a 660-Hz probe from a subject with myringostapediopexia and necrosis of lenticular process of the incus. (Note: rate of pressure change = +28 daPa/s.) The pressure interval marked "W" contains only the peaks due to a regular W-shaped pattern as can be deduced from the phase angle tympanogram. Reprinted with permission from Van de Heyning, Van Camp, Creten, and Vanpeperstraete (1982).

presence of ossicular discontinuity (or a condition similar to ossicular discontinuity).

As mentioned earlier, not only an excessive number of peaks but also an excessive distance between the outermost peaks of the susceptance or conductance is indicative of ossicular discontinuity. For example, Figure 26 shows the susceptance and conductance tympanograms obtained at 660 Hz for a normal middle ear having a normal tympanic membrane, a normal middle ear with a scarred tympanic membrane, and an ear with suspected ossicular discontinuity. Although the tympanometric pattern is W-shaped in all three cases, only the case with ossicular discontinuity has a distance between the outermost susceptance and conductance peaks that exceeds 75 daPa. Margolis and Shanks (1985) obtained similar findings for their case with ossicular discontinuity.

Thus, tympanograms obtained using high-frequency probe tones are useful for identifying ears with mass-loaded systems related to the presence of ossicular discontinuity. Some of the overlap among the tympanometric patterns (e.g., tympanogram for an otosclerotic ear with healed

tympanic-membrane perforation or flaccid tympanic membrane and that for an ear with a normal tympanic membrane and ossicular discontinuity) for the 220-Hz probe tone as shown in Figures 22 and 23 and Table V can be resolved by using high-frequency probe tones which are sensitive to the presence of ossicular discontinuity. Recall that tympanogram 1 in Figures 22 and 23 can be associated with ossicular discontinuity, normal middle ears, and otosclerosis. Also recall that the range of static-acoustic middle-ear admittance values in ears with ossicular discontinuity is between 0.76 and >3.66 acoustic mmhos. This range partially overlaps with those for normal middle ears and ears with otosclerosis. Thus, a tympanogram observed in normal middle ears can be found also in ears with otosclerosis or ossicular discontinuity. If tympanogram 1 is present without an air–bone gap, it can be assumed that the tympanogram represents a normal middle ear. If there is a significant air–bone gap, then it is desirable to obtain the susceptance and conductance tympanograms at 660 Hz. If there is an excessive number of peaks or an excessive distance between the outermost susceptance or conductance peaks, the results are consistent with the presence of ossicular discontinuity; otherwise, the results are consistent with the presence of otosclerosis.

The use of the 660-Hz probe tone can resolve other overlapping tympanometric patterns at 220 Hz. For example, tympanometric pattern 3 shown in Figures 22 and 23 can be obtained in ears with otosclerosis with a flaccid tympanic membrane (atrophic tympanic membrane or healed tympanic-membrane perforation), ears with ossicular discontinuity, or normal middle ears with flaccid tympanic membranes. Tympanometric pattern 3 obtained using an absolute acoustic-immittance device and the 220-Hz probe tone is distinguished from tympanometric pattern 1 on the basis of the static-acoustic middle-ear admittance value. Therefore, if the tympanometric peak pressure is within normal limits but the static-acoustic middle-ear admittance exceeds the range for normal middle ears, the tympanogram is classified as a type 3 pattern. If the tympanometric peak pressure and the static-acoustic middle-ear admittance value are within normal limits, the tympanogram is classified as a type 1 pattern. If there is no significant air–bone gap, the type 3 pattern reflects a normal middle ear with a flaccid tympanic membrane or healed tympanic-membrane perforation.

For the type 3 tympanometric pattern with air-bone gaps, differentiation between an ear with otosclerosis and a flaccid tympanic membrane and an ear with ossicular discontinuity can be made only on the basis of the tympanogram obtained with the 660-Hz probe tone. The ear with ossicular discontinuity will have a 660-Hz tympanogram that shows an excessive number of peaks or an excessive distance between the outermost susceptance or conductance peaks. The ear with otosclerosis and a flaccid tympanic

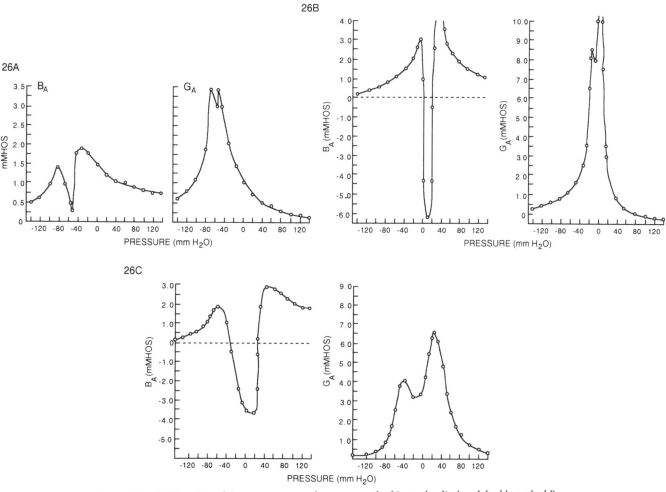

Figure 26 (A) Mean B_A and G_A tympanograms for two normal subjects who displayed double-peaked B_A and G_A tympanograms. The probe frequency is 660 Hz. (B) B_A and G_A tympanograms for one subject who had a large atrophic scar on the tympanic membrane. The probe frequency is 660 Hz. (C) B_A and G_A tympanograms for one subject with a suspected congenital ossicular discontinuity. The probe frequency is 660 Hz. Reprinted with permission from Margolis and Popelka (1977).

membrane or healed tympanic-membrane perforation will yield one of the normal 660-Hz tympanometric patterns as defined by Shanks (1984).

Figure 27 shows the tympanograms obtained with the 220-Hz probe tone and an absolute acoustic-immittance device from an ear with confirmed otosclerosis and an abnormally high static acoustic middle-ear admittance related to a flaccid tympanic membrane and from an ear with confirmed ossicular discontinuity. Type 3 tympanometric patterns were obtained for both ears. When the susceptance and conductance tympanograms were obtained using the 660-Hz probe tone and an absolute acoustic-immittance device, different tympanometric patterns were obtained for the two ears. Figure 28 shows the 660-Hz tympanometric patterns for the two ears. As can be seen in Figure 28, an excessive number of peaks were obtained in the susceptance tympanogram (Figure 28A) and conductance tympanogram (Figure 28B) in the ear with ossicular discontinuity.

Inspection of Figure 28 also reveals that the normal 3B–3G pattern (Figure 28C and D) was obtained in the ear with otosclerosis and a flaccid tympanic membrane.

Feldman (1976) reported that in cases of combined eardrum pathology and other middle-ear pathologies, the tympanometric pattern will reflect the most lateral pathology. For example, ears with multiple middle-ear pathologies such as an ear with a healed tympanic-membrane perforation and otosclerosis will yield the type 3 tympanometric pattern with the 220-Hz probe tone, reflecting the presence of a healed perforation rather than the otosclerosis. Feldman's finding applies in cases in which the medial pathology is a stiffening one, such as otosclerosis, but not in cases in which the medial pathology is a loosening one, such as ossicular discontinuity. The following case illustrates this point. A 60-year-old female was seen for a complete audiologic evaluation following stapes surgery. Figure 29 shows the admittance tympanograms (220-Hz and 660-Hz probe

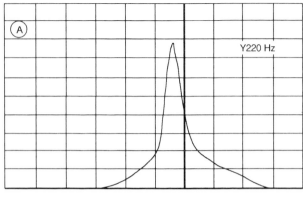

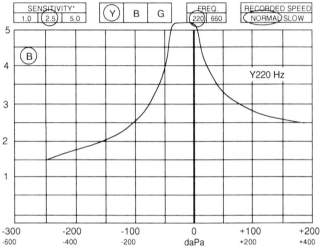

Figure 27 Tympanograms obtained using an absolute acoustic-immittance device with the 220-Hz probe tone. (A) Admittance tympanogram from an ear with otosclerosis and a flaccid tympanic membrane or healed perforation of the tympanic membrane. (B) Admittance tympanogram from an ear with confirmed ossicular discontinuity.

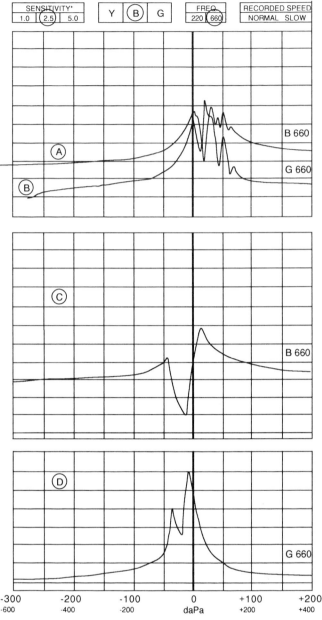

Figure 28 Tympanograms obtained using an absolute acoustic-immittance device with the 660-Hz probe tone. (A) The susceptance tympanogram from the ear with ossicular discontinuity. (B) The conductance tympanogram from the ear with ossicular discontinuity. (C) The susceptance tympanogram from the ear with otosclerosis and a flaccid tympanic membrane or healed perforation of the tympanic membrane. (D) The conductance tympanogram from the ear with otosclerosis and a flaccid tympanic membrane or healed perforation of the tympanic membrane.

tones) and audiogram for this case. Figures 29A, B, and C show the 220-Hz admittance tympanogram, the 660-Hz susceptance tympanogram, and the 660-Hz conductance tympanogram, respectively, for the left ear, obtained with an absolute acoustic-immittance device. Figure 29A reveals the type 3 tympanometric pattern, consistent with the presence of a flaccid tympanic membrane or healed tympanic-membrane perforation. Figures 29B and C reveal the 3B–3G tympanometric pattern, consistent with the presence of a normal middle ear. Figure 29D reveals that significant air–bone gaps were absent in the left ear. Thus, the findings are consistent with a normal left middle ear having a healed tympanic-membrane perforation. The healed tympanic-membrane perforation probably was related to the ear surgery. Two years later, the patient reported a sudden decrease in the hearing sensitivity of the operated ear. Figure 30 shows the audiogram and 660-Hz

conductance and susceptance tympanograms (obtained with an absolute acoustic-immittance device). Figures 30A, B, and C show the left-ear 660-Hz susceptance tympanogram, the left-ear 660-Hz conductance tympanogram, and the audiogram, respectively. Figure 30B shows an excessive

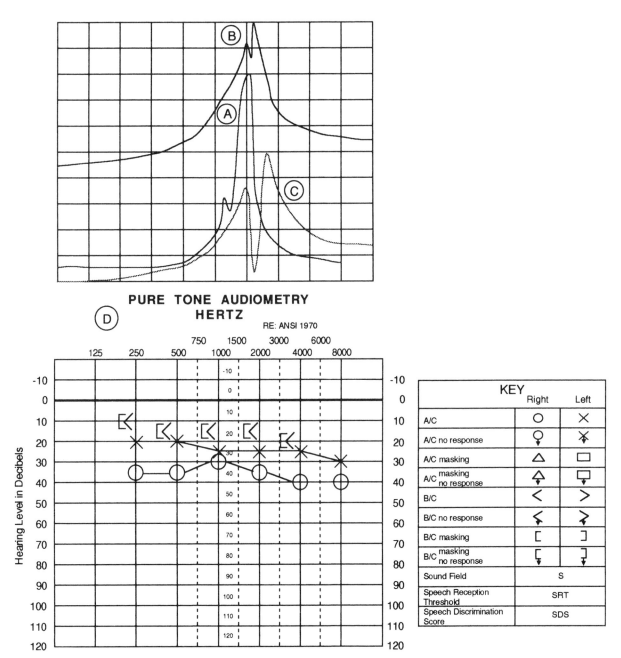

Figure 29 The poststapedectomy tympanograms obtained using an absolute acoustic-immittance device
for the left ear of a patient and audiogram. (A) Admittance tympanogram for the 220-Hz probe tone.
(B) Susceptance tympanogram obtained with the 660-Hz probe tone. (C) Conductance tympanogram for
the 660-Hz probe tone. (D) Post-stapedectomy audiogram (left ear operated on).

number of conductance peaks and Figure 30A shows a
distance between the outermost extreme greater than
100 daPa consistent with the presence of ossicular discontinuity. Figure 30C reveals significant left-ear air–bone gaps
which were greatest at the high frequencies, as expected in
cases of ossicular discontinuity. Surgery revealed the
presence of a dislocated stapes prosthesis in the left ear.

The following example further illustrates the clinical utility of tympanometry using high- as well as low-frequency
probe tones. A 24-year-old male who sustained a concussion (2 years prior to the audiologic evaluation) had a
profound sensorineural or mixed hearing impairment in the
right ear (the bone-conduction thresholds exceeded the limits of the audiometer). Figure 31 shows the results of audiologic assessment for this case. The findings based on just
the presence of the type 3 tympanometric pattern for the

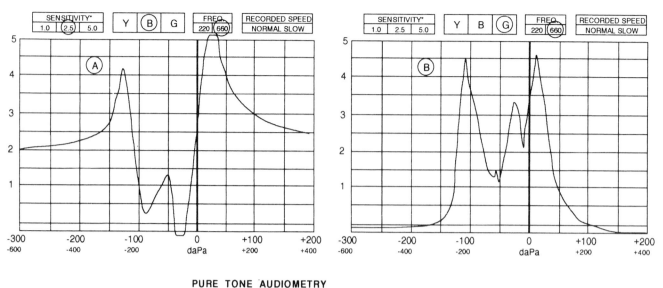

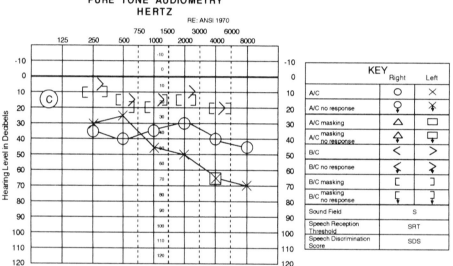

Figure 30 The tympanograms obtained from an absolute acoustic-immittance device with the 660-Hz probe tone and audiogram for subject in Figure 29, two years after the stapedectomy following a complaint of sudden hearing loss in the left ear. (A) The left-ear susceptance tympanogram. This susceptance tympanogram is abnormal since the outermost extrema are separated by more than 100 daPa. (B) The left-ear conductance tympanogram. This conductance tympanogram is abnormal since there are more than three extrema. (C) Audiogram. Note that the left ear, which previously was essentially normal hearing, has developed a conductive hearing loss.

220-Hz probe tone and the audiogram could lead an audiologist to conclude that the patient demonstrated a profound sensorineural hearing impairment and a flaccid tympanic membrane or healed tympanic-membrane perforation. This conclusion is erroneous. The 660-Hz tympanograms revealed an excessive number of conductance peaks, consistent with ossicular discontinuity (suggesting that the audiogram represented a mixed hearing impairment with unseen air–bone gaps beyond the audiometric limits related to the ossicular discontinuity, rather than sensorineural hearing impairment). Exploratory surgery confirmed the presence

of ossicular discontinuity. Figure 32 shows the postoperative audiometric findings. Inspection of Figure 32 reveals an improvement in the air-conduction thresholds of at least 20–30 dB. As a result of the tympanoplasty, some hearing was restored to the patient.

The presence of the type 2 tympanometric pattern (shown in Figures 22 and 23 for the 220-Hz probe tone) is consistent with the presence of ossicular fixation, including otosclerosis, some cases of external otitis, or sclerotic scarring of the tympanic membrane with hyalination from recurrent otitis media or the aging process (tympanosclero-

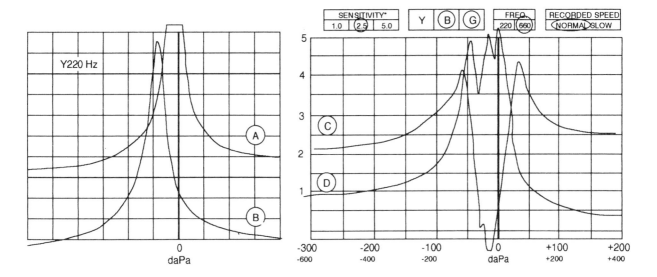

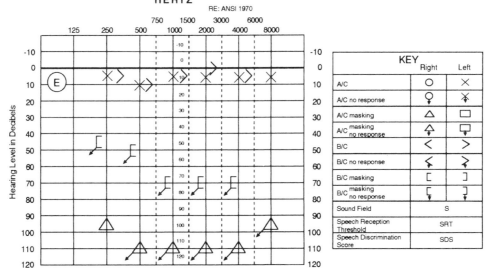

Figure 31 The tympanograms obtained with an absolute acoustic-immittance device for the right ear and an audiogram for a patient who sustained a concussion. (A) The admittance tympanogram obtained with a 220-Hz probe tone when the outer ear is included in the measurement. High static-acoustic admittance of the middle ear is seen in this tympanogram. (B) The admittance tympanogram obtained with a 220-Hz probe tone when the outer ear is excluded from the measurement. High static-acoustic admittance of the middle ear is seen in this tympanogram. (C) The susceptance tympanogram obtained with the 660-Hz probe tone. This susceptance tympanogram is a normal 5-B pattern. (D) The conductance tympanogram obtained with the 660-Hz probe tone. This conductance tympanogram is abnormal since it has more than 3 extrema. (E) The audiogram. Note that there is a profound hearing impairment in the right ear.

sis). When an absolute acoustic-immittance device is employed, the type 2 tympanogram can be distinguished from the type 1 tympanogram only on the basis of the static-acoustic middle-ear admittance. That is, if the tympanometric peak pressure and the static-acoustic middle-ear admittance are within normal limits, the tympanogram is the type 1 pattern. On the other hand, if the tympanometric peak pressure is within normal limits but the

static-acoustic middle-ear admittance is below the range for normal middle ears, the tympanogram is the type 2 pattern. Ossicular fixation can be differentiated from the other pathologies associated with the type 2 tympanometric pattern on the basis of the presence of air–bone gaps and a tympanic membrane which appears normal otoscopically.

The presence of the type 4 tympanometric pattern for the 220-Hz probe tone is consistent with the presence of

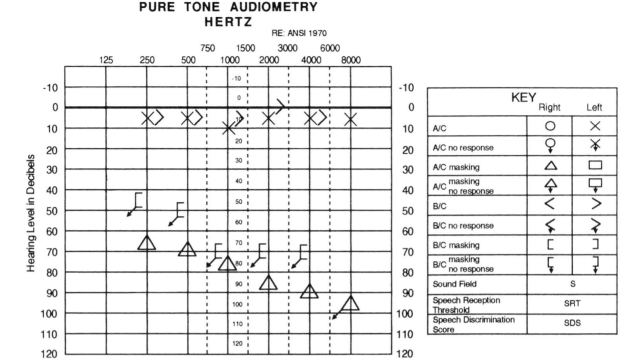

Figure 32 The audiogram for the patient in Figure 31 (history of concussion) following reconstructive surgery for ossicular discontinuity. Note the improvement in hearing sensitivity in the right operated ear.

middle-ear effusion, some cases of advanced otosclerosis, some cases of large middle-ear tumor, perforated tympanic membrane, or the probe being held against the outer-ear canal wall. Shanks (1984) found that when 1 cm³ of water was added to fresh human temporal bones, the susceptance and conductance tympanograms for the 660-Hz probe tones showed notching which was not present in fresh human temporal bones free of water. If this finding is substantiated in clinical cases of middle-ear effusion, then this notching in the 660-Hz susceptance or conductance tympanogram may be the basis for differentiating between ears with extreme ossicular fixation and ears with middle-ear effusion when a type 4 tympanometric pattern is obtained for the 220-Hz probe tone.

The type 5 tympanometric pattern (with tympanometric peak pressure < 100 daPa in children or < −50 daPa in adults) shown in Figures 22 and 23 for the 220-Hz probe tone is consistent with negative middle-ear pressure indicative of Eustachian-tube dysfunction with or without ossicular fixation or discontinuity (depending on the results of high-frequency tympanometry). The reader should recall that this tympanogram type does not preclude the presence of middle-ear effusion.

The previous discussion concerning Table V shows that if tympanometric type 1, 3, or 5 is obtained, high-frequency tympanometry should be employed to differentiate between ossicular fixation and ossicular discontinuity.

D. COMBINING STATIC-ACOUSTIC MIDDLE-EAR ADMITTANCE AND TYMPANOMETRY TO RESOLVE SPECIAL CASES

1. Use of High-Frequency Probe-Tone Tympanometry to Resolve Overlap between Groups in Static-Acoustic Middle-Ear Admittance

The recent introduction of high-frequency probe tones in tympanometry substantially resolves the overlap in the static-acoustic middle-ear admittance between the normal and pathologic middle ears and among the pathologic groups. The following example illustrates this phenomenon. Figures 33A, B, and C show the 220-Hz admittance tympanogram, the 660-Hz susceptance tympanogram, and the 660-Hz conductance tympanogram, respectively. Figure 33A reveals that the 220-Hz admittance tympanogram and the static acoustic middle-ear admittance value of 1.15 acoustic mmhos are within normal limits. (Tables I and III reveal that a static-acoustic middle-ear admittance of 1.15 acoustic mmhos is within the range for normal middle ears and is also within the range for ears with ossicular discontinuity.) Nevertheless, Figures 33B and C show the tympanometric pattern consistent with ossicular discontinuity, a condition that was surgically confirmed.

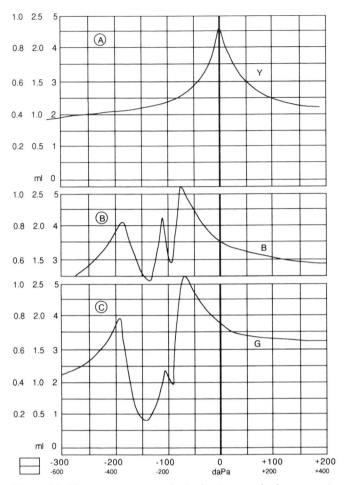

Figure 33 The tympanograms obtained using an absolute acoustic-immittance device from an ear with ossicular discontinuity. (A) The admittance tympanogram obtained with the 220-Hz probe tone. This tympanogram has a normal pattern. (B) The susceptance tympanogram obtained with the 660-Hz probe tone. This susceptance tympanogram is abnormal because the outermost extrema are separated by more than 100 daPa. (C) The conductance tympanogram obtained with the 660-Hz probe tone. This conductance tympanogram is abnormal since there are more three extrema.

2. STATIC-ACOUSTIC EAR-CANAL ADMITTANCE WITH DEEP TYMPANOGRAMS OBTAINED WITH A RELATIVE ACOUSTIC-IMMITTANCE DEVICE

The tympanometric amplitude directly yields the static-acoustic middle-ear admittance only when absolute but not relative acoustic-immittance devices are employed. A deep tympanogram for the 220-Hz probe tone and a relative acoustic-immittance device can be obtained in ears with small ear-canal volumes and normal static-acoustic middle-ear admittance as well as in ears with normal ear-canal volumes and large static-acoustic middle-ear admittance. Shanks (1984) reported that small ear-canal volumes can result in deep tympanograms. A small-static acoustic ear-canal admittance can occur also when the probe tip is in-

serted deep into the ear canal. (A large static-acoustic ear-canal admittance can be obtained with shallow insertion of the probe tip, especially when a large probe tip is used to seal the canal.)

Figure 34 shows two deep 220-Hz admittance tympanograms obtained with a relative acoustic-immittance device. In Figure 34A, the static-acoustic middle-ear admittance is 0.8 acoustic mmho and the static-acoustic ear-canal admittance is 0.4 acoustic mmho. In Figure 34B, the static-acoustic middle-ear admittance is large—2.9 acoustic mmhos—whereas the static-acoustic ear-canal admittance is 0.7 mmho. The tympanogram in Figure 34A was obtained from an ear with a small external ear-canal volume. The tympanogram in Figure 34B was obtained from an ear with confirmed ossicular discontinuity. In summary, deep tympanograms obtained with relative acoustic-immittance devices in some cases can be related to small static-acoustic ear-canal admittance. In such cases with a small static-acoustic ear-canal admittance yielding a deep tympanogram, the static-acoustic middle-ear admittance can differentiate between a normal middle ear with a normal tympanic membrane on the one hand, and on the other hand, (a) ossicular discontinuity with a normal tympanic membrane, (b) flaccid tympanic membrane or tympanic membrane with a healed perforation and an otherwise normal middle ear, or (c) ossicular discontinuity with a flaccid tympanic membrane or a membrane with a healed perforation.

E. ACOUSTIC-REFLEX TESTING

The acoustic reflex is the contraction of the stapedius muscle of the middle-ear in response to an acoustic activating signal. This contraction can be monitored by recording the resultant change in the acoustic immittance of the middle ear. The change in the acoustic immittance of the middle ear as a result of stapedius-muscle contraction forms the basis for the acoustic-reflex threshold and acoustic-reflex decay tests.

The stapedius muscle is enclosed in a bony canal on the posterior wall of the tympanic cavity. The muscle arises from the long canal. Its tendon emerges into the middle ear through the pyramidal eminence of the bony canal and then inserts into the neck of the stapes. When it contracts, the stapedius muscle moves the stapes downward and outward.

The acoustic-reflex center is situated in the superior olivary complex of the brainstem (see Figure 35). There are four acoustic-reflex arcs, two ipsilateral and two contralateral (Borg, 1973). One ipsilateral acoustic-reflex arc consists of (a) the primary auditory neuron of the eighth cranial nerve (the afferent or sensory neuron) from the haircells of the cochlea to the ventral cochlear nuclei, (b) the second-order neuron from the ventral cochlear nuclei through the trapezoid body to the ipsilateral facial-nerve nuclei, and

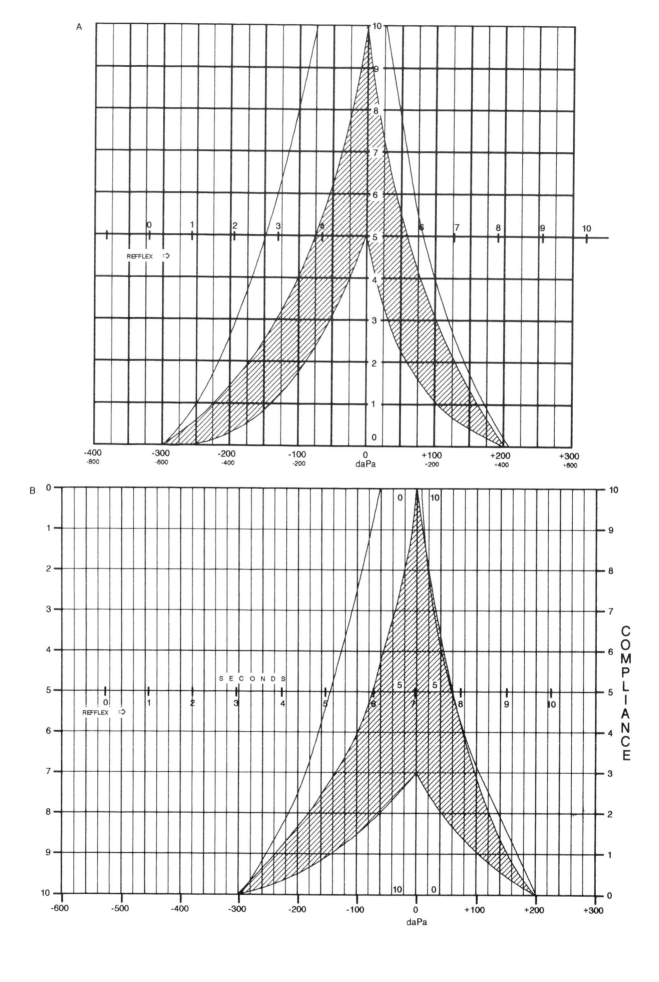

BRAINSTEM

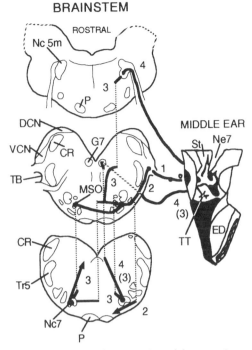

Figure 35 Neuronal organization of the acoustic stapedius (St) and tensor tympani (TT) reflexes as shown in three transverse sections through the rabbit brainstem. The middle ear is shown schematically in posterior view. Solid lines represent nerve tracts. Dotted lines show the connections between the sections. The acoustic stapedius-muscle reflex: The first neuron (1), the primary acoustic neuron from the hair cells to the cochlear nucleus, has contact with the second-order neuron (2) in the ventral cochlear nucleus (VCN). The second neuron (2) passes through the trapezoidal body (TB) and has contact directly with the ipsilateral stapedius-muscle motor neurons in the motor nucleus of the seventh cranial nerve (N. VII, 4,3). Via interneurons (3) in or near the medial superior olive (MSO), it relays to the ipsilateral and contralateral facial nerve. The motor neuron (3 or 4) follows the facial nerve to the stapedius muscle in the middle ear. The tensor tympani muscle reflex: The first-order (1) and second-order (2) neurons follow the same course as for the acoustic stapedius (St) reflex. There are no direct connections from the second-order neuron to the motor nucleus of the fifth cranial nerve (Nc5m). The motor neuron (4) follows the mandibular branch of the trigeminal nerve to the tensor tympani (TT) in the middle ear. Eardrum (ED); pyramidal tract (P); restiform body (CR); dorsal cochlear nucleus (DCN); internal geniculum of the seventh cranial nerve (G7); spinal trigeminal tract (Tr 5); nucleus of the seventh cranial nerve (Nc 7). Reprinted with permission from Borg (1973).

(c) the third-order neuron (the facial nerve) from the ipsilateral facial-nerve nuclei to the ipsilateral stapedius muscle. The other ipsilateral acoustic-reflex arc consists of (a) the primary auditory neuron of the eighth cranial nerve to the ipsilateral ventral cochlear nuclei, (b) the second-order neuron from the ipsilateral ventral cochlear nuclei to the ipsilateral superior olivary complex, (c) the third-order neuron from the ipsilateral superior olivary complex to the ipsilat-

eral facial-nerve nuclei; and (d) the fourth-order neuron from the ipsilateral facial-nerve nuclei to the ipsilateral stapedius muscle.

One contralateral acoustic-reflex arc has (a) the first-order neuron (primary auditory neuron of the eighth cranial nerve) to the ipsilateral ventral cochlear nuclei, (b) the second-order neuron from the ipsilateral ventral cochlear nuclei to the ipsilateral superior olivary complex, (c) the third-order neuron from the ipsilateral superior olivary complex to the contralateral facial-nerve nuclei, and (d) the fourth-order neuron from the contralateral facial-nerve nuclei to the contralateral stapedius muscle. The other contralateral acoustic-reflex arc has (a) the first-order neuron (primary auditory neuron of the eighth cranial nerve) from the haircells of the cochlea to the ipsilateral ventral cochlear nuclei, (b) the second-order neuron from the ipsilateral ventral cochlear nuclei to the contralateral superior olivary complex, (c) the third-order neuron from the contralateral superior olivary complex to the contralateral facial-nerve nuclei, and (d) the fourth-order neuron from the contralateral facial-nerve nuclei to the contralateral stapedius muscle.

Recall that the acoustic-immittance device is calibrated so that it is balanced whenever the sound-pressure level in the ear is 85 dB. Thus, if it is necessary to increase the energy presented to the ear in order to balance the meter, that is, send 85 dB to the tympanic membrane, then it would follow that the device is looking at a large cavity which has less impedance. On the other hand, if the cavity is small so the impedance is high, then the sound-pressure level would be decreased by decreasing the voltage from the source to attain the 85 dB needed to balance the meter. When a high-intensity sound that elicits the acoustic reflex is introduced to the ear, the volume of the middle ear decreases since the stapedius muscle pulls the tympanic membrane inward and stiffens the middle ear. Consequently, the acoustic reflex results in an increase in the middle-ear impedance which is indicated by a needle deflection on the immittance readout of the device.

1. CONTRALATERAL ACOUSTIC-REFLEX THRESHOLD

The threshold of the acoustic reflex is operationally defined as the lowest stimulus intensity level which causes a just-noticeable change in the acoustic immittance of the middle ear (or its components), resulting from contraction of the stapedius muscle; this acoustic-immittance change is time-locked with the stimulus. Recall that the acoustic reflex occurs bilaterally even when acoustic stimulation is unilateral. Thus, the acoustic-reflex threshold (ART) in a

Figure 34 (A) The 220-Hz admittance tympanogram for an ear with a small external auditory meatus. (B) The 220-Hz admittance tympanogram

for an ear with surgically confirmed ossicular discontinuity.

particular ear can be monitored in the ear contralateral as well as ipsilateral to the ear receiving the activating stimulus. The majority of studies on the ART have dealt with the contralateral ART, in which auditory stimulation is presented through an earphone to one ear and the immittance change is monitored in the opposite ear, since the contralateral ART, unlike the ipsilateral ART, is relatively free of artifacts and calibration problems. As shall be discussed later, recent investigators have developed techniques to control artifacts and resolve calibration problems associated with the ipsilateral ART.

a. Calibration of Stimulus Intensity

The ART can be specified in terms of dB SPL, dB HL, or dB SL. If a 1000-Hz tone elicits an acoustic reflex at 87 dB SPL but not 86 dB SPL, then the ART is 87 dB SPL. Since the correction factor for audiometric zero (ANSI, S3.6–1969) is 7 dB for TDH-49 earphones at this frequency, the ART can also be specified as 80 dB HL. In both cases, the ART is specified in terms of the physical level of the activator. An alternative approach is to express the ART as the level above an individual's threshold of hearing in sensation level (dB SL). For example, consider an ART of 80 dB HL in three patients with hearing threshold levels of 0, 20, and 35 dB HL at a particular frequency. In these cases, the ARTs occur at sensation levels of 80, 60, and 45 dB, respectively.

b. Sensitivity of the Electroacoustic-Immittance Device

The amount (magnitude) of acoustic-immittance change associated with the activator intensity level is greatest at levels well above the ART and decreases as the stimulus intensity level decreases. The ART is actually the intensity level corresponding to the smallest measurable electroacoustic-immittance change. Based on the normal range of ART values that will be discussed later, the logical and practical implication is that the electroacoustic-immittance device must be sensitive enough to resolve ARTs in response to BBN activators with intensity levels as low as approximately 60 dB SPL.

Typically, ARTs are measured on the basis of visual monitoring of the needle deflection on the meter of the electroacoustic-immittance device or retrospective analysis of a strip-chart recording or oscilloscope recording. The meter deflection approach is frequently employed clinically whereas the strip-chart or oscilloscope recording approach is more commonly employed in research. The clinical usage of the latter method, however, has increased in recent years. Other monitoring approaches include the use of a computer to record and calculate immittance changes during activator presentation, and the use of computerized averaging techniques. Except for visual inspection of the immittance meter, each of the monitoring approaches permits the use of an event marker which enables the clinician to determine whether the response was time-locked with the stimulus.

In the graphic approaches, a run of stimuli is adminis-

tered in which intensity increases in 1- or 2-dB increments from well below the anticipated ART. The ART is then easily and reliably estimated by inspecting the record for the smallest acoustic-immittance change or the smallest change exceeding a criterion value, such as 0.01 or 0.02 mmho, that is time-locked with the activator presentation, as shown in Figure 36. The visual detection approach has two limitations. First, the clinician must make an "on-the-spot" decision regarding whether or not a particular meter deflection actually was an acoustic-reflex response. Second, related to the first limitation, is the lack of consistency in criteria for the amount of needle deflection on the meter that constitutes an acoustic-reflex response. For example, some studies use the criterion of the "smallest reliably detectable" needle-movement approach and other studies use the criterion of needle deflection of at least one meter unit. Inherent in the visual monitoring of minimal needle deflection on the meter is the tendency to adjust one's criterion according to the moment-to-moment fluctuations in background activity and the limitations imposed by the ballistics of the meter. Also, the "one-unit deflection" approach often results in ARTs biased upward and is based on the erroneous assumption that these arbitrary units are linear or equivalent in actual acoustic-immittance values between tests. (This assumption is upheld, however, for calibrated meters whose units are in absolute units, e.g., mmhos.) The graphic approaches overcome these limitations.

The activator increment size also influences the sensitivity of the electroacoustic-immittance device. The overwhelming majority of clinical research is based on the use of 5-dB increments, just as the traditional audiologic tests are. On the other hand, most laboratory studies have employed 1- or 2-dB increments. The experimental studies based on 1- or 2-dB step size yield lower mean ARTs with smaller standard deviations and between-study variability than the clinical studies based on the 5-dB step size. At this time, normative data are available for the 1-dB and 5-dB step size. There is limited pathologic data for the 1-dB step size. Before a recommendation can be made to use the 1-dB step size under clinical conditions, further research is needed on ARTs from pathologic ears using the 1-dB step size.

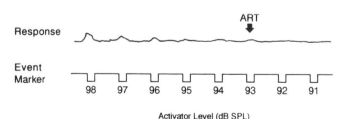

Figure 36 Acoustic-reflex threshold is defined as the lowest activator level at which there is a detectable immittance change from baseline. This change should be timelocked to the activator (shown by the event marker); activator levels above ART should also result in a (generally) larger immittance change. Reprinted with permission from Gelfand (1984).

c. Effect of Frequency

In general, persons with normal hearing thresholds without any pathology of the auditory mechanism or nervous system have ARTs of approximately 85–100 dB for SPL for pure tones between 250 and 4000 Hz. There is some evidence to indicate that the middle frequencies in this range have somewhat better (lower) ARTs than the extreme frequencies in the range. Clinical acoustic-reflex threshold testing is done for the 500-, 1000-, and 2000-Hz tonal activators. The 4000-Hz tonal activator is not routinely employed for ART testing since the ART for the 4000-Hz activator is often elevated or absent in young, normal-hearing persons because of acoustic-reflex adaptation within the first second of activator stimulation (Gelfand, 1984; Gonay, Dutillieux, & Metz, 1974). The normal ARTs for wide-spectrum stimuli, for example, BBN, are approximately 20 dB below the normal ARTs for tonal activators. (A BBN signal is a white noise shaped by the frequency response of the transducer, generally an audiometer earphone and cushion.) The use of the difference between the ARTs of the tonal BBN activators to predict hearing sensitivity will be discussed later.

The test–retest differences in the ART are remarkably small, usually test than 2 dB when high-resolution recording methods are employed. There also tends to be good agreement in the ARTs across clinical as well as laboratory studies. Discrepancies of up to 10 dB between the ARTs for BBN activators reported in the clinical literature and those reported in the experimental literature have been noted. These discrepancies are related to the differences in measurement technique and to the slow growth function of the acoustic reflex for the BBN activator.

d. Low-Level ARTs

Substantially lower ARTs are obtained when facilitating tones are employed. A facilitating tone is one that is presented to the ear at a level just below the ART for the facilitator. The presence of a facilitator results in a reduction in the ART for a test tone with respect to the ART obtained without the addition of the facilitator to the acoustic-reflex activator. Lower-than-expected ARTs have also been reported using computer averaging of ARTs (essentially to improve the signal-to-noise ratio), although this is not a finding common to most studies that have employed computer averaging techniques.

e. Diagnostic Applications

Cochlear Pathology Metz (1946) reported that the ARTs (in dB HL) of cochlear hearing-impaired ears are similar to those of normal-hearing persons. This finding led Metz (1946) to propose that the dB SLs with respect to hearing-threshold levels of cochlear hearing-impaired persons are lower than those of normal-hearing persons. According to Metz (1946), the presence of an ART at a reduced sensation level was indicative of loudness recruitment.

Jerger, Jerger, and Mauldin (1972) reported that in cochlear hearing-impaired ears, as the degree of hearing impairment increases to 85 dB HL, the sensation level of the ART decreases to approximately 25 dB; for cochlear hearing impairment exceeding 85 dB HL, the sensation level of the ART levels off at 25 dB. Jerger *et al.* (1972) concluded that ARTs at sensation levels less than 60 are consistent with cochlear hearing impairment (ARTs ≥ 60 dB SL are consistent with retrocochlear hearing impairment in sensorineural hearing-impaired ears).

The concept of ARTs at reduced sensation levels and the direct relation between magnitude of hearing impairment and decrease in sensation level of the ART in cochlear hearing-impaired ears is not straightforward. That is, cochlear hearing-impaired persons with mild and even, in some cases, moderate hearing impairment often do not have ARTs at reduced sensation levels. Also, persons with severe or worse degree of hearing impairment often have ARTs at SLs exceeding 25 dB (i.e., they have ARTs in dB HL which are higher than those for normal-hearing persons).

The early research showing that the ARTs of cochlear hearing-impaired and normal-hearing persons are essentially equal in dB HL was generally based on samples which lacked significant representation from persons with greater than moderate degree of hearing impairment, so the elevation in ART with substantial impairment was not observed (Alberti & Kristensen, 1970; Beedle & Harford, 1973; Jepsen, 1963; Jerger, 1970; Jerger, Jerger, & Mauldin, 1972; Metz, 1946; Peterson & Liden, 1972). The subsequent research, based on subjects with a wide range of degree of hearing loss, reveals that the tonal ARTs are essentially unaffected by the hearing loss, that is, they are similar to those for normal-hearing persons for hearing losses not exceeding approximately 50–55 dB HL; beyond 50–55 dB HL, the ART increases directly with the degree of hearing loss (Gelfand, Piper, & Silman, 1983; Holmes & Woodford, 1977; Keith, 1979; Martin & Brunette, 1980; Norris, Stelmachowicz, & Taylor, 1974; Popelka, 1981; Silman & Gelfand, 1979, 1981a; Silman, Popelka, & Gelfand, 1978b; Silman, Gelfand, Howard, & Showers, 1982).

Figure 37 shows the mean ARTs, standard deviations, and the 90th percentiles as a function of hearing loss at 500, 1000, and 2000 Hz (Silman & Gelfand, 1981a). The 90th percentile levels establish the upper limits for ARTs for cochlear hearing losses as a function of the magnitude of the hearing loss at 500, 1000, and 2000 Hz. Gelfand *et al.* (1983) obtained similar findings. Olsen, Bauch, & Harner (1983) reported that 97% of their 30 cochlear-impaired ears had ARTs that did not exceed the 90th percentile levels reported by Silman and Gelfand (1981a). Sanders (1984) found that 93% to 98% (depending upon the activator frequency) of his group of 133 cochlear-impaired ears had ARTs below the 90th percentile levels established by Silman and Gelfand (1981a).

108

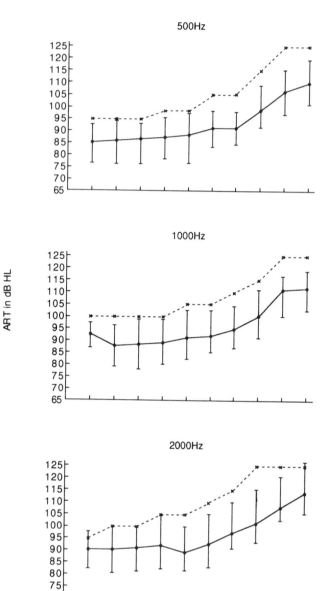

Figure 37 The acoustic-reflex thresholds for 500-, 1000-, and 2000-Hz activating signals as a function of hearing loss. The solid lines connect means (+ one standard deviation) and the broken lines connect the 90th percentile points. Reprinted with permission from Silman and Gelfand (1981a).

The hearing threshold levels at frequencies adjacent to the activator frequency also influence the ART (Gelfand *et al.*, 1983). The effect of the hearing loss at frequencies adjacent to the activator frequency is small but becomes more significant when the hearing loss at the activator frequency exceeds approximately 50 dB HL. This influence should be considered when there is an unexplainable elevation or absence of the ART.

The ART for BBN activators increases as a function of

the magnitude of hearing loss up to 60 dB HL (Handler & Margolis, 1977; Jerger, Hayes, Anthony, & Mauldin, 1978; Keith, 1977; Margolis & Fox, 1977; Peterson & Liden, 1972; Popelka, 1981; Popelka, Margolis, & Wiley, 1976; Silman & Gelfand, 1979, 1981b; Silman *et al.*, 1978, 1982). There are no further increases in the ART for the BBN activator with increases in the magnitude of the hearing loss beyond 60 dB HL (Popelka, 1981).

Retrocochlear Pathology Anderson, Barr, and Wedenberg (1970) reported that elevated ARTs were characteristic of ears with retrocochlear pathology (eighth nerve and/or cerebellopontine angle site). Several other investigators confirmed the finding of pathologically elevated or absent acoustic reflexes in ears with retrocochlear pathology (Frank, May, & Jannetta, 1978; Hayes & Jerger, 1980; Jerger, Harford, Clemis, & Alford, 1974c; Johnson, 1977; Mangham, Lindeman, & Dawson, 1980; Olsen, Stach, & Kurdziel, 1981; Olsen *et al.*, 1983; Sanders, 1984; Sanders, Josey, & Glasscock, 1974; Sheehy & Inzer, 1976; Silman, Gelfand, & Chun, 1978a; Thomsen & Terkildsen, 1975). Researchers disagreed, however, on the level of the ART to be considered the cutoff point for elevation consistent with retrocochlear pathology. For example, Anderson *et al.* (1970) initially considered the cutoff point to be 95 dB HL and later considered the cutoff point to be 105 dB HL. A high false-positive rate has been associated with the criteria established by Anderson and his colleagues (Chiveralls, 1977). Silman and Gelfand (1981a) proposed that ARTs exceeding their 90th percentile levels established on persons with a wide range of magnitude of cochlear hearing impairment might be considered consistent with retrocochlear pathology.

Olsen *et al.* (1983) applied the Silman and Gelfand (1981a) 90th percentile levels to their group of 30 subjects with surgically confirmed cerebellopontine angle tumors. They found that 83% of their retrocochlear-impaired subjects had elevated ARTs exceeding the 90th percentile levels for at least one activator frequency. In 57% of their tumor patients, the ARTs were elevated beyond the 90th percentile levels for at least two activating frequencies. The ARTs exceeded the 90th percentile levels for 21 of their tumor patients for the 500-Hz activator, for 20 of their tumor patients for the 1000-Hz activator, and for 25 of their patients for the 2000-Hz activator.

Sanders (1984) also evaluated the 90th percentile levels for ARTs in their group of 129 ears with confirmed acoustic tumor. They reported that the ART for at least one activator exceeded the 90th percentile levels in 76% of their tumor patients. The sensitivity rates were 67, 69, and 74% for the 500-, 1000-, and 2000-Hz activators, respectively. The false-alarm rates were 7, 2, and 5% for the 500-, 1000-, and 2000-Hz tonal activators, respectively. Sanders (1984) reported that the Silman and Gelfand (1981a) 90th percentile measure was characterized by a higher sensitivity and lower false-alarm rate that the criteria of Metz (1952), Jerger *et al.* (1972), and Anderson *et al.* (1970).

Based on the findings of Silman and Gelfand (1981a), Gelfand *et al.* (1983), Olsen *et al.* (1983), and Sanders (1984), we recommend that persons be considered at risk for retrocochlear pathology if the ART at any activating frequency (500, 1000, or 2000 Hz) exceeds the Silman and Gelfand (1981a) 90th percentile levels, provided conductive pathology is ruled out and provided that the same result is obtained upon retest. (Whenever an abnormally elevated ART is obtained, the clinician should immediately retest after adjusting the earphones and repositioning the probe tip since our clinical experience shows that, in many cases, the ART returns to below the 90th percentile levels after these maneuvers are carried out.)

Research done on normal-hearing and cochlear-impaired ears suggests that larger interaural ART differences, that is, 15 dB or more, may be suggestive of retrocochlear pathology (Chiveralls, 1977; Chiveralls, FitzSimons, Beck, & Kernohan, 1976; Mangham *et al.*, 1980). The large interaural ART measure must be evaluated on a group of retrocochlear-impaired ears before its use can be recommended.

Central Nervous System Disorders Most of the literature on the contralateral ART in pathologies medial to the cochlea deals with eighth-nerve and extra-axial sites of dysfunction. The ART also may be affected by lesions medial to these sites or within the central nervous system proper. Most investigations deal with the effects of intra-axial brainstem lesions and neuropathologies such as multiple sclerosis. The contralateral acoustic reflexes are affected when the trapezoid body of the brainstem or both superior olivary complexes are disordered. The contralateral ART for one ear is abnormal if the pathology affects the superior olivary complex on the earphone-ear side or the facial-nerve nuclei on the probe side.

Some neuropathies affect the contralateral ART. Several researchers have shown that the ART may be elevated unilaterally or bilaterally in patients with multiple sclerosis, particularly during exacerbation (Bosatra, Russolo, & Poli, 1976; Colletti, 1975b; Stephens & Thornton, 1976). As a group, it appears that patients with myasthenia gravis have increased ARTs prior to drug therapy in comparison with ARTs measured after drug therapy. It is clear, however, that the presence of a normal ART does not rule out the presence of neuropathy such as multiple sclerosis or myasthenia gravis.

There is disagreement in the literature regarding the effect of more rostral pathology (midbrain and auditory cortex). Downs and Crum (1980), who investigated three patients with cortical pathology, reported that the ART was decreased because of the loss of central inhibitory influences on the reflex. On the other hand, Jerger and Jerger (1981) and Gelfand and Silman (1982), whose study was based on

14 patients with cortical pathology, reported that the ARTs are unaffected by cortical pathology. Our clinical experience supports the findings of Jerger and Jerger (1981) and Gelfand and Silman (1982).

Conductive Pathology The contralateral ART is elevated or absent when the earphone is on the conductive-impaired ear and is generally absent when the probe is in the conductive-impaired ear. The elevation or absence of the contralateral ART when the earphone is on the conductive hearing-impaired ear results from the attenuation of the activator intensity because of the air–bone gaps created by conductive pathology. Jerger *et al.* (1974a) demonstrated that the probability of obtaining the contralateral acoustic reflex falls to 50% (earphone on the conductive-impaired ear) when there is an air–bone gap of 27 dB (collapsed across the frequencies between 500 and 4000 Hz) in the stimulated ear. This is the predicted result considering that the conductive hearing impairment reduces the sound-pressure level reaching the cochlea. That is, even if the person's sensory status is normal, that is, the bone-conduction thresholds are 0 dB HL, a 27-dB air–bone gap would raise the mean ART levels to about 112–119 dB HL and the 90th percentile levels to approximately 122–127 dB HL. Since the maximum activator intensity employed in the Jerger *et al.* (1974a) study was 110 dB HL, it is not surprising that at least half of the contralateral acoustic reflexes are absent with air–bone gaps of this magnitude. If the maximum activator intensity was 125 dB HL, as is common in current electroacoustic-immittance devices, instead of 110 dB HL, the probability of absent acoustic reflexes for a 27-dB air–bone gap would be somewhat lower than the 50% reported by Jerger *et al.* (1974a).

The contralateral ART is absent when the probe is in the conductive-impaired ear because the conductive pathology causes the ear to become excessively stiff or flaccid, preventing the observation of an acoustic-immittance change resulting from contraction of the stapedius muscle. Jerger *et al.* (1974a) reported that the contralateral acoustic reflex is absent in 50% of the cases when the probe ear has an air–bone gap of only 5 dB.

Since there is an effect on the ART when the earphone is on the conductive-impaired ear and when the probe is in the conductive-impaired ear, the following commonly occur in cases of unilateral conductive pathology: (a) bilaterally absent acoustic reflexes or, (b) an absent acoustic reflex when the good ear is stimulated and an elevated ART when the pathologic ear is stimulated. In cases of bilateral conductive pathology, the acoustic reflexes are generally absent bilaterally.

In cases of conductive pathology solely due to negative middle-ear pressure, the contralateral acoustic reflex often can be elicited, even with the probe in the conductive-impaired ear, if the ear-canal pressure is adjusted to equal the tympanometric peak pressure. When the ear-canal pressure is adjusted in this manner, the ART obtained with the probe in the conductive-impaired ear is often only slightly elevated; with the earphone on the conductive-impaired ear, the contralateral ART is normal.

The exception to the general rule of absence of the acoustic reflex when the probe is in the conductive-impaired ear occurs in cases of ossicular discontinuity medial, not lateral, to the insertion of the stapedius on the stapes. That is, in cases of ossicular discontinuity in which the connection is maintained between the insertion point of the stapedius muscle on the stapes and the eardrum, the contralateral ART is present with the probe in the affected ear. It may be present either at normal or elevated levels, depending on how intact the connection is between the stapedius muscle and the stapes. Typical examples of ossicular discontinuity yielding a contralateral reflex when the probe is in the affected ear include a fracture of the stapes medial to the insertion of the stapedial muscle and cases in which adhesions between the stapes and manubrium of the malleus bridge the gap left by a destroyed incus. When the earphone is on the affected ear, the ART is either elevated or absent due to the air–bone gap resulting from the ossicular discontinuity. Such cases often present the seemingly paradoxical picture (in ears with unilateral conductive hearing impairment) of absence of the ART when the earphone is on the pathologic ear with large air–bone gaps but presence of the ART at normal levels when the probe is in the pathologic ear.

f. Effect of Sex, Aging, and Drugs

The ARTs for males are essentially similar to those for females (Jerger et al., 1972; Osterhammel & Osterhammel, 1979; Silverman, Silman, & Miller, 1983).

Certain drugs can affect the ART. Research findings show that moderate blood concentrations of ethanol can result in up to 7 dB elevation in the mean ART for BBN activators and up to approximately 5 dB elevation for narrow-band noise (NBN) and tonal activators. The prevalence of absent acoustic reflexes is greater in alcoholics than nonalcoholics (Spitzer & Ventry, 1980). In general, there is great intersubject variability in the degree of elevation of the ART resulting from alcohol (Bauch & Robinette, 1978; Cohill & Greenberg, 1977). Barbiturates such as secobarbital and pentobarbital and antipsychotic agents such as chlorpromazine can also cause an elevation in the ART (although there is great intersubject variability on the size of the drug effect). Clinicians should obtain a drug history in all patients with abnormal acoustic-reflex responses.

The results of Osterhammel and Osterhammel (1979) showed that aging essentially has no effect on the tonal ARTs. On the other hand, Jerger et al.'s (1978) retrospective data from a large group of normal-hearing clinical subjects revealed a decrease in the tonal ARTs with increasing age but no age-related changes for the BBN ART. Several laboratory studies (Gelfand & Piper, 1981; Silman,

1979; Silverman et al. 1983; Wilson, 1981) demonstrated no difference between the tonal ARTs of young and older adults but did show that the BBN ARTs are elevated by approximately 8–10 dB among older subjects when compared with the younger adult subjects. Silverman et al. (1983) showed that the age effect for the BBN activator is obscured when clinical rather than laboratory techniques are employed. Studies which have employed statistical analysis have shown that the tonal ARTs are unaffected by age and the BBN ARTs are elevated by age.

2. THE IPSILATERAL ACOUSTIC-REFLEX THRESHOLD

To elicit the ipsilateral acoustic reflex, both the probe tone and activating signals are presented through the probe tube. This is in contrast to the contralateral acoustic reflex, for which the activating signal is presented through the earphone and the probe tone is presented through a tube. For the ipsilateral acoustic reflex, the same ear serves as both the stimulus ear (ear receiving the activating signal) and the probe ear (ear in which the acoustic-reflex response is monitored). Because the activating and probe signals are presented through the same tube, the ipsilateral acoustic reflex, unlike the contralateral acoustic reflex, is characterized by certain artifacts and calibration problems.

a. Advantages

According to Green and Margolis (1984), ipsilateral acoustic-reflex measurement is superior to contralateral acoustic-reflex measurement in the following ways.

1. The status of one ear does not affect acoustic-reflex assessment in the other ear. For example, in cases of unilateral conductive pathology, the integrity of the eighth nerve cannot be assessed in the good ear by contralateral acoustic-reflex measurement since the presence of a conductive loss in the probe ear will obliterate the acoustic reflex. By ipsilateral acoustic-reflex measurement, however, the ART can be measured in the good ear without the contaminating influence of the conductive loss in the other ear. Similarly, in cases of unilateral atresia, contralateral acoustic-reflex information cannot be obtained for the good ear because of the atresia in the probe ear; ipsilateral acoustic-reflex information, however, can be obtained for the good ear since both the eliciting and probe tones are presented in that ear.

2. Acoustic-reflex information can be obtained in cases of collapsed ear canals. With bilateral collapsed ear canals, a bilateral conductive hearing loss is obtained, the tympanograms are normal bilaterally, and the contralateral acoustic reflexes are bilaterally absent. If the clinician is not alert to the possibility of collapsed ear canals, he or she may interpret the findings as consistent with bilateral conductive pathology (making the patient

an excellent candidate for a stapedectomy!). If the patient is tested using ipsilateral acoustic-reflex measurement techniques, normal ARTs will be obtained, causing the clinician to suspect the presence of collapsed ear canals.

3. Acoustic-reflex testing can be done on children who refuse to submit to the contralateral acoustic-reflex testing because of the earphones.

b. Disadvantages

There are several inherent problems in ipsilateral acoustic reflex measurement. These problems include artifacts, inability to calibrate intensity in dB HL, and reduced maximum output intensities.

Artifacts As stated previously, in ipsilateral acoustic-reflex measurement, the probe tone and eliciting signals are presented through the same tube. Under certain conditions, the probe tone and eliciting signals interact acoustically, resulting in a change in sound-pressure level of the probe tone, and consequently in needle deflection, which could be mistakenly interpreted as reflecting a change in the middle-ear acoustic immittance. There are two commonly known artifacts which can affect ipsilateral acoustic-reflex measurement: the additive and subtractive (eardrum) artifacts (Kunov, 1977; Lutman, 1980; Lutman & Leis, 1980).

The probe-tone energy reflected at the eardrum is passed through a microphone, converted into electrical energy, and then passed through a filter. The additive artifact occurs when some of the eliciting-signal energy, also reflected at the eardrum, is picked up by the microphone and passed through the filter along with the probe tone. The passing-through of the eliciting-signal energy will result in an increase in the voltage passed through the filter. This increase in voltage resulting from the addition of the eliciting-signal energy to the probe-tone energy resembles an increase in the probe-tone voltage resulting from acoustic-reflex contraction. The additive artifact can be observed in hard-wall and membranous cavities and therefore in the human ear, which resembles a membranous cavity. The probability of obtaining the additive artifact increases as the frequency of the eliciting stimulus approaches the frequency of the probe tone. The artifact is generally observed as the intensity of the eliciting stimulus approaches the expected ART levels in normal-hearing persons.

The intensity levels (in dB SPL) at which the additive artifact occurs in a 2-cm³ cavity are generally incorporated in the electroacoustic-immittance devices. For example, a light flashes at the intensity levels at which the additive artifact occurs, alerting the clinician not to go above these levels. The reading on the attenuator dial may underestimate the true sound-pressure level in the total-ear cavity in cases in which the total-ear volume is smaller than the 2-cm³ coupler, since the sound-pressure level in a cavity is inversely related to the cavity volume, as shown in Figure 38. Thus, the additive artifact may be obtained at attenua-

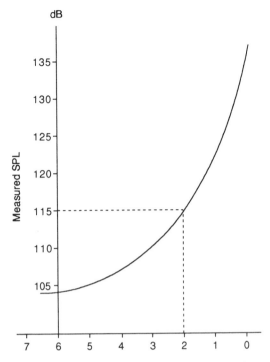

Figure 38 Actual sound pressure levels (SPL) in hard-walled cavity for constant amplitude stimulus. (Calibrated for 115 dB SPL in 2-cc cavity at 20°C and 760 mm Hg.) Reprinted with permission from Madsen North America, Inc.

tor readings below those specified by the manufacturer in persons with total-ear volumes smaller than 2 cm³ because the increased sound-pressure level developed in the ear reflects the energy from the attenuator dial and the energy developed in a smaller-than-2-cm³ cavity. For example, when testing infants and small children who have total-ear volumes as small as 0.5 cm³, the additive artifact may be obtained at levels up to 20 dB below the dial readings yielding artifacts in a 2-cm³ cavity according to the manufacturer of the particular electroacoustic-immittance device. The clinician will assume that the needle-deflection at these low attenuator dial readings represents a true reflex rather than an artifact since they occur at levels below those which the manufacturer says will yield the additive artifact. We recommend that clinicians establish the attenuator readings yielding additive artifacts in hard-wall cavities ranging in size from 0.5 to 5.0 cm³ for different probe tones and activators. The clinician should start with the smallest cavity and work up to the largest volume cavity. If no additive artifacts are seen with the smallest cavity, the clinician does not need to check the other cavities for artifacts.

The subtractive (eardrum) artifact results when two signals, f_1 and f_2, are presented in a nonlinear system such as a membranous cavity like the human ear. Some of the energy from f_1 and f_2 will be distributed over newly formed components that are equal to the sums and differences of the fundamentals. During ipsilateral acoustic-reflex testing, the f_1 and f_2 signals represent the probe and eliciting signals, respectively. Energy will be taken from f_1 and f_2 and redistributed over the newly formed complex sound. The reduction in sound-pressure level of the probe tone will cause a needle deflection in a direction opposite to that usually obtained for the acoustic reflex, resembling the needle deflection associated with a decrease in acoustic impedance which sometimes results from acoustic-reflex contraction. The instrument manuals for electroacoustic-immittance devices do not specify the minimum intensity levels yielding subtractive artifacts in membranous cavity for each of the activating signals. Therefore, the clinician should establish these minimum attenuator dial readings for each of the activating and probe signals in membranous cavities (syringe with a thick membrane as a base) varying in size from 0.5 to 5.0 cm³. (The clinician should be sure to establish these levels at the tympanometric peak pressure.)

The additive and subtractive artifacts can be monitored on an oscilloscope. The latency of an artifact can be established by mixing the probe with the activating stimulus in a hardwall cavity and increasing the intensity of the activating stimulus until a detectable change in the base-line sound-pressure level of the probe tone is observed on the scope. The clinician can then calculate the latency between the onset of the eliciting stimulus and the onset of the deflection in the probe baseline. Usually this latency is close to 0 ms. The latency of the acoustic-reflex is generally not below 40 ms at the highest intensities (Bosatra, Russolo, & Silverman, 1984). Therefore, if the latency of the response is similar to that measured for the artifact, then the clinician is dealing with an artifact rather than with an acoustic-reflex response. If the presence of an artifact has been established according to the latency, then the direction of the deflection will indicate whether the artifact is subtractive or additive, that is, upward deflection is obtained for additive artifacts and downward deflection is obtained for subtractive artifacts. The clinician should recall that either an increase or decrease in immittance can be obtained with acoustic-reflex contractions, so a negative deflection does not necessarily indicate the presence of a subtractive artifact unless the latency is close to 0 ms (although it is more likely to be an artifact than an acoustic-reflex response). We recommend that the oscilloscope technique be employed or establishing the minimum artifact levels for the various cavities.

Calibration of Intensity in dB SPL The calibration of intensity level for the ipsilateral acoustic reflex is done in a 2-cm³ rather than in the 6-cm³ coupler employed for calibration of intensity level in clinical audiometers. Consequently, the intensity levels for the acoustic reflex are reported in dB SPL rather than the dB HL used for the contralateral acoustic reflex. Therefore, the ipsilateral ARTs cannot be directly compared with the contralateral ART. Several investigators have attempted to overcome this

limitation by applying a correction factor to the ipsilateral ART values. Table VI shows the correction factors to be added to the ipsilateral ART when comparing the ipsilateral ARTs (dB SPL) to the contralateral ARTs (converted from dB HL to dB SPL). After the correction factors in Table VI are added to the ipsilateral ARTs (dB SPL), the derived, equivalent SPL values can be easily converted to equivalent dB HL values so the 90th percentiles can be applied to the ipsilateral ARTs. Research is needed to validate the application of the 90th percentile to the ipsilateral ARTs in this manner.

Reduced Maximum Output Intensity Levels Because of the additive and subtractive artifacts, the maximum output levels for the ipsilateral acoustic reflex are reduced significantly in comparison with those for the contralateral ARTs. In general, the output intensity levels for most devices, especially those without multiplexing circuits, do not exceed 95–105 dB SPL (depending on frequency) for ipsilateral acoustic-reflex measurement. The reduced maximum output affects the ability to do ipsilateral acoustic-reflex measurement in persons with hearing impairment, particularly those with significant cochlear hearing impairment, since, in these cases, the ipsilateral ART may occur at SPLs beyond the maximum output intensity levels.

c. Interpretation

The means and SDs for the ipsilateral ARTs in normal-hearing persons are shown in Table VII. From this table, the clinician can determine the range representing the 5th to 95th percentile reflecting the expected ipsilateral ARTs for persons with normal hearing-threshold levels. Table VII

Table VI Mean differences and 95% confidence intervals (CIs) in coupler sound pressure levels (dB) for earphone and probe stimuli producing equal reflex response[a,b]

Instrument	Frequecy (Hz)				
	500	1000	2000	3000	4000
Amplaid 702					
Mean	1.7	−0.7	4.7	—	8.2
95% CI	±2.9	±2.6	±2.2	—	±2.4
Danplex D175					
Mean	2.0	3.1	2.8	—	8.4
95% CI	±2.5	±1.2	±2.9	—	±3.5
Grason–Stadler 1723					
Mean	3.1	0.9	3.2	—	10.3
95% CI	±1.6	±0.9	±2.5	—	±3.8
Kamplex AZ2					
Mean	5.8	3.7	4.2	2.0	—
95% CI	±3.0	±1.0	±2.9	±3.4	—
Madsen ZO 73					
Mean	4.3	2.4	3.5	—	—
95% CI	±2.1	±1.5	±1.9	—	—

[a] Reprinted with permission from Lutman (1980).
[b] 9-A Coupler minus 2 cc coupler data.

Table VII   Behavioral Air-Conduction Thresholds and Ipsilateral Acoustic-Reflex Thresholds for Tones and Broad-Band Noise (BBN)

	Frequency (Hz)						
	250	500	1000	2000	4000	8000	BBN
Behavioral thresholds							
N	253	253	253	253	253	253	—
Mean	2.9	1.2	−0.5	−0.7	2.4	5.6	—
SD	5.3	4.4	4.7	4.8	6.0	6.3	—
90% NR	−5/10	−5/5	−10/5	−10/5	−5/10	−5/15	—
Ipsilateral reflex thresholds							
N	—	248	248	247	55	—	248
Mean (HL)	—	79.9	82.0	86.2	87.5	—	64.6
Mean (SL)	—	78.9	81.5	85.6	85.1	—	—
SD	—	5.0	5.2	5.9	3.5	—	6.9
90% NR	—	72/90	75/90	77/95	80/90	—	55/75

   [a] Adapted from Wiley, Oviatt, and Block (1987), with permission.
   [b] The number of ears (N), mean, standard deviation (SD), and 90% normal range (90% NR) are included for each measure. The 90% NR (5–95%) defines the upper and lower limit that includes 90% of the respective values. All data are presented in terms of hearing level (HL). Reflex thresholds also are referenced in sensation level (SL) relative to behavioral thresholds at each signal frequency. Standard deviations for acoustic-reflex thresholds are based on HL measures.

also reveals that the ipsilateral ARTs are obtained at lower dB HLs (when converted from dB SPL to dB HL) than contralateral ARTs. The fact that the ipsilateral ARTs are lower than the contralateral ARTs reflects the fact that the ipsilateral pathways are shorter than the contralateral pathways for the acoustic reflex.

No data concerning the relation between magnitude of hearing loss and the ipsilateral ART in persons with cochlear hearing impairment are available. Since the research on the contralateral ARTs show that the ARTs increase with hearing loss beyond approximately 50 dB HL, it is reasonable to expect a similar finding for the ipsilateral ART.

The ipsilateral ART is absent in ears with conductive pathology when the reflex is monitored in the ear with the conductive hearing loss. This result is similar to what is found for the contralateral ART.

In general, elevated (relative to the upper limit of the 90% normal range in Table VII) or absent ARTs in persons with hearing-threshold levels not exceeding approximately 50 dB HL with no air–bone gaps may be consistent with retrocochlear pathology in the ear with the affected ipsilateral ART. When the ARTs are elevated or absent in persons with sensorineural hearing loss exceeding 50 dB HL, differentiation between cochlear and retrocochlear pathology cannot be made.

The ipsilateral ARTs in persons with central auditory pathology at levels rostral to the superior olivary complex are assumed to be similar to those for persons with intact eighth nerves, normal middle ears, and hearing-threshold levels not exceeding 50 dB HL.

In persons with facial-nerve pathology medial to the insertion of the nerve on the stapedius muscle, the ipsilateral ART is generally either elevated or absent in the ear with the pathology.

d. Ipsilateral and Contralateral ART Patterns

The ipsilateral and contralateral ARTs should be classified as normal, elevated, or absent. It is useful, for diagnostic purposes, to compare the ipsilateral ART patterns with the contralateral ART patterns. Several ipsilateral vs. contralateral ART patterns that are observed for various pathologies follow (provided that ipsilateral artifacts are ruled out).

1. A contralateral ART which is absent or elevated for only one ear with an ipsilateral ART which is absent or elevated in the same ear. This is consistent with severe to profound cochlear hearing impairment or retrocochlear (eighth-nerve or extra-axial brainstem) pathology in the stimulus ear. For example, absent right contralateral and ipsilateral acoustic reflexes and normal left contralateral and ipsilateral acoustic reflexes are consistent with the presence of severe to profound cochlear hearing impairment or retrocochlear (eighth-nerve or extra-axial brainstem) pathology in the right ear.

2. Contralateral ARTs which are elevated or absent bilaterally with normal ipsilateral ARTs, bilaterally. This pattern is consistent with pathology of the trapezoid body or pathology affecting both superior olivary complexes either directly or indirectly. For example, elevated right and left contralateral ARTs with normal right and left ipsilateral ARTs are consistent with pathology of the trapezoid body or pathology affecting the right and left superior olivary complexes directly or indirectly.

3. A contralateral ART which is elevated or absent for only one ear with an ipsilateral ART which is absent or elevated for only the opposite ear. This pattern is consistent with an abnormality of the stapedius muscle or facial nerve medial to the insertion on the stapedius muscle in the ear which serves as the probe ear when abnormal ARTs are obtained. For example an elevated right contralateral ART, normal left contralateral ART, normal right ipsilateral ART, and elevated left ipsilateral ART are consistent with left stapedius muscle abnormality or left facial-nerve abnormality medial to the insertion on the stapedius muscle.

4. An elevated or absent contralateral ART for only one ear with normal ipsilateral ARTs bilaterally. This pattern is consistent with pathology of the superior olivary complex on the side yielding the abnormal contralateral ART. For example, an absent right contralateral ART with a normal left contralateral ART and normal right and left ipsilateral ARTs is consistent with pathology of the right superior olivary complex.

5. Bilaterally absent or elevated contralateral acoustic reflexes with an ipsilateral ART which is absent or elevated in only one ear. This pattern is consistent with any one of the following pathologies: conductive pathology in the ear yielding the abnormal (generally absent) ipsilateral ART, large acoustic tumor directly or indirectly involving the facial nerve in the ear with the affected ipsilateral ART; pathology of the trapezoid body or pathology directly or indirectly affecting both superior olivary complexes, with cochlear hearing impairment exceeding 50 dB HL in the ear with the affected ipsilateral ART; pathology of the trapezoid body or pathology directly or indirectly affecting both superior olivary complexes, with conductive pathology in the ear with the affected ipsilateral ART; pathology of the trapezoid body or pathology directly or indirectly affecting both superior olivary complexes, with eighth-nerve or extra-axial brainstem pathology in the ear with the affected ipsilateral ART; pathology of the trapezoid body or pathology directly or indirectly affecting both superior olivary complexes, with stapedius muscle abnormality or facial-nerve pathology medial to the insertion on the stapedius muscle in the ear with the affected ipsilateral ART. For example, bilaterally absent contralateral acoustic reflexes with an absent right ipsilateral acoustic reflex and a normal left ipsilateral ART are consistent with (a) conductive pathology in the right ear; (b) a large acoustic tumor pressing on the facial nerve on the right side; (c) pathology of the trapezoid body or pathology directly or indirectly affecting both superior olivary complexes, with cochlear, retrocochlear, or conductive pathology in the right ear; or (d) right stapedius-muscle abnormality or right facial-nerve

abnormality medial to the insertion on the stapedius muscle with pathology of the trapezoid body or pathology indirectly or directly affecting both superior olivary complexes.

6. Bilaterally absent or elevated contralateral and ipsilateral acoustic reflexes. This pattern is consistent with bilateral conductive, severe to profound cochlear, or retrocochlear pathology; brainstem pathology involving a large area of the medulla including both superior olivary complexes and cochlear nuclei; or bilateral stapedius-muscle or facial-nerve pathology (medial to the insertion on the stapedius muscle). For example, absent right and left contralateral and ipsilateral acoustic reflexes are consistent with bilateral conductive, severe to profound cochlear, retrocochlear (eighth-nerve or extra-axial), stapedius-muscle, or facial-nerve (medial to the insertion on the stapedius muscle) pathology, or brainstem pathology affecting a large area of the medulla including the right and left superior olivary complexes and cochlear nuclei.

Figure 39 illustrates these six patterns.

3. ACOUSTIC-REFLEX ADAPTATION

Adaptation of the acoustic reflex is defined as the decrease in acoustic-reflex magnitude during sustained acoustic stimulation. During contralateral acoustic-reflex adaptation testing, the stimulus is presented to one ear and the acoustic-reflex magnitude is monitored in the contralateral ear. During ipsilateral acoustic-reflex adaptation testing, the stimulus is presented to one ear and the acoustic-reflex magnitude is monitored in the same ear.

a. Contralateral Acoustic-Reflex Adaptation

Normal Ears Figure 40 shows the contralateral acoustic-reflex adaptation in normal-hearing ears for five tonal activators presented at three sensation levels (relative to the contralateral ART). The data in this figure are normalized so the point of maximum impedance change is assigned a value of 100%. The other points represent the impedance changes as percentages of the maximum impedance change. Three conclusions can be drawn from this figure. First, the rate of acoustic-reflex adaptation increases as frequency increases, that is, the amount of decrease in acoustic-reflex magnitude per second increases as the frequency of the tonal activator increases. For example, the adaptation rate is significantly slower for 500- and 1000-Hz activating signals than for the higher frequency activators. Second, the onset of acoustic-reflex adaptation occurs earlier for high-frequency activators than for low-frequency activators. Note that, whereas acoustic-reflex magnitude decayed by 50% within 10 s or less at the higher frequencies, the decay in acoustic-reflex magnitude was negligible even when acoustic stimulation was sustained

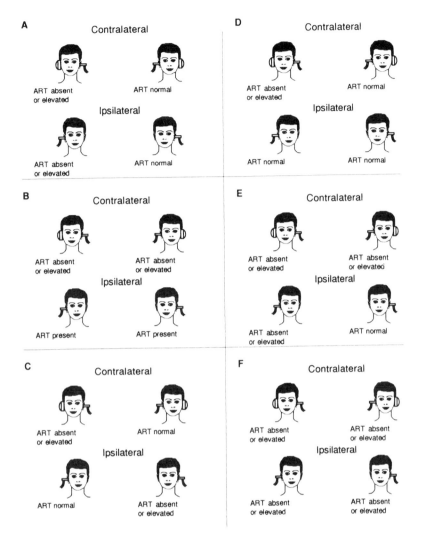

Figure 39 The various contralateral and ipsilateral ART patterns. The ART is described for the stimulated ear, regardless of the mode of elicitation (i.e., contralateral or ipsilateral). (A) A case in which the contralateral ART is absent or elevated for only one ear and the ipsilateral ART is absent or elevated in the same ear. (B) A case in which the contralateral ARTs are elevated or absent bilaterally, with normal ipsilateral ARTs, bilaterally. (C) A case in which the contralateral ART is elevated or absent for only one ear and the ipsilateral ART is elevated or absent for only the opposite ear. (D) A case with an elevated or absent contralateral ART for only one ear with normal ipsilateral ARTs bilaterally. (E) A case with bilaterally absent or elevated contralateral acoustic reflexes with an ipsilateral ART which is absent or elevated in only one ear. (F) A case with bilaterally absent or elevated contralateral and ipsilateral acoustic reflexes.

over a period of 100 s at the lower activating frequencies. Third, the onset and rate of acoustic-reflex adaptation does not vary with intensity level of the activator. Wilson, Shanks, and Lilly (1984) showed that, at lower intensity levels where the acoustic-reflex magnitude is small, the onset of conductance acoustic-reflex adaptation is essentially the same as the onset of susceptance acoustic-reflex adaptation. At higher levels, however, the onset of the conductance acoustic-reflex adaptation occurs later than that of susceptance acoustic-reflex adaptation.

The clinical procedure for acoustic-reflex adaptation assessment is based on the technique employed by Anderson, Barr, and Wedenberg (1969). Anderson *et al.* monitored the amplitude of the acoustic-reflex response while a 500- or 1000-Hz tonal activator is presented for 10 s at 10 dB SL relative to the ART. They considered abnormal acoustic-reflex adaptation to be present if the acoustic-reflex magnitude decayed by at least 50% within the first 5 s for both tonal activators. Several researchers consider acoustic-reflex adaptation to be abnormal if there is 50% or more decay in acoustic-reflex magnitude within 10 s rather than within the first 5 s for either the 500- or 1000-Hz activa-

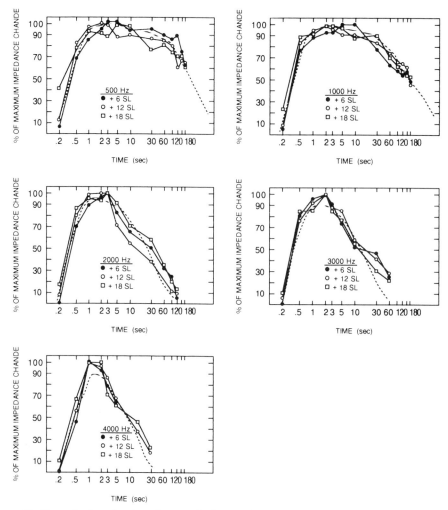

Figure 40 Normalized median impedance at the five test frequencies as a function of time. Ordinate is expressed in percentage of maximum impedance change. Suprathreshold level (re: reflex thresholds) is the parameter. The dashed lines are calculated. Reprinted with permission from Kaplan, Gilman, and Dirks (1977).

tor (Jerger *et al.*, 1974c; Olsen, Noffsinger, & Kurdziel, 1975).

Cochlear Pathology Anderson *et al.*'s (1969, 1970) classic study indicates that, in general, persons with cochlear hearing impairment do not demonstrate abnormal acoustic-reflex decay. Nevertheless, the research findings show that there is faster acoustic-reflex adaptation in persons with cochlear hearing impairment than in normal ears (Chiveralls *et al.*, 1976) but faster acoustic-reflex adaptation in retrocochlear-impaired ears than cochlear-impaired ears (Cartwright & Lilly, 1976).

Olsen *et al.* (1975) reported that 8% of their 50 patients with noise trauma and 14% of their 50 patients with Meniere's disease had at least 50% decay in acoustic-reflex magnitude over the course of 10 s at 500 and/or 1000 Hz. Olsen *et al.* (1981) obtained similar findings. They found that, of their 58 patients with Meniere's disease, 26% had abnormal acoustic-reflex adaptation with the 10-s tech-

nique whereas 22% had abnormal acoustic-reflex adaptation with the 5-s technique at 500 and/or 1000 Hz. They also found that the false-positive rate decreased from 22 to 5% when acoustic-reflex adaptation was considered only at 500 Hz rather than at both 500 and 1000 Hz (using the 5-s technique). Nevertheless, this restriction in frequency resulted in a decrease in the hit rate of the acoustic-reflex adaptation measure. Olsen *et al.* (1983) reported that the false-positive rate for the acoustic-reflex adaptation measure was 10% in their group of 30 nontumor patients. Sanders (1984) reported that only 3% of his 134 cochlear-impaired ears had abnormal acoustic-reflex adaptation using the 5-s technique. Thus, the higher false-positive rates reported by Olsen and his colleagues may reflect the fact that they employed smaller sample sizes than Anderson *et al.* (1969) and Sanders (1984).

Eighth-Nerve Pathology The classic studies by Anderson *et al.* (1969, 1970) revealed that abnormal acoustic-reflex adaptation is characteristic of retrocochlear-impaired ears. This finding was substantiated by several investigators (Bergenius, Borg, & Hirsch, 1983; Jerger et al., 1974c; Mangham et al. 1980; Olsen et al., 1975, 1981, 1983; Sanders, 1984; Sanders, Josey, Glasscock, & Jackson, 1981; Sheehy & Inzer, 1976; Silman et al. 1978a; Thomsen & Terkildsen, 1975).

Olsen et al. (1975) reported that 21% of their 28 patients with confirmed eighth-nerve lesions had abnormal acoustic-reflex adaptation at 500 or 1000 Hz using the 10-s technique. Acoustic-reflex decay testing was possible in only 9 of the 23 cases, since the acoustic reflexes were absent in 68% of the cases. Using the criterion of absent acoustic reflexes or abnormal acoustic-reflex adaptation at 500 or 1000 Hz, the hit rate was 86%. Olsen et al. (1981) obtained similar findings in their investigation of 58 patients with confirmed eighth-nerve lesions. They found that 31% had at least 50% decay in acoustic-reflex magnitude within 10 s at 500 and/or 1000 Hz and 28% had at least 50% decay in acoustic-reflex magnitude within the first 5 s at 500 and/or 1000 Hz. Abnormal acoustic-reflex decay within the first 5 s at 500 Hz was present in 21% of the cases; only 2 of the 58 patients had abnormal acoustic-reflex decay at only 1000 Hz. Thus, abnormal acoustic-reflex adaptation at 500 Hz is a stronger indication of retrocochlear pathology than that at 1000 Hz. Because the hit rate is improved when both frequencies are assessed, and the false-alarm rate is not substantially increased by the use of two rather than one frequency, we recommend that acoustic-reflex adaptation testing be done at both 500 and 1000 Hz. Similarly, we recommend that acoustic-reflex adaptation testing be done using the 10-s rather than the 5-s technique. Nevertheless, the presence of abnormal acoustic-reflex adaptation within the first 5 s is a stronger indication of retrocochlear pathology than abnormal acoustic-reflex adaptation within 10 s (and after the first 5 s). Using the criterion of absent acoustic reflexes or abnormal acoustic-reflex adaptation within the first 5 or 10 s at 500 and/or 1000 Hz, 95% of patients with eighth-nerve lesions were correctly identified. Olsen et al. (1983) investigated acoustic-reflex decay using the 5-s technique in 30 patients with confirmed cerebellopontine angle tumor (matched by pairs in degree and configuration of hearing loss with a group of 30 nontumor subjects). They reported that acoustic-reflex adaptation was abnormal in 23% of their patients at 500 and/or 1000 Hz. In all of these cases, however, the acoustic-reflex decay measure was a second indicator of retrocochlear pathology since the ART was elevated beyond the 90th percentile levels at 500, 1000, and/or 2000 Hz. Sanders (1984) found that the acoustic-reflex adaptation measure (using the 5-s technique) identified an additional 9% of the 129 ears with confirmed acoustic tumors beyond those identified by just the ART measure. Using the criterion of ARTs elevated beyond the

90th percentile levels for ARTs or abnormal acoustic-reflex adaptation, 85% of the acoustic-tumor ears were correctly identified.

Table VIII, from Wilson et al. (1984), shows the sensitivity rates reported by various investigators for the acoustic-reflex adaptation measure with the 5-s and 10-s technique. This table demonstrates that acoustic-reflex adaptation testing cannot be done in a large proportion of persons with retrocochlear pathology since the acoustic reflexes are absent in approximately 41–63% of these cases.

Very little research concerning the effect of stimulus intensity level on the sensitivity of the acoustic-reflex adaptation measure has been done. According to Mangham et al. (1980), who measured acoustic-reflex adaptation in terms of a time constant (time from the onset of the acoustic-reflex response to 63% of the peak acoustic-reflex magnitude), both the sensitivity and specificity of the acoustic-reflex adaptation measure were higher for the 20-dB SL than the 10-dB SL presentation level. Further research is needed on the effect of reflex-activator level on acoustic-reflex adaptation in cochlear and retrocochlear ears before recommendations can be made regarding the clinical feasibility of higher stimulus presentation levels in acoustic-reflex adaptation testing.

Other Pathologies Abnormal acoustic-reflex adaptation has been reported in persons with certain demyelinating diseases such as multiple sclerosis, and brainstem disorders including intra-axial brainstem pathology (Alberti & Kristensen, 1976; Anderson et al., 1969; Jerger & Jerger, 1977; Stephens & Thornton, 1976). Abnormal acoustic-reflex adaptation has also been observed in persons with

Table VIII Comparison of Eighth-Nerve Lesion Studies

Study	Criteria (sec)	N	Absent reflexes (%)	Abnormal adaptation (%)	False-negative rate (%)
Anderson et al. (1969)	5	17	41.2	58.8	0
Hirsch and Anderson (1980)	5	97	59.8	23.7	16.5
Bergenius et al. (1983)	5	21	42.9	19.1	38.0
Sanders et al. (1981)	5	149	56.4	22.2	21.4
Hirsch and Anderson (1980)	10	97	59.8	33.0	7.2
Jerger et al. (1974c)	10	30	63.3	13.3	23.4
Sheehy and Inzer (1976)	10	24	45.8	33.3	20.9

[a] Reprinted with permission from Wilson, Shanks, and Lilly (1984).

disorders of the efferent part of the acoustic-reflex arc (facial nerve or stapedius muscle). For example, Wilson *et al.* (1984) observed abnormal acoustic-reflex adaptation when the probe was in the affected ear of patients with Bell's palsy during the stage in which the palsy subsides. Neuromuscular diseases such as myasthenia gravis are also associated with abnormal acoustic-reflex adaptation (observed when the probe is in the affected ear) for activators having durations prolonged beyond 10 s (Blom & Zakrisson, 1974; Kramer, Ruth, Johns, & Sanders, 1981).

b. Ipsilateral Acoustic-Reflex Adaptation

The results of recent investigations on ipsilateral acoustic-reflex adaptation indicate that, in normal subjects, the decay in acoustic-reflex magnitude is less than 50% over a 10-s period (Alberti, Fria, & Cummings, 1977; Oviatt & Kileny, 1984). Nevertheless, the amount of ipsilateral acoustic-reflex adaptation is slightly greater than that of contralateral adaptation in normal subjects. This trend becomes increasingly apparent the more the stimulus duration is increased beyond 10 s. Oviatt and Kileny (1984) reported that abnormal ipsilateral but not contralateral acoustic-reflex adaptation (greater than 50% decay in acoustic-reflex magnitude) over a 10-s period occurred in 2 of their 4 subjects with cochlear hearing impairment. In general, whenever abnormal contralateral acoustic-reflex adaptation was present, abnormal ipsilateral acoustic-reflex adaptation was also present. They concluded that research is needed to determine whether separate ipsilateral acoustic-reflex adaptation norms are necessary in order to be able to classify the ipsilateral acoustic-reflex adaptation as normal or abnormal.

Silverman, Silman, Gelfand, and Lutolf (1986) and Silman, Silverman, Gelfand, Lutolf, and Lynn (1988) reported the presence of abnormal acoustic-reflex adaptation (contralateral and ipsilateral) when the probe was in the affected ear of two normal-hearing subjects with confirmed facial-nerve pathology. In both of these subjects, the ipsilateral and contralateral ARTs were present at levels below the 90th percentiles for the ART. These results suggest that when abnormal contralateral acoustic-reflex adaptation is detected, clinicians should consider doing ipsilateral acoustic-reflex adaptation testing in order to better differentiate between pathologies affecting the afferent part of the acoustic-reflex arc and pathologies affecting the efferent part of the acoustic-reflex arc, particularly when the ipsilateral and contralateral ARTs are normal.

4. Prediction of Hearing Loss from the ART

Several researchers have used ART measurements to predict hearing impairment. This nonbehavioral, noninvasive, inexpensive technique is clinically useful to predict hearing sensitivity in the difficult-to-test who cannot be assessed by traditional audiometry. The underlying principle in prediction of hearing impairment from the ART is the decreased difference between the tonal ARTs and BBN ART in persons with sensorineural hearing impairment. The Niemeyer and Sesterhenn (1974) and Jerger, Burney, Mauldin, and Crump (1974b) methods were based on the assumption that the difference between the tonal ARTs and the BBN ART decreased linearly as the magnitude of the hearing impairment increased. These methods and the modifications of the Jerger *et al.* (1974b) method are characterized by high false-positive rates ranging from 25–40% (Keith, 1977; Margolis & Fox, 1977; Schwartz & Sanders, 1976). The high false-positive rates are related to the following factors.

1. Niemeyer and Sesterhenn (1974) and Jerger *et al.* (1974b) did not control for age. Several studies show that the noise–tone difference is decreased as a function of age (Gelfand & Piper, 1981; Silman, 1979; Silverman *et al.*, 1983).

2. The Niemeyer and Sesterhenn (1974) method and the Jerger *et al.* (1974b) method were based on the assumption that the noise–tone difference decreases as the magnitude of the hearing loss increases. Research indicates that this assumption holds only for mild-to-moderate hearing impairment up to 40–50 dB HL. Further increases in the hearing impairment results in an elevation of the ART for the tonal but not BBN activator. Thus, the noise–tone difference increases with increases in the magnitude of hearing impairment beyond 50 dB HL.

Popelka *et al.* (1976) and Popelka (1981) attempted to overcome the limitations of the methods developed by Niemeyer and Sesterhenn (1974) and Jerger *et al.* (1984b) with their bivariate-plot method. In this method, the ARTs are used to predict whether or not a hearing impairment is present. This is in contrast to the methods of Niemeyer and Sesterhenn (1974) and Jerger *et al.* (1974b), in which the *magnitude* of the hearing impairment was predicted from the ARTs. In the classic bivariate-plot method, two acoustic-reflex quantities which increase as the hearing impairment increases are plotted as coordinates on a bivariate graph. The ART for a single tonal activator or the average of the ARTs for three tonal activators is represented on the ordinate. The ratio of the ART for a noise activator (broad band, high-, or low-pass) to the ART for a tonal activator (or the average of the ARTs for several tonal activators, most commonly 500, 1000, and 2000 Hz) is represented on the abscissa. In order to construct the bivariate plot, a group of young normal-hearing subjects are tested and their ART data are plotted on the graph. Two line segments are then drawn, one vertical and one diagonal with a slope of -1.0 such that at least 90% of the data from the normal-hearing subjects are located within the delineated (left) region of the graph as shown in Figure 41. The normal-hearing region should not be large enough to include any obvious "out-

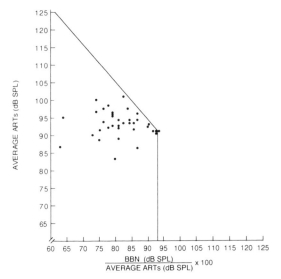

Figure 41 Illustration of the traditional bivariate plot as described by Popelka (1981). The ordinate represents the average of the ARTs for the 500-, 1000-, and 2000-Hz tonal activators and the abscissa represents the ratio of the ART for the BBN activator to the average of the ARTs for the 500-, 1000-, and 2000-Hz tonal activators multiplied by 100. The line segments were drawn after plotting the data points for the normal-hearing ears. The line segments consist of the vertical segment and a diagonal segment with a slope of −1.0. The line segments were drawn so that at least 90% (here, 97%) of the data points for the normal-hearing ears were located to the left of them. Reprinted with permission from Silman, Gelfand, Piper, Silverman, and Van Frank (1984a).

liers," since their inclusion will elevate the false-negative rate. The miss rate can be determined by obtaining ART data from a group of hearing-impaired subjects whose pure tone averages (PTAs) are known to exceed 32 dB HL, plotting these data on the graph along with the data from the normal-hearing subjects, and then determining the percentage of hearing-impaired ears which fall in the normal-hearing region. The false-positive rate is obtained by determining the percentage of normal-hearing ears which fall into the hearing-impaired region.

The hit rate of the classical bivariate procedure is approximately 90% and the false-alarm rate is approximately 5% in children (Silman *et al.* 1984a). The hit and false-alarm rates are improved slightly when 1-dB or 2-dB increments are used with a strip-chart recorder to measure the ARTs instead of 5-dB increments with visual inspection of needle deflection. The hit rate is decreased markedly, approaching chance level, however, when the sample includes persons with mild and high-frequency sensorineural hearing impairment (which occurs much more frequently in adults than children) and persons more than 44 years of age (Silman *et al.*, 1984a). This finding is unsurprising since the ART for the BBN activator in persons with mild and/or high-frequency hearing impairment or in normal-hearing older

adults (more than 44 years of age) is elevated (Silman & Gelfand, 1979; Silman, Silverman, Showers, & Gelfand, 1984b; Silverman *et al.*, 1983).

The predictive accuracy of the classical bivariate-plotting procedure in adults with mild or high-frequency hearing impairment can be improved by (a) excluding the data from persons more than 44 years of age, (b) plotting the data points from the hearing-impaired as well as the normal-hearing ears before the line segments are drawn, and (c) drawing the line segments so that the hit rate is maximized without incurring a large false-alarm rate, that is, the vertical and diagonal lines should be adjusted so that 90% or more of the mild and high-frequency (as well as significant) hearing-impaired ears fall in the hearing-impaired region (Silman *et al.*, 1984a,b). This modified bivariate graph is then used for prediction of the presence of a hearing impairment (of any magnitude, including high-frequency hearing impairment). That is, the ARTs from a patient are plotted on this bivariate graph. If the point falls in the left region, the patient is assumed to have normal hearing thresholds through 4000 Hz. If the point falls in the right region, the person is assumed to have hearing impairment.

Neither the classical nor modified bivariate-plotting procedure should be employed with persons more than 44 years of age. The classical bivariate-plotting procedure should be employed with children and the modified bivariate-plotting procedure should be employed with adults less than 44 years of age.

Silman *et al.* (1984b) developed criteria for the identification of hearing impairment in the over-44-years-of-age group based on the following absolute ART levels: (a) an ART greater than or equal to 105 dB SPL for the 1000- and/or 2000-Hz activator, or (b) an ART greater than 90 dB SPL for the BBN activator. The ARTs were measured under laboratory conditions, that is, 1-dB intensity increments and a strip-chart recorder to record acoustic-immittance changes. They reported that these criteria correctly identified 87% of the significantly hearing-impaired adults and 85% of the normal-hearing adults. The ability to identify mild and/or high-frequency hearing impairment, however, approached the chance level.

Wallin, Mendez-Kurtz, and Silman (1986) evaluated the ART criteria developed by Silman *et al.* (1984b) in the older adult population using routine clinical procedures for ART measurement, that is, 5-dB intensity increments and visual monitoring of the needle deflection. Their sample included 126 ears from 83 subjects between 45 and 84 years of age. Wallin *et al.* (1986) reported that 90% of their ears with significant hearing impairment were identified as having at least a mild or high-frequency hearing impairment. The predictive accuracy for the mild and/or high-frequency hearing-impaired ears remained problematic; approximately half of these ears had ARTs not exceeding these criteria and the other half had ARTs meeting these criteria. The predictive accuracy for the normal-hearing ears was 93%. Thus, the findings of Silman *et al.* (1984b) and Wallin *et al.* (1986) suggest that these ART criteria can be employed as a screening device to identify the presence of hearing impairment in difficult-to-test adults who are more than 44 years of age. The clinician should bear in mind that, with this technique, approximately 50% of the mild and/or high-frequency hearing-impaired ears will be misidentified.

A potentially promising technique for prediction of hearing impairment is reflex modulation Reiter, 1981; Reiter, Goetzinger, & Press, 1981). Reflex modulation is the inhibition of a cutaneous reflex, such as the air-puff elicited eyeblink reflex, with preliminary auditory stimulation. Preliminary studies have been done with small samples of difficult-to-test subjects and normal-hearing adults. Further large sample research on hearing-impaired and normal hearing persons is required to evaluate the clinical usefulness of this approach.

5. Biphasic Acoustic Reflex

Generally, acoustic-reflex contraction results in an increase in the acoustic impedance of the middle ear. Occasionally, in certain normal ears with loose coupling between the stapes and the oval window, acoustic-reflex contraction results in a decrease, rather than increase, of the acoustic impedance of the middle ear because of the decrease in the resistive component during acoustic-reflex contraction. Two biphasic acoustic-reflex patterns are shown in Figure 42. In many normal ears, a small, transitory decrease at stimulus onset precedes the large impedance increase (see Figure 42A). Another biphasic pattern in normal ears has been reported for high-frequency probe tones, for example, 660 Hz. This pattern shows a brief impedance decrease at stimulus onset followed by another brief impedance decrease at stimulus offset (see Figure 42B) (Bennett & Weatherby, 1979; Creten, Vanpeperstraete, Van Camp, & Doclo, 1976; Van Camp, Vanpeperstraete, Creten, & Vanhuyse, 1975). According to Bennett and Weatherby (1979), the biphasic pattern seen in normal ears, which is shown in Figure 41B, first occurs at the reversing frequency—the lowest probe-tone frequency at which the net change in acoustic impedance during acoustic-reflex contraction is a net decrease in the acoustic impedance because of the substantial decrease in the resistive component and minimal increase in the reactance component. The reversing frequency is approximately 625 Hz in normal adults (Bennett & Weatherby, 1979). Bennett and Weatherby (1979) also reported that the biphasic pattern shown in Figure 42B was present in 21% of their 50 normal ears. Point A in the biphasic pattern (shown in Figure 42B), obtained at stimulus onset, results from a large decrease in the acoustic resistance of the middle ear and an small increase in the acoustic stiffness reactance of the middle ear; point B, obtained while the stimulus is still on, reflects an increase in the acoustic stiffness reactance that is greater in absolute magnitude than the decrease in acoustic resistance; point C, obtained at the offset of the stimulus, results from a large decrease in the acoustic resistance and a small increase in the acoustic stiffness reactance (Bennett & Weatherby, 1979).

Flottorp and Djupesland (1970) were the first to report the presence of the biphasic acoustic reflex in otosclerotic ears. This biphasic reflex has the pattern shown in Figure 42B. The presence of this particular biphasic acoustic-reflex pattern in some otosclerotic ears has been attributed to changes in the elastic properties of the stapes and annular ligament where partial fixation of the footplate of the stapes has occurred (Bel, Causse, Michaux, Cezard, Canut, & Tapon, 1976). When the biphasic pattern occurs in otosclerotic ears, it occurs at all probe-tone frequencies (Bennett & Weatherby, 1979). The mechanism underlying the biphasic pattern in otosclerotic ears is different than that in normal-hearing ears. That is, point A, at stimulus onset, reflects a small increase in the acoustic resistance and a large decrease in the acoustic stiffness reactance; point B reflects the return of the acoustic resistance and acoustic stiffness reactance values to the baseline values while the stimulus is still on; point C, occurring at stimulus offset, reflects a small increase in the acoustic resistance and a large decrease in the acoustic stiffness reactance (Bennett & Weatherby, 1979). This biphasic pattern has also been reported for ears with osteogenesis imperfecta, congenital fixation of the stapes, or Cogan's syndrome (Djupesland, Flottorp, Hansen, & Sjaastad, 1974).

F. ACOUSTIC-IMMITTANCE TESTING IN INFANTS

The characteristics of the outer and middle ear in neonates differ from those in adults. In neonates, the osseous portion of the external ear canal is not developed so the infant ear is highly compliant in comparison with the adult ear. Also, the tympanic ring is not fully developed until the end of the first year. The outer- and middle-ear volume in infants is smaller than that in adults. Consequently, the immittance patterns seen in infants are different than those seen in

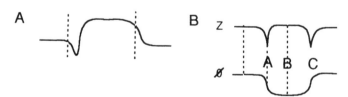

Figure 42 (A) The time course of the acoustic reflex in a normal ear. Note the negative deflection at the onset. Adapted from Jerger (1975). (B) Biphasic reflex at 800-Hz probe tone from a normal ear. Point A is the onset peak, point B is the center component and point C is the offset peak. Adapted from Bennett (1984).

adults. Also, these anatomical differences are the basis for the high false-negative rate for tympanometry with respect to the identification of middle-ear effusion in neonates.

1. TYMPANOMETRY
a. Normal Ears

The findings of early tympanometric studies in normal neonates indicate that single-peaked or notched tympanograms for the 220-Hz probe tone are obtained when only the impedance vector is measured (Bennett, 1975; Correa & Konow, 1978; Keith, 1973, 1975; Poulsen & Tos, 1978; Zarnoch & Balkany, 1978). Himmelfarb, Popelka, and Shanon (1979) noted the importance of obtaining resistance and reactance tympanograms in addition to the impedance tympanograms in neonates. Several investigators reported that more than 90% of the neonates studied demonstrate notched (W-shaped) susceptance or conductance tympanograms for the 220-Hz probe tone; for the 660-Hz probe tone, neonates have single-peaked, flat, or rising susceptance and/or conductance tympanograms (Cannon, Smith, Reece, & Thebo, 1974; Sprague, et al., 1985). These

tympanometric findings in normal neonates contrast with those in adults, who generally demonstrate single-peaked susceptance and conductance tympanograms at 220 Hz and notched tympanograms at 660 Hz.

As mentioned earlier, notched tympanograms occur (a) when the acoustic reactance is stiffness controlled but its absolute value is smaller than that of the acoustic resistance near ambient pressure and is greater than that of the acoustic resistance at extreme pressures in the susceptance tympanogram, or (b) when the acoustic reactance is mass controlled near ambient ear-canal pressure and stiffness controlled at extreme pressures in the admittance, susceptance, and conductance tympanograms. Based on the second principle, Sprague et al. (1985) concluded that the neonate ear is mass dominated at 220 Hz since most of their infants had susceptance tympanograms with the notch below the baseline at 220 Hz. Since most of the neonates had single-peaked susceptance and conductance tympanograms at 660 Hz, Sprague et al. concluded that the neonate ear was stiffness dominated at 660 Hz. Figure 43 shows the susceptance and conductance tympanograms for the 220-

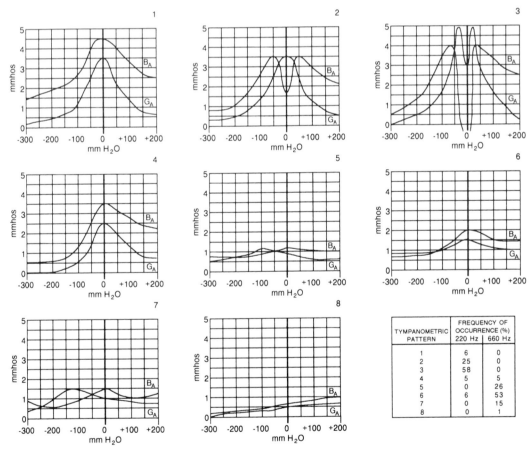

Figure 43 Tympanometric patterns observed for both the 220-Hz and 660-Hz probe tones in neonates. Frequency of pattern occurrence by probe is calculated at the bottom of the figure. Reprinted with permission from Sprague, Wiley, and Goldstein (1985).

Hz and 660-Hz probe tones. As can be seen from this figure, most infants have notched susceptance and/or conductance tympanograms at 220 Hz and single-peaked susceptance and/or conductance tympanograms at 660 Hz.

Since the neonate ear is stiffness dominated at 660 Hz, Sprague et al. (1985) suggested that the 660-Hz probe tone was best for detecting middle-ear effusion. In contrast, Margolis and Shanks (1985) advocated the use of low probe-tone frequencies such as 220 Hz for the detection of middle-ear effusion in neonates. Based on the tympanometric findings by Himmelfarb et al. (1979), Margolis and Shanks concluded that the introduction of positive air-pressure during tympanometry was associated with a distention of the ear-canal walls and consequently an increase in the ear-canal volume and, therefore, the susceptance of the ear canal at 220 Hz; this increase in outer-ear susceptance at 220 Hz is multiplied threefold for the 660-Hz probe tone since the acoustic susceptance is directly proportional to the product of probe frequency and volume. Since the outer-ear volume and susceptance is exaggerated at 660-Hz, the estimate of the middle-ear volume and susceptance at this probe-tone frequency will be artifactually reduced, making the 660-Hz probe tone less sensitive for the detection of middle-ear effusion. The controversy regarding the ideal probe-tone frequency for the detection of middle-ear effusion indicates that the clinical application of tympanometry in neonates is not as well defined as in adults. Further research is necessary to resolve this controversy.

b. Abnormal Ears

Many neonates with middle-ear effusion demonstrate normal tympanograms for the 220-Hz probe tone (Paradise et al., 1976; Zarnoch & Balkany, 1978). This finding was attributed to the flaccidity of the ear-canal walls in neonates resulting in distention of the walls in accordance with the pressure changes.

Several investigators reported that the prevalence of otitis media in normal term neonates is low (Klein, 1978; Tos et al., 1984; Zarnoch & Balkany, 1978). Otitis media occurs frequently in normal infants following the neonatal period (after 28 days of age) (Klein, 1978; Zarnoch & Balkany, 1978). There is a high prevalence of middle-ear effusion in preterm infants and neonates, and infants and neonates in the intensive care unit (NICU) (Balkany, Berman, Simmons, & Jafek, 1978; Jaffe, Hurtado, & Hurtado, 1970; Paradise, 1980). This high prevalence in the NICU is related to intubation for assisted ventilation, tube feeding, and constant supine positioning (Balkany et al., 1978; Paradise, 1980).

Because of the high prevalence of normal tympanograms in neonates and infants less than 2 months of age with middle-ear effusion, and the low rate of otitis media in normal term neonates, it is recommended that routine screening tympanometry not be done in this population unless suspicion of middle-ear pathology exists; when such

suspicion exists, acoustic-reflex testing should be done as well as tympanometry (which has a low false-positive rate with respect to middle-ear effusion) since a normal tympanogram will not rule out middle-ear effusion in this population and since acoustic-reflex testing with high-frequency probe tones is sensitive to the presence of middle-ear effusion. Further research is needed on ways to improve the clinical feasibility of tympanometry in this population. Since there is a high incidence of middle-ear effusion in the NICU and since there is a high false-negative rate but low false-positive rate for tympanometry with respect to middle-ear effusion, it is recommended that both acoustic-reflex testing using high-frequency probe tones and tympanometry be done when screening neonates and infants from the NICU. Again, the presence of a normal tympanogram will not rule out the presence of middle-ear effusion. Infants with normal or abnormal middle ears who are at least 2 months of age have tympanometric patterns resembling those of adults (Margolis & Popelka, 1975; Zarnoch & Balkany, 1978). Therefore, tympanometry can be employed with confidence as a screening or diagnostic tool in infants at least 2 months of age.

2. ACOUSTIC-REFLEX TESTING
a. Contralateral

There is a high percentage of absent contralateral acoustic reflexes for the 220-Hz probe tone in neonates. For example, Sprague et al. (1985) reported that only 49% of their neonates had acoustic reflexes for the broad-band noise activator and only 34% had acoustic reflexes for the 1000-Hz activator when stimuli were presented through insert receivers and calibrated in a 2-cm³ coupler. Mc-Millan, Bennett, Marchant, and Shurin (1985) reported that the contralateral acoustic reflexes for the 220-Hz probe tone were present in 5% of the normal neonates for the 500-Hz activator, 9% for the 1000-Hz activator, 20% for the 2000-Hz activator, and 14% for the 4000-Hz activator when stimuli were presented under earphones. Other investigators have obtained similar findings (Bennett, 1975; Keith, 1973; Keith & Bench, 1978; Stream, Stream, Walker, & Breningstall, 1978). When the contralateral acoustic reflexes are present in neonates for the 220-Hz probe tone, they are generally present at elevated levels (Abahazi & Greenberg, 1977; Himmelfarb, Shanon, Popelka, & Margolis, 1978).

Weatherby and Bennett (1980) showed that the ART decreases with increasing probe-tone frequency in neonates. Bennett and Weatherby (1982) reported that the contralateral ARTs in neonates approximate those in adults when the 1200-Hz probe-tone frequency is employed. Mc-Millan et al. (1985) reported that the contralateral acoustic reflexes for the 660-Hz probe tone were present in 38–63% of neonates, depending upon the tonal activator.

The proportion of neonates with acoustic reflexes (us-

Table IX Normative Contralateral Acoustic-Reflex Threshold Data in Neonates for the 1000-Hz Tonal and Broadband Noise Activators[a]

Mode and investigator	Probe tone (Hz)	Activator frequency (Hz)	Range (dB SPL)	Median (dB SPL)	Mean (dB SPL)	SD
Under earphones						
Weatherby & Bennett	660	BBN	62–80[b]	70		
Under insert receivers						
Sprague *et al.*	220	1000	80–110		92.2	8.9
	220	BBN	45–105		70.0	14.3
	660	1000	70–110		89.1	11.0
	660	BBN	45–110		70.1	17.4

[a] Data obtained under earphones and insert receivers for the 220-Hz and 660-Hz probe tones, as reported by Sprague, Wiley, and Goldstein (1985) and Weatherby and Bennett (1980).
[b] 5th to 95th percentiles.

ing high-frequency probe tones) is higher for the broadband noise signal than for tonal activators. For example, Weatherby and Bennett (1980) obtained contralateral acoustic reflexes for the BBN activator in 88% of neonates when the probe-frequency was 2000 Hz, 68% when the probe frequency was 500 Hz, 42% when the probe-frequency was 400 Hz, and 0% at 220 Hz. Sprague *et al.* (1985) reported that the contralateral acoustic reflexes for the BBN activator at 660 Hz were present in 88% of their normal neonates. The mean and median ARTs and their ranges for the BBN and the 1000-Hz tonal activators and the 220- and 660-Hz probe-tone frequencies when the activating stimuli are presented through earphones and insert receivers are shown in Table IX.

Theoretically, if the contralateral ART for the BBN activator is present bilaterally, the presence of conductive and severe-to-profound sensorineural hearing loss can be ruled out bilaterally. If the contralateral ART for the BBN activator is absent, it is recommended that the clinician attempt to determine the ART for the 500-, 1000-, or 2000-Hz activator.

b. Ipsilateral

As mentioned earlier in the section on the ipsilateral acoustic reflex, the sound-pressure levels of ipsilateral activating stimuli are calibrated in a 2-cm³ rather than the 6-cm³ coupler used to calibrate the intensity of the contralateral activating stimuli. The volume of the outer ear in infants is significantly smaller than in adults. Therefore, the sound-pressure level developed in the ear-canal of infants for a given dial reading will be greater than that developed in a 2-cm³ coupler. (In adults, the sound-pressure level developed in the ear canal for a given dial reading approximates that developed in a 2-cm³ coupler.) Table X shows the mean sound-pressure levels associated with a 0-dB dial reading as measured in a 2-cm³ coupler (manufacturer's specification) and as measured in the ear canals (real-ear measurement) of 95 ears from 51 neonates and 20 adults. Since the real-ear dB SPLs for the ipsilateral activators are higher in neonates than adults and since the 2-cc coupler

values are close to the real-ear values in adults, underestimation of the ipsilateral ARTs may occur in neonates when activating signals are calibrated in a 2-cc coupler. Therefore, the ipsilateral ARTs in infants should be interpreted with respect to their presence vs. absence rather than absolute level until standardization for the calibration for ipsilateral acoustic reflexes in infants is established.

Very little research is available on the ipsilateral ART in infants, and studies differ in the method of calibrating the sound-pressure levels of the activating stimuli. For example, Sprague *et al.* (1985) calibrated the sound-pressure levels of the ipsilateral activating stimuli in a 2-cm³ coupler. McMillan *et al.* (1985) obtained real-ear measurements of the sound-pressure levels of the ipsilateral activating stimuli. The results of a limited number of studies on the ipsilateral acoustic reflexes in infants show that there is a higher percentage of acoustic reflexes with ipsilateral than contralateral stimulation and of ipsilateral acoustic reflexes us-

Table X Measured Sound Pressure Levels for Ipsilateral Activators Compared With the Grason–Stadler 1723 Otoadmittance Meter Specifications[a]

Activator (Hz)	Manufacturer's specifications	Mean sound pressure level at 0 dB HL dial reading	
		Measured Levels	
		Neonates	Adults
500	14.0	15.5	11
		SD = 1.9	SD = 0.7
1000	7.0	16.2[b]	8.8
		SD = 4.0	SD = 1.6
2000	5.0	30.0[b]	8.2
		SD = 4.8	SD = 2.7
4000	−3.0	9.0	9.5
		SD = 2.8	SD = 2.4

[a] Reprinted with permission from McMillan, Bennett, Marchant, and Shuring (1985).
[b] Combined across first and second studies. Large SD due to higher levels in second study, possibly due to subjects' younger age and smaller canal volumes.

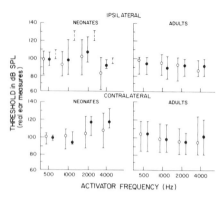

Figure 44 Acoustic-reflex thresholds in neonates and adults. Open circles are the medians and ranges at 660 Hz; closed circles are the medians and ranges at 220 Hz; the dashes are the upper equipment limit ranges in neonates. Reprinted with permission from McMillan, Bennett, Marchant, and Shurin (1985).

ing the 660-Hz probe tone than of ipsilateral acoustic reflexes using the 220-Hz probe tone (McMillan *et al.*, 1985; Sprague *et al.*, 1985). Figure 44 shows the medians and ranges for the real-ear ipsilateral and contralateral ARTs in neonates and adults (McMillan *et al.*, 1985).

G. RELATION BETWEEN OTOSCOPY AND ACOUSTIC IMMITTANCE

Tympanometry has proven to be superior to routine otoscopy in correctly predicting the absence or presence of middle-ear effusion. For example, Swogger and Brenman (1975) reported a predictive accuracy of 97% for tympanometry and only 87% for otoscopy, when the presence or absence of middle-ear effusion was established by myringotomy performed immediately after the tympanometric and otoscopic measurements on 150 ears of 75 children between the ages of 3 months and 3 years. Similar findings were obtained by Rosenberg, Brenman, and Rosenberg (1978) who examined the predictive accuracy of tympanometry and otoscopy on 150 ears of 75 patients under 2 years of age with bilateral myringotomies. Tympanometry correctly predicted the absence or presence of middle-ear effusion in 93%; otoscopy correctly predicted the absence or presence of middle-ear effusion in 84%.

Two factors underlie the false-negative rate for otoscopy with respect to the identification of middle-ear effusion.

1. Otoscopic assessment relies on subjective assessment of the position, color, translucency, vascularity, and mobility of the tympanic membrane. Therefore, the clinical experience will introduce interphysician variability in otoscopic assessment (Stool, 1984). This point is illustrated in the study by Roeser *et al.* (1978), who reported poor interexaminer agreement for routine otoscopy on children. For example, agreement between tympanometry and otoscopy on a

population of 30 ears with type C tympanograms was 47% for an otolaryngologist with 10 years of clinical experience and 73% for a pediatrician with 7 years of clinical experience.

2. When determining the mobility of the tympanic membrane using a rubber bulb, the physician, in cases of complete middle-ear effusion, may apply excessive pressure on the bulb, forcing some movement of the tympanic membrane leading to the erroneous conclusion that the tympanic membrane is almost normal (Stool, 1984).

Some small perforations cannot be identified with routine otoscopy. These small perforations can be identified with acoustic-immittance testing. Acoustic-immittance findings consistent with the presence of a tympanic-membrane perforation include flat tympanogram, large physical volume, or the inability to establish or maintain a seal during tympanometry.

In adults, there is good agreement between the otoscopic findings and the tympanometric peak pressure. Several investigators determined the cutoff tympanometric peak pressure in adults which separates normal ears from ears with negative middle-ear pressure on the basis of otoscopic findings (Holmquist & Miller, 1972; Peterson & Liden, 1972).

In children, however, there is a lack of agreement between the otoscopic findings and the tympanometric peak pressure. For example, in the study by Roeser *et al.* (1978) on children, 27 of the 39 ears with tympanometric peak pressures between −100 and −200 daPa were otoscopically normal. Investigators who attempted to define the normal tympanometric peak-pressure range in children established the tympanometric peak-pressure limits on the basis of nonmedical criteria such as the range of tympanometric peak pressures associated with the absence of the acoustic reflex, the range of peak pressures encompassing 90% of the sample, or the range of peak pressures associated with significant air–bone gaps (Brooks, 1969; Jerger, 1970; Liden & Renvall, 1978; Renvall & Liden, 1978). Also, as already mentioned in the section on pressure, artifacts associated with the AGC circuitry in electroacoustic-immittance devices, the introduction of negative pressure in the ear canal during tympanometric assessment when there is retraction of the tympanic membrane, and the flaccidity of the tympanic membrane exaggerate the tympanometric peak pressure; this exaggeration is more significant in children than in adults since the former commonly have transient negative middle-ear pressure.

The advantage of tympanometry over otoscopy is apparent in disorders such as ossicular discontinuity and ossicular fixation, which can often be identified when comparing low-frequency probe-tone tympanograms with high-frequency probe-tone tympanograms, as discussed earlier in this chapter.

Otoscopy, but not tympanometry, is capable of detecting retraction pockets in the pars flaccida which can result in an acquired cholesteatoma (Stool, 1984). Otoscopy is superior to tympanometry using the 220-Hz probe tone in the identification of middle-ear masses not involving the ossicular chain. (Of course, middle-ear masses involving the ossicular chain can be detected with tympanometry using the 220-Hz probe tone.) Research is needed on the accuracy of otoscopy and tympanometry with high-frequency probe tones in the identification of middle-ear masses not involving the ossicular chain.

H. DETECTING MIDDLE-EAR EFFUSION IN CHILDREN

In the previous section (II.B.) on pressure, it was mentioned that the middle-ear pressure in children is often exaggeratedly negative because children often have negative middle-ear pressure which is artifactually made more negative during the tympanometric procedure (for determining the typanometric peak pressure). It is important to differentiate between this artifactually exaggerated negative middle-ear pressure which does not coexist with middle-ear effusion and nonartifactually exaggerated negative middle-ear pressure coexisting with middle-ear effusion which may have adverse effects on speech-language function, academic achievement, and health.

Because of the problem of recording an artifactually exaggerated negative middle-ear pressure in some children with negative middle-ear pressure during tympanometry, recent reports (ASHA Committee on Audiologic Evaluation-Working Group on Acoustic Immittance Measurement, 1989) suggest elimination of the tympanometric peak pressure for detection of middle-ear effusion. Margolis and Heller (1987) and the ASHA Committee on Audiologic Evaluation-Working Group on Acoustic Immittance Measurement (1989) recommended using the tympanometric gradient and static-acoustic middle-ear admittance in place of the tympanometric peak pressure for identification of middle-ear effusion. ASHA (1989) proposed that a tympanometric gradient >150 daPa or static-acoustic middle-ear admittance <0.2 mmhos (with ear-canal volume measured at +200 daPa) is consistent with middle-ear effusion. ASHA (1989) further proposed that acoustic-immittance screening be done using an absolute acoustic-immittance device. These ASHA (1989) proposed guidelines have not been clinically evaluated until very recently (Silman & Silverman, 1990).

As well as recommending the elimination of the tympanometric peak-pressure measure, ASHA (1989) also recommended the abolition of the acoustic-reflex measure based on the high false-positive rates associated with acoustic-immittance screening protocols involving the acoustic reflex such as the ASHA (1979) screening protocol

(Lous, 1983; Roush & Tait, 1985). Reasons for the high false-positive rates for the acoustic-immittance screening protocols based solely on the contralateral acoustic reflex in children include the following:

1. The status of the earphone ear affects whether an acoustic reflex will be monitored in the probe ear;

2. Collapsed ear canals are associated with absent or elevated acoustic reflexes;

3. A maturation effect is present for the contralateral acoustic reflex whereby the contralateral acoustic-reflex thresholds are elevated in children as compared with young adults; and

4. Ninety-five percent of the children with absent middle-ear effusion but with minimal eardrum abnormalities investigated by Hall and Weaver (1979) have contralateral acoustic reflexes for the tonal activators present at levels less than or equal to 107 dB HL.

Reasons for the high false-positive rates for screening protocols based solely on the ipsilateral acoustic-reflex threshold measure include the following:

1. The cutoff level of the 105 dB SPL is excessively low. This level was selected by ASHA (1979) to avoid possible artifacts and because commercial instrumentation available at that time had low maximum output intensities for ipsilateral acoustic-reflex assessment.

2. A maturation effect may be present for the ipsilateral acoustic reflex, similar to that for the contralateral acoustic reflex. Although this effect has not yet been investigated with respect to the ipsilateral reflex, this effect must be considered as a potential factor in the high false-positive rates associated with acoustic-reflex screening in children.

Even before the ASHA (1989) proposed guidelines, the ipsilateral acoustic-reflex measure tended not to be used for acoustic-immittance screening because studies showed that additive and subtractive artifacts can occur during ipsilateral acoustic-reflex measurement even at levels below 105 dB SPL (Kunov, 1977; Lutman, 1980; Lutman & Leis, 1980). Also, many commercially available acoustic-immittance screening devices in the early to mid 1980s had the capacity for contralateral but not ipsilateral acoustic-reflex threshold assessment.

Fiellau-Nikolajsen (1983) conducted a longitudinal study on the acoustic-immittance findings in 88 ears of 44 children with and without middle-ear effusion at myringotomy. The following acoustic-immittance criteria for middle-ear effusion were evaluated: (a) tympanometric-peak pressure <= −100 daPa or flat tympanogram, (b) tympanometric-peak pressure <= −200 daPa or flat tympanogram, (c) flat tympanogram, (d) flat tympanogram on the one hand or, on the other hand, tympanometric peak pressure $<= -100$ daPa together with an absent ipsilateral acoustic reflex for the 1000-Hz tonal activator at 100 dB SPL. According to Fiellau-Nikolajsen (1983), a flat tympanogram is one with either an absent tympanometric peak pressure or a gradient less than or equal to 0.1. Gradient was defined as the ratio AG—the distance from the tympanometric peak to the horizontal line intersecting the tympanogram such that the pressure interval between the intersection points is 100 daPa—to AC—the maximal height at the tympanometric peak. Table XI shows the sensitivity and specificity of these acoustic-immittance parameters with respect to middle-ear effusion. As can be seen from this table, criterion "d" (IV in Table XI) was associated with the highest combined sensitivity (96%) and specificity (98%). The low specificity for criterion "a" (I in Table XI) reaffirms our contention stated earlier in Sections II,B,3 and II,B,4 that negative tympanometric peak pressure as an isolated criterion is associated with a high false-positive rate with respect to middle-ear effusion. Since Fiellau-Nikolajsen's (1983) study was done using a relative acoustic-immittance device, the findings cannot be generalized to absolute acoustic-immittance devices.

Silman and Silverman (1990) evaluated the effectiveness of the ASHA (1989) proposed procedure adjusted for the pump speed of 50 daPa/s. As ASHA (1989) recommended the obtaining of normative data whenever other combinations of ear-canal correction and/or pump speed are employed, Silman and Silverman (1990) obtained 90% ranges for static-acoustic middle-ear admittance and tympanometric gradient using the pump speed of 50 daPa/s; similar to ASHA (1989), equivalent ear-canal volume was estimated at +200 daPa using an absolute acoustic-immittance device. The normative sample was composed of 42 ears of 42 subjects ranging in age from 3 to 10 years. Based on this normative sample, the 90% range (5th to 95th

percentile) for static-acoustic middle-ear admittance was 0.35 to 1.25 mmhos and the 90% range (5th to 95th percentile) for tympanometric gradient, as defined by the ASHA (1989) proposed guidelines, was 55 to 180 daPa.

Since tympanometric peak pressure and the ipsilateral acoustic reflex were measures excluded in the ASHA (1989) proposed guidelines, Silman and Silverman (1990) also evaluated the sensitivity and specificity of these measures in the middle-ear effusion and control group samples. The tympanometric peak pressure was considered to be significantly negative if it was less than or equal to -100 daPa (Jerger, 1970). The ipsilateral acoustic reflex was considered to be abnormal if it was absent at 1000 Hz at 110 dB HL (117 dB SPL) for the Grason-Stadler 1723 acoustic-immittance device. This level controlled for the effects of maturation and minimal eardrum abnormalities.

Silman and Silverman's (1990) middle-ear effusion sample was composed of 82 ears and 54 subjects ranging in age from 3 to 11 years. The control sample was composed of 53 ears of 53 subjects ranging in age from 3 to 10 years. Middle-ear effusion was established based on micro-otoscopy and pneumatic otoscopy performed by otolaryngologists with at least 10 years of experience. Acoustic-immittance measurements were accomplished using a Grason-Stadler 1723 absolute acoustic-immittance device with a multiplexing circuit to eliminate additive and subtractive artifacts during ipsilateral acoustic-reflex assessment. This device also has a high output level (117 dB SPL) for ipsilateral acoustic-reflex measurement. Data were collected prospectively.

With respect to the total sample of ears with middle-ear effusion, the sensitivity was 89% and 92.5% for the tympanometric peak-pressure and ipsilateral acoustic-reflex measures, respectively as compared with 81.5% for the ASHA (1989) proposed guidelines. With respect to the middle-ear subgroup having a hearing-threshold level

Table XI Validation of Tympanometric Diagnosis of Middle-Ear Effusion in Relation to Findings for 88 Myringotomies in 44 Three-Year-Old Children (Study G)[a]

		Middle-ear effusion seen on tympanogram						
		YES		NO				
		Seen at myringotomy		Seen at myringotomy				
		YES	NO	YES	NO	Sensitivity	Specificity	Accuracy
I	Middle-ear pressure ≤ -100 mm H$_2$O, or flat curve	44	15	2	27	96%	64%	81%
II	Middle-ear pressure ≤ -200 mm H$_2$O, or flat curve	42	5	4	37	91%	88%	90%
III	Flat curve	38	0	8	42	83%	100%	91%
IV	Flat curve, or pressure ≤ -100 mm H$_2$O comb, with absent middle-ear reflexes	44	1	2	41	96%	98%	97%

[a] Reprinted with permission from Fiellau-Nikolajsen (1983).

> 20 dB HL at 1000, 2000, and/or 4000 Hz, the sensitivity was 98% and 93% for the tympanometric peak-pressure and ipsilateral acoustic-reflex measures, respectively as compared with 93% for the ASHA (1989) proposed guidelines. With respect to the middle-ear effusion subgroup having hearing-threshold levels <= 20 dB HL at 1000, 2000, and 4000 Hz, the sensitivity dropped to 79% for the tympanometric peak-pressure measure but remained high (94.5%) for the ipsilateral acoustic-reflex measure as compared with the low sensitivity of 63% for the ASHA (1989) proposed guidelines. With respect to the control group, the specificity was slightly higher for the tympanometric peak-pressure and ipsilateral acoustic-reflex measures (83% for the former and 84% for the latter) than for the ASHA (1989) proposed guidelines (79%). The striking finding is the markedly increased sensitivity for the ipsilateral acoustic-reflex measure as compared with the ASHA (1989) proposed guidelines and tympanometric peak-pressure measure in the middle-ear subgroup with normal-hearing thresholds.

Silman and Silverman (1990) also evaluated the sensitivity and specificity of (a) the combined nonASHA (1989) measures whereby middle-ear effusion suspected if there was a significantly negative tympanometric peak pressure less than or equal to −100 daPa and the ipsilateral acoustic reflex was absent at 1000 Hz, and (b) a modification of the ASHA (1989) proposed guidelines whereby middle-ear effusion was suspected if the ASHA (1989) proposed guidelines were failed and the ipsilateral acoustic reflex was absent at 1000 Hz. With respect to the total sample of middle-ear effusion ears, the sensitivity was 75.5% for the modified ASHA guidelines and 84% for the combined nonASHA (1989) measures as compared with 81.5% for the ASHA (1989) proposed guidelines. With respect to the middle-ear effusion subgroup having a hearing-threshold level > 20 dB HL at 1000, 2000, and/or 4000 Hz, the sensitivity was 88% for the modified ASHA guidelines and 91% for the combined nonASHA (1989) measures as compared with 93% for the ASHA (1989) proposed guidelines. With respect to the middle-ear effusion subgroup having hearing-threshold levels <= 20 dB HL at 1000, 2000, and 4000 Hz, the sensitivity was 58% for the modified ASHA guidelines and 79% for the combined nonASHA measures as compared with 63% for the ASHA guidelines. With respect to the control group, the specificity was 94% for the modified ASHA guidelines and 92% for the combined nonASHA measures compared with 79% for the ASHA (1989) proposed guidelines.

If acoustic-immittance screening is performed in conjunction with audiometric hearing screening, then audiometric screening will detect middle-ear effusion ears with poorer than 20 dB HL thresholds at 1000, 2000, and/or 4000 Hz but will miss middle-ear effusion ears with hearing-threshold levels less than or equal to 20 dB HL at these

frequencies. The most important, middle-ear effusion group then, for evaluation of acoustic-immittance screening procedures, is the middle-ear effusion subgroup having hearing-threshold levels <= 20 dB HL at 1000, 2000, and 4000 Hz. For this group, when comparing the ASHA (1989) with the modified ASHA guidelines and the combined nonASHA measures, highest sensitivity was obtained for the combined nonASHA measures; specificity was markedly higher for the modified ASHA and combined nonASHA measures than the ASHA (1989) proposed guidelines.

Silman and Silverman (1990) then evaluated the effectiveness of failing either the modified ASHA procedure or the combined nonASHA measures. That is, failure of the ASHA (1989) proposed guidelines together with absence of the ipsilateral acoustic reflex at 1000 Hz or, on the other hand, having a significantly negative tympanometric peak press <= −100 daPa together with absence of the ipsilateral acoustic reflex at 1000 Hz. With respect to the total sample of middle-ear effusion ears, the sensitivity was 90% as compared with 75.5% for the modified ASHA method, 84% for the combined nonASHA measures, and 81.5% for the ASHA (1989) proposed guidelines. With respect to the subgroup of middle-ear effusion ears having hearing-threshold levels >20 dB HL at 1000, 2000, and/or 4000 Hz the sensitivity was 91% as compared with 88% for the modified ASHA method, 91% for the combined nonASHA measures, and 93% for the ASHA (1989) proposed guidelines. With respect to the subgroup of ears with middle-ear effusion having hearing-threshold levels <= 20 dB HL at 1000, 2000, and 4000 Hz, the sensitivity was 89.5% as compared with 58% for the modified ASHA method, 79% for the combined nonASHA measures, and 63% for the ASHA (1989) proposed guidelines. With respect to the control group, the specificity was 92.5% as compared with 94% for the modified ASHA method, 92% for the combined nonASHA measures, and 79% for the ASHA (1989) proposed guidelines. Note that screening based on both the modified ASHA method and the combined nonASHA measures yields higher sensitivity for a total middle-ear effusion group, approximately equal sensitivity for the middle-ear subgroup with greater than 20 dB HL at 1000, 2000, or 4000 Hz, markedly higher sensitivity for the middle-ear subgroup with <= 20 dB HL at 1000, 2000, and 4000 Hz, and markedly higher specificity than the ASHA (1989) proposed guidelines. Also, acoustic-immittance screening based on the modified ASHA (1989) method and the combined nonASHA measures yields a markedly higher sensitivity than the modified ASHA procedure or the combined nonASHA measures and a specificity that is approximately equal to the modified ASHA procedure as well as the combined nonASHA guidelines. Therefore, it appears that for the middle-ear subgroup with hearing-threshold levels <= 20 dB HL, the modified ASHA procedure and the combined nonASHA measures supplement each other with respect to identification of ears with middle-ear effusion. That is, the modified ASHA guidelines miss ears with middle-ear effusion which have significantly negative tympanometric peak pressure together with an absent ipsilateral acoustic reflex but also have normal tympanometric gradient and static-acoustic middle-ear admittance. On the other hand, the combined nonASHA measures miss ears with middle-ear effusion which have abnormal tympanometric gradient or static-acoustic admittance but which also have normal tympanometric peak pressure.

Based on Silman and Silverman's (1990) findings using an absolute acoustic-immittance device, middle-ear effusion should be suspected if the ASHA (1989) proposed guidelines are failed and the ipsilateral acoustic reflex at 1000 Hz is absent or, on the other hand, if the tympanometric peak pressure is less than or equal to −100 daPa and the ipsilateral acoustic reflex at 1000 Hz is absent. Silman and Silverman's (1990) findings highlight the effectiveness of the tympanometric peak pressure and ipsilateral acoustic-reflex measures in combination for the detection of middle-ear effusion. The sensitivity and specificity of the combined tympanometric peak pressure and ipsilateral acoustic-reflex measures are greater than those of either the tympanometric peak-pressure measure or the ipsilateral acoustic-reflex measure. Silman and Silverman's (1990) findings support the earlier classical studies by Jerger (1970) and Jerger et al. (1974a) which showed that middle-ear effusion is best predicted by a combination of rather than a single acoustic-immittance parameter and that middle-ear effusion may be present in cases of negative tympanometric peak pressure with normal static-acoustic middle-ear admittance. Based on Fiellau-Nikolajsen's (1983) findings using a relative acoustic-immittance device, middle-ear effusion should be suspected if (a) the tympanometric peak pressure is absent or the tympanometric gradient is less than or equal to 0.1, or (b) tympanometric peak pressure is less than or equal to −100 daPa and the ipsilateral acoustic reflex is absent at 1000 Hz at 100 dB SPL.

Although these procedures were developed for the purpose of mass screenings, these recommended screening protocols can also be employed by the clinician within the context of a complete, diagnostic, audiologic evaluation for the purpose of identification of middle-ear effusion in children between 2 months and 10 years of age.

I. ASSESSMENT OF EUSTACHIAN-TUBE FUNCTION

Several researchers have stated that Eustachian-tube dysfunction is a precursor of middle-ear effusion (Bluestone & Beery, 1976; Bluestone & Cantekin, 1981; Cantekin, Beery, & Bluestone, 1977). According to Bluestone (1980), abnormal function of the Eustachian tube can result from obstruction or abnormal patency. Functional obstruction reflects persistent Eustachian-tube collapse because of increased tubal compliance or an inadequate opening mechanism. This occurs commonly in children because their Eustachian tubes are characterized by less stiff cartilages and less efficient tensor veli palatini muscles than those of adults. In cases of functional obstruction of the Eustachian tube, there is a lack of intermittent active opening of the tube. Opening of the tube occurs when negative middle-ear pressure develops, resulting in a pressure gradient between the nasopharynx and middle ear such that there is sufficiently positive pressure in the nasopharynx (relative to the middle ear) to force open the Eustachian tube. This ventilation mechanism is characteristic of many children with normal middle ears (Beery et al., 1973). Bluestone (1980) refers to this functional obstruction of the Eustachian tube as atelectasis. Intrinsic mechanical obstruction of the Eustachian tube results from inflammation of the tube (Bluestone, 1980). Extrinsic mechanical obstruction of the Eustachian tube results from nasopharyngeal tumors or enlarged adenoids (Bluestone, 1980). A Eustachian tube is considered abnormally patent if it is constantly open, even at rest.

Eustachian-tube testing has been done to identify abnormal Eustachian-tube function, to differentiate functional obstruction from mechanical obstruction, and to differentiate obstruction from abnormal patency. Medical management of the patient may depend on whether the obstruction is functional or mechanical. Serial Eustachian-tube testing in cases with tympanostomy tubes may provide information concerning when tubal function returns to normal, thereby guiding the physician in determining when the tubes should be removed. Eustachian-tube testing has also been done to monitor Eustachian-tube functioning following cleft-palate repair, adenoidectomy, and elimination of nasal and nasopharyngeal inflammation (Bluestone, Paradise, Beery, & Wittel, 1972; Bluestone, Cantekin, & Beery, 1975; Bluestone, Cantekin, & Beery, 1977). Holmquist (1968) and Siedentop, Tardy, and Hamilton (1968) used the Eustachian-tube results in patients with chronic perforation of the tympanic membrane to predict the success of myringoplastic surgery.

Eustachian-tube testing has not gained clinical acceptance in most clinical settings (Givens & Seidemann, 1984; Riedel, Wiley, & Block, 1987). Normative data in children are lacking. Normative data in adults were lacking until recently (Riedel et al., 1987). Standardized protocols and procedures were unavailable until the recent report by Riedel et al. (1987). These normative data and standardized protocols in adults have not yet been applied to pathological ears so the sensitivity, specificity, and efficiency of these Eustachian-tube tests remain unknown. Therefore, until research is done on pathological ears in adults and children and normative data are obtained in children, Eustachian-tube testing should not be a part of routine acoustic-immittance assessment.

We suggest that, if Eustachian-tube testing is done, it should be done only as an elective procedure or upon the physician's request in adults, for example, in cases of middle-ear effusion to help differentiate functional from mechanical obstruction, tympanostomy tubes, cleft-palate repair, adenoidectomy, elimination of nasal and nasopharyngeal inflammation, and tympanoplasty.

1. PROTOCOL AND PROCEDURES

a. Valsalva

Riedel et al. (1987) suggested that a baseline admittance tympanogram for the 220-Hz probe tone be obtained for the Valsalva maneuver. The patient is then instructed to pinch the nares and inflate the cheeks through forced expiration with the mouth closed until the ears feel full. The patient is then asked to release the nose and to refrain from swallowing. Another admittance tympanogram is then obtained for the 220-Hz probe tone. Riedel et al. (1987) reported that the 95% confidence interval in adults with normal middle-ear function for the shift in tympanometric peak pressure during this maneuver was 47 to 79 daPa; in 94%, the shift in tympanometric peak pressure (>2 daPa) was in the positive direction. Riedel et al. (1987) suggested that, if the purpose is to confirm tubal functioning (opening), then a shift in either direction should be accepted. By this criterion, 98% demonstrated a shift in tympanometric peak pressure. The greatest shift in tympanometric peak pressure was induced with this procedure, as opposed to the Toynbee, Inflation, and Deflation procedures. Riedel et al. (1987) considered the Valsalva procedure to be the best for producing reliable and interpretable results in adults with normal middle ears.

b. Toynbee

Riedel et al. (1987) suggested that a baseline admittance tympanogram for the 220-Hz probe tone be obtained for the Toynbee maneuver. The patient is then asked to swallow while pinching the nares. Afterward, the patient is to release the nares and not swallow. Another admittance tympanogram is recorded. The 95% confidence interval in adults for the shift in tympanometric peak pressure was −26 to −4 daPa. Thus, a smaller shift was seen for this procedure than for the Valsalva. In 67% of the patients, the shift in tympanometric peak pressure was in the negative direction. A shift (>2 daPa) was seen in 96% of the patients. Riedel et al. (1987) concluded that, although the Toynbee procedure could be used to establish tubal functioning (opening) reliably, it was an unreliable measure for inducing negative middle-ear pressure in order to equilibrate abnormal positive middle-ear pressure.

c. Inflation

Riedel et al. (1987) suggested obtaining a baseline admittance tympanogram for the 220-Hz probe tone for the inflation maneuver. Ear-canal pressure is then increased to

+400 daPa. The patient is then asked to swallow several times with water. Another tympanogram is then recorded. The 95% confidence interval for the shift in tympanometric peak pressure using this procedure was −6 to 0 daPa. Because the shift in tympanometric peak pressure was so small, Riedel et al. (1987) concluded that the inflation procedure lacked usefulness as a test of Eustachian-tube function. With the inflation procedure, a shift (>2 daPa) in the expected negative direction was obtained in 83% of the subjects. This procedure was the least successful of the Eustachian-tube procedures evaluated by Riedel et al. (1987) in yielding a significant tympanometric peak-pressure shift or producing a shift in the negative direction.

Bluestone (1980) recommended the following inflation procedure in cases with nonintact tympanic membranes.

1. Ear-canal pressure is increased until the pressure indicator deflects in the direction back to 0 daPa (indicating the forced opening of the Eustachian tube).
2. If the pressure indicator does not return to 0 daPa, the patient is then asked to swallow. The clinician then observes whether the pressure indicator returns to 0 daPa. If the patient is unable to equilibrate the pressure completely, then it is assumed that the patient has Eustachian-tube dysfunction.

d. Deflation

The same procedure as for the inflation procedure is employed except that, in the ear-canal, pressure is decreased to −400 daPa rather than increased to +400 daPa. Similarly, if the deflation procedure is employed in ears with nonintact tympanic membranes, the same procedure as for the inflation procedure is employed (Bluestone, 1980) except that the ear-canal pressure is decreased rather than increased until the pressure indicator deflects toward 0 daPa. Riedel et al. (1987) reported that the 95% confidence interval for the shift in tympanometric peak pressure with this deflation procedure was 12 to 18 daPa. In 90%, the shift was in the expected positive direction. Similar to the inflation procedure, the deflation procedure produced only a small shift in the tympanometric peak pressure.

J. PROPOSED CLASSIFICATION OF ACOUSTIC-IMMITTANCE RESULTS WITH RESPECT TO MIDDLE-EAR FUNCTIONING

In his classical paper, Jerger (1970) categorized the tympanometric results into five types. Type A, similar to Type 1 in Figure 22, represents tympanograms having the point of greatest acoustic admittance within +100 daPa with a large, inverted-V shape. Type A tympanograms were considered to be characteristic of normal middle ears. Type As, similar to Type 2 in Figure 22, represents a shallower version of the Type A tympanogram. Type As tympanograms were often associated with ears having ossicular fixation. Type Ad tympanograms, similar to Type 3 in Figure 22, represent tympanograms in which the positive and negative sides of the inverted V do not meet. Type Ad tympanograms were associated with ossicular discontinuity or flaccid tympanic membranes. Type B tympanograms, similar to Type 4 in Figure 22, represented tympanograms without a tympanometric peak pressure. Type B tympanograms were associated with a fluid-filled middle ear or one with massive ossicular fixation. Type C, similar to pattern 5 in Figure 2, reflects tympanograms having a shape like that of Type A but with a peak admittance at pressures below −100 daPa. Type C tympanograms were associated with negative middle-ear pressure resulting from Eustachian-tube dysfunction.

Jerger's (1970) classifications were based on the use of a relative acoustic-immittance device and the 220-Hz probe tone. As shown throughout this chapter, tympanograms generally cannot be interpreted adequately unless more than one acoustic-immittance component is recorded and more than one probe tone is employed (i.e., one high-frequency and one low-frequency probe tone) and the tympanograms are interpreted in light of the tympanometric gradient, the static acoustic middle-ear admittance, and contralateral and ipsilateral acoustic-reflex thresholds.

As mentioned earlier, because of the overlap in the static acoustic middle-ear admittance between the pathological and normal ears, the problems related to the middle-ear pressure in children, and the contribution of the 660-Hz susceptance and conductance tympanograms in resolving these problems, the following classification system is proposed. The proposed classification system is based on the findings for the 220-Hz probe tone unless otherwise specified.

1. INFANTS FROM BIRTH TO 2 MONTHS OF AGE

Regardless of the tympanometric peak pressure, and provided the tympanogram is not flat, if the contralateral or ipsilateral acoustic reflex is present for the 1000-Hz tonal activator or BBN activator and for the 220-Hz or 660-Hz probe tone, then the results are consistent with normal middle-ear functioning.

Either of the following is consistent with the presence of middle-ear effusion: (a) absence of the contralateral and ipsilateral acoustic reflexes for the 1000-Hz tonal and BBN activator for the 220-, 660-, and 1000-Hz (if available) probe-tone frequencies and tympanometric peak pressure more negative than −100 daPa, or (b) flat tympanogram. Middle-ear effusion cannot be ruled out if the ipsilateral and contralateral acoustic reflexes for both probe tones are absent and the tympanometric peak pressure is greater than or equal to −100 daPa.

2. CHILDREN BETWEEN 2 MONTHS AND 10 YEARS OF AGE

If the tympanometric pattern is type 1 and the ipsilateral (probe in the ear under investigation) acoustic reflex is

present for the 1000-Hz tonal activator, the results should be considered as consistent with the absence of middle-ear effusion regardless of the tympanometric gradient or static-acoustic middle-ear admittance. The selection of −100 daPa as the cutoff point for normal middle-ear pressure in children is essentially based on the finding by Jerger (1970) and Fiellau-Nikolajsen (1983) that negative middle-ear pressure less than (more negative than) −100 daPa may be associated with middle-ear effusion depending on whether other acoustic-admittance measures are abnormal.

If the tympanometric pattern is type 5 the ipsilateral (probe in ear with negative tympanometric peak pressure) acoustic reflex for the 1000-Hz tonal activator is present and air-bone gaps are absent, then these results should be considered as possibly consistent with Eustachian-tube dysfunction; a child with these results should be considered to be at low-risk for middle-ear effusion.

For an absolute acoustic-immittance device with a pump speed of 50 daPa/s and equivalent ear-canal volume estimated at +200 daPa, any one or more of the following is consistent with the presence of middle-ear effusion provided that tympanic-membrane perforation, cerumen in the ear canal, and technical factors are ruled out: (a) tympanometric gradient > 180 daPa or < 55 daPa or static-acoustic middle-ear admittance < 0.35 mmho together with an absent ipsilateral acoustic reflex at 1000 Hz at 117 dB SPL, or (b) tympanometric peak pressure <= −100 daPa together with an absent ipsilateral acoustic reflex at 1000 Hz at 117 dB SPL.

For a relative acoustic-immittance device, any one or more of the following should be considered as consistent with middle-ear effusion: (a) absent tympanometric peak pressure or a tympanometric gradient less than or equal to 0.1, or (b) tympanometric peak pressure less than or equal to −100 daPa and the ipsilateral acoustic reflex is absent at 1000 Hz.

If the tympanometric pattern is type 2, contralateral ART for the 1000-Hz tonal activator (probe in the ear with the type 2 tympanometric pattern) is absent, ipsilateral acoustic reflex for the 1000-Hz tonal activator (probe in the ear with the type 2 tympanometric pattern) is absent, and significant air-bone gaps are present, then the results are consistent with ossicular fixation. If information concerning the air-bone gaps cannot be obtained, then the presence of significant sensorineural hearing impairment must be ruled out.

If the tympanometric pattern is type 1 or 3, the susceptance and conductance tympanograms for the 660-Hz probe tone are abnormal with respect to Vanhuyse et al.'s (1975) criteria, and significant air–bone gaps are present, these results are consistent with ossicular discontinuity. If the contralateral ART is present at normal or elevated levels for the 1000-Hz tonal activator (probe in the ear with the abnormal tympanograms), then the results are consistent with the presence of ossicular discontinuity medial to the site of insertion of the stapedius muscle in the ear with the abnormal tympanograms. If the contralateral ART is absent for the 1000-Hz tonal activator, (probe in the ear with the abnormal tympanograms), then the results are consistent with the presence of ossicular discontinuity lateral to the site of insertion of the stapedius muscle in the ear with the abnormal tympanograms. If the acoustic-immittance device does not permit obtaining 660-Hz susceptance and conductance tympanograms, then a type 1 or 3 tympanogram with significant air–bone gaps should be considered consistent with the presence of either ossicular discontinuity or ossicular fixation (with a flaccid tympanic membrane or membrane with a healed perforation in the case of the type 3 tympanometric pattern).

If the tympanometric pattern is type 1 or 3, the susceptance and conductance tympanograms for the 660-Hz probe tone are normal according to Vanhuyse et al.'s (1975) criteria, the contralateral ART is elevated or absent for the 1000-Hz tonal activator (probe in the ear with the type 1 or 3 tympanogram), the ipsilateral ART for the 1000-Hz tonal activator is absent (probe in the ear with the type 1 or 3 tympanometric pattern), and significant air–bone gaps are present, then the results are consistent with both ossicular fixation (and a flaccid tympanic membrane or membrane with healed perforation in the case of type 3 tympanometric pattern) in the ear with the type 1 or 3 tympanometric pattern.

If the tympanometric pattern is type 3, and significant air–bone gaps are absent, then the results are consistent with the presence of a flaccid tympanic membrane or a tympanic membrane with a healed perforation and an otherwise normal middle ear.

Although only the 1000-Hz tonal activator is recommended for classification of middle-ear function in children, the audiologist is encouraged to obtain the ARTs for all tonal activators (500-, 1000-, and 2000-Hz) for interpretation of disorders other than middle-ear disorders.

3. ADULTS

If the tympanometric pattern is type 1, the contralateral ARTs for the 500-, 1000-, and 2000-Hz activators are present at normal levels bilaterally, the ipsilateral ARTs for the tonal activators are present, and no significant air–bone gaps are present, then the results are consistent with normal middle-ear functioning.

If the tympanometric pattern is type 5, contralateral ARTs are elevated or absent for the tonal activators (probe in the ear with the negative tympanometric peak pressure), and ipsilateral ARTs for the tonal activators are elevated or absent, (probe in the ear with the negative tympanometric peak pressure), then the results are consistent with Eustachian-tube dysfunction with or without middle-ear effusion.

If the tympanometric pattern is type 4, the results are consistent with middle-ear effusion provided that the presence of tympanic-membrane perforation, cerumen in the ear canal, and technical factors have been ruled out.

If the tympanometric pattern is type 2, contralateral ARTs for the tonal activators are elevated or absent (probe in the ear with the type 2 pattern), the ipsilateral ARTs for the tonal activators are elevated or absent, (probe in the ear with the type 2 pattern), and significant air–bone gaps are present, then the results are consistent with ossicular fixation.

If the tympanometric pattern is type 1 or 3, the susceptance and conductance tympanograms for the 660-Hz probe tone are abnormal with respect to Vanhuyse et al.'s (1975) criteria, and significant air–bone gaps are present, then the results are consistent with ossicular discontinuity. If the contralateral ARTs are present at normal or elevated levels for the tonal activators (probe in the ear with the abnormal tympanograms), then the results are consistent with the presence of ossicular discontinuity medial to the site of insertion of the stapedius muscle in the ear with the abnormal tympanograms. If the contralateral ARTs are absent for the tonal activators (probe in the ear with the abnormal tympanograms), then the results are consistent with the presence of ossicular discontinuity lateral to the site of insertion of the stapedius muscle in the ear with the abnormal tympanograms.

If the tympanometric pattern is type 1 or 3, susceptance and conductance tympanograms for the 660-Hz probe tone are normal according to Vanhuyse et al.'s (1975) criteria, contralateral ARTs are elevated or absent for the tonal activators (probe in the ear with the type 1 or 3 pattern), ipsilateral ARTs for the tonal activators are absent or elevated, (probe in the ear with the type 1 or 3 tympanometric pattern), and significant air–bone gaps are present, then the results are consistent with ossicular fixation (with a flaccid tympanic membrane or tympanic membrane with a healed perforation in the case of the type 3 pattern) in the ear with the air-bone gaps. If the acoustic-immittance device does not permit obtaining 660-Hz susceptance and conductance tympanograms, then a type 1 or 3 tympanometric pattern, elevated or absent contralateral acoustic-reflex thresholds for the tonal activators (probe in the ear with the air-bone gaps), absent ipsilateral acoustic reflexes for the tonal activators (probe in the ear with the air-bone gaps), and significant air–bone gaps are consistent with the presence of either ossicular discontinuity or ossicular fixation (with a flaccid tympanic membrane or membrane with a healed perforation in the case of the type 3 tympanometric pattern) in the ear with the air-bone gaps.

If the tympanometric pattern is type 3, and significant air–bone gaps are absent, then the results are consistent with the presence of a flaccid tympanic membrane or a tympanic membrane with a healed perforation and an otherwise normal middle ear.

So far we have discussed acoustic-immittance findings for a single isolated middle-ear disorder such as middle-ear effusion, ossicular discontinuity, or ossicular fixation. When two or more middle-ear disorders are present in the same ear, the interpretation becomes more complex. When a type 5 tympanometric pattern is present with significant air-bone gaps, the presence of dual middle-ear pathology should be ruled out using high-frequency tympanometry. Of course, when high-frequency tympanometry is abnormal, the clinician will not be able to determine whether the negative tympanometric peak pressure is consistent with middle-ear effusion or negative middle-ear pressure without middle-ear effusion based on the acoustic reflex since the acoustic reflex will be absent because of the other pathology—the ossicular discontinuity. When high-frequency tympanometry is normal, on the other hand, differentiation cannot be made among Eustachian-tube dysfunction in isolation and combined Eustachian-tube dysfunction with ossicular fixation.

K. MEDICAL REFERRAL IN CASES OF SUSPECTED MIDDLE-EAR PATHOLOGY

Infants should be referred for otolaryngologic followup if any of the following findings are obtained: (a) flat tympanogram, (b) absence of all tonal and BBN activators at the 220-Hz, 660-Hz, and 1000-Hz (if available) probe-tone frequencies, for ipsilateral and contralateral stimulation.

Children between 2 months and 10 years of age should be referred for acoustic-immittance re-evaluation in 3 months, if no medical complaints were present, otoscopic inspection did not reveal any unusual findings, no significant air-bone gaps were present and any one or more of the following acoustic-immittance results were obtained at the initial evaluation: For a relative acoustic-immittance device, (a) absent tympanometric peak pressure or a tympanometric gradient less than or equal to 0.1, or (b) tympanometric peak pressure less than or equal to −100 daPa and an absent ipsilateral acoustic reflex at 1000 Hz; for an absolute acoustic-admittance device, (a) tympanometric gradient > 180 daPa (or static-acoustic middle-ear admittance < 0.35 mmho) together with an absent ipsilateral acoustic reflex at 1000 Hz, or (b) tympanometric peak pressure <= −100 daPa together with an absent ipsilateral acoustic reflex at 1000 Hz. If these results persist after the acoustic-immittance re-evaluation performed 3 months after the initial acoustic-immittance evaluation, the child should be referred for an otolaryngologic evaluation. Monitoring (acoustic-immittance re-evaluation) in such cases is recommended since several investigators (Fiellau-Nikolajsen, 1983; Liden & Renvall, 1980; Thomsen, Tos, Hancke, & Melchiors, 1982; Tos, 1980) reported that most cases of middle-ear effusion in young children spontaneously resolve over time.

Children between 2 months and 10 years of age should be referred for trimonthly acoustic-immittance re-evaluations over a 1-year period if the tympanometric peak pressure is less than −200 daPa and the ipsilateral acoustic reflex is present for the 1000-Hz tonal activator. As mentioned earlier, Tos *et al.* (1984) reported that persistent negative tympanometric pressure less than −200 daPa is directly related to irreversible eardrum abnormalities. If the tympanometric peak pressure is less than −200 daPa (and the ipsilateral acoustic reflex is present at 1000 Hz) at the acoustic-immittance re-evaluation performed 1 year after the initial acoustic-immittance evaluation, the child should be referred for an otolaryngologic evaluation.

Children between 2 months and 10 years of age should be referred for otolaryngologic followup regardless of the acoustic-immittance findings if medical ear-related complaints are present, there is a recent history of middle-ear problems, otoscopic inspection reveals unusual findings, or significant air-bone gaps are present.

Older children more than 10 years of age and adults should be referred for otolaryngologic followup if any 1 or more of the following are obtained for absolute or relative acoustic-immittance devices: (a) tympanometric peak pressure less than −50 daPa with absent or elevated ipsilateral acoustic reflexes for the tonal activators and absent or elevated contralateral acoustic reflexes for the tonal activators (probe ear in the ear with the negative tympanometric peak pressure); (b) flat tympanogram; (c) significant air-bone gaps; (d) medically related ear, nose, or throat complaints; (e) recent history of middle-ear problems; or (f) unusual findings upon otoscopic inspection.

REFERENCES

Abahazi, D. A., & Greenberg, H. J. (1977). Clinical acoustic reflex threshold measurements in infants. *J. Speech Hear. Res., 42,* 514–519.

Alberti, P. W. R., & Jerger, J. F. (1974). Probe-tone frequency and the diagnostic value of tympanometry. *Arch. Otolaryngol., 99,* 206–210.

Alberti, P. W. R., & Kristensen, R. (1970). The clinical application of impedance audiometry. *Laryngoscope, 80,* 735–746.

Alberti, P. W. R., & Kristensen, R. (1976). The clinical application of impedance audiometry. In J. Northern (Ed.), *Selected readings in impedance audiometry,* pp. 61–68. New York: American Electromedics.

Alberti, P. W. R., Fria, J., & Cummings, F. (1977). The clinical utility of ipsilateral stapedius reflex tests. *J. Otolaryngol., 6,* 466–472.

American National Standards Institute (1970). American National Standard specifications for audiometers (ANSI S3.6–1969). New York: American National Standards Institute.

American National Standards Institute (1987). American National Standard specifications for instruments to measure aural acoustic impedance and admittance (ANSI S3.39–1987). New York: American National Standards Institute

American Speech–Language–Hearing Association, Committee on Audiologic Evaluation—Working Group on Acoustic Immittance Measurement (1989). Draft: Guidelines for screening for hearing impairment and middle ear disorders. *Asha, 32,* 71–77.

American Speech–Language–Hearing Association, Subcommittee on Impedance Measurement of the Committee on Audiologic Evaluation (1979). Guidelines for acoustic immittance screening of middle-ear function. *Asha, 27,* 49–52.

Anderson, H., Barr, B., & Wedenberg, E. (1969). Intra-aural reflexes in retrocochlear lesions. In C. A. Hamberger & J. Wersall (eds.), *Nobel symposium 10, Disorders of the skull base region*, pp. 48–54. Stockholm: Almquvist & Wikell.

Anderson, H., Barr, B., & Wedenberg, E. (1970). Early diagnosis of VIIIth-nerve tumours by acoustic reflex tests. *Acta Otolaryngol., 262*, 232–237.

Balkany, T., Berman, S., Simmons, M., & Jafek, B. (1978). Middle ear effusions in neonates. *Laryngoscope, 88*, 398–405.

Bauch, C. D., & Robinette, M. S. (1978). Alcohol and the acoustic reflex: Effects of stimulus spectrum, subject variability, and sex. *J. Am. Aud. Soc., 4*, 104–112.

Beedle, R. K., & Harford, E. R. (1973). A comparison of acoustic reflex and loudness growth in normal and pathological ears. *J. Speech Hear. Res., 16*, 271–281.

Beery, Q. C., Andrus, W. S., Bluestone, C. D., & Cantekin, E. I. (1973). Tympanometric pattern classification in relation to middle ear effusions. *Ann. Otol., 84*, 56–64.

Beery, Q. C., Bluestone, C. D., Andrus, W. E., & Cantekin, E. I. (1975). Tympanometric pattern classification in relation to middle ear effusions. *Ann. Otol. Rhinol. Laryngol., 84*, 56–64.

Bel, J., Causse, P., Michaux, P., Cezard, R., Canut, T., & Tapon, J. (1976). Mechanical explanation of the on–off effect (diphasic impedance change) in otospongiosis. *Audiol., 15*, 128–140.

Bennett, M. (1975). Acoustic impedance bridge measurements with the neonate. *Br. J. Audiol., 9*, 117–124.

Bennett, M. (1984). Impedance concepts relating to the acoustic reflex. In S. Silman (ed.), *The acoustic reflex: Basic principles and clinical applications*, pp. 35–61. New York: Academic Press.

Bennett, M. J., & Weatherby, L. A. (1979). Multiple probe frequency acoustic reflex measurements. *Scand. Audiol., 8*, 233–239.

Bennett, M. J., & Weatherby, L. A. (1982). Newborn acoustic reflexes to noise and pure-tone signals. *J. Speech Hear. Res., 25*, 383–387.

Bergenius, J., Borg, E., & Hirsch, A. (1983). Stapedius reflex test, brainstem audiometry and optovestibular tests in diagnosis of acoustic neurinomas. *Scand. Audiol., 12*, 3–9.

Blom, S., & Zakrisson, J. E. (1974). The stapedius reflex in the diagnosis of myasthenia gravis. *J. Neurolog. Sci., 21*, 71–76.

Bluestone, C. D. (1980). Assessment of Eustachian tube function. In J. Jerger & J. L. Northern (eds.), *Clincal impedance audiometry*, 2d ed., pp. 83–108. Acton, Massachusetts: American Electromedics Corporation.

Bluestone, C., & Beery, Q. (1976). Concepts of the pathogenesis of middle ear effusion. *Ann. Otol. Rhinol. Laryngol., 85*, 182–186.

Bluestone, C. D., & Cantekin, E. (1981). Panel on experiences with testing Eustachian tube function tests. *Ann. Otol. Rhinol. Laryngol., 90*, 552–562.

Bluestone, C. D., Paradise, J., Beery, Q., & Wittel, R. (1972). Certain effects of cleft palate repair on Eustachian tube function. *Cleft Palate J., 9*, 183–193.

Bluestone, C. D., Beery, Q. C., & Paradise, J. L. (1973). Audiometry and tympanometry in relation to middle ear effusions in children. *Laryngoscope, 83*, 594–604.

Bluestone, C. D., Cantekin, E., & Beery, Q. (1975). Certain effects of adenoidectomy on Eustachian tube ventilatory function. *Laryngoscope, 83*, 113.

Bluestone, C. D., Cantekin, E., & Beery, Q. (1977). Effect of inflammation on the ventilatory function of the Eustachian tube. *Laryngoscope, 87*, 493.

Borg, E. (1973). On the neuronal organization of the acoustic middle ear reflex. A physiological and anatomical study. *Brain Res., 49*, 101–123.

Bosatra, A., Russolo, M., & Poli, P. (1976). Oscilloscopic analysis of the stapedius muscle reflex in brain stem lesions. *Arch. Otolaryngol., 102*, 284–285.

Bosatra, A., Russolo, M., & Silverman, C. A. (1984). Acoustic-reflex latency: State of the art. In S. Silman (ed.), *The acoustic reflex: Basic principles and clinical applications*, pp. 301–328. New York: Academic Press.

Brooks, D. N. (1968). An objective method of detecting fluid in the middle ear. *Int. Audiol., 7*, 280–286.

Brooks, D. N. (1969). The use of the electro-acoustic impedance bridge in the assessment of the middle ear function. *J. Int. Audiol., 8*, 563–569.

Brooks, D. N. (1971). A new approach to identification audiometry. *Audiology, 10*, 334–339.

Brooks, D. N. (1980). Impedance in screening. In J. Jerger & J. L. Northern (eds.), *Clinical impedance audiometry*, 2d ed., pp. 164–182. Acton, Massachusetts: American Electromedics Corporation.

Cannon, S. S., Smith, K. E., Reece, C. A., & Thebo, J. L. (1974). Middle-ear measurements in neonates: A normative study [Abstract]. *Asha, 16*, 564.

Cantekin, E., Beery, Q., & Bluestone, C. (1977). Tympanometric patterns found in middle ear effusions. *Ann. Otol. Rhinol. Laryngol., 86*, 16–20.

Cantekin, E., Bluestone, C., Fria, T., Stool, S., Berry, Q., & Sabo, D. (1980). Identification of otitis media with effusion in children. *Ann. Otol. Rhinol. Laryngol. Suppl. 68, 89*, 190–195.

Cartwright, D., & Lilly, D. (1976). A comparison of acoustic-reflex decay patterns for patients with cochlear and VIIIth-nerve disease. Paper presented at the annual convention of the American Speech–Language–Hearing Association, Houston, Texas.

Chiveralls, K. (1977). A further examination of the use of the stapedius reflex in diagnosis of acoustic neuroma. *Audiology, 16*, 331–337.

Chiveralls, K., FitzSimons, R., Beck, G. B., & Kernohan, H. (1976). The diagnostic significance of the acoustic reflex. *Brit. J. Audiol., 10*, 122–128.

Cohill, E. N., & Greenberg, H. J. (1977). Effects of ethyl alcohol on the acoustic reflex threshold. *J. Am. Aud. Soc., 2*, 121–123.

Colletti, V. (1975a). Methodologic observations on tympanometry with regard to the probe tone frequency. *Acta Otolaryngol., 80*, 54–60.

Colletti, V. (1975b). Stapedius reflex abnormalities in multiple sclerosis. *Audiology, 14*, 63–71.

Colletti, V. (1977). Multifrequency tympanometry. *Audiology, 16*, 278–287.

Correa, A., & Konow, W. (1978). La impedanciometria en el recien nacedo [English abstract]. *Revista Otorhinolaringologica, 39*, 16–18.

Creten, W. L., Vanpeperstraete, P. M., Van Camp, K. J., & Doclo, J. R. (1976). An experimental study on diphasic acoustic reflex patterns in normal ears. *Scand. Audiol., 5*, 3–8.

Creten, W. L., Van Camp, K. J., Maes, M. A., & Vanpeperstraete, P. M. (1981). On the diagnostic value of phase angle tympanograms. *Audiology, 17*, 97–107.

Creten, W. L., Van de Heyning, P. H., & Van Camp, K. J. (1985). Immittance audiometry: Normative data at 220 and 660 Hz. *Scand. Audiol., 14*, 115–121.

Dempsey, C. (1975). Static compliance. In J. Jerger (ed.), *Handbook of clinical impedance audiometry*, pp. 71–84. Dobbs Ferry, New York: American Electromedics Corporation.

Downs, D. W., & Crum, M. A. (1980). The hyperactive acoustic reflex: Four case studies. *Arch. Otolaryngol., 106*, 401–404.

Djupesland, G., Flottorp, G., Hansen, E., & Sjaastad, O. (1974). Cogan's syndrome: The audiological picture. *Arch. Otolaryngol., 99*, 218–225.

Elner, A. S., Ingelstedt, & Ivarsson, A. (1971). The elastic properties of the tympanic membrane. *Acta Otolaryngol., 72*, 397–403.

Feldman, A. S. (1975). Acoustic impedance immittance measurements. In L. J. Bradford (ed.), *Physiological measures of the audio-vestibular system*, pp. 87–145. New York: Academic Press.

Feldman, A. S. (1976). Tympanometry—Procedures, interpretation and variables. In A. S. Feldman & L. A. Wilber (eds.), *Acoustic impedance and admittance: The measurement of middle ear function*, pp. 103–155. Baltimore: Williams & Wilkins.

Fiellau-Nikolajsen, M. (1983). Tympanometry and secretory otitis media. *Acta Otolaryngol. Suppl., 394*, 1–73.

Flottorp, G., & Djupesland, G. (1970). Diphasic impedance change and its applicability to clinical work. *Acta Otolaryngol., 263*, 200–204.

Frank, T., May, M., & Jannetta, P. J. (1978). Acoustic neurinoma in a child: A case study. *J. Speech Hear. Dis., 43*, 506–512.

Gelfand, S. A. (1984). The contralateral acoustic-reflex threshold. In S. Silman (ed.), *The acoustic reflex: Basic principles and clinical applications*, pp. 137–183. New York: Academic Press.

Gelfand, S. A., & Piper, N. (1981). Acoustic reflex thresholds in young and elderly subjects with normal hearing. *J. Acoust. Soc. Am., 69*, 295–297.

Gelfand, S. A., & Silman, S. (1982). Acoustic reflex thresholds in brain damaged patients. *Ear Hear., 3*, 93–95.

Gelfand, S. A., Piper, N., & Silman, S. (1983). Effects of hearing levels at the activator and other frequencies upon the expected levels of the acoustic reflex threshold. *J. Speech Hear. Dis., 48*, 11–17.

Givens, G., & Seidemann, M. (1984). Acoustic immittance testing of the Eustachian tube. *Ear. Hear., 5*, 297–299.

Gonay, P., Dutillieux, D., & Metz, T. (1974). La dynamique de la contraction du muscle de etrier en fonction de l'age. *Rev. Electrodiagnostic-Therapie, 11*, 17–22.

Grason–Stadler (1973). *Otoadmittance handbook 2: A guide to users of the Grason–Stadler Model 1720 otoadmittance meter.* Concord, Massachusetts: Grason–Stadler.

Green, K. W., & Margolis, R. H. (1984). The ipsilateral acoustic reflex. In S. Silman (ed.), *The acoustic reflex: Basic principles and clinical applications*, pp. 275–299. New York: Academic Press.

Hall, J. W., & Weaver, T. (1979). Impedance audiometry in a young population: The effect of age, sex, and tympanogram abnormalities. *J. Otolaryngol., 3*, 210–221.

Handler, S. D., & Margolis, R. H. (1977). Predicting hearing loss from stapedial reflex thresholds in patients with sensorineural impairment. *Ann Otol. Rhinol. Laryngol., 84*, 425–431.

Harford, E. R. (1980). Tympanometry. In J. Jerger & J. L. Northern (eds.), *Clinical impedance audiometry*, 2d ed., pp. 40–64. Acton, Massachusetts: American Electromedics Corporation.

Hayes, D., & Jerger, J. (1980). The effect of degree of hearing loss on diagnostic test strategy. *Arch. Otolaryngol., 106*, 266–268.

Himmelfarb, M. Z., Shanon, E., Popelka, G. R., & Margolis, R. H. (1978). Acoustic reflex evaluation in neonates. In S. E. Gerber & G. T. Mencher (eds.), *Early diagnosis of hearing loss*, pp. 109–123. New York: Grune & Stratton.

Himmelfarb, M. Z., Popelka, G. R., & Shanon, E. (1979). Tympanometry in normal neonates. *J. Speech Hear. Res., 22*, 179–191.

Hirsch, A., & Anderson, H. (1980). Audiologic test results in 96 patients with tumors affecting the eighth nerve. *Acta Otolaryngol. Suppl., 369*, 1–26.

Holmes, D. W., & Woodford, C. M. (1977). Acoustic reflex threshold and loudness discomfort level: Relationships in children with profound hearing losses. *J. Am. Aud. Soc., 2*, 193–196.

Holmquist, J. (1968). The role of the Eustachian tube in myringoplasty. *Acta Otolaryngol., 66*, 289–295.

Holmquist, J., & Miller, J. (1972). Eustachian tube evaluation using the impedance bridge. In D. Rose & L. Keating (eds.), *Mayo Foundation impedance symposium*, pp. 297–308. Rochester, Minnesota: Mayo Foundation.

Jaffe, B. F., Hurtado, F., & Hurtado, E. (1970). Tympanic membrane mobility in the newborn (with seven months follow up). *Laryngoscope, 80*, 36–48.

Jepsen, O. (1963). Middle-ear muscle reflexes in man. In J. Jerger (ed.), *Modern developments in audiology*, pp. 193–239. New York: Academic Press.

Jerger, J. (1970). Clinical experience with impedance audiometry. *Arch. Otolaryngol., 92*, 311–324.

Jerger, J. (1975). Diagnostic use of impedance measures. In J. Jerger (ed.), *Handbook of clinical impedance audiometry*, pp. 149–174. Dobbs Ferry, New York: American Electromedics.

Jerger, J., Jerger, S., & Mauldin, L. (1972). Studies in impedance audiometry. I. Normal and sensorineural ears. *Arch. Otolaryngol., 96*, 513–523.

Jerger, J., Anthony, L., Jerger, S., & Mauldin, L. (1974a). Studies in impedance audiometry. III. Middle ear disorders. *Arch. Otolaryngol., 99*, 165–171.

Jerger, J., Burney, P., Mauldin, L., & Crump, B. (1974b). Predicting hearing loss from the acoustic reflex. *J. Speech Hear. Dis., 39*, 11–22.

Jerger, J., Harford, E., Clemis, J., & Alford, B. (1974c). The acoustic reflex in eighth nerve disorders. *Arch. Otolaryngol., 99*, 409–413.

Jerger, J., Hayes, D., Anthony, L., & Mauldin, L. (1978). Factors influencing prediction of hearing level from the acoustic reflex. *Maico Monogr. Contemp. Audiol., 1*, 1–20.

Jerger, S., & Jerger, J. (1977). Diagnostic value of crossed vs. uncrossed acoustic reflexes. *Arch. Otolaryngol., 103*, 445–453.

Jerger, S., & Jerger, J. (1981). *Auditory disorders: A manual for clinical evaluation.* Boston: Little, Brown.

Jerger, S., Jerger, J., Mauldin, L., & Segal, P. (1974). Studies in impedance audiometry for children less than six years old. *Arch. Otolaryngol., 99*, 1–9.

Johnson, E. W. (1977). Auditory test results in 500 cases of acoustic neuroma. *Arch. Otolaryngol., 103*, 152–158.

Kaplan, H., Gilman, S., & Dirks, D. D. (1977). Properties of acoustic reflex adaptation. *Ann. Otol. Rhinol. Laryngol., 86*, 348–356.

Keith, R. W. (1973). Impedance audiometry with neonates. *Arch. Otolaryngol., 97*, 465–467.

Keith, R. W. (1975). Middle-ear function in neonates. *Arch. Otolaryngol., 101*, 376–379.

Keith, R. W. (1977). An evaluation of predicting hearing loss from the acoustic reflex. *Arch. Otolaryngol., 103*, 419–424.

Keith, R. W. (1979). Loudness and the acoustic reflex: Cochlear-impaired listeners. *J. Am. Aud. Soc., 5*, 65–70.

Keith, R. W., & Bench, R. J. (1978). Stapedial reflex in neonates. *Scand. Audiol., 7*, 188–191.

Klein, J. O. (1978). Epidemiology of otitis media. In E. R. Harford, F. H. Bess, C. D. Bluestone, & J. O. Klein (eds.), *Impedance screening for middle ear disease in children*, pp. 11–16. New York: Grune & Stratton.

Koebsell, K. A., Margolis, R. H. (1986). Tympanometric gradient measured from normal preschool children. *Audiology, 25*, 149–157.

Kramer, L. D., Ruth, R. A., Johns, M. E., & Sanders, D. B. (1981). A comparison of stapedial reflex fatigue with repetitive stimulation and single-fiber EMG in myasthenia gravis. *Ann. Neurol., 9*, 531–536.

Kunov, H. (1977). The "eardrum artifact" in ipsilateral reflex measurements. *Scand. Audiol., 6*, 163–166.

Liden, G., & Renvall, U. (1978). Impedance audiometry for screening middle ear disease in school children. In E. R. Harford, F. H. Bess, C. D. Bluestone, & J. O. Klein (eds.), *Impedance screening for middle ear disease in children*, pp. 197–206. New York: Grune & Stratton.

Liden, G., & Renvall, U. (1980). Impedance and tone screening of school-children. *Scand. Audiol., 9*, 121–126.

Liden, G., Harford, E., & Hallen, O. (1974). Tympanometry for the diagnosis of ossicular disruption. *Arch. Otolaryngol., 99*, 23–29.

Lous, J. (1983). Three impedance screening programs on a cohort of seven-year-old children. *Scand. Audiol. Suppl., 17*, 60–64.

Lutman, M. E. (1980). Real-ear calibration of ipsilateral acoustic reflex stimuli from five types of impedance meters. *Scand. Audiol., 9*, 137–145.

Lutman, M. E., & Leis, B. R. (1980). Ipsilateral acoustic reflex artifacts measured in cadavers. *Scand. Audiol., 9*, 33–39.

McCandless, G. A., & Thomas, G. K. (1974). Impedance audiometry as a screening procedure for middle ear disease. *Trans. Am. Acad. Ophthal-*

mol. Otolaryngol. ORL, 78, 98–102.

McMillan, P. M., Bennett, M. J., Marchant, C. D., & Shurin, P. (1985). Ipsilateral and contralateral acoustic reflexes in neonates. Ear Hear., 6, 320–324.

Madsen Electronics. Model ZO73 electro-acoustic impedance meter: Operator's manual. Buffalo, New York: Madsen Electronics.

Mangham, C. A., Lindeman, R. C., & Dawson, W. R. (1980). Stapedius reflex quantification in acoustic tumor patients. Laryngoscope, 90, 242–250.

Margolis, R. H. (1978). Tympanometry in infants: State of the art. In E. R. Harford, F. H. Bess, C. D. Bluestone, & J. O. Klein (eds.), Impedance screening for middle ear disease in children, pp. 41–56. New York: Grune & Stratton.

Margolis, R. H. (1981). Fundamentals of acoustic immittance. Appendix A. In G. R. Popelka (ed.), Hearing assessment with the acoustic reflex, pp. 117–143. New York: Grune & Stratton.

Margolis, R. H., & Fox, C. M. (1977). A comparison of three methods for predicting hearing loss from acoustic reflex thresholds. J. Speech Hear. Res., 20, 241–253.

Margolis, R. H., & Heller, J. W. (1987). Screening tympanometry: Criteria for medical referral. Audiol., 26, 197–208.

Margolis, R. H., & Popelka, G. R. (1975). Static and dynamic acoustic impedance measurements in infant ears. J. Speech Hear. Res., 18, 435–443.

Margolis, R. H., & Popelka, G. R. (1977). Interactions among tympanometric variables. J. Speech Hear. Res., 20, 447–462.

Margolis, R. H., & Shanks, J. E. (1985). Tympanometry. In J. Katz (ed.), Handbook of clinical audiology, 2d ed., pp. 438–475. Baltimore: Williams & Wilkins.

Margolis, R. H., Osguthorpe, J. D., & Popelka, G. R. (1978). The effects of experimentally produced middle-ear lesions on tympanometry in cats. Acta Otolaryngol., 86, 428–436.

Margolis, R. H., Van Camp, J., Wilson, R. H., & Creten, W. L. (1985). Multifrequency tympanometry in normal ears. Audiology, 24, 44–53.

Marquet, J., Van Camp, K. J., Creten, W. L., Decraemer, W. F., Wolff, H. B., & Schepens, P. (1973). Topics in physics and middle ear surgery. Acta Otolaryngol. Belgica, 27, 139–319.

Martin, F. N., & Brunette, G. W. (1980). Loudness and the acoustic reflex. Ear Hear., 1, 106–108.

Metz, O. (1946). The acoustic impedance measured on normal and pathologic ears. Acta Otolaryngol. Suppl., 63, 1–254.

Metz, O. (1952). Threshold of reflex contractions of muscles of middle ear and recruitment of loudness. Arch. Otolaryngol., 55, 536–543.

Niemeyer, W., & Sesterhenn, G. (1974). Calculating the hearing threshold from the stapedius reflex threshold for different sound stimuli. Audiology, 13, 421–427.

Norris, T. W., Stelmachowicz, P. G., & Taylor, D. J. (1974). Acoustic reflex relaxation to identify sensorineural hearing impairment. Arch. Otolaryngol., 99, 194–197.

Olsen, W. O., Noffsinger, D., & Kurdziel, S. A. (1975). Acoustic reflex and reflex decay. Arch. Otolaryngol., 101, 622–625.

Olsen, W. O., Stach, B. A., & Kurdziel, S. A. (1981). Acoustic reflex decay in 10 seconds and in 5 seconds for Meniere's disease patients and for VIIIth nerve tumor patients. Ear Hear., 2, 180–181.

Olsen, W. O., Bauch, C. D., & Harner, S. G. (1983). Application of Silman and Gelfand (1981) 90th percentile levels for acoustic reflex thresholds. J. Speech Hear. Dis., 48, 330–332.

Osterhammel, D., & Osterhammel, P. (1979). Age and sex variations for the normal stapedial reflex thresholds and tympanometric compliance values. Scand. Audiol., 8, 153–158.

Oviatt, D. L., & Kileny, P. (1984). Normative characteristics of ipsilateral acoustic reflex adaptations. Ear Hear., 5, 145–152.

Paradise, J. L. (1980). Otitis media in infants and children. Pediatrics, 65, 917–943.

Paradise, J. L., & Smith, C. L. (1978). Impedance screening for preschool children: State of the art. In E. R. Harford, F. H. Bess, C. D. Bluestone, & J. O. Klein (eds.), Impedance screening for middle ear disease, pp. 113–123. New York: Grune & Stratton.

Paradise, J. L., Smith, C. G., & Bluestone, C. D. (1976). Tympanometric detection of middle ear effusion in infants and young children. Pediatrics, 58, 198–210.

Peterson, J. L., & Liden, G. (1972). Some static characteristics of the stapedial muscle reflex. Audiology, 11, 94–114.

Popelka, G. R. (ed.) (1981). Hearing assessment with the acoustic reflex. New York: Grune & Stratton.

Popelka, G. R., Margolis, R. H., & Wiley, T. L. (1976). Effect of activating signal bandwidth on acoustic reflex thresholds. J. Acoust. Soc. Am., 59, 153–159.

Porter, T. A. (1974). Otoadmittance measurements in a residential deaf population. Am. Ann. Deaf, 119, 47–52.

Porter, T., & Winston, M. (1973). Methodological aspects of admittance measurements of the middle ear. J. Aud. Res., 13, 172–177.

Poulsen, G., & Tos, M. (1978). Screening tympanometry in newborn infants during the first six months of life. Scand. Audiol., 7, 159.

Reiter, L. A. (1981). Experiments re: Clinical application of reflex modulation audiometry. J. Speech Hear. Res., 24, 92–98.

Reiter, L. A., Goetzinger, C. P., & Press, S. E. (1981). Reflex modulation: A hearing test for the difficult-to-test. J. Speech Hear. Dis., 46, 262–266.

Renvall, U., & Holmquist, J. (1976). Tympanometry revealing middle-ear pathology. Ann. Otol. Rhinol. Laryngol. Suppl. 25, 85, 209–215.

Renvall, U., & Liden, G. (1978). Clinical significance of reduced middle ear pressure in school children. In E. R. Harford, F. H. Bess, C. D. Bluestone, & J. O. Klein (eds.), Impedance screening for middle ear disease in children, pp. 189–196. New York: Grune & Stratton.

Renvall, U., Liden, G., Jungert, S., & Nilsson, E. (1975). Impedance audiometry in the detection of secretory otitis media. Scand. Audiol., 4, 119–124.

Riedel, C. L., Wiley, T. L., & Block, M. G. (1987). Tympanometric measures of Eustachian tube function. J. Speech Hear. Res., 30, 207–214.

Roberts, M. E. (1976). Comparative study of pure tone, impedance, and otoscopic hearing screening methods. Arch. Otolaryngol., 102, 690–694.

Roeser, R. J., Soh, J., Dunckel, D. C., & Adams, R. M. (1978). Comparison of tympanometry and otoscopy in establishing pass/fail referral criteria. In E. R. Harford, F. H. Bess, C. D. Bluestone, & J. O. Klein (eds.), Impedance screening for middle ear disease in children, pp. 135–144. New York: Grune & Stratton.

Roush, J., & Tait, C. A. (1985). Pure-tone and acoustic immittance screening of pre-school aged children: An examination of referral criteria. Ear Hear., 6, 245–250.

Sanders, J. W. (1984). Evaluation of the 90th percentile levels for acoustic reflex thresholds. Paper presented at the Annual Convention of the American Speech–Language–Hearing Association, San Francisco, California.

Sanders, J. W., Josey, A. F., & Glasscock, M. E. (1974). Audiologic evaluation in cochlear and eighth nerve disorders, Arch. Otolaryngol., 100, 282–289.

Sanders, J. W., Josey, A., Glasscock, M., & Jackson, C. (1981). The acoustic reflex test in cochlear and eighth nerve pathology ears. Laryngoscope, 91, 787–793.

Schwartz, D. M., & Sanders, J. W. (1976). Critical bandwidth and sensitivity prediction in the acoustic stapedial reflex. J. Speech Hear. Dis., 41, 244–255.

Shanks, J. E. (1984). Tympanometry. Ear Hear., 5, 268–280.

Shanks, J. E., & Lilly, D. J. (1981). An evaluation of tympanometric estimates of ear canal volume. J. Speech Hear. Res., 24, 557–566.

Shanks, J. E., & Wilson, R. H. (1986). Effects of direction and rate of ear-canal pressure changes on tympanometric measures. J. Speech

Hear. Res., 29, 11–19.

Shaw, E. A. G. (1980). The acoustics of the external ear. In G. A. Studebaker & I. Hochberg (eds.), *Acoustical factors affecting hearing aid performance,* pp. 32–51. Baltimore: University Park Press.

Sheehy, J. L., & Inzer, B. E. (1976). Acoustic reflex test in neuro-otologic diagnosis: A review of 24 cases of acoustic tumors. *Arch. Otolaryngol., 102,* 647–653.

Siedentop, K., Tardy, M., & Hamilton, L. (1968). Eustachian tube function. *Arch. Otolaryngol., 88,* 66–75.

Silman, S. (1979). The effects of aging on the acoustic reflex thresholds. *J. Acoust. Soc. Am., 66,* 735–738.

Silman, S., & Gelfand, S. A. (1979). Prediction of hearing levels from acoustic reflex thresholds in persons with high-frequency hearing losses. *J. Speech Hear. Res., 22,* 697–707.

Silman, S., & Gelfand, S. A. (1981a). The relationship between magnitude of hearing loss and acoustic reflex threshold levels. *J. Speech Hear. Dis., 46,* 312–316.

Silman, S., & Gelfand, S. A. (1981b). Effect of sensorineural hearing loss on the stapedius reflex growth function in the elderly. *J. Acoust. Soc. Am., 69,* 1099–1106.

Silman, S., Gelfand, S. A., & Chun, T. H. (1978a). Some observations in a case of acoustic neuroma. *J. Speech Hear. Dis., 43,* 459–466.

Silman, S., Popelka, G. R., & Gelfand, S. A. (1978b). Effect of sensorineural hearing loss on acoustic stapedius reflex growth functions. *J. Acoust. Soc. Am., 64,* 1406–1411.

Silman, S., Gelfand, S. A., Howard, J. C., & Showers, T. J. (1982). Clinical application of the bivariate plotting procedure in the prediction of hearing loss. *Scand. Audiol., 11,* 115–124.

Silman, S., Gelfand, S. A., Piper, N., Silverman, C. A., & Van Frank, L. (1984a). Prediction of hearing loss from the acoustic-reflex threshold. In S. Silman (ed.), *The acoustic reflex: Basic principles and clinical applications,* pp. 187–223. New York: Academic Press.

Silman, S., Silverman, C. A., Showers, T. J., & Gelfand, S. A. (1984b). The effect of age on prediction of hearing loss with the bivariate plotting procedure. *J. Speech Hear. Res., 27,* 12–19.

Silman, S., Silverman, C. A., Gelfand, S. A., Lutolf, J., & Lynn, D. J. (1988). Ipsilateral acoustic-reflex adaptation testing in detection of facial-nerve pathology: Three case studies. *J. Speech Hear. Dis., 53,* 378–382.

Silman, S., & Silverman, C. A. (1990). Tympanometry and otitis media. Paper presented at the conference, Implications of otitis media, October 19, 1990, Manhattan Eye, Ear & Throat Hospital, New York, N.Y.

Silverman, C. A., Silman, S., Gelfand, S. A., & Lutolf, J. J. (1986). The efferent acoustic-reflex adaptation pattern. Paper presented at the Annual Convention of the American Speech–Language–Hearing Association, Detroit, Michigan.

Silverman, C. A., Silman, S., & Miller, M. H. (1983). The acoustic reflex threshold in aging ears. *J. Acoust. Soc. Am., 73,* 248–255.

Spitzer, J. B., & Ventry, I. M. (1980). Central auditory dysfunction among chronic alcoholics. *Arch. Otolaryngol., 106,* 224–229.

Sprague, B. H., Wiley, T. L., & Goldstein, R. (1985). Tympanometric and acoustic-reflex studies in neonates. *J. Speech Hear. Res., 28,* 265–272.

Stephens, S., & Thornton, A. (1976). Subjective and electrophysiologic tests in brain-stem lesions. *Arch. Otolaryngol., 102,* 608–613.

Stool, S. E. (1984). Medical relevancy of immittance measurements. *Ear Hear., 5,* 309–313.

Stream, R., Stream, K., Walker, J., & Breningstall, G. (1978). Emerging characteristics of the acoustic reflex in the neonate. *Otolaryngol. Head Neck Surg., 86,* 628–636.

Swogger, J. R., & Brenman, A. K. (1975). Tymps and tubes for tots. Paper presented at the Annual Convention of the American Speech and Hearing Association, Washington, D.C.

Terkildsen, K., & Scott-Nielsen, S. (1960). An electroacoustic imped-

ance measuring bridge for clinical use. *Acta Otolaryngol., 72,* 33ʳ 346.

Thomsen, J., & Terkildsen, K. (1975). Audiological findings in 125 cases of acoustic neuroma. *Acta Otolaryngol., 80,* 353–361.

Thomsen, J., Tos, M., Hancke, A. B., & Melchiors, H. (1982). Repetitive tympanometric screenings in children followed from birth to age four. *Acta Otolaryngol. Suppl., 386,* 155–157.

Tos, M. (1980). Spontaneous improvement of secretory otitis media and impedance screening. *Arch. Otolaryngol., 106,* 345–349.

Tos, M., Stangerup, S. E., Holm-Jensen, S., & Sorensen, C. H. (1984). Spontaneous course of secretory otitis and changes of the eardrum. *Arch. Otolaryngol., 110,* 281–289.

Turner, R. G., Shepard, N. T., & Frazer, G. J. (1984). Clinical performance of audiological and related diagnostic tests. *Ear Hear., 5,* 187–194.

Van Camp, K. J., Vanpeperstraete, P. M., Creten, W. L., & Vanhuyse, V. J. (1975). On irregular acoustic reflex patterns. *Scand. Audiol., 4,* 227–232.

Van Camp, K. J., Vanhuyse, V. J., Creten, W. L., & Vanpeperstraete, P. M. (1978). Impedance and admittance tympanometry. II. Mathematical approach. *Audiology, 17,* 108–119.

Van Camp, K. J., Creten, W. L., Vanpeperstraete, P. M., & Van de Heyning, P. H. (1980). Tympanometry—Detection of middle ear pathologies. *Acta Otorhinolaryngol., 34,* 574–583.

Van Camp, K. J., Creten, W. L., Van de Heyning, P. H., Decraemer, W. F., & Vanpeperstraete, P. M. (1983). A search for the most suitable immittance components and probe tone frequency in tympanometry. *Scand. Audiol., 12,* 27–34.

Van Camp, K. J., Margolis, R. H., Wilson, R. H., Creten, W. L., & Shanks, J. E. (1986). *Principles of tympanometry.* ASHA Monograph No. 24. Rockville, Maryland: American Speech–Language–Hearing Association.

Van de Heyning, P. H., Van Camp, K. J., Creten, W. L., & Vanpeperstraete, P. M. (1982). Incudo-stapedial joint pathology: A tympanometric approach. *J. Speech Hear. Res., 25,* 611–617.

Vanhuyse, V. J., Creten, W. L., & Van Camp, K. J. (1975). On the W-notching of tympanograms. *Scand. Audiol., 4,* 45–50.

Wallin, A., Mendez-Kurtz, L., & Silman, S. (1986). Prediction of hearing loss from acoustic reflex thresholds in the older adult population. *Ear Hear., 7,* 400–404.

Weatherby, L., & Bennett, M. (1980). The neonatal acoustic reflex. *Scand. Audiol., 9,* 103–110.

Wiley, T. L., & Block, M. G. (1979). Static acoustic-immittance measurements. *J. Speech Hear. Res., 22,* 677–696.

Wiley, T. L., Oviatt, D. L., & Block, M. G. (1987). Acoustic immittance measures in normal ears. *J. Speech Hear. Res., 30,* 161–170.

Wilson, R. H. (1981). The effects of aging on the magnitude of the acoustic reflex. *J. Speech Hear. Res., 24,* 406–414.

Wilson, R. H., Shanks, J. E., & Kaplan, S. K. (1984). Tympanometric changes at 226 and 678 Hz across ten trials and for two directions of ear-canal pressure change. *J. Speech Hear. Res., 27,* 257–266.

Wilson, R. H., Shanks, J. E., & Velde, T. M. (1981). Aural acoustic-immittance measurements: Inter-aural differences. *J. Speech Hear. Dis., 46,* 413–421.

Wilson, R. H., Shanks, J. E., & Lilly, D. J. (1984). Acoustic-reflex adaptation. In S. Silman (ed.), *The acoustic reflex: Basic principles and clinical applications,* pp. 329–386. New York: Academic Press.

Zarnoch, J. M., & Balkany, T. J. (1978). Tympanometric screening of normal and intensive care unit newborns: Validity and reliability. In E. R. Harford, F. H. Bess, C. D. Bluestone, & J. O. Klein (eds.), *Impedance screening for middle-ear disease in children,* pp. 69–79. New York: Grune & Stratton.

Zwislocki, J., & Feldman, A. S. (1970). *Acoustic impedance of pathological ears.* ASHA Monograph No. 15. Rockville, Maryland: American Speech and Hearing Association.

CHAPTER 4

FUNCTIONAL HEARING IMPAIRMENT

When a patient presents with intratest and/or intertest discrepancies during audiologic assessment that cannot be accounted for by any known organic cause, the condition is termed functional hearing loss (Chaiklin & Ventry, 1963). Upon resolution of a functional hearing loss, normal-hearing thresholds or an organic hearing loss remain. Prior to resolution of the functional hearing loss in the latter case, the hearing threshold levels are exaggerated—there was a functional component or overlay superimposed on an organic deficit. Other terms used synonymously with functional hearing loss include pseudohypacusis, nonorganic hearing loss, hysterical deafness, psychogenic hearing loss, malingering, and exaggerated hearing loss. Chaiklin and Ventry (1963) prefer the term "functional hearing loss" since it allows for the possibility that in the future some organic condition can be found to explain the test discrepancies. Martin (1985) and Rintelmann (1979) prefer the term "pseudohypacusis" (literally, false hearing loss) which is the shortened form of the term "pseudoneural hypacusis" (Brockman & Hoversten, 1960).

The audiologist has no procedure for determining whether there is an unconscious or a conscious basis for the nonorganic hearing loss and should not attempt to specify the basis of the functional hearing loss. Terms which lack implications regarding the nature of the loss (unconscious or conscious), such as pseudohypacusis, nonorganic hearing loss, and functional hearing loss, are preferred.

Malingering is a term used to refer to the conscious exaggeration of hearing loss. The diagnosis of malingering can be made only upon patient confession of falsification of hearing loss.

The terms "psychogenic" or "hysterical" hearing loss have been used to refer to hearing loss with an unconscious basis. According to Goldstein (1966), psychogenic hearing loss is proven only if the patient presents with a hearing loss on conventional, behavioral audiologic tests, has better hearing threshold levels as revealed through hypnosis or electrophysiologic tests, has a clinical history consistent with the presence of a hearing loss, and has improved hearing threshold levels after the psychological problem has

been resolved. Since there have not been reports of any psychogenic hearing loss which meets these criteria, Goldstein (1966) concluded that psychogenic hearing loss does not not exist and that all functional hearing loss has a conscious basis. Therefore, all persons with functional hearing loss are malingerers.

Ventry (1968), who presented a case study of a patient with unilateral psychogenic hearing loss, disagreed with the criteria for psychogenic hearing loss developed by Goldstein (1966). He suggested that psychogenic hearing loss refers to hearing loss having an apparent psychogenic origin, and its unconscious or conscious basis is irrelevant.

The issue of differentiating between malingerers (who do not confess to falsification of the hearing loss) and those with psychogenic hearing loss remains unresolved.

I. PREVALENCE

A. ADULTS

The prevalence of functional hearing loss in veterans increased markedly after World War II. According to Johnson, Work, and McCoy (1956), the prevalence of functional hearing loss in veterans increased from 11 to 45% over a 10-year period after World War II. Johnson *et al.* attributed this increase to the inadequate techniques for identification of functional hearing loss, the increase in compensation awards, and increased public awareness of functional hearing loss and, in some cases, inadequate counseling at the initial hearing-test session. In recent years, the prevalence of functional hearing loss in veterans has decreased. Schwartz (in Rintelmann, 1979), found that approximately 2% of veterans seen in 1978 at the Walter Reed Hospital Audiology and Speech Center had functional hearing loss. The senior author has obtained a similar estimate of functional hearing loss in veterans at the Veterans Administration Medical Center in East Orange, New Jersey. Rintelmann (1979) attributed the decreased prevalence of functional hearing loss in veterans to improved audiologic techniques, audiologic training, and experience.

The prevalence of functional hearing loss now approximates that in the general population. In the general population, the prevalence of functional hearing loss has been estimated to be between 1 and 5% (Kinstler, 1971; Zwislocki, 1963).

An increase in the prevalence of functional hearing loss is a recent trend in industrial settings. Following the Occupational Safety and Health Act of 1970, which recognized the hazardous effects of excessive noise exposure with respect to hearing loss and the responsibility of employers to safeguard the hearing of their workers, the number of compensation claims for occupational hearing loss has increased. Barelli and Ruder (1970), for example, reported that 24% of workers who filed compensation claims had functional hearing loss. Alberti (1970) reported that the number of claims in the Province of Ontario following the Workman's Compensation Act in the early 1950s increased dramatically. Alberti, Morgan, and Czuba (1978) reported that functional hearing loss was present in approximately 15 to 20% of persons filing compensation claims for hearing impairment related to excessive noise exposure on the job site. Thus, the prevalence of functional hearing loss is increased in populations characterized by a high rate of medicolegal claims for compensation for loss of hearing resulting from excessive noise exposure.

B. CHILDREN

Doerfler (1951) reported that the prevalence of functional hearing loss in children was negligible in 74% of audiologic centers, between 1 and 5% in 21% of audiologic centers, and greater than 5% in 7% of audiologic centers responding to a survey. These findings have been substantiated by other investigators. For example, Berk and Feldman (1958) reported that functional hearing loss was present in 3% of children seen at the Pittsburgh Eye and Ear Hospital. Leshin (1960) found that 2.5% of 1902 children who failed hearing screenings had functional hearing loss. Dixon and Newby (1959) reported evaluating only 40 children with functional hearing loss over a 2-year period at the San Francisco Hearing and Speech Center. Campanelli (1963) reported that functional hearing loss was present in 4.8% of 860 children who failed school hearing screenings and received audiologic follow-up. Based on the review of audiologic records, Stein (1966) found that functional hearing loss was present in 3.5% of children less than 18 years old. Berger (1965) observed a seasonal fluctuation in the prevalence rate of functional hearing loss in children, with greater rates in late winter or early spring, times during which otitis media is especially prevalent.

Functional hearing loss occurs three times as frequently in girls than boys (Brockman & Hoversten, 1960; Calvert,

Moncur, Smith, & Snyder, 1961; Dixon & Newby, 1959). The basis for this predilection for females is unknown.

Berger (1965) suggested that functional hearing loss typically occurs in children with academic difficulties and a recent ear infection. He also observed that many nonorganic visual problems were present in children with functional hearing loss.

II. BEHAVIORAL SIGNS

Various behaviors have been associated with functional hearing loss, for example, (a) exaggerated attempts to lipread with constant visual fixation on the face; (b) exaggerated attempts to hear as evidenced, for example, by tilting one's head so that the ear is more directly in line with the speech signal; (c) complaint of inability to hear accompanied by the request that communication occur through written messages; (d) unfamiliarity with the operation of a hearing aid belonging to the functionally hearing-impaired person; (e) the use of a hearing aid with a dead battery belonging to the functionally hearing-impaired person; (f) apparent nervousness and anxiety; and (g) apparent discrepancy between the clinical history and the articulation and voice qualities (Fournier, 1958; Johnson et al., 1956; Thorne, 1960). In general, such behaviors represent an exaggeration of the perceived behaviors of the organic hearing impaired. A commonly observed behavior in children with functional hearing loss is the ability to carry on a conversation easily in an informal setting. Some researchers have suggested drastic methods to uncover functional hearing loss in children such saying softly, "button your pants" or "you dropped your money." These behaviors are not diagnostic of functional hearing loss since many persons with organic hearing loss demonstrate these behaviors. The presence of these behaviors, however, should alert the clinician to the possibility of a functional hearing loss.

A physiologic response, the aural–palpebral reflex (an eyeblink or an eyelid tightening when the eyes are closed), in response to an unexpected intense sound has been considered by some investigators to be a sign of functional hearing loss (Fournier, 1958). This response cannot be considered a reliable measure of functional hearing loss since the aural–palpebral reflex does not always occur in normal-hearing persons, is a suprathreshold response which therefore is less likely to occur as the magnitude of the hearing loss increases, and habituates with repeated presentations.

III. INDICATORS WITHIN ROUTINE AUDIOLOGIC TESTS

A. TEST–RETEST RELIABILITY

Lack of intertest or intratest reliability is a sign of functional hearing loss (Heller, 1955; Newby, 1958; Watson & Tolan, 1949). Several investigators have reported that intratest reliability (as indicated by repeat measurement during the test session) of pure-tone threshold measurement is within ±5 dB in normal-hearing and organic hearing-impaired persons (Carhart & Jerger, 1959; Chaiklin, Ventry, & Barrett, 1961; Witting & Hughson, 1940).

Ventry and Chaiklin (1965a) reported that a test–retest difference of at least 15 dB at 1000 Hz was present in 11% of functional-hearing-loss ears; if four rather than two measurements at 1000 Hz were made, then a test–retest difference of at least 15 dB was present in 66% of persons with functional hearing loss. Ventry and Chaiklin suggested that the sensitivity of the test–retest measure could be increased by the use of an ascending approach for the first threshold measurement and a descending approach for the repeat threshold measurement at a particular frequency. Carhart and Jerger (1959) and Harris (1958) reported that the use of an ascending or descending approach to pure-tone threshold determination does not affect pure-tone test–retest reliability in persons with organic hearing loss. Harris (1958) found that persons with functional hearing loss have substantial differences between the ascending and descending pure-tone thresholds. Nevertheless, several investigators have reported that many persons with functional hearing loss have good test–retest reliability on pure-tone threshold tests (Berger, 1965; Campanelli, 1963; Lehrer, Hirschenfang, Miller, & Radpour, 1964; Shepherd, 1965).

The clinician should be cautioned that some persons with organic hearing loss, particularly central auditory pathology, may have large test–retest differences. In such patients, pure-tone thresholds are often difficult to obtain. Also, the presence of tinnitus may yield test–retest differences which often can be minimized with the use of pulsed tones.

MODIFIED PURE-TONE THRESHOLD
MEASUREMENT METHODS
a. Variable Intensity Pulse-Count Method
Modifications of the threshold-determination technique have been suggested for the detection of functional hearing loss and the assessment of true hearing sensitivity in children. Ross (1964) developed a technique, a variation of that suggested by Newby (1958, p. 1), called the Variable Intensity Pulse Count Method (VIPCM). The child is told that a test of counting ability is being given. A sequence of 1 to 6 tones above the admitted threshold is presented until reliably accurate results are obtained. Then, the sequences of tones are presented so that some of the tones in the particular sequence are below the admitted threshold. If the child reported hearing the correct number of tones, it is assumed that the child must have heard the tones below as well as above the threshold. Thus, for each sequence of tones presented, a variable number of tones below the threshold are interspersed with those above the threshold. The true threshold of the child can be obtained in this manner. Ross reported that the thresholds obtained using the VIPCM method were consistent with the SRTs.

b. Yes–No Method
Another modification of the threshold-determination technique for use with children suspected of functional hearing loss is the "yes–no" method, in which tones are presented using the ascending approach and the child is instructed to say "yes" when the tone is heard and "no" when the tone is not heard (Frank, 1976; Miller, Fox, & Chan, 1968). It is assumed that, whether the response is "yes" or "no," either response indicates that the child heard the tone if the response is time-locked with the stimulus. This technique is appropriate for children who are not yet intellectually mature enough to appreciate the basis of this test.

B. INTERAURAL ATTENUATION OF AIR- AND BONE-CONDUCTION TONES

Another sign of functional hearing loss is the absence of a shadow curve. The range of interaural attenuation values for air-conduction tones ranges from 40 to 85 dB (Chaiklin, 1967; Liden, Nilsson, & Anderson, 1959; Zwislocki, 1953), with values at the lower end of the range present at the low frequencies and values at the higher end of the range present at the high frequencies. Therefore, an interaural unmasked air-conduction threshold difference of 85 dB or more may be indicative of functional hearing loss.

Similarly, the interaural attenuation values of bone-conduction signals can be as large as 20 dB, particularly at the high frequencies (Feldman, 1961; Liden et al., 1959; Sanders & Rintelmann, 1964; Studebaker, 1964; Zwislocki, 1953). Therefore, interaural unmasked bone-conduction threshold differences of 25 dB or more should alert the clinician to the possibility of a functional hearing loss.

C. POOR BONE-CONDUCTION THRESHOLD LEVELS

Another sign of functional hearing loss is the presence of bone-conduction thresholds substantially poorer than the air-conduction thresholds (Johnson et al., 1956). Since bone-conduction threshold testing measures the integrity of only part of the auditory system beginning with the inner ear whereas air-conduction testing measures the integrity of the entire auditory system beginning with the outer ear, bone-conduction thresholds cannot be poorer than air-conduction thresholds, at least in theory. Nevertheless, because of factors such as calibration, placement of the bone oscillator, and the applied force of the oscillator on the mastoid or forehead, slightly worse values may sometimes be obtained for bone-conduction than air-conduction thresholds. Therefore, bone-conduction thresholds poorer than air-conduction thresholds by at least 20 dB should be considered a sign of functional hearing loss.

D. FALSE-ALARMING

Feldman (1962) observed that persons with functional hearing loss fail to false-alarm during the silent periods of pure-tone testing. That is, they fail to respond during the silent periods between tonal presentations. This failure to false-alarm is in contrast with the behavior of persons with organic hearing loss, who often false-alarm during the silent period between tonal presentations. Chaiklin and Ventry (1965) reported that only 14% of the nonfunctional-hearing-loss group as opposed to 88% of the functional-hearing-loss group failed to false-alarm during the silent periods of pure-tone testing. Chaiklin and Ventry employed 1-min silent periods as well as the routine silent periods between tonal presentations to detect the presence or absence of false-alarms.

E. ERROR RESPONSES DURING SRT AND MONOSYLLABIC PB-WORD SPEECH-RECOGNITION ASSESSMENT

Several investigators have reported that persons with functional hearing loss often repeat only half of the stimulus bisyllable given during speech-recognition threshold (SRT) testing (Brockman & Hoversten, 1960; Fournier, 1958; Johnson et al., 1956; Thorne, 1960) (See Chapter 2 for further details on SRT testing.) Since both parts of the spondee represent complete words, the half-stimulus response is a whole-word response, for example, "play" for "playground." Chaiklin and Ventry (1965) reported that the half-stimulus response error during SRT testing occurred in 46% of their functional-hearing-loss subjects and only 9% of their nonfunctional-hearing-loss subjects.

Chaiklin and Ventry (1965) found that functionally hearing-impaired subjects were more likely to make no-response errors and response errors consisting of a monosyllabic word not containing part of the stimulus than organic-hearing-loss subjects. On the basis of this finding, they constructed a spondee-error index (SERI) calculated as

$$\text{SERI} = (\text{NRE} - \text{OS} - \text{SL})/\text{TE} \times 100$$

where NRE is the number of no-response errors, OS is the number of one-syllable errors—either the half-stimulus or other one-syllable error—, SL is the spondee from the stimulus list, and TE is the total number of errors. Chaiklin and Ventry (1965) reported that a score exceeding 85 was obtained by 73% of the functional-hearing-loss subjects and by 17% of their nonfunctional-hearing-loss subjects. When the measure was applied to new groups of functional-hearing-loss and nonfunctional-hearing-loss subjects, the SERI measure had a hit rate of 85% and a false-alarm rate of 13%.

Engelberg (1978) and Campbell (1965) suggested that failure to respond to the "easy" (more intelligible) spondaic and monosyllabic PB words during SRT or monosyllabic speech-recognition testing along with correct responses to the more "difficult" (less intelligible) spondaic and monosyllabic PB words during SRT or monosyllabic speech-recognition testing were indicative of functional hearing loss.

F. SRT–PTA DISCREPANCY

Carhart (1952) was the first to report that the SRT is usually lower than the pure-tone average (PTA) in persons with functional hearing loss. This finding was subsequently substantiated by other investigators (Brockman & Hoversten, 1960; Chaiklin, Ventry, Barrett, & Skalbeck, 1959; Fournier, 1958; Glorig, 1954; Newby, 1958). Ventry and Chaiklin (1965a) considered an SRT–PTA discrepancy of 12 dB or more to be indicative of functional hearing loss. The SRT is compared with the 3-frequency PTA when the speech-frequency thresholds do not differ by more than 5 dB. A 2-frequency PTA (best 2 of the 3 speech frequencies) is compared with the SRT when the thresholds at 2 of the speech frequencies differ by 10 dB or more. In cases of sharply sloping losses with at least a 25-dB drop between 500 and 1000 Hz, an SRT–PTA discrepancy of more than 25 dB is considered to be consistent with functional hearing loss.

The SRT–PTA discrepancy was found by Ventry and Chaiklin (1965a) to have a hit rate of 70%. Ventry and Chaiklin (1965a) considered the SRT–PTA discrepancy to be the best measure for detection of functional hearing loss of the four measures evaluated: SRT–PTA discrepancy, pure-tone test–retest measure, pure-tone Stenger, and speech Stenger. Alberti et al. (1978) considered an SRT–PTA discrepancy greater than 10 dB to be indicative of functional hearing loss. They reported that the SRT–PTA discrepancy had a hit rate of 62% for their group of 121 functional-hearing-loss subjects and a false-alarm rate of 3% for their group of 475 nonfunctional-hearing-loss subjects. Rintelmann and Harford (1963) found that the SRT–PTA discrepancy was present in 100% of their group of 10 children with functional hearing loss; the SRTs in these cases were within normal limits or close to normal. Conn, Ventry, and Woods (1972) reported that the SRT–PTA discrepancy can be increased in normal-hearing persons with simulated hearing loss if the SRT is measured using the ascending rather than descending approach.

Several investigators have proposed that persons with functional hearing loss employ a mental loudness yardstick against which the loudness of signals can be compared (Doerfler & Stewart, 1946; Fournier, 1958; Glorig, 1954). Ventry (1976) felt that the loudness yardstick hypothesis was supported by the findings of Conn et al. (1972) and Barrett (1959) that persons with simulated hearing loss employ a loudness reference to guide their responses in audiologic testing. This loudness reference is employed either on a conscious (Goldstein, 1966) or unconscious (Hopkinson, 1967; Ventry, 1968) basis. Research has shown that, at equal SPLs above threshold, the loudness of speech and pure tones is equal (Mendel, Sussman, Merson, Naeser, & Minifie, 1969). Ventry (1976) suggested that this fact was essential to understanding the basis of the SRT–PTA discrepancy in functional hearing loss.

Another fact essential to understanding the basis of the SRT–PTA discrepancy, according to Ventry (1976), was the calibration of speech vs. pure tones. The audiometer is calibrated so that the audiometric zero for speech is 20 dB relative to 20 μPa as opposed to 7 dB relative to 20 μPa for the 1000-Hz air-conducted signal. Therefore, equivalent thresholds for speech and pure tones at the speech frequencies in dB SPL result in lower dB HL values for speech than for pure tones.

Ventry (1976) suggested that, if a loudness reference criterion is employed during pure-tone and speech testing, speech and pure tones are equally loud at equal SPLs, and the thresholds are measured in dB HL, then an SRT–PTA discrepancy will result. Martin (1978) suggested that the SRT–PTA discrepancy is based on the relation between the loudness of speech and the loudness of its low-frequency components. As shown by the equal-loudness contours, the loudness of the low frequencies grows faster than that of the mid frequencies (speech frequencies). This hypothesis was supported by the findings of McLennan and Martin (1976).

Monro and Martin (1977) reported that knowledge about the SRT–PTA discrepancy and practice adversely affected the sensitivity of the measure to simulated hearing loss to a greater extent than the test–retest ascending–descending measure, the pure-tone Stenger, and the pure-tone delayed auditory feedback (DAF) test.

G. SPEECH-RECOGNITION TESTING WITH MONOSYLLABIC PB WORDS

Some investigators have suggested presenting the monosyllabic PB words employed during speech-recognition assessment at low sensation levels relative to the admitted SRT when testing persons with suspected functional hearing loss (Hopkinson, 1978; Olsen & Matkin, 1978) (See Chapter 5 for further details on suprathreshold speech-recognition assessment.) High speech-recognition scores at these low sensation levels may be indicative of the presence of exaggerated SRTs since they are generally expected at levels of 30–40 dB SL relative to the SRT. Gold, Lubinsky, and Shahar (1981) found that their group of functionally hearing-impaired young adults had speech-recognition scores that, on average, were significantly higher than those of normal-hearing persons at 5, 10, and 15 dB SL relative to the SRT. The largest differences between groups were obtained at the lowest sensation level (5 dB). One shortcoming of this measure of functional hearing loss is that some persons with organic hearing loss attain high speech-recognition scores at low sensation levels.

H. AUDIOLOGIC CONFIGURATION

The configuration of the pure-tone audiogram has been employed to identify patients with functional hearing loss. The saucer audiogram was previously thought to be a sign of functional hearing loss (Carhart, 1958; Doerfler, 1951; Goetzinger & Proud, 1958; Johnson et al., 1956). Some researchers suggested that the flat audiogram is also indicative of functional hearing loss (Fournier, 1958; Semenov, 1947). Chaiklin et al. (1959) provided evidence suggesting that the saucer audiogram is unlikely to be diagnostic of functional hearing loss and functional hearing loss is not characterized by a particular pure-tone configuration. Ventry and Chaiklin (1965b) analyzed the pure-tone configuration of 64 persons with functional hearing loss and 36 persons with nonfunctional hearing loss. They found that the saucer and flat audiometric configuration had a low incidence of occurrence in both the functional and nonfunctional groups. Ventry and Chaiklin (1965b) also observed that the functional overlay at 4000 and 8000 Hz was decreased in comparison with the overlay at low frequencies. They suggested that the presence of loudness recruitment at the high frequencies was probably responsible for the decreased magnitude of the functional overlay in that frequency region.

Gelfand and Silman (1985) analyzed the records of adults with resolved bilateral functional hearing loss to determine if the configuration of the functional overlay was related to that of the resolved hearing-threshold levels. The magnitude of the functional overlay was essentially similar across frequencies when the resolved hearing sensitivity was normal or near normal. When the resolved hearing-threshold levels were consistent with a high-frequency hearing loss, the magnitude of the functional overlay was markedly decreased at the impaired high frequencies relative to the low frequencies. When the resolved hearing-threshold levels were consistent with a moderate or severe hearing loss, the magnitude of the functional overlay decreased gradually as frequency increased. Gelfand and Silman suggested that these findings indicate that persons with functional hearing loss use a mental target loudness to guide their responses during pure-tone threshold assessment. They also suggested that decreased magnitude of functional overlay was expected at frequencies where recruitment is commonly present, that is, at the high-frequency region.

The functional indicators in routine, audiologic tests cannot be considered functional signs unless other variables have been ruled out, such as equipment malfunction (e.g., inadequate connection of transducers into the jack panel, partial break in the cable, mechanical clicks with stimulus presentation, misplaced or absent test or masking signal, nonlinearity of the attenuator, poor calibration), excessive ambient noise, patient artifacts (e.g., short attention span, tinnitus, diplacusis or pitch distortion, collapsed canals), or inappropriate test materials or procedures (e.g., poor instructions, word lists with vocabulary unfamiliar to the patient, inappropriate pure-tone test procedures, inappropriate masking, and tactile thresholds interpreted wrongly as bone-conduction thresholds in some cases of severe or worse hearing impairment) (Lloyd & Kaplan, 1978).

IV. SPECIAL BEHAVIORAL TESTS

A. SENSORINEURAL ACUITY LEVEL

The sensorineural acuity level (SAL) test developed by Jerger and Tillman (1960) was designed as an alternative to bone-conduction threshold measurement. It is a modification of the Rainville Technique (Rainville, 1955) in which masking is presented through the bone-conduction oscillator and the amount of masking required to cause a shift in the air-conduction threshold is measured. With the SAL technique, broad-band noise (2 V) is presented through the bone-conduction oscillator placed on the forehead. The difference between the air-conduction thresholds with and without masking is the SAL shift for that individual. The individual SAL shift is then subtracted from the average SAL shift for a group of normal-hearing subjects to yield the SAL threshold which is comparable to the bone-conduction threshold.

Problems with the SAL technique include underestimation of the cochlear reserve in subjects with conductive hearing loss since the absence of the occlusion effect results in a smaller shift in the air-conduction thresholds resulting from the noise. (Feldman, 1961; Siedentorp, Kapple, & Derbyshire, 1966; Tillman, 1963). The noise causes an increased shift in air-conduction thresholds in some sensorineural hearing-impaired persons, particularly the elderly, resulting in decreased SAL thresholds in these persons. (Feldman, 1961; Siedentorp et al., 1966; Tillman, 1963).

Rintelmann and Harford (1963) employed the SAL test to identify (presbycusis) in a group of 10 school children. They found that, in all of the subjects, there was a gap between the voluntary admitted thresholds and the SAL thresholds before the functional hearing loss was resolved. This finding was termed the "Air–Sal" gap. Thus, the presence of an Air–Sal gap is an indication of functional hearing impairment and the bone-conduction thresholds are assumed to be at least as good as the SAL thresholds.

The SAL test has also been used with spondaic words rather than pure tones (Bailey & Martin, 1963; Bragg, 1962; Rintelmann & Johnson, 1970). Little has been reported regarding the effectiveness of the speech SAL test in detecting functional hearing loss.

B. LOMBARD AND SIDETONE-AMPLIFICATION EFFECTS

The Lombard voice reflex refers to the change in vocal intensity resulting from the presence of noise. According to Egan (1971), Lombard (1911) developed the Lombard test based on his observations that persons with sensorineural hearing loss have increased vocal intensity and are unable to monitor their voice and normal-hearing persons increase their vocal intensity in noisy situations.

The Lombard test involves the sudden presentation of noise to a patient reading aloud or answering questions and noting any changes in vocal intensity. The noise is presented to both ears, either successively or simultaneously, with greater changes in vocal intensity associated with the latter than with the former procedure in normal-hearing persons. When the noise is applied unilaterally, only a small increase in vocal intensity is observed. The superiority of binaural over monaural has been reported by several investigators (Egan, 1967; Taylor, 1949; Waldron, 1960). Bilateral simultaneous masking causes an increase in vocal intensity in both normal-hearing and unilaterally hearing-impaired persons. Unilateral hearing impairment can be detected through the use of successive (alternate) masking, since the presence of masking in the impaired ear will not result in a vocal intensity increase. With bilateral hearing loss, the vocal intensity does not increase regardless of the method of masking. Conductive hearing loss must be ruled out before employing this test, since persons with conductive hearing loss can monitor their voices through bone-conducted feedback. Lombard also cautioned against the use of this technique in persons with partial hearing loss since the magnitude of the hearing loss is inversely related to the amount of vocal intensity change.

Lombard's observations concerning vocal intensity increases in noise and the direct relation between noise levels and vocal intensity levels were substantiated by several investigators (Black, 1950; Brown & Brandt, 1971; Charlip & Burk, 1969; Dreher & O'Neil, 1957; Egan, 1967; Hanley & Steer, 1949; Korn, 1954; Waldron, 1960). The Lombard effect is also dependent on the spectral composition of the noise (Black, 1950; Egan, 1967; Pickett, 1958). Black (1951) supported Lombard's hypothesis that an increase in the vocal intensity in noise resulted from the speaker's attempt to monitor his or her own voice.

The sidetone-amplification effect is related to the Lombard effect. Both have in common a change in vocal intensity. In the sidetone-amplification effect, however, the change in vocal intensity occurs as a result of receiving the feedback from one's own voice at an amplified level rather than as a result of the presence of the noise (Lightfoot & Morrill, 1949). Garber, Siegell, Pick, & Alcorn (1979) found that those noise signals that adversely affect speech intelligibility are the signals that most enhance the sidetone-amplification and Lombard effects.

Pe

"Page 142, first column, third paragraph: "presbycusis" should read pseudohypacusis."

A functional hearing loss is confirmed if bilateral simultaneous masking results in increased vocal intensity and alternate (successive) masking results in increased vocal intensity regardless of the ear receiving the noise. With unilateral masking, the noise is placed in the bad ear and a functional hearing loss is confirmed if there is an increase in vocal intensity. If the Lombard voice reflex occurs at noise intensity levels below the admitted voluntary thresholds, the test is positive. Binaural application of the noise results in larger vocal intensity changes than monaural noise.

The patient reads aloud a passage into a microphone while wearing earphones which transmit the noise into one or both ears. If the microphone output is fed into the volume unit (VU) meter of the audiometer, the intensity levels can be monitored (Simonton, 1965). Harris (1965) suggested noise and talkback intensity levels so that the former is at 0 dB and the latter peaks at 0 on the VU meter. Then the intensity of the noise is gradually increased until a meter deflection beyond the 0 point on the VU meter is observed.

The Lombard and sidetone-amplification tests have not gained popularity for the following reasons:

1. They do not enable threshold estimation but merely detect the presence of functional hearing loss.
2. They are characterized by large intertest and intratest variability in the magnitude of the vocal-intensity changes in noise.
3. Some persons are resistant to the effects of the noise.

C. DOERFLER–STEWART TEST

The Doerfler–Stewart test (Doerfler & Stewart, 1946) was one of the earliest tests for the detection of functional hearing loss. The purpose of the test is to detect the presence of bilateral functional hearing loss. Nevertheless, the test has also been administered in the monaural mode in order to detect the presence of unilateral functional hearing loss. The basic principle of the Doerfler–Stewart (D-S) test is the disruption by noise of the loudness yardstick employed by functional-hearing-loss subjects to present consistent audiologic results. The more the noise and procedure confuses the patient, the more effective the test in detecting the presence of functional hearing loss. The procedure is as follows.

1. Obtain SRT_1 using the binaural ascending mode.
2. Calculate the $SRT_1 + 5$ dB value.
3. Introduce 0 dB HL of noise, bilaterally, and increase the noise intensity in 5-dB steps until the patient can no longer repeat the spondaic words presented at the $SRT_1 + 5$ dB level. This level of noise is called the noise interference level (NIL).
4. Continue presenting the spondaic words at the $SRT_1 + 5$ dB level with the noise increasing above NIL in 5-dB steps until a noise level equivalent to NIL + 20 dB is reached. One spondaic word per noise level is presented.

5. With the noise level at NIL + 20 dB, present spondaic words, one per level, with the intensity of speech decreasing in 5-dB steps until the level equivalent to $SRT_1 - 15$ dB is reached.
6. With the speech at the $SRT_1 - 15$ dB level, decrease the noise in 10-dB steps, giving one spondaic word per level, until the NIL is reached and then decrease in 5-dB steps until the lower limit of the audiometer is reached.
7. Repeat step 1 to get the SRT_2.
8. Obtain the noise-detection threshold (NDT) using the binaural ascending mode and 5-dB increments.
9. Calculate the following difference measures: (a) $SRT_1 - SRT_2$, (b) $SRT_1 - NDT$, (c) $SRT_2 - NDT$, (d) $SRT_1 + 5 - NIL$, and (e) $NDT - NIL$.
10. Compare the results with the normative values. The D–S test is positive for functional hearing loss if at least two of the difference measures exceed the upper limit of the normal range (Ventry & Chaiklin, 1965a).

The noise should be a sawtooth noise (Doerfler & Stewart, 1946) which is psychologically more disruptive than other noises (Doerfler & Epstein, 1956).

Doerfler and Epstein (1956) stated that a positive result on the NDT − NIL and/or the $SRT_1 + 5 - NIL$ measure is more significant than a positive result on the other difference measures. They felt that the number of positive measures was not as significant as the particular measure on which the positive response was obtained.

Menzel (1960) reported a hit rate of 58% for the D-S test. Ventry and Chaiklin (1965a) reported a hit rate of 38% and a false-alarm rate of 28%. When the criterion of two or more positive difference scores or a positive result on the NDT − NIL or $SRT_1 + 5 - NIL$ measure was employed, the hit rate was 42% and the false-alarm rate was 50%. The measures with the lowest false-alarm rates were the $SRT_1 - NDT$ and the $SRT_2 - NDT$ measures, contrary to the findings reported by Doerfler and Epstein (1956). Ventry and Chaiklin (1965a) obtained new normative data and compared the findings in the functional subjects against these new norms. Using the criterion that the D–S test was positive if two or more difference scores based on the new normative data were positive, the hit rate was 65% and the false-alarm rate was 17%. Thus, the use of the new normative data improved the sensitivity and specificity of the test.

Hattler and Schuchman (1971) reported that they were unable to administer the D–S test to approximately 65% of their 225 subjects with functional hearing loss. For the group consisting of the persons to whom the D–S test could be administered, the hit rate was 77% and the false-alarm rate was 20%.

Martin and Hawkins (1963) modified the D–S test and employed pure tones rather than spondaic words as the stimuli. The only measures which had to be obtained were the tonal threshold (T_1), $T_1 + 5$, NIL, and T_2. The difference scores calculated and compared against the normative data included $T_1 - T_2$ and NIL $- T_1 + 5$. Pang-Ching (1970) developed a "tone-in-noise" test similar to the Martin and Hawkins (1963) modification.

D. STENGER TEST

1. PURE-TONE STENGER

Stenger (1900, 1907) developed the Stenger test, which employed two matched-frequency tuning forks held at various distances from the ears of the subject. The basis of this test, the Stenger effect, is the following phenomenon. If two tones of the same frequency which differ in intensity are presented, one to each ear of a subject, the subject will hear the tone only in the ear receiving the signal at the greater sensation level. Other researchers developed modifications of the tuning-fork procedure (Firestone, 1934; Russell, 1934). The Stenger test was adopted for use with an audiometer and earphones (Ballantyne, 1960; Guttman, 1928).

The Stenger test is best administered while doing basic pure-tone threshold determination so the subject is less aware that the Stenger test is being administered. The instructions for the Stenger test should not differ from those given for pure-tone audiometry. Two tones are presented, one above the threshold of the good ear and one below the admitted threshold of the poor ear. If the subject fails to indicate that the tone is heard, the test is positive for functional hearing loss. The failure to respond indicates that the tone is heard at a higher sensation level in the bad than in the good ear.

Most investigators suggest a presentation level of 5-10 dB SL in the good ear (Davis & Silverman, 1960; Goetzinger & Proud, 1958; Newby, 1958; O'Neill & Oyer, 1966; Ventry, 1962). Various starting levels in the bad ear have been proposed, such as 0 dB HL, 40 dB HL (Goetzinger & Proud, 1958), 10 dB SL relative to the good-ear threshold (O'Neill & Oyer, 1966), and at equal dB HLs in the two ears (Ventry, 1962).

Altshuler (1970) described the methods of test presentation in terms of three categories. The first category includes those Stenger procedures which attempt to detect only the presence of functional hearing loss rather than establish the true thresholds. These methods involve the presentation of tones at only one level, for example, near the threshold in the good ear and at 40 dB HL in the poor ear. Failure to respond is indicative of a functional hearing loss in the bad ear.

The second category includes those Stenger procedures which attempt to estimate thresholds in the functionally hearing-impaired ear. The following procedure exemplifies a method in this category.

1. Present a tone to the better and poorer ears, for example, at 10 dB SL relative to the better ear hearing threshold level, bilaterally. The tones should be presented in a manner similar to that employed during routine pure-tone audiometry. The patient should indicate that the tone is heard (in the good ear).
2. Increase the intensity in the poor ear in 5-dB increments. The patient should continue to indicate that a tone is heard (in the good ear). If the Stenger is negative, the patient continues to signal hearing a tone (initially in the good ear and, later on, when the SL in the bad ear exceeds that in the good ear, in the bad ear). If the subject fails to respond at some intensity below the admitted voluntary threshold, the Stenger test is positive, that is, the tone was heard at a higher SL in the bad than good ear. Presumably, the patient is not "letting on" that the tone is heard in the bad ear and is unaware of the tone in the good ear. This method has been employed by several investigators (Azzi, 1950; Feldman, 1962; Fournier, 1958; Menzel, 1965; Newby, 1958; Ventry & Chaiklin, 1965a).

Some investigators have employed a descending approach (Fournier, 1958; Goetzinger & Proud, 1958; Menzel, 1965; Portmann & Portmann, 1961) as follows.

1. Present a tone to the good ear near threshold and to the poor ear at a high intensity. The test is negative if the patient responds, indicating that the tone is heard (in the bad ear). The test is positive if the patient fails to respond, signaling that the SL of the tone in the bad ear exceeds that in the good ear.
2. Decrease the intensity in the bad ear, in 5-dB increments. The tones should be presented in a manner similar to that employed during routine pure-tone audiometry. If the Stenger test continues to be negative, the patient will continue responding—to the poor ear initially at levels above the voluntary admitted threshold levels and then to the good ear when the SL in the good ear exceeds that in the bad ear. The Stenger is positive if, initially, there is no response but then a response occurs for the tone in the good ear when the intensity decreases to a certain point, indicating the level has been reached at which the SL in the good ear exceeds that in the bad ear.

Whether the ascending or descending approach is employed, the test is positive if a response alteration occurs at levels at least 15 dB below the voluntary admitted threshold (Ventry & Chaiklin, 1965a). The lowest intensity level at which response alteration occurs has been termed the minimum contralateral interference level (Martin, 1985). The behavioral threshold is estimated to be within 10–20 dB of the minimum contralateral interference level (provided the tone is presented to the good ear at 10 dB SL).

The third category includes those Stenger procedures which employ a fadeout technique. With the ascending approach, some patients continue to respond to the tone in the good ear even when the SL in the bad ear exceeds that in the good ear because they have "figured out the test" and realize that there must also be a tone in the good ear. If the tone from the good ear is withdrawn while the tone in the bad ear is continued and the patient continues to respond as if the tone is heard in the good ear, the result is positive, provided that the intensity of the tone does not permit cross-hearing. The tone can be either abruptly withdrawn or slowly attenuated in the good ear (Davis & Silverman, 1960; Newby, 1958; O'Neill & Oyer, 1966; Ventry & Chaiklin, 1965a; Watson & Tolan, 1949).

The Stenger test is most successful when it is employed in persons presenting with a substantial unilateral hearing loss. It is less effective in cases of asymmetrical bilateral hearing loss. Ventry and Chaiklin (1965a) observed that the likelihood of a positive result in a patient with a functional hearing loss was directly related to the size of the interaural threshold difference or the magnitude of the functional overlay in the poorer ear. They felt the test was most sensitive when there was an interaural difference of at least 40 dB.

The authors have observed, from their personal experience, that the likelihood of obtaining a positive Stenger test in cases presenting with asymmetrical bilateral hearing loss depends on the size of the functional overlay in the poorer ear relative to that in the good ear. For example, if a patient has an organic deficit of 50 dB in the good ear and a functional overlay of 50 dB superimposed on an organic deficit of 50 dB in the bad ear, a positive Stenger test result may be obtained when the sensation level in the bad ear exceeds that in the good ear. On the other hand, if there is a functional hearing loss in both ears, a negative Stenger test result may be obtained if the functional overlay in the good ear is greater than that in the bad ear. For example, consider a patient with a true hearing threshold of 0 dB and a functional overlay of 50 dB in the good ear and a true hearing threshold of 50 dB with a functional overlay of 40 dB in the bad ear; a 60 dB HL sound is presented to the two ears. The 60 dB sound is at a higher SL in the good ear than in the bad ear. Thus, a negative Stenger test would result. Even if the sound intensity in the bad ear is increased to 80 dB (10 dB below the admitted threshold in the bad ear), the tone in the good ear (at 60 dB) would still be heard at a higher sensation level than the tone in the bad ear, and there would be a negative Stenger test. When a patient presents with a bilateral asymmetrical hearing loss, it cannot be known in advance whether there is a functional hearing loss in one or both ears or, in the latter case, which ear has the larger functional overlay. Therefore, although a positive Stenger result would be indicative of a functional hearing loss in cases of bilateral asymmetrical hearing loss, a functional hearing loss in such cases cannot be ruled out by a negative Stenger test result.

The following true case illustrates the point that a functional hearing loss cannot be ruled out if a negative Stenger is obtained. The patient is a 47-year-old male with an asymmetrical hearing loss. Table I shows the audiologic data obtained for audiologic testing 3 years apart. At the initial visit, the speech-recognition threshold was in agreement with the pure-tone average, bilaterally. The results of the pure-tone Stenger test administered at 1000 Hz was negative. At the second visit, 3 years later, air-conduction thresholds in both ears were substantially increased. Again, the pure-tone Stenger test at 1000 Hz was negative. Nevertheless, functional hearing loss was suspected this time since the speech-recognition threshold was markedly better than the pure-tone average, bilaterally. Interestingly, the

Table I Air-Conduction Thresholds, Speech-Recognition Thresholds (SRTs), Speech-Recognition Scores (PB), and Acoustic-Reflex Thresholds (ARTs) for the 500-Hz, 1000-Hz, and 2000-Hz Activators[a]

Time of test and ear tested	Frequency (Hz)						SRT	PB (%)	Acoustic-reflex threshold (dB HL)		
	250	500	1000	2000	4000	8000			500 Hz	1000 Hz	2000 Hz
Initial visit											
Right	45	50	55	45	75	90	55	88	80	90	90
Left	5	0	0	5	10	25	10	92	85	85	90
Three years later (before counseling)											
Right	85	90	95	90	110+	90+	65	88	85	85	90
Left	50	55	60	65	70	90+	25	88	80	85	85
Three years later (after counseling)											
Right	55	50	60	60	90	90+	45	96	85	85	90
Left	5	5	10	0	15	45	10	88	80	85	85

[a] Tests were done on the right and left ears at the initial audiologic test, the repeat audiologic test three years later before counseling the patient regarding the inter- and intra-test descrepancies, and the audiologic retest three years later after counseling the patient.

acoustic-reflex thresholds, which remained essentially constant since the first visit, were below the admitted air-conduction thresholds for the right ear. The patient was counseled regarding the intratest and intertest discrepancies. When the testing was repeated immediately after counseling, the air-conduction thresholds and speech-recognition thresholds in both ears improved, becoming similar to those obtained at the initial visit. Bone-conduction thresholds are not shown since these were always within 10 dB of the air-conduction thresholds. The functional overlay in the poorer ear was smaller than that in the better ear at the Stenger test frequency, accounting for the negative Stenger result at the second visit.

We recommend the use of a screening pure-tone Stenger at test frequencies where the interaural difference in air-conduction thresholds is at least 40 dB. With the screening technique employed, for example, in many Veterans Administration Medical Centers, the tone is presented in the good ear at 10 dB SL relative to the good-ear threshold and the tone is also simultaneously presented in the bad ear at 10 dB below the admitted threshold of the bad ear. If the patient responds, the result is negative. If there is no response, the result is positive. If the result is negative, the tone is then withdrawn from the good ear while the tone is continued in the bad ear. If the hand is now lowered, the result is negative. If the hand continues to be raised, the result is positive. Once a positive result is established, the technique described earlier for estimating the air-conduction thresholds in the bad ear can be employed (i.e., start at 10 dB SL relative to the good-ear air-conduction threshold, bilaterally).

Altshuler (1970) suggests that the speech frequencies are likely to be most sensitive to functional hearing loss. Since recruitment is often present above 2000 Hz and the interaural attenuation value is reduced below 500 Hz. Altshuler (1970) recommends the use of pulsed rather than continuous tones since the bad ear may adapt to the continuous tone. Azzi (1950) reported that pulsed tones were preferable since they prevent the subject from becoming aware of the step increases in intensity.

One problem which can invalidate the Stenger test is the presence of diplacusis (Menzel, 1965; Newby, 1958; Nober, 1966; Watson & Tolan, 1949). Chaiklin and Ventry (1963), however, suggested that, if pitch differences are small, the Stenger effect can overcome the diplacusis. When diplacusis is present, the speech Stenger should be employed. Another problem which can invalidate the pure-tone Stenger is recruitment in the good ear. The problem of recruitment is essentially not a factor if only candidates with unilateral hearing loss are tested. To minimize the problem of recruitment, low sensation levels for tonal presentation in the better ear have been suggested (Altshuler, 1970; Menzel, 1965).

Several investigators have reported that listener sophistication affects the Stenger-test results. On the other hand, other investigators have reported that listener sophistication does not affect the test. Monro and Martin (1977) found that listener sophistication effects on the Stenger test results are negligible in adults with simulated hearing loss. On the other hand, Martin and Shipp (1982) found that increased practice and sophistication affect the sensitivity of the Stenger test.

Chaiklin and Ventry (1965) reported that the pure-tone Stenger was positive in 43% of the functionally hearing-impaired ears tested. Hattler and Schuchman (1971) reported a hit rate of 48% in their group of 225 persons with functional hearing loss and found that the Stenger test had the poorest hit rate when compared with the LOT and D–S tests. On the other hand, Kinstler, Phelan, and Lavender (1972) reported a sensitivity of 83% for the pure-tone Stenger in a group of 31 adults with functional hearing loss. Peck and Ross (1970) found the sensitivity rate for the pure-tone Stenger to be 100% in their group of 35 subjects with simulated total unilateral hearing loss. The difference in the sensitivity rates reported by various investigators is probably related to intersubject variability in hearing sensitivity. Thus, higher hit rates are expected when the test is administered on persons with substantial unilateral hearing loss.

2. SPEECH STENGER

The speech Stenger is similar to the pure-tone Stenger except that speech—most commonly spondaic words—rather than pure-tone stimuli are employed (Johnson *et al.*, 1956; Taylor, 1949; Watson & Tolan, 1949). When spondaic words are employed as the stimuli, the instructions are similar to those given during SRT testing. The recommended sensation level in the better ear is 15 dB. Johnson *et al.* (1956) suggested increasing the task difficulty and thereby confusing the patient by instructing the patient to raise the hand on the side of the head that the speech is heard and to repeat the words. It is preferable to administer the speech Stenger rather than the pure-tone Stenger if diplacusis is present or there is a possibility that the two tones presented do not have the same frequency, leading to a beating tone. The speech Stenger cannot be employed in cases in which the speech-recognition is markedly poorer in the bad than in the good ear, leading to awareness of the two signals.

Ventry and Chaiklin (1965a) reported that the speech Stenger was positive in 40% of their functional-hearing-loss subjects. Like the pure-tone Stenger, it is most effective when interaural differences exceed 40 dB. Martin and Shipp (1982) found that listener sophistication resulted in elevated response alteration levels, leading to an overestimation of the SRT.

E. BEKESY (AUTOMATIC) AUDIOMETRY

Jerger and Herer (1961) evaluated more than 600 audiograms administered over a three-year period and observed that a unique Bekesy configuration characterized three cases with functional hearing loss. The Bekesy tracings for these three cases revealed that the tracking for continuous (C) tones was at lower levels than for interrupted (I) tones. (See Chapter 5 for more details concerning Bekesy testing.) Resnick and Burke (1962) obtained similar findings in their group of patients with functional hearing loss, that is, the Bekesy tracings of persons with functional hearing loss differed substantially from the clinically established Bekesy Type I–IV patterns.

Stein (1963) reported a hit rate of 57% for their 30 patients with functional hearing loss; unclassifiable tracings were obtained in 30%. Thus, if either Type V (C-tracking lower than I-tracking) or unclassifiable tracings were considered signs of functional hearing loss, the hit rate was 87%.

Price, Shepherd, and Goldstein (1965) identified a Bekesy audiogram as Type V if at least a 5-dB difference between the tracings was present, with the C tracing better than the I tracing, over any 1 min of a 2- or 3-min fixed-frequency tracing. They found a false-alarm rate of 6% in their normal-hearing subjects. Hopkinson (1965) reported a false-alarm rate of 48% in her group of 52 conductive hearing-impaired ears. She employed the criterion of at least a 5-dB separation between the C and I tracings for the identification of functional hearing loss. Stark (1966) reported a false-alarm rate of approximately 5% in a group of 61 children with normal hearing and approximately 8% in a group of 52 children with sensorineural hearing loss. Rintelmann and Harford (1967) suggested that the criterion for the Type V pattern was based on too narrow a separation. This criterion, therefore, might at least partially account for the high false-alarm rates reported previously.

Rintelmann and Harford (1967) evaluated the sweep and fixed-frequency Bekesy tracings from 33 patients with functional hearing loss in order to derive a clinically useful definition of the Type V pattern. They defined a Bekesy audiogram as Type V if the C tracing was tracked at lower SPLs than the I tracing by at least 10 dB (measured at the midpoints of the excursions) over at least two octaves. The separation between the C and I tracings typically includes the mid-frequency region. The C and I tracings do not overlap and there is a peak separation of at least 15 dB at some point. They concluded that sweep-frequency Bekesy audiograms were preferable to fixed-frequency Bekesy audiograms for the assessment of functional hearing loss. Ventry (1971) supported the use of the criteria developed by Rintelmann and Harford (1967) for the identification of Type V Bekesy audiograms. Using these criteria to establish

the Type V pattern, Rintelmann and Harford (1967) reported that the hit rate for their group of 33 functional-hearing-loss subjects was 76%; the false-alarm rate was 0% for their group of 32 normal-hearing persons, 2% for their group of 50 conductive hearing-loss patients, and 3% for their group of sensorineural hearing-impaired subjects.

Rintelmann and Carhart (1964) suggested that the Type V pattern occurs in persons who simulate hearing impairment because of the use of a loudness reference gauge for determining when to respond to the signals. Pulsed tones are tracked at higher intensity levels since they are less loud than continuous tones. Melnick (1967) employed a procedure which did not rely on long-term memory. His findings suggested that each subject develops his or her own loudness gauge for responding to signals. Hattler (1968) found that the tracking levels were inversely related to the duty cycle and were independent of other temporal parameters such as duration and repetition rate. This finding lent support for the theory which attributed the Type V pattern to the differential effects of memory on the tracking of C and I tones.

1. LENGTHENED OFF-TIME

One modification of the Bekesy test which has been developed is the LOT (Lengthened Off-Time) fixed-frequency Bekesy audiogram. Hattler (1970) compared the effectiveness of the conventional 200-ms on-time, 200-ms off-time pulsed signal with that of the lengthened off-time pulsed signal (200-ms on-time, 800-msec off-time) in identifying functional hearing loss. Hattler reported that the Type V pattern based on pulsed signals with the conventional off-time was present in only 40% of the group of functional-hearing-loss subjects. In contrast, the Type V pattern based on pulsed tones with the LOT was present in 95% of the group of functional-hearing-loss subjects. The results were considered indicative of functional hearing loss if the LOT tracking was at least 5.5 dB poorer than the C or standard I trackings. The false-alarm rate was 0% for the standard and LOT methods in a group of organic hearing-impaired subjects. Hattler and Schuchman (1970) obtained similar findings for the LOT test. In contrast, Citron and Reddell (1976) reported a hit rate of only 50% for the LOT test in their group of 14 functional-hearing-loss ears. Behnke and Lankford (1976) found low false-alarm rates in children 7 1/2 to 10 1/2 years of age for the LOT test at 1000, 2000, and 4000 Hz; the false-alarm rate was increased, however, at 500 Hz.

Martin and Monro (1975) demonstrated that increased Bekesy test sophistication and practice in persons with simulated hearing loss is associated with a decreased likelihood of a Type V pattern in Bekesy fixed-frequency tracings, particularly for the standard off-time pulsed signal as compared with the LOT signal. Modifications of Bekesy audiometry employing variations in on-time also have been developed (Dean, Wright, & Valerio, 1976).

2. Bekesy Ascending/Descending Gap Evaluation

Hood, Campbell, and Hutton (1964) developed the Bekesy ascending/descending gap evaluation (BADGE) test to improve the sensitivity of the Bekesy test to functional hearing loss. This test was based on fixed-frequency Bekesy tracings. With the BADGE test, a 1-min continuous ascending (CA) tracing is obtained with the starting level at -20 dB HL; a 1-min pulsed ascending (PA) tracing is obtained with the starting level below threshold; a 1-min pulsed descending (PD) tracing is also obtained with the starting level at 40–60 dB SL relative to the PA threshold.

Hood *et al.*'s (1964) results revealed that in their group of 27 organic hearing-impaired veterans, the CA threshold was slightly greater than the PA threshold and there was essentially little or no difference (no gap) between the PA and PD thresholds. On the other hand, in their group of functional-hearing-loss veterans, the CA threshold was lower than the PA threshold. Also, there was a gap between the PA and PD tracings which was greater at the beginning than at the end of the tracing. The hit rate for the gap measure (PA − PD, CA − PD, or CA − PA) was approximately 70%. The false-alarm rate for the gap measure was approximately 30%.

3. Wide Bekesy Excursions

Istre and Burton (1969) suggested that wide Bekesy swings signal the presence of functional hearing loss. It has been shown, however, that slow reaction times and certain personality traits can result in increased Bekesy swing widths (Shepherd & Goldstein, 1968; Suzuki & Kubota, 1966).

F. DELAYED AUDITORY FEEDBACK TEST

1. Pure-Tone Delayed Auditory Feedback

The pure-tone delayed auditory feedback (DAF) test is based on the principle that auditory feedback which is delayed can cause changes in keytapping performance. The subject is asked to tap out a pattern such as "---- --" on an electromechanical key using the index finger. Each tap causes a brief tone to be generated that is fed to a tape recorder, delayed by approximately 200 ms, and then fed through the earphones. If the subject hears the delayed auditory feedback (DAF), the keytapping rhythm is interrupted. If the subject does not hear the DAF, the keytapping rhythm is maintained. According to Ruhm and Cooper (1962), changes in keytapping performance occur even at sensation levels as low as 5 dB. The changes in tapping performance are manifested by a decreased tapping rate, irregular rhythm, increased manual pressure, and errors in

the number of taps required for the pattern. These changes are unaffected by the feedback tone frequency, subject gender, and manual fatigue (Ruhm & Cooper, 1963).

The DAF apparatus was described by Ruhm and Cooper (1964). The key features of the apparatus include an electromechanical key which causes tones (50-ms duration at the mean peak amplitude and 12-msec rise–fall time) to be generated from the audiometer when the key is tapped, a delay feature so the tone generated when the key is tapped is not instantly fed through the earphones worn by the subject, the use of a visual shield to prevent the subject from observing his or her hand and the key, and a means of monitoring the keytapping performance. The keytapping performance can be measured by feeding the output of the audiometer to a monitor earphone or a loudspeaker, an oscilloscope, or a graphic level strip-chart recorder. Because the tones employed in DAF audiometry are much briefer than those employed in behavioral pure-tone audiometry, the DAF and behavioral thresholds are not equivalent. Ruhm and Cooper (1964) suggest that a subtraction correction factor (rounded to the nearest 5-dB step) be applied to the hearing-level dial reading. The subtraction correction factor can be derived by obtaining the median difference between the behavioral thresholds for 50-ms and at least 200-ms duration tones.

Cooper, Stokinger, and Billings (1976) developed criteria for the interpretation of the pure-tone DAF. An absolute time error was significant if the difference between the mean time required to tap the pattern for the simultaneous auditory feedback condition differed from that under the DAF condition by at least 116.3 ms. The relative time error was significant if the absolute time error divided by the mean simultaneous auditory feedback time was greater than or equal to 5%. The pattern error was significant if the number of DAF pattern deviations minus the number of simultaneous pattern deviations was greater than or equal to 1.

Ruhm and Cooper (1964) evaluated the effectiveness of the pure-tone DAF procedure in a group of normal-hearing adults who had one ear plugged, a group of organic hearing-impaired veterans, and a group of functionally hearing-impaired veterans. The DAF results were compared with the results of electrodermal audiometry. Five patterns were tapped under the control condition. Then the audiometer dial was set at 0 dB and DAF was given to the subject. If no changes in performance occurred, the intensity was increased by 6 dB. This procedure, in which control and DAF conditions were employed at each intensity level, was continued until the lowest intensity level was obtained at which a change in keytapping behavior occurred or until approximately five intensity increases were made without tapping changes. When a change in the keytapping behavior was observed, the intensity was decreased by 6 dB and the procedure repeated at the new level. The intensity is then increased in 2-dB steps, with the procedure repeated at each level, until the lowest level at which changes in tapping patterns occur is obtained. The lowest intensity level at which keytapping changes occurred in at least two of the three ascending runs was recorded as 5 dB SL. From this number, 10 dB is subtracted (5 dB since the change occurs at 5 dB SL and a 5-dB correction factor for the signal duration). The threshold is obtained in this manner for each of the audiometric speech frequencies.

The DAF results were in agreement with the electrodermal audiometry results for the organic, normal-hearing plugged, and functional-hearing-loss groups. Ruhm and Cooper (1964) suggested, therefore, that the DAF procedure, like electrodermal audiometry, represented an objective, valid, and rapid procedure for the audiologic assessment of persons with functional hearing loss. Moreover, the DAF procedure was successfully employed in those who could not be conditioned with electrodermal audiometry. They cautioned that the arm of the subject should be stationary on the table. Otherwise changes in keytapping behavior may not be observed until much higher sensation levels are reached. One drawback of the DAF procedure is that some persons are incapable of tapping the "---- --" pattern. In such cases, a simpler tapping pattern should be given. The procedure cannot be employed in those who are unable or unwilling to repeatedly tap a pattern.

Alberti (1970) reported that the pure-tone DAF threshold occurs at levels between 5 and 15 dB SL relative to the behavioral pure-tone threshold although levels as high as 40 dB SL have been encountered. The pure-tone DAF was successful in establishing thresholds in 78% of his group of 32 patients with functional hearing loss. The test could not be used in persons who could not or would not establish a tapping rhythm, those who complained of stiffness and pain in their fingers, and those who could not understand what was expected of them.

Ruhm and Cooper (1962) reported that a delay time of 200 msec was the most effective one for producing changes in tapping performance at sensation levels of 5–10 dB. In 1963, they found that practice did not affect DAF performance. Test sophistication did affect DAF performance, but only at levels above 5 dB SL. Cooper and Stokinger (1976), however, reported that if practice was carried out at high sensation levels (+15 and +30 dB) keytapping behavior for DAF at low sensation levels (−6, 0, and +6 dB) was less likely to result in keytapping performance changes. Therefore, they recommended against the use of practice in administering the DAF test. Monro and Martin (1977) reported that the sensitivity of the pure-tone DAF test could be decreased with listener sophistication and practice; in their sample of persons with simulated hearing loss, the hit rate decreased from 93 to 67% as a result of listener sophistication and practice. Nonetheless, Martin and Shipp (1982) reported that listener sophistication and prac-

tice at low DAF intensity levels did not affect DAF performance. Robinson and Kasden (1973) found the DAF test to be effective in the evaluation of functional hearing loss.

Cooper *et al.* (1976) developed criteria for absolute and relative time and pattern error. Using these criteria, the test was successful in establishing thresholds at 1000 Hz in 90% of the normal-hearing subjects. Billings and Stokinger (1975) reported that the pure-tone DAF enabled threshold determination in 88% of 100 patients receiving medicolegal evaluation. Citron and Reddell (1976) reported that the pure-tone DAF enabled threshold determination in 87% of 86 patients receiving the DAF test. The remaining 13% either did not exhibit changes in keytapping performance or could not tap the pattern. Of the patients identified as having functional hearing loss, 57% had DAF thresholds which were better than the thresholds obtained by conventional behavioral audiometry. Cooper, Stokinger, and Billings (1977) found that the pure-tone DAF enables threshold determination in persons with hearing impairment as well as normal-hearing persons.

2. SPEECH DELAYED AUDITORY FEEDBACK

The effects of DAF of one's own voice upon one's speech were first observed by Black (1951) and Lee (1950). These investigators reported that the DAF of one's own voice results in changes in vocal rate and intensity. With the speech DAF test, the subject is asked to read a passage aloud. The speech is picked up by a microphone, tape-recorded, and then fed back through the earphones after a delay. The intensity of the feedback is adjusted until the lowest level is found which results in changes in vocal rate or intensity. Typically, such changes include hesitation, repetition, and a decrease in vocal rate, or dysfluent behavior. Some people speed up their reading rate. A stop watch is employed to measure changes in rate. Changes in vocal intensity can be monitored on a VU meter. More complex but accurate means of monitoring the vocal changes have been developed (McGranahan, Causey, and Studebaker, 1960).

Some investigators suggest obtaining another reading without DAF after readings with DAF have been completed in order to provide another baseline for comparison with the DAF results. Also, some investigators have suggested the use of a simultaneous auditory feedback condition— feedback without delay—to provide a better baseline for comparison with the DAF condition. Hanley and Tiffany (1954) reported that the post-DAF reading was faster than the pre-DAF reading. A change of 3 s from the no-DAF condition to the DAF condition is considered significant. In general, this change in reading rate first occurs at a level within 10 dB of the SRT. Hanley and Tiffany (1954) reported that a delay time of 0.18 s was the most effective one for the speech DAF test. With this delay, a change of at least

8% in reading rate is observed when the DAF test is administered at 20–30 dB SL relative to the SRT.

Harford and Jerger (1959) reported that changes in vocal intensity and rate occurred at lower sensation levels in hearing-impaired than normal-hearing listeners. It has also been reported that changes in vocal intensity and rate do not occur in some persons and that the levels at which the changes occur are variable. Thus, the speech DAF test has never gained popularity as a test for the assessment of functional hearing loss.

V. ELECTROPHYSIOLOGIC TESTS

A. ACOUSTIC-REFLEX THRESHOLDS

Investigators have reported that the acoustic-reflex thresholds are present at lower than expected hearing threshold levels in persons with functional hearing loss (Alberti, 1970; Feldman, 1963; Lamb and Peterson, 1967). Jepsen (1953) reported that the acoustic-reflex thresholds of three patients with functional hearing loss were similar to those for normal-hearing subjects. Feldman (1963) found that the impedance change from the acoustic reflex was equivalent in both ears of a patient with a unilateral functional hearing loss. Terkildsen (1964) suggested that the presence of acoustic-reflex thresholds at or below the behavioral pure-tone thresholds signal the presence of functional hearing loss.

Gelfand and Piper (1984) presented the acoustic-reflex thresholds corresponding to the deciles between the 10th and 90th deciles for normal-hearing and cochlear-impaired adults. They suggested that either the 10th or 20th decile be used to determine the presence of a functional hearing loss. That is, a person with an acoustic-reflex threshold below that associated with the 10th percentile is at risk for functional hearing loss. The 10th percentiles of the acoustic-reflex thresholds and their ranges as a function of hearing-loss magnitude and activator frequency are shown in Table II (See Chapter 3 for further details on the acoustic-reflex thresholds.) This table reveals that the presence of functional hearing loss should be suspected in a person with a hearing loss of 70–75 dB at 500 Hz and an acoustic-reflex threshold of 85 dB HL at the same activator frequency. Future research on the applicability of the 10th percentiles of the acoustic-reflex thresholds in the detection of functional hearing loss is needed.

Silman, Gelfand, Piper, Silverman, and Van Frank (1984a) suggested that the modified bivariate-plotting procedure (Silman, Silverman, Showers, & Gelfand, 1984b) can be used to estimate hearing sensitivity in persons with functional hearing loss. (See Chapter 3 for a description of the modified bivariate-plotting procedure.) They plotted

Table II The 10th Percentiles of the Acoustic-Reflex Thresholds as a Function of Hearing-Threshold Level for the 500-Hz, 1000-Hz, and 2000-Hz Activators[a]

dB HL	Activator Frequency (Hz)		
	500	1000	2000
≤25	75	80	80
30–35	75	80	80
40–45	80	80	85
50–55	85	80	85
60–65	90	90	85
70–75	92.5	95	95
80–85	96	102	100
≥90	[b]	100	101

[a] From Gelfand and Piper (1984).
[b] Not calculated because of small sample size.

the data for 17 functional-hearing-loss cases. All of the ears that fell in the hearing-loss region were found, after resolution of the functional component, to have at least a mild hearing loss exceeding a pure-tone average of 29 dB HL or a high-frequency hearing loss. Of the 8 functional-hearing-loss cases that fell in the normal-hearing region, only 12.5% (1 case) had a hearing loss exceeding 30 dB HL. Thus, the hearing sensitivity was accurately predicted in 16/17 or 93% of the functional-hearing-loss cases.

B. ELECTRODERMAL AUDIOMETRY

The psychogalvanic reflex refers to the decrease in skin resistance following a change in emotional state. In electrodermal audiometry (EDA), electrodes are placed on the fingertips so changes in electrical resistance resulting in changes in current flow can be recorded. An electrical shock, the unconditioned stimulus, is paired with the conditioned stimulus, the tone, until conditioning occurs, that is, the skin resistance changes with tonal presentation. The electrodermal threshold for the tone, the lowest intensity level at which skin resistance changes are observed, is then determined. EDA has been employed with both speech and pure-tone signals (Burk, 1958; Chaiklin et al., 1961; Doerfler & McClure, 1954).

EDA was formerly a widely used test for assessment of functional hearing loss. It used to be required for veterans seeking compensation for service-connected hearing loss. The test has since been abandoned because it involves the use of electric shocks. Knox (1978) reported that the safety standards of the American National Standards Institute, the National Laboratories Standards Institute, and Underwriters Laboratories preclude the application of electrical current to the body in excess of 5 μA, which is less than that employed in EDA. Also, the Underwriters Laboratories

Medical and Dental Equipment Standard (1974) requires that equipment attached to the patient be capable of providing isolation to a surge of 2500 V. Conventional audiometers do not meet this standard. For these reasons, EDA has been abandoned. In 1977, audiologists in the Veterans Administration were ordered to cease administering EDA using shock as the conditioning stimulus. The test, however, can be administered using a non-noxious conditioning stimulus.

C. AUDITORY-EVOKED POTENTIALS

1. Brainstem Auditory-Evoked Potentials

Sanders and Lazenby (1983) assessed the effectiveness of brainstem auditory-evoked potentials (BAEP) assessment in persons with functional hearing loss. (See Chapter 7 for further details regarding BAEP testing.) They recorded the BAEPs for clicks and, in some cases, the SN10 response to 500-Hz tone pips in four persons with functional hearing loss.

In an adult with a unilateral functional hearing loss following an automobile accident, the BAEP at 75 dBnHL revealed normal morphology and absolute, interwave, and interaural latencies; wave V was recorded in the functional ear at levels as low as 25 dBnHL. The audiogram obtained following BAEP testing revealed substantially improved thresholds in the functionally hearing-impaired ear compared with the pre-BAEP audiogram, although functional signs were still present.

The BAEP for clicks at 85 dBnHL was also recorded in a young veteran with a bilateral functional hearing loss following excessive noise exposure. Normal absolute, interwave, and interaural latencies were obtained bilaterally; wave V was present at levels as low as 30 dBnHL in the right ear and 35 dBnHL in the left ear. The post-BAEP audiogram revealed improved hearing threshold levels bilaterally compared with the pre-BAEP audiogram, that is, normal hearing-threshold levels in the right ear and essentially normal hearing thresholds with a notch at 4000 Hz in the left ear.

Case 3 was a 13-year-old female with a unilateral functional hearing loss following an influenza infection. A conductive component was present in the better ear. BAEP testing, done 4 months after the initial audiologic assessment, revealed normal absolute, interwave, and interaural latencies and normal morphology for clicks presented at 80 dBnHL, bilaterally. The post-BAEP audiogram revealed normal-hearing sensitivity, bilaterally.

Case 4 was a young female veteran who had received a medical discharge from military service because of a whiplash injury. She complained of a hearing loss resulting from noise exposure during basic training and 6 months of work as an airplane mechanic. She presented with a bilateral

severe functional hearing loss. The BAEPs obtained for clicks presented at 80 dBnHL revealed normal absolute, interwave, and interaural latencies and normal morphology, bilaterally. Wave V was present for intensities as low as 20 dBnHL in the right ear and 10 dBnHL in the left ear. To assess low-frequency hearing sensitivity, the SN10 for a 500-Hz tone pip was obtained which was also present at 20 dBnHL bilaterally. The post-BAEP audiogram revealed normal-hearing thresholds, bilaterally.

Sanders and Lazenby concluded that the BAEP technique was successful for the identification of functional hearing loss and the estimation of true hearing sensitivity in persons with functional hearing loss. The BAEP test apparently served to motivate functional-hearing-loss patients to present improved hearing threshold levels in the post-BAEP test. According to Sanders and Lazenby, an important factor influencing the voluntary return to improved behavioral thresholds post-BAEP assessment was the instruction prior to BAEP testing which stressed that the "hearing nerve and brain waves will respond automatically to the sound and that the computer will then tell us exactly how well they can hear" (p. 297). Also, the clinicians performing the BAEP test and/or post-BAEP audiogram differed from those who did the pre-BAEP audiogram to allow the patient to "save face."

As mentioned previously in Chapter 5, a drawback of BAEP testing in estimating the hearing sensitivity is that a normal BAEP threshold can be obtained in some persons with a hearing loss in the 500–6000 Hz frequency region with a normal-hearing threshold at 8000 Hz (Glattke, 1983; Stapells, Picton, Perez-Abalo, Read, & Smith, 1985).

The clinician should suspect the presence of a functional hearing loss if the BAEP threshold is obtained at low intensities such as 30 dBnHL. The clinician should recall, however, that normal BAEP thresholds can be obtained in persons with significant hearing loss throughout the frequency range, with a normal hearing threshold level at only one isolated high frequency. When a normal BAEP threshold is obtained, the clinician should consider the possibility of a hearing loss affecting some but not all of the high frequencies. The use of tonebursts as stimuli to improve the ability to predict the hearing threshold levels has drawbacks. That is, these stimuli are associated with spectral splatter throughout the frequency range and a loss of waveform clarity. Therefore, the tonebursts lack frequency specificity. If a normal BAEP threshold for the click is obtained, the audiologist should use tonebursts in notched noise if the instrumentation is available. Otherwise, the audiologist should consider other audiologic data such as the acoustic-reflex thresholds, or agreement between the speech-recognition threshold and pure-tone average.

BAEP testing is valid in the assessment of functional hearing loss if the admitted hearing-threshold levels are elevated beyond normal levels at all frequencies and the BAEP can be obtained at levels below the admitted behavioral threshold levels. The following case illustrates this point. The patient was a 26-year-old male who claimed a total left-ear hearing loss immediately following a motor vehicle accident, with occasional dizziness, nausea, and tinnitus. Table III shows the audiologic data for this patient. Note the absence of a shadow audiogram and the presence of the acoustic-reflex thresholds below the admitted threshold levels in the left ear. Figure 1 shows the ipsilateral and contralateral BAEPs for the right and left ears for the 40 dBnHL click. Note that the left BAEP is present at a low intensity compared with the admitted pure-tone threshold levels. Note that there is only a 0.06 ms interaural wave V latency difference, supporting the possibility of normal hearing-threshold levels in the left ear. Although in this case the presence of the acoustic-reflex thresholds at levels below the admitted hearing levels indicate the presence of a functional hearing loss, the clinical value of BAEP testing in the assessment of functional hearing loss is increased when the acoustic-reflex is absent because of a slight conductive pathology.

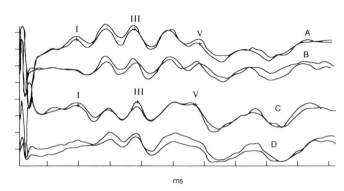

Figure 1 The BAEPs for the 26-year-old male with a unilateral functional hearing loss in the left ear. The BAEPs were obtained for a click stimulus at 40 dBnHL at a repetition rate of 11.7/s. (A) The test–retest ipsilateral BAEPs for the left ear. (B) The test–retest contralateral BAEPs for the left ear. (C) The test–retest ipsilateral BAEPs for the right ear. (D) The test–retest contralateral BAEPs for the right ear. Courtesy of Janet Zarnoch, St. Francis Hospital, Jersey City, New Jersey.

2. LATE AUDITORY-EVOKED POTENTIAL

The evoked cortical response has been employed to assess hearing sensitivity in persons with functional hearing loss. For example, Alberti (1970) reported that cortical evoked response testing was successful in estimating pure-tone hearing-threshold levels in 20 of 21 persons with functional hearing loss. Cortical evoked potentials testing could not be done in 1 of the 21 persons with functional hearing loss who continually moved his head in a way that disrupted the electrode attachment. McCandless and Lentz (1968) obtained similar findings.

Because of the variability in the late auditory-evoked potential with changes in alertness and attention, the late auditory-evoked potentials test is not clinically feasible for measurement of true hearing sensitivity in persons with functional hearing loss.

3. MIDDLE-LATENCY AUDITORY-EVOKED POTENTIAL

Musiek and Donnelly (1983) present a case with high-frequency organic hearing loss and exaggerated hearing-threshold levels in the mid frequencies. The BAEP for the click yielded thresholds consistent with high-frequency hearing loss. The middle-latency auditory-evoked potential for the 1000-Hz tone pip was present at 35 dBnHL, compared with the behavioral threshold of 60 dB HL. Musiek and Donnelly suggested that the middle-latency auditory-evoked potentials are more valuable than the BAEPs in some instances since they provide evidence of auditory function at relatively high rostral levels of the auditory pathway.

The tone bursts employed in middle-latency response testing have a longer rise–fall and plateau time than those used for BAEP testing. The tonebursts used for middle-latency response testing typically have a 3-ms rise–fall time

Table III Air-Conduction Thresholds, Unmasked Bone-Conduction Thresholds, Speech-Recognition Thresholds (SRTs), Speech-Recognition Scores, and Contralateral and Ipsilateral Acoustic-Reflex Thresholds for the Right and Left Ears in a Patient with a Unilateral Functional Hearing Loss

Test and ear	Frequency (Hz)					
	250	500	1000	2000	4000	8000
Air-conduction threshold						
Right	20	20	10	10	10	10
Left	NR[a]	NR	NR	NR	NR	NR
Unmasked bone-conduction threshold	30	25	15	15	20	
Contralateral acoustic-reflex threshold						
Right		100	100	NR		
Left		100	105	NR		
Ipsilateral acoustic-reflex threshold						
Right				NR	NR	
Left				NR	NR	

Ear	SRT (db HL)	Speech-recognition score[b] (%)
Right	10	100
Left	NR	NR

[a] No response to the output of the audiometer.
[b] Speech-recognition scores are at 40 dB SL with respect to SRT.

with a 2-ms plateau, compared with those for BAEP testing which typically have a 2-ms rise–fall time with a 1-ms plateau. Therefore, the tonebursts used in middle-latency response testing have greater frequency specificity than those used in BAEP testing. Moreover, middle-latency responses are larger in amplitude than the BAEPs. Therefore, the middle-latency responses can be observed nearer the behavioral threshold than the BAEPs (Wolf, Vivion, & Goldstein, 1979). Data are lacking on the middle-latency responses in persons with cochlear hearing loss. Moreover, the middle-latency response demonstrates maturational effects to a considerably greater degree than the BAEPs (Kraus, Smith, Reed, Stein, & Cartee, 1985). Therefore, the use of middle-latency response testing for the assessment of functional hearing loss cannot be recommended at this time.

4. ELECTROCOCHLEOGRAPHY

The drawbacks of electrocochleography using tone pips are similar to those of BAEPs with respect to frequency selectivity. Moreover, sensitive electrocochleography recordings are obtained using an invasive transtympanic approach which requires anesthesia. For these reasons, therefore, electrocochleography is not a promising tool for the routine clinical assessment of functional hearing loss.

VI. UNCOMMONLY EMPLOYED TESTS

Other audiologic tests have been employed to detect functional hearing loss. For example, Falconer (1966) developed a lip-reading test which consisted of lists of monosyllabic homophonous words. The patient is told that the examiner wishes to measure his or her lip-reading ability. The lists are presented, first with auditory stimuli in addition to the visual stimuli. The intensity is decreased successively on subsequent word lists until only visual cues are given. The test is based on the principle that correct repetition can occur only if the auditory stimuli are heard. The speech-recognition threshold is estimated from the articulation (gain) test.

Another test, called the FIT (Fusion Inferred Test), was developed by Bergman (1964) for the detection of pseudo-hypacusis. The test is similar to the Stenger test in that two tones are presented, one to each ear, and the intensity in the test ear is increased until there is a response alteration. The response alteration level is the lowest intensity level at which the listener reports a change in lateralization of the tone. The response alteration level was found to occur within 5 dB of the threshold.

Calearo (1957) developed the switched speech test. The test is based on the principle that at low interruption rates (1–4/s) using a 50% duty cycle, speech-recognition performance is poor but increases as the interruption rate in-

creases. If a person has an organic unilateral hearing loss, the speech-recognition performance at relatively low switching rates is poor. If a person has a functional hearing loss, the speech-recognition performance is substantially better than would be expected since the patient is presumably confused about which ear received which portions of the message.

The swinging story test involves the telling of a story, parts of which are delivered to the good ear (e.g., 10 dB SL relative to the SRT), and parts of which are delivered to the bad ear (e.g., 10 dB below SRT). If the patient repeats parts of the story presented to the bad ear, it is assumed that the patient heard the story at levels below the voluntary admitted thresholds. Martin (1985) suggests having the theme of the story change as the story is switched from one ear to the other or is presented bilaterally. He feels this switching in story theme makes it more difficult for the patient to recall which portions went to which ear(s).

VII. COUNSELING

Counseling a patient with functional hearing loss can be a means of obtaining improved, more valid thresholds. Ventry, Trier, and Chaiklin (1965) counseled their functional-hearing-loss patients by informing them of their test discrepancies, allowing the patient to offer an explanation for these discrepancies and, if the patient does not then volunteer any explanation, suggesting that the patient may have misunderstood the instructions, been inattentive, or have waited too long before responding to the stimuli. The counseling was done in a nonthreatening, nonhostile manner. This counseling technique is similar to that employed by Johnson et al. (1956). Ventry et al. (1965) reported that 56% of their patients who were counseled in this manner demonstrated resolution of the functional hearing loss.

We do not recommend the use of intimidation to obtain resolution of functional hearing loss. The clinician should make it as easy as possible for the patient to change his or her behavior in a face-saving manner. If the functional hearing loss cannot be resolved, the report should indicate that the test results are invalid because of the presence of test discrepancies which are then described. If the functional hearing loss is resolved within the test session, the report should simply describe the hearing sensitivity without reference to the functional behaviors. If normal hearing sensitivity has been estimated in a child who presented with a functional hearing loss, the parents should be counseled regarding the true hearing sensitivity and be advised "not to treat the child as though he had a hearing loss, not to give him preferential seating in the classroom, not to discuss hearing at all, and certainly not to confront the child with his 'deception' or accuse him of lying" (Berger, 1965; p.

456). It may be appropriate, in some cases of unresolved functional hearing loss, to recommend follow-up counseling by a mental health professional.

VIII. RECOMMENDATIONS

Indicators that should alert the clinician regarding the possibility of functional hearing loss are (a) behavioral signs, (b) bone-conduction thresholds worse than air-conduction thresholds by more than 20 dB, (c) false-alarm responses, (d) half-stimulus responses during speech-recognition threshold testing, and (e) excessively large interaural attenuation values for air- or bone-conduction threshold testing.

Strong audiologic tests and measures of functional hearing loss which can be obtained during routine audiologic assessment are (a) test–retest reliability, (b) SRT–PTA discrepancy, and (c) acoustic-reflex thresholds below the 10th percentile levels. The pure-tone or speech Stenger test is also a strong measure in cases of unilateral or asymmetrical functional hearing loss. In cases of bilateral asymmetrical functional hearing loss, a negative Stenger result is inconclusive and a positive Stenger test is indicative of functional hearing loss.

If there are signs of functional hearing loss present but negative results are obtained on the strong tests or measures of functional hearing loss, the audiologist should consider the use of the following special tests which are not generally done during routine audiologic assessment: BAEP testing (see Chapter 7), the bivariate-plot procedure (see Chapter 3), or sweep-frequency Bekesy or LOT fixed-frequency Bekesy testing.

The only reliable and valid technique for the estimation of hearing-threshold level at a given frequency in cases of unilateral (or asymmetrical) functional hearing loss is the pure-tone Stenger test.

A functional hearing loss is considered resolved if, upon a repeated audiologic evaluation, there is good test–retest reliability, good SRT–PTA agreement, and acoustic-reflex thresholds present at levels above the 10th percentiles (provided no conductive pathology is present).

REFERENCES

Alberti, P. (1970). New tools for old tricks. *Ann. Otol. Rhinol. Laryngol., 79,* 800–807.

Alberti, P. W., Morgan, P. P., & Czuba, I. (1978). Speech and pure-tone audiometry as a screen for exaggerated hearing loss in industrial claims. *Acta Otolaryngol., 85,* 328–331.

Altshuler, M. W. (1970). The Stenger phenomenon. *J. Commun. Dis., 3,* 89–105.

Aplin, D. Y., & Kane, J. M. (1985a). Variables affecting pure tone and speech audiometry in experimentally simulated hearing loss. *Br. J. Audiol., 19,* 219–228.

Aplin, D. Y., & Kane, J. M. (1985b). Personality and experimentally simulated hearing loss. *Br. J. Audiol., 19,* 251–255.

Azzi, A. (1950). Le prove per svelare la simulazione di sordita. *Riv. Audiol. Prat., 1,* 22–23.

Bailey, H. A. T., Jr., & Martin, F. N. (1963). A method for predicting postoperative SRT. *Arch. Otolaryngol., 77,* 177–180.

Ballantyne, J. C. (1960). *Deafness.* Boston: Little, Brown.

Barelli, P. A., & Ruder, L. (1970). Medico-legal evaluation of hearing problems. *Eye, Ear, Nose, Throat Month., 49,* 398–405.

Barrett, L. S. (1959). *Threshold relationships in simulated hearing loss.* Ph.D. Thesis, Stanford, California: Stanford University.

Behnke, C. R., & Lankford, J. E. (1976). The LOT test and school-age children. *J. Speech Hear. Dis., 41,* 498–502.

Berger, K. (1965). Nonorganic hearing loss in children. *Laryngoscope, 75,* 447–457.

Bergman, M. (1964). The FIT test. *Arch. Otolaryngol., 80,* 440–449.

Berk, R. L., & Feldman, A. S. (1958). Functional hearing loss in children. *N. Engl. J. Med., 259,* 214–216.

Billings, B. L., & Stokinger, T. E. (1975). A comparison of pure-tone thresholds as measured by delayed feedback audiometry, electrodermal response audiometry, and voluntary response audiometry. *J. Speech Hear. Res., 18,* 754–756.

Black, J. W. (1950). Some effects upon voice of hearing tones of varying intensity and frequency while reading. *Speech Monogr., 17,* 95–98.

Black, J. W. (1951). The effect of delayed side-tone upon vocal rate and intensity. *J. Speech Hear. Dis., 16,* 56–60.

Bragg, V. C. (1962). Measurement of sensorineural acuity level using spondee words. Paper presented at the Annual Convention of the American Speech and Hearing Association, New York.

Brockman, S. J., & Hoversten, H. G. (1960). Pseudoneural hypacusis in children. *Laryngoscope, 70,* 825–839.

Brown, W., & Brandt, J. (1971). Effects of auditory masking on vocal intensity and intraoral air pressure during sentence production. *J. Acoust. Soc. Am., 49,* 1903–1905.

Burk, K. W. (1958). Traditional and psychogalvanic skin response audiometry. *J. Speech Hear. Res., 1,* 275–278.

Calearo, C. (1957). Detection of malingering by periodically switched speech. *Laryngoscope, 67,* 130–136.

Calvert, D. R., Moncur, J. P., Smith, D. W., & Snyder, J. (1961). Nonorganic hearing loss in school-age children. *The Voice, 10,* 6–11.

Campanelli, P. A. (1963). Simulated hearing loss in school children following identification audiometry. *J. Aud. Res., 3,* 91–108.

Campbell, R. (1965). An index of pseudo-discrimination loss. *J. Speech Hear. Res., 8,* 77–84.

Carhart, R. (1952). Speech audiometry in clinical evaluation. *Acta Otolaryngol., 41,* 18–42.

Carhart, R. (1958). Audiometry in diagnosis. *Laryngoscope, 68,* 253–279.

Carhart, R., & Jerger, J. F. (1959). Preferred method for clinical determination of pure-tone thresholds. *J. Speech Hear. Dis., 24,* 330–345.

Chaiklin, J. B. (1967). Interaural attenuation and cross-hearing in air-conduction audiometry. *J. Aud. Res., 7,* 413–424.

Chaiklin, J. B., & Ventry, I. M. (1963). Functional hearing loss. In J. Jerger (ed.), *Modern developments in audiology,* pp. 76–125. New York: Academic Press.

Chaiklin, J. B., & Ventry, I. M. (1965). Patient errors during spondee and pure-tone threshold measurement. *J. Aud. Res., 3,* 219–230.

Chaiklin, J. B., Ventry, I. M., Barrett, L. S., & Skalbeck, G. S. (1959). Pure-tone threshold patterns observed in functional hearing loss. *Laryngoscope, 69,* 1165–1179.

Chaiklin, J. B., Ventry, I. M., & Barrett, L. S. (1961). Reliability of conditioned GSR pure-tone audiometry with adult males. *J. Speech Hear. Res., 4,* 269–280.

Charlip, W. S., & Burk, K. W. (1969). Effects of noise on selected speech parameters. *J. Commun. Dis., 2,* 212–219.

Citron, E., III, & Reddell, R. C. (1976). A comparison of EDR, LOT, pure-tone DAR, and conventional pure-tone threshold audiometry for medico-legal audiological assessment. *Arch. Otolaryngol., 102,* 204–206.

Conn, M., Ventry, I. M., & Woods, R. W. (1972). Pure-tone average and spondee threshold relationships in simulated hearing loss. *J. Aud. Res., 12,* 234–239.

Cooper, W. A., Jr., & Stokinger, T. E. (1976). Pure tone delayed auditory feedback: Effects of prior experience. *J. Am. Aud. Soc., 1,* 164–168.

Cooper, W. A., Jr., Stokinger, T. E., & Billings, B. L. (1976). Pure tone delayed auditory feedback: Development of criteria of performance deterioration. *J. Am. Aud. Soc., 1,* 192–196.

Cooper, W. A., Jr., Stokinger, T. E., & Billings, B. L. (1977). Pure tone delayed auditory feedback: Effect of hearing loss on disruption of tapping performance. *J. Am. Aud. Soc., 3,* 102–107.

Davis, H., & Silverman, S. (1960). *Hearing and deafness.* New York: Holt, Rinehart, and Winston.

Dean, L. A., Wright, H. N., & Valerio, M. W. (1976). Brief-tone audiometry in pseudohypacusis. *Arch. Otolaryngol., 102,* 621–626.

Dixon, F. F., & Newby, H. A. (1959). Children with nonorganic hearing problems. *Arch. Otolaryngol., 70,* 619–623.

Doerfler, L. S. (1951). Psychogenic deafness and its detection. *Ann. Otol. Rhinol. Laryngol., 60,* 1045–1048.

Doerfler, L. G., & Epstein, A. (1956). The Doerfler-Stewart (D–S) test for functional hearing loss. Unpublished monograph. Washington, D.C.: Veterans Administration.

Doerfler, L. G., & McClure, C. (1954). The measurement of hearing loss in adults by galvanic skin response. *J. Speech Hear. Dis., 19,* 184–189.

Doerfler, L. G., & Stewart, K. (1946). Malingering and psychogenic deafness. *J. Speech Hear. Dis., 11,* 181–186.

Dreher, J., & O'Neil, J. (1957). Effects of ambient noise on speech intelligibility for words and phrases. *J. Acoust. Soc. Am., 29,* 1320–1323.

Egan, J. J. (1967). *Psychoacoustics of the Lombard voice reflex.* Unpublished Ph.D. Thesis: Cleveland, Ohio: Case Western Reserve University.

Egan, J. J. (1971). The Lombard reflex: Historical perspective. *Arch. Otolaryngol., 92,* 310–312.

Engelberg, M. W., (1978). Functional hearing level. *Otolaryngol. Clin. N. Am., 11,* 741–757.

Falconer, G. (1966). A "lipreading test" for nonorganic deafness. *J. Speech Hear. Dis., 31,* 241–247.

Feldman, A. S. (1961). Problems in the measurement of bone conduction. *J. Speech Hear. Dis., 26,* 39–44.

Feldman, A. S. (1962). Functional hearing loss. *Maico Audiological Library Series, Rep. 7.*

Feldman, A. S. (1963). Impedance measurements at the eardrum as an aid to diagnosis. *J. Speech Hear. Res., 6,* 315–327.

Firestone, C. (1934). A test for simulation of deafness. *Laryngoscope, 44,* 211–218.

Fournier, J. E. (1958). The detection of auditory malingering. *Trans. Beltone Instit. Hear. Res., Rep. 8.*

Frank, T. (1976). Yes–no test for nonorganic hearing loss. *Arch. Otolaryngol., 102,* 162–165.

Garber, S. F., Siegel, G. M., Pick, H., Jr., & Alcorn, S. R. (1979). The influence of selected masking noises on Lombard and sidetone amplification effects. *J. Speech Hear. Res., 19,* 523–535.

Gelfand, S. A., & Piper, N. (1984). Acoustic reflex thresholds: Variability and distribution effects. *Ear Hear., 5,* 228–234.

Gelfand, S. A., & Silman, S. (1985). Functional hearing loss and its relationship to resolved hearing levels. *Ear Hear., 6,* 151–158.

Glattke, T. J. (1983). *Short-latency auditory evoked potentials. Fundamental bases and clinical applications.* Baltimore: University Park Press.

Glorig, A. (1954). Malingering. *Ann. Otol. Rhinol. Laryngol., 63,* 802–814.

Goetzinger, G., & Proud, G. (1958). Deafness: Examination techniques for evaluating malingering and psychogenic disabilities. *J. Kans. Med. Soc., 59,* 95–101.

Gold, S., Lubinsky, R., & Shahar, A. (1981). Speech discrimination scores at low sensation levels as possible index of malingering. *J. Aud. Res., 21,* 137–141.

Goldstein, R. (1966). Pseudohypacusis. *J. Speech Hear. Dis., 31,* 341–352.

Guttman, J. (1928). A new method of determining unilateral deafness and malingering. *Laryngoscope, 38,* 56–71.

Hanley, T. D., & Steer, M. (1949). Effect of level of distracting noise upon speaking rate, duration, and intensity. *J. Speech Hear. Dis., 14,* 363–368.

Hanley, C. N., & Tiffany, W. R. (1954). An investigation into the use of electromechanically delayed side tone in auditory testing. *J. Speech Hear. Dis., 19,* 367–374.

Harford, E. R., & Jerger, J. F. (1959). Effects of loudness recruitment on delayed speech feedback. *J. Speech Hear. Res., 2,* 361–368.

Harris, D. A. (1958). A rapid and simple technique for the detection of nonorganic hearing loss. *Arch. Otolaryngol., 68,* 758–760.

Harris, J. D. (1965). Speech audiometry. In A. Glorig (ed.), *Audiometry: Principles and practices,* pp. 141–169. Baltimore: Williams & Wilkins.

Hattler, K. W. (1968). The Type V Bekesy pattern: The effects of loudness memory. *J. Speech Hear. Res., 11,* 567–575.

Hattler, K. W. (1970). Lengthened off-time: A self-recording screening device for nonorganicity. *J. Speech Hear. Dis., 35,* 113–122.

Hattler, K. W., & Schuchman, G. I. (1971). Efficiency of the Stenger, Doerfler-Stewart, and lengthened off-time Bekesy tests. *Acta Otolaryngol., 72,* 252–267.

Heller, M. F. (1955). *Functional otology.* New York: Springer.

Hood, W. H., Campbell, R. A., & Hutton, C. L. (1964). An evaluation of the Bekesy ascending descending gap. *J. Speech Hear. Res., 7,* 123–132.

Hopkinson, N. T. (1965). Type V Bekesy audiograms: Specification and clinical utility. *J. Speech Hear. Dis., 30,* 243–251.

Hopkinson, N. (1967). Comment on pseudohypacusis. *J. Speech Hear. Dis., 32,* 293–294.

Hopkinson, N. T. (1978). Speech tests for presbycusis. In J. Katz (ed.), *Handbook of clinical audiology,* 2d ed., pp. 291–303. Baltimore: Williams & Wilkins.

Istre, C. O., & Burton, M. (1969). Automatic audiometry for detecting malingering. *Arch. Otolaryngol., 90,* 326–332.

Jepsen, O. (1953). Intratympanic muscle reflexes in psychogenic deafness (impedance measurement). *Acta Otolaryngol. Suppl., 109,* 61–69.

Jerger, J., & Tillman, T. (1960). A new method for the clinical determination of sensorineural acuity level (SAL). *Arch. Otolaryngol., 71,* 948–955.

Jerger, J., & Herer, G. (1961). An unexpected dividend in Bekesy audiometry. *J. Speech Hear. Dis., 26,* 390–391.

Johnson, K. O., Work, W. P., & McCoy, G. (1956). Functional deafness. *Ann. Otol. Rhinol. Laryngol., 65,* 154–170.

Kinstler, D. B. (1971). Functional hearing loss. In L. E. Travis (Ed.), *Handbook of speech pathology,* pp. 375–398. New York: Appleton-Century-Crofts.

Kinstler, D. B., Phelan, J. G., & Lavender, R. W. (1972). The Stenger and speech Stenger tests in functional hearing loss. *Audiology, 11,* 187–193.

Knox, A. W. (1978). Electrodermal audiometry. In J. Katz (ed.), *Handbook of clinical audiology,* pp. 304–310. Baltimore: Williams & Wilkins.

Korn, T. (1954). Effect of physiological feedback on conversational noise reduction in rooms. *J. Acoust. Soc. Am., 26,* 793–794.

Kraus, N., Smith, D. I., Reed, N. L., Stein, L. K., & Cartee, C. L. (1985). Auditory middle latency responses in children: Effects of age and diagnostic category. *Electroencephalogr. Clin. Neurophysiol., 62,* 343–351.

Lamb, L. E., & Peterson, J. L. (1967). Middle ear reflex measurements in pseudohypacusis. *J. Speech Hear. Dis., 32,* 46–57.

Lee, B. (1950). Some effects of side-tone delay. *J. Acoust. Soc. Am., 22,* 639–640.

Lehrer, N. D., Hirschenfang, S., Miller, M. H., & Radpour, S. (1964). Nonorganic hearing problems in adolescents. *Laryngoscope, 74,* 64–70.

Leshin, G. J. (1960). Childhood nonorganic hearing loss. *J. Speech Hear. Dis., 25,* 290–292.

Liden, G., Nilsson, G., & Anderson, H. (1959). Narrow band masking with white noise. *Acta Otolaryngol., 50,* 116–124.

Lightfoot, C., & Morrill, S. (1949). Loudness of speaking: The effect of the intensity of the sidetone upon the intensity of the speaker. Joint Project Rept. No. 4. Bureau of Medicine and Surgery, U.S. Navy Project No. 001.053.

Lloyd, L. L., & Kaplan, H. (1978). *Audiometric interpretation: A manual of basic audiometry.* Baltimore: University Park Press.

Lombard, E. (1911). Le signe de l'elevation de la voix. *Annls. Mal. Oreille Larynx, 37,* 101–119.

McCandless, G. A., & Lentz, W. E. (1968). Amplitude and latency characteristics of the auditory evoked response at low sensation levels. *J. Aud. Res., 8,* 273–282.

McGranahan, L. M., Causey, D., & Studebaker, G. (1960). Delayed side tone audiometry (Abstract). *Asha, 2,* 357.

McLennan, R. O., & Martin, F. N. (1976). On the discrepancy between the speech reception threshold and the pure-tone average in nonorganic hearing loss. Poster session at the Annual Convention of the American Speech and Hearing Association, Houston, Texas.

Martin, F. N. (1978). Pseudohypacusis perspectives and pure tone tests. In J. Katz (ed.), *Handbook of clinical audiology,* 2d ed., pp. 276–290. Baltimore: Williams & Wilkins.

Martin, F. N. (1985). The pseudohypacusic. In J. Katz (ed.), *Handbook of clinical audiology,* 3d ed., pp. 742–765. Baltimore: Williams & Wilkins.

Martin, F. N., & Hawkins, R. R. (1963). A modification of the Doerfler–Stewart method for the detection of non-organic hearing loss. *J. Aud. Res., 3,* 147–150.

Martin, F. N., & Monro, D. A. (1975). The effects of sophistication on Type V Bekesy patterns in simulated hearing loss. *J. Speech Hear. Dis., 40,* 508–513.

Martin, F. N., & Shipp, D. B. (1982). The effects of sophistication on three threshold tests for subjects with simulated hearing loss. *Ear Hear., 3,* 34–36.

Medical and Dental Equipment Standard, UL 544, effective September 30, 1974. Melville, New York: Underwriters Laboratories, Inc.

Melnick, W. (1967). Comfort level and loudness matching for continuous and interrupted signals. *J. Speech Hear. Res., 10,* 99–109.

Mendel, M., Sussman, M., Merson, R., Naeser, M., & Minifie, F. (1969). Loudness judgments of speech and non-speech stimuli. *J. Acoust. Soc. Am., 46,* 1556–1561.

Menzel, O. J. (1960). Clinical efficiency in compensation audiometry. *J. Speech Hear. Dis., 25,* 49–54.

Menzel, O. J. (1965). The Stenger test. *Eye, Ear, Nose, Throat Month., 44,* 21–25.

Miller, A. L., Fox, M. S., & Chan, G. (1968). Pure tone assessment as an aid in detecting suspected non-organic hearing disorders in children. *Laryngoscope, 78,* 2170–2176.

Monro, D. A., & Martin, F. N. (1977). Effects of sophistication on four tests for nonorganic hearing loss. *J. Speech Hear. Dis., 42,* 528–534.

Musiek, F. E., & Donnelly, K. (1983). Clinical applications of the (auditory) middle latency responses—An overview. *Sem. Hear., 4,* 391–401.

Newby, H. A. (1958). *Audiology: Principles and practice.* New York: Appleton-Century-Crofts.

Nober, E. (1966). Psychogenic auditory problems in adults. In R. Rieber & R. Brubaker (eds.), *Speech pathology,* pp. 94–99. Amsterdam: North-Holland.

Noble, W. (1987). The conceptual problem of 'functional hearing loss.' *Brit. J. Audiol., 21,* 1–3.

Olsen, W. O., & Matkin, N. D. (1978). Differential audiology. In D. E. Rose (ed.), *Audiological assessment,* pp. 368–419. Englewood Cliffs, New Jersey: Prentice Hall.

O'Neill, J. J., & Oyer, H. J. (1966). *Applied audiometry.* New York: Dodd, Mead.

Pang-Ching, G. (1970). The tone-in-noise test: A preliminary report. *J. Aud. Res., 10,* 322–327.

Peck, J. E., & Ross, M. (1970). A comparison of the ascending and the descending modes for the administration of the pure-tone Stenger test. *J. Aud. Res., 10,* 218–220.

Pickett, J. M. (1958). Limits of direct communication in noise. *J. Acoust. Soc. Am., 30,* 278–281.

Portmann, M., & Portmann, C. (1961). *Clinical audiometry.* Springfield, Illinois: Thomas.

Price, L. L., Sheperd, D. C., & Goldstein, R. (1965). Abnormal Bekesy tracings in normal ears. *J. Speech Hear. Dis., 30,* 139–144.

Rainville, M. J. (1955). Nouvelle methode d'assourdissement pour le releve des courbes de conduction osseuse. *J. Franc. Oto-laryngol., 4,* 851–859.

Resnick, D. M., & Burke, K. S. (1962). Bekesy audiometry in non-organic auditory problems. *Arch. Otolaryngol., 76,* 38–41.

Rintelmann, W. F. (1979). Pseudohypacusis. In W. F. Rintelmann (ed.), *Hearing assessment,* pp. 379–424. Baltimore: University Park Press.

Rintelmann, W. F., & Carhart, R. (1964). Loudness tracking by normal hearers via Bekesy audiometer. *J. Speech Hear. Res., 7,* 79–93.

Rintelmann, W., & Harford, E. (1963). The detection and assessment of pseudohypacusis among school children. *J. Speech Hear. Dis., 28,* 141–152.

Rintelmann, W. F., & Harford, E. R. (1967). Type V Bekesy pattern: Interpretation and clinical utility. *J. Speech Hear. Res., 10,* 733–744.

Rintelmann, W. F., & Johnson, K. R. (1970). Comparison of pure-tone versus speech sensorineural acuity level (SAL) test. Paper presented at the Annual Convention of the American Speech and Hearing Association, New York.

Robinson, M., & Kasden, S. D. (1973). Clinical application of pure tone delayed auditory feedback in pseudohypacusis. *Eye, Ear, Nose, Throat Month., 52,* 91–93.

Ross, M. (1964). The variable intensity pulse count method (VIPCM) for the detection and measurement of the pure-tone thresholds of children with functional hearing losses. *J. Speech Hear. Dis., 29,* 477–482.

Ruhm, H. B., & Cooper, W. A., Jr. (1962). Low sensation level effects of pure-tone delayed auditory feedback. *J. Speech Hear. Res., 5,* 185–193.

Ruhm, H. B., & Cooper, W. A., Jr. (1963). Some factors that influence pure-tone delayed auditory feedback. *J. Speech Hear. Res., 6,* 223–237.

Ruhm, H. B., & Cooper, W. A., Jr. (1964). Delayed feedback audiometry. *J. Speech Hear. Dis., 29,* 448–455.

Russell, R. D. (1934). Detection of simulated deafness. *Laryngoscope, 44,* 201–210.

Sanders, J. W., & Lazenby, P. B. (1983). Auditory brain stem response measurement in the assessment of pseudohypacusis. *Am. J. Otol., 4,* 292–299.

Sanders, J. W., & Rintelmann, W. F. (1964). Masking in audiometry: Clinical evaluation of three methods. *Arch. Otolaryngol., 80,* 541–556.

Schwartz, D. M. (1979). Cited in W. F. Rintelmann (ed.), *Hearing assessment*, p. 382. Baltimore: University Park Press.

Semenov, H. (1947). Deafness of psychic origin and its response to narcosynthesis. *Trans. Am. Acad. Opthalmol. Oto-Laryngol., 51*, 326–248.

Shepherd, D. C. (1965). Non-organic hearing loss and the consistency of behavioral auditory responses. *J. Speech Hear. Res., 8*, 149–163.

Shepherd, D. C., & Goldstein, R. (1968). Intrasubject variability in amplitude of Bekesy tracings and its relation to measures of personality. *J. Speech Hear. Res., 11*, 523–535.

Siedentorp, K. H., Kapple, H., & Derbyshire, A. J. (1966). Auditory threshold determination. *Arch. Otolaryngol., 83*, 35–38.

Silman, S., Gelfand, S. A., Piper, N., Silverman, C. A., & Van Frank, L. (1984a). Prediction of hearing loss from the acoustic-reflex threshold. In S. Silman (ed.), *The acoustic reflex: Basic principles and clinical applications*, pp. 187–223. New York: Academic Press.

Silman, S., Silverman, C. A., Showers, T., & Gelfand, S. A. (1984b). The effect of age on prediction of hearing loss with the bivariate plotting procedure. *J. Speech Hear. Res., 27*, 12–19.

Simonton, K. M. (1965). Audiometry and diagnosis. In A. Glorig (ed.), *Audiometry: Principles and practice*, pp. 185–206. Baltimore: Williams & Wilkins.

Stapells, D. R., Picton, T. W., Perez-Abalo, M., Read, M., & Smith, A. (1985). Frequency specificity in evoked potential audiometry. In J. T. Jacobson (ed.), *The auditory brainstem response*, pp. 147–177. San Diego: College-Hill Press.

Stark, E. W. (1966). Jerger types in fixed-frequency Bekesy audiometry with normal and hypacusic children. *J. Aud. Res., 6*, 135–140.

Stein, L. (1963). Some observations on Type V Bekesy tracings. *J. Speech Hear. Res., 6*, 339–348.

Stein, L. K. (1966). Functional hearing problems in children. Maico Audiological Library Series, 4, Rep. 10.

Stenger, P. (1900). An attempt to objectively identify unilateral deafness, making allowances for difficulty in hearing tuning forks in the middle frequencies. *Arch. Ohrenheilk., 50*, 197.

Stenger, P. (1907). Similation and dissimulation of ear diseases and their identification. *Deutsch. Med. Wochenschr., 33*, 970–973.

Studebaker, G. A. (1964). Clinical masking of air- and bone-conducted stimuli. *J. Speech Hear. Dis., 29*, 23–35.

Suzuki, T., & Kubota, K. (1966). Normal width in tracing on Bekesy audiogram. *J. Aud. Res., 6*, 91–96.

Taylor, G. L. (1949). An experimental study of tests for the detection of auditory malingering. *J. Speech Hear. Dis., 14*, 119–130.

Terkildsen, K. (1964). Clinical application of impedance measurements with a fixed frequency technique. *Int. Audiol., 3*, 123–128.

Thorne, B. (1960). Psycho-Tell: An aid in the estimate of functional auditory disorders. *Arch. Otolaryngol., 72*, 626–630.

Tillman, T. W. (1963). Clinical applicability of the SAL test. *Arch. Otolaryngol., 78*, 36–47.

Ventry, I. M. (1962). Relative efficiency of tests used to detect functional hearing loss. *Internat. Audiol., 1*, 145–150.

Ventry, I. M. (1968). A case for psychogenic hearing loss. *J. Speech Hear. Dis., 33*, 89–92.

Ventry, I. M. (1971). Bekesy audiometry in functional hearing loss: A case study. J. Speech Hear. Dis., 36, 125–141.

Ventry, I. M. (1976). Pure tone–spondee relationships in functional hearing loss. *J. Speech Hear. Dis., 41*, 16–22.

Ventry, I. M., & Chaiklin, J. B. (1965a). The efficiency of auditory measures used to identify functional hearing loss. *J. Aud. Res., 3*, 196–211.

Ventry, I. M., & Chaiklin, J. B. (1965b). Evaluation of pure-tone audiogram configurations used in identifying adults with functional loss. *J. Aud. Res., 3*, 212–218.

Ventry, I. M., Trier, T. R., & Chaiklin, J. B. (1965). Factors related to persistence and resolution of functional hearing loss. *J. Aud. Res., 3*, 231–240.

Waldron, D. L. (1960). *The Lombard voice reflex: An experimental study*. Unpublished Ph.D. Thesis. Stanford, California: Stanford University.

Watson, L. A., & Tolan, T. (1949). *Hearing tests and hearing instruments*. Baltimore: Williams & Wilkins.

Witting, E. G., & Hughson, W. (1940). Inherent accuracy of a series of repeated clinical audiograms. *Laryngoscope, 50*, 259–269.

Wolf, K. E., Vivion, M. C., & Goldstein, R. (1979). Middle components of the AER at high and low audiometric frequencies. Paper presented at the biennial symposium of the International Electric Response Audiometry Study Group, Santa Barbara, California.

Zwislocki, J. (1953). Acoustic attenuation between ears. *J. Acoust. Soc. Am., 25*, 742–759.

Zwislocki, J. (ed.) (1963). *Critical evaluation of methods of testing and measurement of nonorganic hearing impairment*. Report of the Working Group 36, NAS-NRC Committee on Hearing, Bioacoustics and Biomechanics.

CHAPTER 5

TRADITIONAL AUDIOLOGIC SITE-OF-LESION TESTS

The audiologic test battery was initially developed for the purpose of differentiating between cochlear and retro-cochlear (eighth-nerve and extra-axial brainstem) etiologies of unilateral or asymmetrical sensorineural hearing impairment. The traditional tests used in the audiologic "site-of-lesion" test battery included Alternate Binaural Loudness Balance (ABLB), Short Increment Sensitivity Index (SISI), tone-decay, speech-recognition, Bekesy, acoustic-reflex threshold and decay (see Chapters 3 and 9), and electronystagmography (see Chapters 8 and 9). More recently, brainstem auditory-evoked potentials (BAEPs) were added to the site-of-lesion battery (see Chapters 7 and 9).

Fowler (1936) developed the ABLB test but Dix, Hall-pike, and Hood (1948) were the first to establish the utility of this test with respect to the differential diagnosis of eighth-nerve and cochlear lesions. Schubert (1944) was the originator of the tone-decay test and Bekesy (1947) developed the Bekesy audiometer. The clinical applications of these tests became apparent after Reger and Kos (1952) described a drift in the continuous-tone tracing in a patient with eighth-nerve pathology and Kos (1955) reported marked adaptation in a patient with eighth-nerve pathology. Jerger (1960) classified the Bekesy patterns and established their significance with respect to auditory site of lesion. Hood (1955) and then Carhart (1957) and others developed the clinical tone-decay tests. Schuknecht and Woellner (1955) and Walsh and Goodman (1955) were among the first to observe very markedly reduced speech-recognition scores in patients with eighth-nerve pathology and normal-hearing threshold levels. Jerger and Jerger (1971) observed the phenomenon of rollover in speech-recognition in patients with eighth-nerve pathology, an observation that served as the basis for the rollover index. Metz (1946) developed the electromechanical bridge and was the first to make clinical measurements of acoustic immittance. Anderson, Barr, and Wedenberg (1969) were among the first to observe elevated acoustic-reflex thresholds and acoustic-reflex decay in patients with eighth-nerve pathology. In the 1970s, electronystagmography (tests of oculomotor function and balance) became popular for eval-

uation of dizzy patients to determine if a lesion existed in the vestibular pathway and the site of the lesion (if present). Brainstem auditory-evoked potentials were first described by Jewett and Williston (1971) and Sohmer and Feinmesser (1970). But Starr and Achor (1975) were among the first to demonstrate the ability of BAEPs to detect disorders of the auditory nervous system from the eighth-nerve to the brainstem levels.

Soon after the advent of the audiologic site-of-lesion battery, extraordinary strides in medical technology were made, such as the development of computerized axial tomography so acoustic tumors could be detected earlier, before hearing loss occurred. Consequently, referrals for audiologic follow-up were made at an earlier stage of development of the tumor (Sanders, 1984). The audiologic site-of-lesion tests were then administered not only to persons with unilateral or asymmetrical sensorineural hearing impairment but also to persons with normal-hearing threshold levels with eighth-nerve signs such as balance disorders (vertigo or unsteadiness), tinnitus, difficulty understanding speech, or aural pressure or fullness. Signs that are generally found later on in the course of acoustic-tumor development include paresthesia of the face, anesthesia of the face, and facial weakness or paralysis. Other symptoms of cerebello-pontine angle tumors may include headaches, ataxia, and vomiting. A person who is at low risk for retrocochlear pathology does not demonstrate any of these eighth-nerve signs and does not have unilateral or asymmetrical sensori-neural hearing impairment. A person who is considered at high risk for retrocochlear pathology is one with unilateral or asymmetrical sensorineural hearing impairment or one who manifests one of the eighth-nerve signs.

Jerger (1973), and more recently Miller (1985), stressed the following limitation of site-of-lesion testing. These tests can determine site but not type of auditory pathology. Thus, even though acoustic tumors account for 8% of all brain tumors and 78% of all cerebellopontine-angle tumors (Gates, 1976), an eighth-nerve disorder is not necessarily an acoustic tumor. Other disorders which can affect the eighth nerve include viral infection, vascular insult, trauma, multiple sclerosis, cerebellopontine-angle tumors other than acoustic neuromas, acquired luetic hearing loss, etc.

When a retrocochlear impairment causes a deficit on an audiologic site-of-lesion test, the deficit is usually seen ipsilateral to the affected ear. A result that is consistent with a retrocochlear site is considered positive. When the result is inconsistent with a retrocochlear site, it is considered negative. A positive or negative result must be differentiated from a positive or negative score. A positive or negative score may be obtained on the ABLB or SISI tests. As will be shown later in this chapter, however, a positive ABLB or SISI score is consistent with cochlear pathology (negative result) whereas a negative ABLB or SISI score is consistent with retrocochlear pathology (positive result).

The central auditory test battery came into existence after the traditional audiologic site-of-lesion battery. The central auditory test battery was designed to detect intra-axial brainstem and temporal-lobe disorders affecting the central auditory nervous system. Unlike disorders of the cochlea and eighth nerve, central auditory disorders were generally associated with normal pure-tone hearing-threshold levels. But, similar to cochlear and eighth-nerve disorders, central auditory nervous system disorders were associated with a loss in the ability to understand speech. Central auditory testing will be discussed in Chapters 6 and 9.

This chapter will discuss the traditional site-of-lesion tests: speech-recognition, tone-decay, ABLB, SISI, and Bekesy. Acoustic-reflex threshold and decay testing with respect to differential diagnosis of retrocochlear and cochlear pathology was discussed in Chapter 3. The diagnostic aspects of BAEPs with respect to cochlear and retrocochlear pathology will be discussed in Chapter 7. Electronystagmography will be discussed in Chapter 8. In Chapter 9, the concept of the test battery (administration of a combination rather than a single site-of-lesion test) will be addressed more fully and a comparison of the site-of-lesion tests with respect to their hit rates (percentage of retrocochlear-impaired ears with positive results) and false-alarm rates (percentage of cochlear-impaired ears with positive results) will be made.

I. SPEECH-RECOGNITION TESTING

Suprathreshold speech-recognition testing, commonly referred to as speech-discrimination testing, has traditionally been done (a) to estimate the degree of hearing handicap or communicative functioning of the patient, (b) to determine the anatomical site of lesion, (c) to monitor progress in aural rehabilitation, and (d) to assess hearing-aid performance. This chapter will deal only with suprathreshold speech-recognition testing with respect to differential diagnosis (peripheral or eighth-nerve pathology). The applicability of suprathreshold speech-recognition testing with

respect to central pathology will be discussed in Chapter 6. The other applications of suprathreshold speech-recognition testing are beyond the scope of this book.

The traditional term describing the ability to repeat words or other speech stimuli is "speech-discrimination ability." The repetition of speech stimuli, however, is not a discrimination task involving judgements of sameness or difference. Rather, the repetition task involves recognition (Olsen & Matkin, 1979). Wilson and Margolis (1983) suggest further delineating the term "speech recognition" by indicating the speech stimulus employed; an illustration of this suggestion is given by the phrase "word-recognition" or "speech-recognition" for monosyllabic words. In this chapter, the term "suprathreshold speech-recognition testing" or "suprathreshold speech-recognition score" or "ability" shall be used. The acronym SRT will not be used to refer to speech-recognition testing in abbreviated form since it is commonly used to refer to the threshold for speech (see Chapter 2).

A. DEVELOPMENT OF THE CID W-22s

During World War II, research on suprathreshold speech-recognition testing was centered upon the assessment of communication equipment such as the telephone using live-voice presentation. Most of the seminal work in this area was done at the Psychoacoustic Laboratory at Harvard University. Egan (1948) constructed 20 "equivalent" Harvard phonetically balanced lists of 50 monosyllabic words (PAL PB-50s) from previously developed Harvard Psychoacoustic Laboratory speech lists so they met the following criteria:

1. The test items consisted of commonly used monosyllabic words.
2. The average difficulty of each list was equivalent to that of the other lists.
3. The range of difficulty of each list was equivalent to that of the other lists.
4. The phonetic composition (with respect to speech sounds in the initial, medial, and final position) of one list was equivalent to that of the other lists.
5. The phonetic composition of each list represented a normal sampling of speech sounds in the English language (phonetic balance).

Phonetic balance (PB) was obtained by having the proportions of speech sounds in each list reflect the relative occurrences of the phonemes in the American English-speaking population as reported by Dewey (1923) in his survey of 100,000 words in newsprint. The lists were too short to completely fulfill the criterion of phonetic balance. Nevertheless, the fact that the PB-50 word lists roughly approximated phonetic balance meant that, in general, speech-sound recognition ability in everyday communica-

Table I   The Twenty PAL PB-50 Word Lists[a]

PB-50 List 1

Are	Death	Fuss	Not	Rub
Bad	Deed	Grove	Pan	Slip
Bar	Dike	Heap	Pants	Smile
Bask	Dish	Hid	Pest	Strife
Box	End	Hive	Pile	Such
Cane	Feast	Hunt	Plush	Then
Cleanse	Fern	Is	Rag	There
Clove	Fold	Mange	Rat	Toe
Crash	Ford	No	Ride	Use (yews)
Creed	Fraud	Nook	Rise	Wheat

PB-50 List 2

Awe	Dab	Hock	Perk	Start
Bait	Earl	Job	Pick	Suck
Bean	Else	Log	Pit	Tan
Blush	Fate	Moose	Quart	Tang
Bought	Five	Mute	Rap	Them
Bounce	Frog	Nab	Rib	Trash
Bud	Gill	Need	Scythe	Vamp
Charge	Gloss	Niece	Shoe	Vast
Cloud	Hire	Nut	Sludge	Ways
Corpse	Hit	Our	Snuff	Wish

PB-50 List 3

Ache	Crime	Hurl	Please	Take
Air	Deck	Jam	Pulse	Thrash
Bald	Dig	Law	Rate	Toil
Barb	Dill	Leave	Rouse	Trip
Bead	Drop	Lush	Shout	Turf
Cape	Fame	Muck	Sit	Vow
Cast	Far	Neck	Size	Wedge
Check	Fig	Nest	Sob	Wharf
Class	Flush	Oak	Sped	Who
Crave	Gnaw	Path	Stag	Why

PB-50 List 4

Bath	Dodge	Hot	Pert	Shed
Beast	Dupe	How	Pinch	Shin
Bee	Earn	Kite	Pod	Sketch
Blonde	Eel	Merge	Race	Slap
Budge	Fin	Move	Rack	Sour
Bus	Float	Neat	Rave	Starve
Bush	Frown	New	Raw	Strap
Cloak	Hatch	Oils	Rut	Test
Course	Heed	Or	Sage	Tick
Court	Hiss	Peck	Scab	Touch

PB-50 List 5

Add	Flap	Love	Rind (rind)	Thud
Bathe	Gape*	Mast	Rode	Trade
Beck	Good	Nose	Roe	True
Black	Greek	Odds	Scare	Tug
Bronze	Grudge	Owls	Shine	Vase (vace)
Browse*	High	Pass	Shove	Watch
Cheat	Hill	Pipe	Sick	Wink
Choose	Inch	Puff	Sly	Wrath
Curse	Kid	Punt	Solve	Yawn
Feed	Lend	Rear	Thick	Zone

*Bake, Drive

PB-50 List 6

As	Deep	Gap	Prig*	Shank
Badge	Eat	Grope	Prime	Slouch
Best	Eyes	Hitch	Pun	Sup
Bog*	Fall	Hull	Pus	Thigh
Chart	Fee	Jag	Raise	Thus
Cloth	Flick	Kept	Ray	Tongue
Clothes	Flop	Leg	Reap	Wait
Cob	Forge	Mash	Rooms	Wasp
Crib	Fowl	Nigh	Rough	Wife
Dad	Gage	Ode	Scan	Writ*

* Beg, Match, Plug

PB-50 List 7

Act	Dope	Jug	Pounce	Siege
Aim	Dose	Knit	Quiz	Sin
Am	Dwarf	Mote*	Raid	Sledge
But	Fake	Mud	Range	Sniff
By	Fling	Nine	Rash	South
Chop	Fort	Off	Rich	Though
Coast	Gasp	Pent	Roar	Whiff*
Comes	Grade	Phase*	Sag	Wire
Cook	Gun	Pig	Scout	Woe
Cut	Him	Plod	Shaft	Woo

* Meet, Shave, Whip

PB-50 List 8

Ask	Cod	Forth	Look	Shack
Bid	Crack	Freak	Night	Slide
Bind	Day	Frock	Pint	Spice
Bolt	Deuce	Front	Queen	This
Bored	Dumb	Guess	Rest	Thread
Calf	Each	Hum	Rhyme	Till
Catch	Ease	Jell	Rod	Us
Chant	Fad	Kill	Roll	Wheeze*
Chew	Flip	Left	Rope	Wig
Clod	Food	Lick	Rot	Yeast

* Horse

PB-50 List 9

Arch	Crowd	Grace	Odd	Than
Beef	Cud*	Hoof	Pact*	Thank
Birth	Ditch	Ice	Phone	Throne
Bit	Flat	Itch	Reed	Toad
Boost	Fluff*	Key	Root	Troop
Carve	Foe	Lit	Rude	Weak
Chess	Fume	Mass	Sip	Wild
Chest	Fuse	Nerve	Smart	Wipe
Clown	Gate	Noose	Spud	With
Club	Give	Nuts	Ten	Year

* Skill, Tax, Tub

PB-50 List 10

Ail	Cue	Gull	Pink	Staff
Back	Daub*	Hat	Plus	Tag
Bash*	Ears	Hurt	Put	Those
Bob	Earth	Jay	Rape*	Thug
Bug	Etch*	Lap	Real	Tree

Champ	Fir	Line	Rip	Valve
Chance	Flaunt	Maze	Rush	Void*
Clothe	Flight	Mope*	Scrub	Wade
Cord	Force	Nudge	Slug	Wake
Cow	Goose	Page	Snipe	Youth

* Died, Dust, Gold, Lock, Rake, Spin

PB-50 List 11

Arc	Doubt	Jab	Pond	Shot
Arm	Drake	Jaunt*	Probe	Sign
Beam	Dull	Kit	Prod	Snow
Bliss	Feel	Lag	Punk	Sprig*
Chunk	Fine	Latch	Purse	Spy
Clash	Frisk*	Loss	Reef	Stiff
Code	Fudge	Low	Rice	Tab
Crutch	Goat	Most	Risk	Urge
Cry	Have	Mouth	Sap	Wave
Dip	Hop	Net	Shop	Wood

* Door, Fist, Skin

PB-50 List 12

And	Cling	Frill	Lash	Rove
Ass*	Clutch	Gnash	Laugh	Set
Ball	Depth	Greet	Ledge	Shut
Bluff	Dime	Hear	Loose	Sky
Cad	Done	Hug	Out	Sod
Cave	Fed	Hunch	Park	Throb
Chafe*	Flog*	Jaw	Priest	Tile
Chair	Flood	Jazz	Reek*	Vine
Chap	Foot	Jolt	Ripe	Wage
Chink	Fought	Knife	Romp	Wove

* Glass, Make, Speed, Teeth

PB-50 List 13

Bat	Few	Jig	Nip	Sled
Beau	Fill	Made	Ought	Smash
Change	Fold	Mood	Owe	Smooth
Climb	For	Mop	Patch	Soap
Corn	Gem	Moth	Pelt	Stead
Curb	Grape	Muff	Plead	Taint
Deaf	Grave	Mush	Price	Tap
Dog	Hack	My	Pug	Thin
Elk	Hate	Nag	Scuff	Tip
Elm	Hook	Nice	Side	Wean

PB-50 List 14

At	Dead	Isle	Prude	Stuff
Barn	Douse	Kick	Purge	Tell
Bust	Dung	Lathe	Quack	Tent
Car	Fife	Life	Rid	Thy
Clip	Foam	Me	Shook	Tray
Coax	Grate	Muss	Shrug	Vague
Curve	Group	News	Sing	Vote
Cute	Heat	Nick	Slab	Wag
Darn	Howl	Nod	Smite	Waif
Dash	Hunk	Oft	Soil	Wrist

PB-50 List 15

Bell	Fact	Less	Pup	Teach
Blind	Flame	May	Quick	That
Boss	Fleet	Mesh	Scow	Time
Cheap	Gash	Mitt	Sense	Tinge
Cost	Glove	Mode	Shade	Tweed
Cuff	Golf	Morn	Shrub	Vile

Dive	Hedge	Naught	Sir	Weave
Dove (duv)	Hole	Ninth	Slash	Wed
Edge	Jade	Oath	So	Wide
Elf	Kiss	Own	Tack	Wreck

PB-50 List 16

Aid	Droop	Kind	Pump	Stress
Barge	Dub	Knee	Rock	Suit
Book	Fifth	Lay	Rogue	Thou
Cheese	Fright	Leash	Rug	Three
Cliff	Gab	Louse	Rye	Thresh
Closed	Gas	Map	Sang	Tire
Crews	Had	Nap	Sheep	Ton
Dame	Hash	Next	Sheik	Tuck
Din	Hose	Part	Soar	Turn
Drape	Ink	Pitch	Stab	Wield

PB-50 List 17

All	Crush	Hence	Past	Sell
Apt	Dart	Hood	Pearl	Ship
Bet	Dine	If	Peg	Shock
Big	Falls	Last	Plow	Stride
Booth	Feet	Ma	Press	Tube
Brace	Fell	Mist	Rage	Vice
Braid	Fit	Myth	Reach	Weep
Buck	Form	Ox	Ridge	Weird
Case	Fresh	Paid	Roam	Wine
Clue	Gum	Pare	Scratch	You

PB-50 List 18

Aims	Chip	Flare	Hush	Sack
Art	Claw	Fool	Lime	Sash
Axw	Claws	Freeze	Lip	Share
Bale	Crab	Got	Loud	Sieve
Bless	Cub	Grab	Lunge	Thaw
Camp	Debt	Gray	Lynch	Thine
Cat	Dice	Grew	Note	Thorn
Chaff	Dot	Gush	Ouch	Trod
Chain	Fade	Hide	Rob	Waste
Chill	Fat	His	Rose	Weed

PB-50 List 19

Age	Chose (choz)	Fond	Notch	Slid
Bark	Crude	Gin	On	Splash
Bay	Cup	God	Paste	Steed
Bough	Dough	Gyp	Perch	Thief
Buzz	Drug	Hike	Raft	Throat
Cab	Dune	Hut	Rote	Up
Cage	Ebb	Lad	Rule	Wheel
Calve (cav)	Fan	Led	Sat	White
Cant	Find	Lose (looz)	Shy	Yes
Chat	Flank	Lust	Sill	Yield

PB-50 List 20

Ace	Duke	Joke	Retch	Slush
Base	Eye	Judge	Robe	Soak
Beard	Fair	Lid	Roost	Souse
Brass	Fast	Mow (mo)	Rouge	Theme
Cart	Flash	Pack	Rout (rowt)	Through
Click	Gang	Pad	Salve	Tile
Clog	Get	Pew	Seed	Walk
Cork	Gob	Puss	Sigh	Wash
Crate	Hump	Quip	Skid	Web
Did	In	Ramp	Slice	Wise

[a] From Egan (1948). Substitutions for the Rush Hughes recording are indicated by an asterisk.

161

tive situations could be assessed. The ability to measure recognition of typical, everyday speech sounds lent the test face validity. Thus, although the PB-50 word lists were originally intended for assessing communications systems, their use in clinical audiologic practice became widespread, and standardized recordings were made. Table I shows the PB-50 word lists. The recordings, however, turned out to be clinically infeasible because of the difficult vocabulary. The recording made by the recorder, Rush Hughes, was a particularly difficult version.

Because the vocabulary of the PB-50s was large and contained unfamiliar words, the criterion of phonetic balance was incompletely satisfied, and good commercial recordings of the PB lists were unavailable, Hirsh, Davis, Silverman, Reynolds, Eldert, and Benson (1952) developed a modified version of the PAL PB-50s, called the Central Institute for the Deaf (CID) W-22s. The criterion of familiar vocabulary was fulfilled by having judges rate the PB-50 words (1000 words) and 80 words not drawn from any familiar source for familiarity. Of the 120 PAL words selected to be in the CID W-22 lists, 112 were rated as most familiar, 7 were rated as fairly familiar, and only 1 was rated as very unfamiliar. Of the 200 words in the W-22 lists, 190 were among the 4000 most common English words according to Thorndike (1932). The distribution of vowels and consonants in the initial and final positions in the W-22 lists were based on the newsprint survey by Dewey (1923) and the business-telephone-call survey by French, Carter, and Koenig (1930). Four W-22 lists, each containing 50 monosyllabic words, were recorded with the carrier phrase "You will say" monitored on the VU meter. The test item following the carrier phrase was spoken "as it would naturally follow in the phrase" (p.329). Six scramblings (A–F) of each list were made. Table II shows the four W-22 word lists.

To examine list equivalency, Hirsh et al. (1952) administered the 24 lists to 15 normal-hearing subjects at 10-dB increments between 20 and 70 dB SPL. The percentage of words correctly identified was plotted as a function of signal intensity in dB SPL for each list (articulation function). The articulation functions for the lists were essentially similar at high intensity levels. Below 40 dB SPL, however, the articulation function for list 1 differed from those for the other lists. Since the average relative intensity of the words was 2.5 dB lower than the words on the other lists, as estimated from the VU meter, the intensity of the words on list 1 was increased by 2 dB relative to the intensity at which the other lists were recorded. Administration of the final version of the W-22 tests at 80 dB and 25 dB SPL to 15 normal-hearing subjects revealed that the four lists were essentially equivalent in difficulty. Comparison of the articulation functions for the W-22s with those for the recorded PB-50s revealed that the former test has a steeper function, and is therefore easier than the latter test. Hirsh et al. (1952)

Table II The Four CID Auditory Test W-22 Lists of Monosyllabic PB Words

List 1	List 2	List 3	List 4
Ace	Ail (ale)	Add (Ad)	Aid
Ache	Air (heir)	Aim	All (awl)
An	And	Are	Am
As	Bin	Ate (eight)	Arm
Bathe	By (buy)	Bill	Art
Bells	Cap	Book	At
Carve	Cars	Camp	Bee (be)
Chew	Chest	Chair	Bread (bred)
Could	Die (dye)	Cute	Can
Dad	Does	Do	Chin
Day	Dumb	Done (dun)	Clothes
Deaf	Ease	Dull	Cook
Earn (urn)	Eat	Ears	Darn
East	Else	End	Dolls
Felt	Flat	Farm	Dust
Give	Gave	Glove	Ear
High	Ham	Hand	Eyes (ayes)
Him	Hit	Have	Few
Hunt	Hurt	He	Go
Isle (aisle)	Ice	If	Hang
It	Ill	Is	His
Jam	Jaw	Jar	In (inn)
Knees	Key	King	Jump
Law	Knee	Knit	Leave
Low	Live (verb)	Lie (lye)	Men
Me	Move	May	My
Mew	New (knew)	Nest	Near
None (nun)	Now	No (know)	Net
Not (knot)	Oak	Oil	Nuts
Or (oar)	Odd	On	Of
Owl	Off	Out	Ought (aught)
Poor	One (won)	Owes	Our (hour)
Ran	Own	Pie	Pale (pail)
See (sea)	Pew	Raw	Save
She	Rooms	Say	Shoe
Skin	Send	Shove	So (sew)
Stove	Show	Smooth	Stiff
Them	Smart	Start	Tea (tee)
There (their)	Star	Tan	Than
Thing	Tare (tear)	Ten	They
Toe	That	This	Through
True	Then	Though	Tin
Twins	Thin	Three	Toy
Yard	Too (two, to)	Tie	Where
Up	Tree	Use (yews)	Who
Us	Way (weigh)	We	Why
Wet	Well	West	Will
What	With	When	Wood (would)
Wire	Yore (your)	Wool	Yes
You (ewe)	Young	Year	Yet

attributed the difference in steepness of the function to the fact that the W-22 test had a smaller vocabulary (200 as opposed to 1000 words) and was therefore more intelligible, and to the fact that the W-22 test recordings of the words were more similar to each other in intensity level.

Test–Retest Reliability and Interlist Equivalency of the CID W-22s

Elpern (1960) obtained a pool of 1490 speech-recognition scores (monaural) for subjects with various types of losses from Veterans Administration Medical Center audiology clinics and compared the means and standard deviations for the four CID W-22 lists. He found that the means and standard deviations for the lists did not differ by more than 5% so he considered the lists essentially equivalent for clinical purposes.

Ross and Huntington (1962) evaluated the test–retest reliability and equivalency of the W-22 lists in a group of 33 subjects with acquired sensorineural hearing losses greater than or equal to 30 dB for at least one of the frequencies between 250 and 4000 Hz. The lists (1C, 2C, 3C, 4C, 1D, 2D, 3D, and 4D) were presented at 30 dB SL relative to the SRT. The results of analysis of variance revealed that the lists differed with respect to the mean level of difficulty. Nevertheless, the differences found between lists 1 and 3, 1 and 4, and 2 and 4, were slight and clinically insignificant. Test–retest reliability coefficients, however, were high, ranging from $r = 0.91$ to $r = 0.95$ (Hagerman, 1976; Loven and Hawkin, 1983).

B. BINOMIAL DISTRIBUTION MODEL

Egan (1948) noted that the intrasubject test–retest differences were masked by the group mean test–retest differences or could not be detected by the use of reliability correlation coefficients, which are dependent on the dispersion of test scores. Another source of test variability was the variability of the test score itself. According to Egan (1948), the test score variability was smallest at the extreme ends of the score range and greatest at the middle of the score range, the variability was inversely related to the length of the test list, and there was a normal error distribution only for the mid-range scores.

Thornton and Raffin (1978) suggested that the variance between test forms could be estimated using a probabilistic model since the responses could be scored as correct or incorrect, the score was in the form of a percentage, and the alternate forms of the speech-recognition tests had an equal number of test items. Since the response to each speech stimulus is independent of those for the other stimuli, Thornton and Raffin contended that the test responses could be evaluated as a binomial distribution.

The simple binomial model is based on sampling theory in which the pool consists of the common monosyllabic PB words, p̃ is the true score in the original pool and the expected score for a randomly selected sample of words from the pool, and n is the number of items in the sample test. Each of the alternate lists can be considered a random sample of stimuli drawn from the larger pool of comon monosyllabic PB words.

Thornton and Raffin (1978) calculated the standard deviations for the binomial distribution for each test score based on the formula SD (%) = $100\{[\bar{R}(1 - \tilde{p})]/n\}^{1/2}$. They compared the SDs for the binomial distribution with the SDs of the subsets of the 50-word CID W-22 lists rescored as two 25-word lists and five 10-word lists. The plot of the measured and binomial distribution standard deviation as a function of the true speech-recognition score for the 10-, 25-, and 50-item lists revealed that the test variability was dependent upon the subject's true score and the number of items (words) in the list. This plot is shown in Figure 1.

To test an obtained difference in test scores against the null hypothesis, the binomial distribution of differences in test scores must be obtained. Since the characteristics of the distribution of differences between binomial variables were not available, Thornton and Raffin (1978) used an arc-sine transform and applied this transform to a Z-table to calculate the limits of critical differences between two scores obtained on lists with an equal number of items. A variance stabilization transformation on test scores was necessary since the variance changes rapidly as the test score approaches 100%. Table III shows the 95% critical differences associated with each percentage score for 100-, 50-, 25-, and 10-item word lists. For example, if the score is 60%, there is a 95% probability that the score on another form of the test would fall between 42–78% on a 50-item test, between 36–80% on a 25-item test, or 20–90% on a 10-item test. Clearly, the smaller the test list, the larger the test–retest difference score needed to exceed the confidence limits. The binomial characteristics of suprathreshold

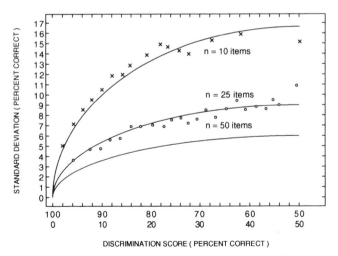

Figure 1 Within-subject standard deviations for 10- and 25-word tests grouped by estimated true scores (50 words). Solid lines show standard deviations of binomial distributions as a function of p̃ (in percentage) for $n = 10, 25$, and 50. Measured standard deviations are shown by X and O, respectively. Reprinted from Thorton and Raffin (1978) with permission.

Table III Lower and Upper Limits of the 95% Critical Differences for Percentage Scores[a]

Score (%)	n = 50	n = 25	n = 10	Score (%)	n = 100[b]
0	0–4	0–8	0–20	50	37–63
2	0–10			51	38–64
4	0–14	0–20		52	39–65
6	2–18			53	40–66
8	2–22	0–28		54	41–67
10	2–24		0–50	55	42–68
12	4–26	4–32		56	43–69
14	4–30			57	44–70
16	6–32	4–40		58	45–71
18	6–34			59	46–72
20	8–36	4–44	0–60	60	47–73
22	8–40			61	48–74
24	10–42	8–48		62	49–74
26	12–44			63	50–75
28	14–46	8–52		64	51–76
30	14–48		10–70	65	52–77
32	16–50	12–56		66	53–78
34	18–52			67	54–79
36	20–54	16–60		68	55–80
38	22–56			69	56–81
40	22–58	16–64	10–80	70	57–81
42	24–60			71	58–82
44	26–62	20–68		72	59–83
46	28–64			73	60–84
48	30–66	24–72		74	61–85
50	32–68		10–90	75	63–86
52	34–70	28–76		76	64–86
54	36–72			77	65–87
56	38–74	32–80		78	66–88
58	40–76			79	67–89
60	42–78	36–84	20–90	80	68–89
62	44–78			81	69–90
64	46–80	40–84		82	71–91
66	48–82			83	72–92
68	50–84	44–88		84	73–92
70	52–86		30–90	85	74–93
72	54–86	48–92		86	75–94
74	56–88			87	77–94
76	58–90	52–92		88	78–95
78	60–92			89	79–96
80	64–92	56–96	40–100	90	81–96
82	66–94			91	82–97
84	68–94	60–96		92	83–98
86	70–96			93	85–98
88	74–96	68–96		94	86–99
90	76–98		50–100	95	88–99
92	78–98	72–100		96	89–99
94	82–98			97	91–100
96	86–100	80–100		98	92–100
98	90–100			99	94–100
100	96–100	92–100	80–100	100	97–100

[a] Values within the range shown are not significantly different from the value shown in the percentage score columns (p > 0.05). Reprinted from Thornton and Raffin (1978) with permission.
[b] If score is less than 50%, find % Score = 100−observed score and subtract each critical difference limit from 100.

speech-recognition tests are not influenced by subject characterics, listening conditions, and type of stimulus; these characteristics only affect the subject's true score.

C. SPEAKER EFFECT

Brandy (1966) showed that even a single talker's repetition of a monosyllabic word list (CID W-22s) under monitored live-voice conditions introduced variability in suprathreshold speech-recognition scores. According to Tillman and Olsen (1973), suprathreshold speech-recognition tests cannot be considered standardized unless recordings are used. Penrod (1979) obtained recordings of four audiologists presenting the W-22s using monitored live voice. The recordings of the four talkers were administered to a group of 30 sensorineural hearing-impaired subjects at a single presentation level. The results revealed that, although the mean scores did not vary with the talker, 43% of the subjects' scores for the talkers differed significantly (were outside the Thornton and Raffin confidence limits). There also appeared to be a talker–listener interaction. Therefore, until recordings are standardized, clinicians should use commercially available recordings whenever possible rather than live voice and should note on the audiogram which recording was used. Furthermore, differences in recordings should be considered whenever test–retest differences occur.

D. DEVELOPMENT OF THE NU-6s

Lehiste and Peterson (1959) concluded that phonetic balance was not possible—only phonemic balance of lists of words was possible. They noted that the PAL PB-50s did not conform strictly to the criterion for phonemic balance so they developed test materials which adhered more strictly to the criterion of phonemic balance. Their test materials consisted of 1263 consonant-vowel-consonant (CNC) monosyllables from the Thorndike and Lorge (1944) list of 30,000 words. Lehiste and Peterson based their criteria for phonemic balance on the frequency of occurrence of phonemes in the initial consonant, nucleus (vowel), and final consonant positions in this group of 1263 words. From this pool of 1263 words, they developed ten lists of CNCs which were phonemically balanced. Peterson and Lehiste (1962) revised their lists to eliminate the less familiar words, resulting in ten revised 50-word CNC lists.

Tillman, Carhart, and Wilber (1963) and Tillman and Carhart (1966) reduced the number of CNC lists from ten to two in order to more precisely meet the criterion of phonemic balance. The recording of these two lists became known as the Northwestern University (NU) Auditory Test No. 4. These two NU-4 lists were later expanded to become four lists recorded with a different male speaker and also with a female speaker. The male speaker version became known as the Northwestern University Auditory Test No. 6-M and the female version became known as the Norwestern University Test No. 6-F. Four scramblings of the four lists were developed. The NU-6 lists are shown in Table IV.

Table IV Northwestern University Auditory Test No. 6[a]

List 1	List 2	List 3	List 4
Bean	Bite	Bar	Back
Boat	Book	Base	Bath
Burn	Bought	Beg	Bone
Chalk	Calm	Cab	Came
Choice	Chair	Cause	Chain
Death	Chief	Chat	Check
Dime	Dab	Cheek	Dip
Door	Dead	Cool	Dop
Fall	Deep	Date	Doll
Fat	Fail	Ditch	Fit
Gap	Far	Dodge	Food
Goose	Gaze	Five	Gas
Hash	Gin	Germ	Get
Home	Goal	Good	Hall
Hurl	Hate	Gun	Have
Jail	Haze	Half	Hole
Jar	Hush	Hire	Join
Keen	Juice	Hit	Judge
King	Keep	Jug	Kick
Kite	Keg	Late	Kill
Knock	Learn	Lid	Lean
Laud	Live	Life	Lease
Limb	Loaf	Luck	Long
Lot	Lore	Mess	Lose
Love	Match	Mop	Make
Met	Merge	Mouse	Mob
Mode	Mill	Name	Mood
Moon	Nice	Note	Near
Nag	Numb	Pain	Neat
Page	Pad	Pearl	Pass
Pool	Pick	Phone	Peg
Puff	Pike	Pole	Perch
Rag	Rain	Rat	Red
Raid	Read	Ring	Ripe
Raise	Room	Road	Rose
Reach	Rot	Rush	Rough
Sell	Said	Search	Sail
Shout	Shack	Seize	Shirt
Size	Shawl	Shall	Should
Sub	Soap	Sheep	Sour
Sure	South	Soup	Such
Take	Thought	Talk	Tape
Third	Ton	Team	Thumb
Tip	Tool	Tell	Time
Tough	Turn	Thin	Tire
Vine	Voice	Void	Vote
Week	Wag	Walk	Wash
Which	White	When	Wheat
Whip	Witch	Wire	Wife
Yes	Young	Youth	Yearn

[a] Reprinted from Tillman and Carhart (1966) with permission.

TEST–RETEST RELIABILITY AND INTERLIST EQUIVALENCY FOR THE NU-6s

The Tillman and Carhart (1966) recording of the NU-6s with a male speaker resulted in good group test–retest reliability and interlist equivalency in normal-hearing persons. Another recording with a male speaker which was produced by Auditec of St. Louis in 1972 was found to have good interlist equivalency (Wilson, Coley, Hanel, & Browning, 1976); in this recording, the carrier phrase is "Say the word . . .". Rintelmann, Schumaier, Jetty, Burchfield, Beasley, Mosher, Mosher, and Penley (1974) made another recording of the NU-6s using a male speaker and also found good interlist equivalency in both normal-hearing and hearing-impaired subjects. In the hearing-impaired subjects, Tillman and Carhart (1966) reported that the results with the Northwestern recording of the NU-6s revealed that interlist equivalency was not as great as for normal-hearing listeners.

Causey, Hermanson, Hood, and Bowling (1983) investigated the reliability and interlist equivalency of the Maryland version of the NU-6 test (recorded with a female speaker) in sensorineural hearing-impaired listeners. Statistical comparison of the mean speech-recognition scores revealed that lists 1, 3, and 4 were equivalent and significantly easier than list 2. Test–retest reliability coefficients (the retest was administered 5 weeks after the initial test) were high, ranging between 0.92 and 0.96 for all lists. Thus, list equivalency must be considered with respect to the particular recording employed. In fact, different recordings of the same list should be considered different suprathreshold speech-recognition tests (Hood & Poole, 1980; Kreul, Bell, & Nixon, 1969) if test–retest differences are outside the confidence limits.

Raffin and Schafer (1980) applied the binomial model to the NU-6s. They presented two 50-word lists to the same ear of each subject at the same sensation level, using the same talker. The two 50-word scores were considered a single 100-word score and rescoring was done for subsets of two 50-word, four 25-word, and ten 10-word lists. The number of retest scores falling outside the 95% critical difference limits (binomial distribution) was determined. The hypothesized proportion of retest scores exceeding the critical difference limits was 0.05. The obtained proportions of retest scores actually falling outside the critical difference limits was 0.0493, 0.0532, and 0.0578 for the 50-word, 25-word, and 10-word lists, respectively. Thus, these results confirm the conclusion that variability among scores is dependent upon the true performance score and the number of items in a list. The results also indicate that the binomial model can be used to evaluate the intersubject variability for the NU-6s as well as any other test, providing the assumptions of the binomial model are met.

E. SYNTHETIC SENTENCE IDENTIFICATION (SSI) TEST

Speaks and Jerger (1965) and Jerger, Speaks, and Trammell (1968) contended that the temporal dimension of speech could not be investigated using single words—longer speech samples were necessary. They also felt that a closed-set (multiple-choice) test rather then an open-set test should be employed in order to control for word familiarity and previous linguistic history. They contended that the traditional, open-set, suprathreshold speech-recognition test required written or spoken responses which were subject to the contaminating influence of the audiologist's sensitivity to the subject's spelling ability or articulation.

Speaks and Jerger (1965) developed synthetic (artificial) sentences for suprathreshold speech-recognition testing under closed-set conditions. Unlike real English sentences, the meaning could not be conveyed by one or two key words. The sequence of words in these synthetic sentences depended on whether they were first, second, or third-order sentences. In the first-order synthetic sentences, the words were selected randomly. In the second-order sentential approximations, the choice of the second word was dependent on the first, the choice of the third word was dependent on the second, and so forth. In the third-order sentential approximations, the third word was dependent on the first and second words, the fourth word was dependent on the second and third words, and so forth. Examples of first-, second-, and third-order sentential approximations are shown in Table V. The SSI test consisted only of third-order sentential approximations of 7-word length. The words were selected from the Thorndike and Lorge (1944) directory of the 1000 most common English words. Table VI shows the third-order sentential approximations comprising the SSI test. The subject, who has a placard with the ten sentences numbered from 1 to 10, is required to respond to the sentence presented by giving the number associated with the sentence on the placard.

Jerger et al. (1968) reported that the SSI in quiet was too easy. They developed a continuous discourse (events of the life of Davy Crockett) which was presented with the synthetic sentences at various message-to-competition ratios (MCRs). The same talker who recorded the sentences recorded the competing speech. At 0 MCR, they found that

Table V Examples of Sentences from the Synthetic Sentence Identification (SSI) Test Showing Different Levels of Approximation to Actual Sentences[a]

Sentence	Approximation level
Due his fit along sick nearly	First
Three came home on any woman can	Second
Agree with him only to find out	Third

[a] Reprinted from Bess (1983) with permission.

Table VI Synthetic Sentences Identification (SSI) Third-Order Sentential Approximations[a]

1. Small boat with a picture has become
2. Built the government with the force almost
3. Go change your car color is red
4. Forward march said the boy had a
5. March around with a care in your
6. That neighbor who said business is better
7. Battle cry and be better than ever
8. Down by the time is real enough
9. Agree with him only to find out
10. Women view men with green paper should

[a] Jerger et al. (1968).

the performance-intensity function for PB words in normal-hearing persons or persons with peripheral hearing loss was essentially the same as that for the SSI except in cases of sloping audiometric configurations. As the audiometric configuration increases in slope, performance on the PB words declines more rapidly than on the SSI. This finding is expected since PB speech-recognition performance is dependent upon hearing sensitivity at high frequencies above 1000 Hz whereas SSI speech-recognition performance is dependent upon hearing sensitivity at low frequencies below 1000 Hz. The disadvantage of the SSI was that the scores were not as stable as those for PB words.

Jerger and Jerger (1974a, 1975a) further refined the SSI test by developing two test mode presentations. In the CCM (contralateral competing message) mode, the SSI is given in one ear and the Davy Crockett competing message is given in the other ear at MCRs of 0, −20, and −40. In the ICM (ipsilateral competing message) mode, the SSI and the Davy Crockett competing message are given in the same ear at MCRs of +10, 0, −10, and −20. Randomizations of the single list of synthetic sentences are given at the various MCRs.

RELIABILITY

Speaks and Jerger (1965) reported that learning and practice effects on the SSI can be minimized using a lengthy (100 item) practice session. Speaks, Jerger, and Jerger (1966) also suggested that practice effects be minimized using 4–6 repetitions of the 10-item list (40–60 practice items). Speaks (1967) suggested having 2 practice trials prior to each test trial. Jerger et al. (1968) and Jerger and Thelin (1968) suggested having 3 practice trials and basing each test score on 30 items.

According to Dubno and Dirks (1983), the high reliability estimates reported by the above investigators may not be accurate for the following reasons:

1. Some of the reliability estimates were obtained for the SSI in the absence of a competing message or other noise.
2. Most of the reliability studies were done on normal-

hearing persons whose performance was degraded by masking and/or filtering rather than hearing-impaired persons.

3. Possible long-term learning effects were not controlled.

4. The elicitation of performance-intensity functions in these reliability studies may have been contaminated by floor and ceiling effects.

Another problem affecting the reliability of the SSI was identified by Martin and Mussell (1979), who reported that identification of just a single word in a synthetic sentence during an acoustic window (pause in the competing message) could result in correct complete sentence identification.

Dubno and Dirks (1983) investigated the reliability of the SSI presented in a background of a noise (cafeteria) which eliminated the acoustic windows in sensorineural hearing-impaired subjects. They employed the adaptive procedure to estimate the signal-to-noise ratio yielding 50% speech-recognition score on the SSI. Dubno and Dirks concluded that the SSI presented in the background of a cafeteria noise is reliable if (a) 3 SSI lists are presented as practice under difficult signal-to-noise ratios, and (b) the test scores are based on responses to at least 30 sentences (large intrasubject differences between trials were obtained).

F. DIAGNOSTIC SIGNIFICANCE OF THE SUPRATHRESHOLD SPEECH-RECOGNITION SCORE FOR A SINGLE PRESENTATION LEVEL

1. Suprathreshold Speech-Recognition Score at the Most Comfortable Loudness Level

Most comfortable loudness (MCL) refers to the intensity level of presentation of auditory stimuli which yields, for the listener, a comfortably loud listening experience. Clemis and Carver (1967) found that the MCL could not reliably be used as the level for obtaining PB_{max} (maximum suprathreshold speech-recognition score). Posner and Ventry (1977), using a different set of instructions for finding MCL, also investigated whether MCL could be used to obtain PB_{max} in sensorineural hearing-impaired subjects. They found that the mean suprathreshold speech-recognition scores obtained at the level selected as most comfortable for loudness and intelligibility were both significantly poorer than the mean PB_{max}. The inter- and intra-subject variability of MCL can be attributed, at least partially, to the fact that MCL is a range of intensities rather than a single intensity level (Dirks & Morgan, 1983). Therefore, we recommend that when a single presentation level is used to measure suprathreshold speech-recognition, 30–40 dB SL rather than MCL should be used.

2. Peripheral Hearing Loss

In general, suprathreshold speech-recognition scores for conductive hearing-impaired ears are high, similar to those for normal-hearing listeners. Table VII shows the suprathreshold speech-recognition scores for conductive and cochlear hearing-impaired ears from Bess (1983). This table also reveals that, as a group, the cochlear hearing-impaired have poorer mean suprathreshold speech-recognition scores than the conductive hearing-impaired. Nevertheless, the range of suprathreshold speech-recognition scores for the conductive and cochlear hearing-impaired ears as well as for the various cochlear pathologies overlap considerably. Because of this larger variability in suprathreshold speech-recognition scores, suprathreshold speech-recognition tests have limited value for differentiating between cochlear and conductive hearing loss and among the various cochlear pathologies.

3. Eighth-Nerve Pathology

Suprathreshold speech-recognition scores obtained with monosyllabic PB words (W-22s or NU-6s) at estimated PB_{max} levels (approximately 30–40 dB SL relative to the SRT) have been used to differentiate between cochlear and retrocochlear ears (Bess, 1983; Johnson, 1977; Olsen, Noffsinger, & Kurdziel, 1975). The score of 30% has commonly been employed as a criterion to distinguish between cochlear and retrocochlear ears. Johnson (1977) reported that 30% of his 418 eighth-nerve tumor patients suprathreshold had speech-recognition scores less than or equal to 30%. Many (44%) of these eighth-nerve tumor cases had scores exceeding 60%. Olsen *et al.* (1975) reported that none of his patients with eighth-nerve tumors had scores below 30%. Moreover, scores do not necessarily exceed 30% in cochlear hearing-impaired ears. Bess (1983) reported that the NU-6 speech-recognition scores ranged from 8–100% in 136 subjects with Meniere's disease.

Table VII Mean Word Recognition Scores (NU #6) Obtained from Various Etiologic Groups[a]

Diagnosis	N	Ears (%)	Mean word recognition (%)	SD	Range (%)
Conductive					
Otitis media	50	62	96	6.8	80–100
Glomus tumor	32	32	93	9.0	60–96
Otosclerosis	25	25	91	6.0	82–100
Sensorineural					
Sudden deafness	19	19	32	32.0	0–100
Meniere's disease	112	136	78	26.0	8–100
Presbycusis	139	208	93	10.0	56–100
Cochlear otosclerosis	9	9	74	9.5	62–88
Acoustic neuroma	105	105	54	34.0	0–100

[a] Reprinted from Bess (1983) with permission.

Bauch, Olsen, and Harner (1983) compared suprathreshold speech-recognition scores for the W-22s in 30 patients with cerebellopontine angle tumors and 30 patients with cochlear pathology. The subjects were matched for degree and configuration of hearing impairment. They found substantial overlap in scores between the two groups. Of the cochlear ears, 27% obtained scores below 30% and more than half of the retrocochlear ears obtained scores greater than 30%. Of the cochlear patients, 20% had poorer scores than their retrocochlear counterparts. The mean suprathreshold speech-recognition scores were 46 and 67% for the retrocochlear and cochlear groups, respectively. Thus, a suprathreshold speech-recognition score below 30% is an insensitive measure of retrocochlear pathology.

Bess (1983) found that the suprathreshold speech-recognition scores for retrocochlear ears decrease as the degree of hearing loss increases. The mean score does not fall below 50% until the hearing loss exceeds 60 dB HL in retrocochlear ears. Moreover, more than 95% of retrocochlear ears with a hearing loss less than 41 dB have scores above 30%. A substantial percentage of those having hearing losses as great as 61–80 dB have suprathreshold speech-recognition scores exceeding 30%.

Since many retrocochlear ears have high suprathreshold speech-recognition scores, many cochlear hearing-impaired ears have low suprathreshold speech-recognition scores, and many cochlear ears matched to retrocochlear ears on the basis of the degree and configuration of hearing loss have poorer suprathreshold speech-recognition scores than their counterparts, there is no compelling reason to do suprathreshold speech-recognition testing at a single presentation level for the purpose of differential diagnosis of cochlear and retrocochlear pathology. Also, suprathreshold speech-recognition testing cannot be employed to differentiate among various cochlear pathologies.

We recommend that those clinicians who do not wish to abandon suprathreshold speech-recognition testing at this time follow the common clinical practice of considering patients with symmetrical audiometric configurations and significant asymmetry between ears in suprathreshold speech-recognition scores outside the 95% confidence limits at risk for retrocochlear pathology. We also recommend, based on Hood and Poole's (1971) finding that the suprathreshold speech-recognition score is minimally affected by cochlear hearing impairment with a magnitude less than or equal to 30 dB, that the clinician consider a patient with a pure-tone average (PTA) less than 30 dB HL and a suprathreshold speech-recognition score below 80% at risk for retrocochlear pathology.

G. DIAGNOSTIC SIGNIFICANCE OF ROLLOVER ON THE PERFORMANCE-INTENSITY FUNCTION

Jerger and Jerger (1971) obtained the performance-intensity (articulation) functions using half-lists of PB-50s in subjects with cochlear hearing impairments, eighth-nerve pathology, and brainstem pathology. They found that the cochlear hearing-impaired subjects had poor PB_{max} scores in the hearing-loss ear and that subjects with eight-nerve pathology had even poorer scores in the pathological ear. Subjects with brainstem lesions had reduced PB_{max} scores in the ear contralateral to the lesion. Nevertheless, there was significant overlap in the PB scores among the groups. When the presence of rollover using the formula

$$RI = (PB_{max} - PB_{min})/PB_{max}$$

where PB_{min} is the minimum suprathreshold speech-recognition score at a level above that yielding PB_{max}, and RI is the rollover index, was evaluated, better separation between the cochlear and retrocochlear ears was obtained. An example of a patient with rollover is shown in Figure 2. Jerger and Jerger's (1971) highest cochlear RI was 0.40 and their lowest eighth-nerve RI index was 0.45. The RIs for the brainstem group overlapped with those for the cochlear and eighth-nerve subjects. In another group of 741 patients with various types of losses (normal-hearing, conductive, mixed, and sensorineural), they found that only 2% had RIs equal to or greater than 0.40. Nine had RIs between 0.5 and 0.59. Eight of these nine cases were sensorineural hearing-impaired ears and one was a mixed hearing-loss ear. The rollover effect also applied for the SSI test. Thus, Jerger and Jerger found rollover present in both cochlear and retro-

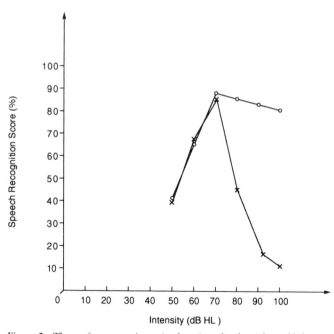

Figure 2 The performance–intensity functions for the right and left ears of a person with bilateral sensorineural hearing impairment. The performance–intensity function for the right ear is indicated by the lines connecting the circles. The performance–intensity function for the left ear is indicated by the lines connecting the Xs. The RI was normal (0.06) for the right ear, consistent with right cochlear pathology but abnormal (0.86) for the left ear, consistent with left retrocochlear pathology.

cochlear ears although the degree of rollover was greater in the latter than former case.

Dirks, Kamm, Bower, and Betsworth (1977) used half-lists of the recorded PAL PB-50s in obtaining performance-intensity (PI) functions in 66 subjects with cochlear and confirmed retrocochlear lesions. About six presentation levels were required to obtain the PI functions, starting at least 10 dB above the speech-recognition threshold. The step size did not exceed 10 dB and was generally about 4–6 dB in the area of PB_{max}. They found that, although the occurrence of very low PB_{max} scores was greater in the retrocochlear than the normal and cochlear groups, there was considerable overlap in scores among the groups, similar to that found by Jerger and Jerger (1971). When the magnitude of the rollover effect was calculated from the formula rollover = $PB_{max} - PB_{min}$, overlap between the groups was decreased but still substantial. Since, as noted by Jerger and Jerger (1971), the magnitude of the rollover effect was influenced by the PB_{max} score, the possible biasing effect of the PB_{max} score was controlled by dividing the difference between PB_{max} and PB_{min} by the PB_{max} score as suggested by Jerger and Jerger (1971). Dirks et al. (1977) reported that the overlap between the cochlear ($N = 59$), and retrocochlear ($N = 5$) groups was almost entirely eliminated when an RI of 0.45 was used to separate retrocochlear from cochlear ears. That is, only one (2%) cochlear-impaired subject, a female with moderate hearing loss and significant acoustic-reflex decay, had an RI exceeding 0.45. Their subjects with retrocochlear pathologies had relatively large tumors (greater than or equal to 2 cm), however, and also showed other signs of retrocochlear impairment such as elevated or absent acoustic reflexes, abnormal adaptation, or the absence of loudness recruitment. Thus, conclusions about the diagnostic utility of the rollover index in the beginning stage of acoustic tumors cannot be drawn soley from the Dirks et al. (1977) study.

Dirks et al. (1977) noted that the magnitude of the RI depended upon how accurately PB_{max} was measured. Since PB_{max} was obtained in a narrow range of intensities in some subjects, the use of a large step size (10 dB) could result in an underestimation of the PB_{max} and thereby decrease the magnitude of the RI. Therefore, they cautioned that small step sizes of 4–6 dB rather than 10 dB should be used when measuring PB_{max}, particularly when scores above 90% are not obtained. Another finding was that PB_{min} was obtained at presentation levels less than or equal to 100 dB HL in all cases. Since the speech-test materials and speaker vary from clinic to clinic, Dirks et al. recommend that each clinic obtain data from cochlear and retrocochlear ears to establish the RI that shall be used to identify retrocochlear-impaired ears.

Bess, Josey, and Humes (1979) reported that an RI of 0.25 was positive for retrocochelar pathology for the Auditec recording of the NU-6s. The RI was below 0.25 in 94% of their 15 cochlear subjects and the RI exceeded 0.25 in 90% of their 30 retrocochlear subjects. Bess (1983) noted that the PI–PB function cannot be obtained when PB_{max} is less than or equal to 30%.

Meyer and Mishler (1985) calculated the RI that was significant for half- and full-lists of the Auditec NU-6 recording in 25 normal-hearing subjects, 19 cochlear hearing-impaired subjects, and 9 retrocochlear subjects. The taped lists were presented at 10, 40, and 60 dB SL, and 90 and 100–105 dB HL. This reduced number of levels was employed in consideration of the need for a clinically feasible test time. There was overlap in the RIs among the three groups. The RIs for the full list ranged from 0–0.22 for the normal group, 0–0.35 for the cochlear group, and 0.02–0.70 for the retrocochlear group. The RI >0.35 best differentiated between the cochlear and retrocochlear ears. For the half-list, the range of RIs was 0–0.20 for the normal group, 0–0.36 for the cochlear, and 0–0.88 for the retrocochlear group. Thus, the half-list RIs are at least as accurate as the full-list RIs even though greater reliability is associated with the full-list PB_{max} than the half-list PB_{max}. The results also revealed that the RI was a more sensitive measure of retrocochlear pathology when the maximum level for establishing the PI function was 100–105 dB HL rather than 90 dB HL as used by many previous investigators.

Meyer and Mishler (1985) found that the RIs for 3 of the 9 retrocochlear ears fell within normal limits. The sensitivity of the RI was 56%, compared with the 65% reported by Jerger and Jerger (1983), 90% reported by Bess et al. (1979), and 100% reported by Dirks et al. (1977). Subject characteristics such as the size and type of tumor may have affected the magnitude of the RI. Whereas the tumors in the Dirks et al. (1977) study were at least 2.0 cm, this study and the Bess et al. (1979) study included ears with tumor sizes less than or equal to 1.7 cm. Bess, Josey, Glasscock, and Wilson (1984) suggested that the RI may be less sensitive in patients with bilateral acoustic tumors from Recklinghausen's disease. In the Meyer and Mishler (1985) study, 3 of the 9 retrocochlear subjects had Recklinghausen's disease.

1. Reliability of the PI Function

Beattie and Warren (1983) found substantial intersubject variability in the slope of the PI function for the CID W-22s in mild-to-moderate sensorineural hearing-impaired subjects. Bettie and Raffin (1985) found that the mean test–retest slopes (based on the 20–80% intelligibility points) of the PI functions for the Auditec recording of the CID W-22s in their group of 20 normal-hearing persons were essentially similar for full-lists and half-lists. Similar findings were obtained for their group of 25 elderly persons with mild-to-moderate sensorineural hearing loss.

Although the test and retest means reported by Beattie and Raffin (1985) revealed the absence of significant slope differences between the normal-hearing and hearing-impaired groups, indicating the lack of a practice effect, there were large individual differences in the slope from test to retest. The standard error of measurement for the slope was approximately 1% per dB in the normal-hearing group for the full- and half-lists. Thus, increasing the number of items did not improve the reliability of the slope measure. The standard error of measurement of the slope for the hearing-loss group was 0.57% per dB. Although the absolute value of the standard error was smaller than for the normal group, the relative error with respect to the mean slope was similar for both groups. That is, the standard error of the mean is approximately 20% of the mean slope for both groups. Because of the considerable individual test–retest variability, the slope has limited usefulness for differentiating between hearing impaired and normal listeners.

2. EFFECT OF AGE

Gang (1976) reported that 6 of 32 male veterans aged 60–84 years had moderate to marked RIs between 0.33 and 0.66 on the CID W-22s. None of the 6, however, showed abnormal adaptation on the tone-decay test. Gang concluded that presbycusis resulted in atrophy of the neural pathway which affected ability to process complex but not tonal signals. He argued against the use of the RI as a diagnostic tool since aging could produce a significant RI. Jerger and Jerger (1976) contended that the RI was site specific rather than tumor specific. "Any disorder of the eighth nerve, whether caused by neoplasm, virus, or aging, should be identified by a diagnostic test that is sensitive to disorders at that site" (p. 557). Jerger and Jerger (1976) reaffirmed the use of the RI as a diagnostic tool.

Dirks *et al.* (1977) obtained PI–PB functions using half-lists of the PB-50s at six presentation levels in 102 patients. Four ears of the 102 patients had RIs equal to or exceeding 0.45. Only one of these four ears had a surgically confirmed tumor. The other ears demonstrated retrocochlear signs on other audiologic tests but radiologic evaluations did not reveal the presence of a space-occupying lesion. These 3 patients were all at least 64 years old. Dirks *et al.* suggested that elderly patients with significant rollover probably have neural presbycusis in which suprathreshold speech-recognition ability is more adversely affected than expected from the magnitude of the pure-tone hearing loss.

The sensitivity of the RI is not high enough to warrant the administration of the PI–PB (or PI–SSI) function in all persons at risk for retrocochlear pathology. We suggest that PI–PB functions be obtained and RIs calculated on those with PTAs less than or equal to 30 dB HL and suprathreshold speech-recognition scores less than 80% at estimated PB_{max} levels to confirm the low estimated PB_{max} score obtained at a single presentation level. We further suggest that a PI–PB function be obtained in persons with symmetrical audiometric configurations if there is asymmetry (outside the 95% confidence limits) between ears on the suprathreshold speech-recognition score obtained at the estimated PB_{max} level, to confirm the observed asymmetry at the single presentation level. In other words, PI–PB (or SSI) testing should be done on all persons with a suprathreshold speech-recognition score at a single level suggestive of retrocochlear pathology to identify those with abnormal RIs who are otherwise at low risk for retrocochlear pathology.

Meyer and Mishler (1985) demonstrated that an adequate PI–PB function can be defined with half-lists at six presentation levels: 10, 40, and 60 dB SL, 90 and 100–105 dB HL. The RI considered positive with respect to retrocochlear pathology ideally should be based on the data for cochlear and retrocochlear ears for a particular recording for a particular clinic. If it is not possible to obtain these data, we suggest that an RI of 0.45 for the W-22s and 0.35 for the NU-6s be considered significant; positive RIs in such cases, however, should be interpreted cautiously. Positive RIs should also be interpreted with caution in elderly persons more than 65 years of age.

H. DIGITIZED SPEECH RECORDINGS

Kamm, Carterette, Morgan, and Dirks (1980) discussed the feasibility of using digitized speech recordings (digital representation of a real-speech waveform) in clinical practice. They recommended the use of digitized recordings for (a) their high signal-to-noise ratio and dynamic range, (b) the presence of zero wow and flutter, (c) the absence of harmonic distortion near the upper signal intensity range and of modulation noise sidebands near the signal, (d) the absence of crosstalk between channels, (e) the presence of a full bandwidth, (f) the lack of amplitude variations resulting from regional changes in magnetization, (g) the absence of print-through or other interaction between adjacent tape layers, and (h) the ability to randomly select speech items. Digitized speech has only recently become commercially available on a few audiometers. Whenever possible, digitized recordings should be used in speech testing.

I. ABBREVIATED WORD LISTS

Runge and Hosford-Dunn (1985) investigated whether suprathreshold word-recognition performance can be measured accurately with a small number of the most difficult items in the CID W-22 word lists. The items were arranged in decreasing order of difficulty on the full 50-word lists. The order of item difficulty was based on the error frequencies reported by Thornton and Raffin (1978). A group of 136 normal-hearing ears and 508 hearing impaired ears (SRTs ranging from 0–75 dB HL, sensorineural, conductive, and mixed) were investigated. Suprathreshold word-recognition scores (the presentation level was usually 40 dB SL relative to the SRT) were calculated for the full list, the first 25 words (half-score on the rank-ordered list), the first 10 words (difficult score on the rank-ordered list), the last 10 words (easy score on the rank-ordered list), and the first

10 words from the original W-22 list. Each of the subtest scores were compared with the full score. Sensitivity, specificity, and efficiency were calculated based on a 90% cutoff value on the full list. Hence, abbreviated-list scores of at least 90% were negative if the full-list score was also above 90% and abbreviated-list scores below 90% were positive if the full-list score was also below 90%. The sensitivity was 99.6% for the half-list, 93% for the difficult subtest, 71% for the first 10 words of the original CID W-22 (random) list, and 38% for the easy subtest. The specificity was 75% for the half-list, 81% for the difficult list, 92% for the random list, and 99% for the easy list. The efficiency was 83% for the half-list, 86% for the difficult list, 83% for the random list, and 74% for the easy list.

Runge and Hosford-Dunn (1985) concluded that abbreviated versions of the CID W-22 word lists can be used to measure suprathreshold word-recognition performance in normal-hearing and hearing-impaired listeners if the modified lists are composed of the more difficult items from the full lists and if strict screening criteria indicate whether additional items need to be administered. They recommend using lists rank-ordered by difficulty and terminating testing after 10 words if no errors occur or after 25 words if there are no more than 4 errors. With a greater number of errors, the full 50-item list should be administered. Runge and Hosford-Dunn (1985) also calculated the hit and false-alarm rates for the abbreviated lists using various pass/fail criteria. False-alarm scores ranged from 10–25% depending upon the list/sublist and pass/fail criteria. They suggested that various strategies could be adopted for lists of varying lengths, depending upon error tolerances judged acceptable by the tester. They suggested that a conservative strategy would be one in which the shortened list is given only to normal-hearing persons.

Runge and Hosford-Dunn (1985) contended that it was defensible to use shortened lists since such lists contain the diagnostic test items. Their results supported the finding of Hagerman (1976) and Thornton and Raffin (1978) that randomly-ordered shortened lists are inadequate because of increased test-score variability. According to Runge and Hosford-Dunn (1985), this is not the case for shortened lists of items rank ordered by difficulty.

The use of abbreviated test lists consisting of difficult items as a screening tool to determine who should receive the full 50-word list is a novel approach. Before this approach can be adopted, however, the results have to be substantiated by other investigators, test–retest reliability and interlist equivalency have to be established, and commercial recordings of the shortened lists of rank-ordered items must be made available.

J. PEDIATRIC POPULATION

Maturation effects on suprathreshold speech-recognition performance are generally not observed beyond 12 years of age (McNamee, 1960; Sanderson-Leepa & Rintelmann, 1976). Therefore, the recommendations made in this chapter can be applied to children more than 12 years of age who do not have a language delay.

The goal of suprathreshold speech-recognition testing in children who are unable to respond appropriately to traditional suprathreshold speech-recognition tests is to determine how well the child can function in everyday listening situations. Traditional suprathreshold speech-recognition tests have been modified for pediatric applications by making the vocabulary more familiar to children and using picture-pointing rather than verbal responses. These modified suprathreshold speech-recognition tests for young children do not have applicability for differential diagnosis.

K. MASKING

Masking of the contralateral ear with speech noise during suprathreshold speech-recognition assessment should be done whenever the crossover level of the speech signal (presentation level minus 40 dB) equals or exceeds any bone- or air-conduction threshold in the nontest ear.

1. INITIAL MASKING

A masking level equal or exceeding initial masking (IM) level (without causing overmasking) can be used to mask the nontest ear during suprathreshold speech-recognition testing. The IM can be derived from the formula

$$IM = \text{crossover level} + \text{largest } ABG_{nt} + MEM$$

where crossover level equals presentation level minus 40 dB of interaural attenuation, the largest ABG_{nt} equals the largest air–bone gap in the nontest ear, and MEM is minimum effective masking for suprathreshold speech-recognition testing. (The procedure for determining MEM for suprathreshold speech-recognition testing is described in Chapter 1.)

2. OVERMASKING

Overmasking during suprathreshold speech-recognition testing may occur if the equation

$$ML_{nt} \geqq BB_t + IA$$

holds, where ML_{nt} is the masking level in the nontest ear, BB_t is the best bone-conduction threshold in the test ear, and IA is the interaural attenuation for air-conduction testing (40 dB). If there is a possibility of overmasking, the suprathreshold speech-recognition test should be repeated without masking. If there is no significant difference in score, the possibility of overmasking can be ruled out. If the masked score is significantly lower than the unmasked score, it cannot be determined whether the decreased masked score results from overmasking or from elimination of the participation of the nontest ear.

3. MAXIMUM MASKING

The maximum amount of masking noise that one can confidently introduce into the nontest ear without resulting in overmasking of the test ear during suprathreshold speech-recognition testing can be derived from the formula

$$MM = BB_t + IA - 5 \text{ dB}$$

where MM is maximum masking, BB_t is the best bone-conduction threshold of the test ear, and IA is the interaural attenuation for air-conduction testing (40 dB).

II. TESTS OF AUDITORY ADAPTATION

Ward (1970), as cited by Green (1978), stated that Lord Rayleigh in 1882 was the first to demonstrate tone decay (adaptation) by air conduction and Corradi in 1890 was the first to demonstrate tone decay by bone conduction. Gradenigo (1893) observed that patients with eighth-nerve pathology were unable to hear a tuning fork vibrating with maximal amplitude for more than a few seconds. He referred to this phenomenon as "functional exhaustibility." Functional exhaustibility was found to be present in ears with cochlear pathology but not to the extent or severity found in cases of eighth-nerve pathology. Schubert (1944), as cited by Morales-Garcia and Hood (1972), was the first to develop a procedure for measuring auditory adaptation at threshold. The procedure involved presenting the tone at 5 dB SL relative to the pure-tone threshold and then increasing the intensity in 5-dB increments whenever the tone faded away, until a plateau was obtained. Schubert (1944) observed that when the procedure was administered to persons with substantial hearing loss, a plateau could not be reached by the time the intensity was raised to the maximum output of the audiometer. He concluded that moderate threshold adaptation was characteristic of end-organ (cochlear) pathology.

Hallpike and Hood (1951) observed that, if a simultaneous loudness balance employing continuous tones was performed in a normal-hearing person with the constant-intensity tone in the test ear presented at 80 dB SL, a loudness match is obtained when the varied-intensity tone in the control ear is at 80 dB SL. If the tone in the control ear is removed and a fatiguing tone is presented continuously in the test ear for at least 3 min, to cause that ear to become fully adapted, followed by a repeat simultaneous loudness balance (with continuous tones) in which the tone in the test ear is again presented at 80 dB SL, a loudness match will be obtained with the varied-intensity tone at 50 dB SL in the control ear. Hallpike and Hood (1951) referred to this loss of sensitivity in response to continuous stimulation as perstimulatory fatigue; this effect is observed during stimulation. If a recovery period is inserted in the test ear between the fatiguing tone and the repeat simultaneous loudness balance, then the loudness match will occur at a sensation

level approximating that in the control ear, depending on the length of the recovery period.

According to Hallpike and Hood (1951), the time course of the perstimulatory fatigue is similar to the adaptation process of the stretch receptor described by Matthews (1931). Matthews (1931) found that application of tension to a stretch receptor of a muscle resulted in a brief burst of impulses (on-effect) followed by a decline in the frequency of impulses over time (adaptation). Adaptation was complete after about 3.5 min of stimulation.

If the tone is removed from the test ear after complete adaptation and then reapplied after a rest period exceeding 1 s, a normal on-effect (initial burst of auditory excitation) occurred but was followed by accelerated adaptation (relapse). Shorter rest periods resulted in diminished or absent on-effects followed by relapse. Hallpike and Hood (1951) suggested that the sense organ impaired by cochlear pathology, as well as the adapted sense organ in a normal-hearing person, exhibits on-effect normalcy (when the rest period between tones is sufficiently long) and relapse to sustained tonal stimulation. The site of the relapse and on-effect mechanisms was posited to be in the cochlear hair-cell receptors, the adapted hair cells in normal-hearing persons and the diseased hair cells in persons with cochlear hearing impairment.

Hood (1955) stated that abnormal adaptation (relapse) was independent of stimulus intensity. Hence, adaptation could be observed at threshold as well as suprathreshold levels. Hood revealed the presence of relapse in persons with cochlear impairment such as Meniere's disease by presenting a tone at 5 dB SL relative to the pure-tone threshold and asking the subject to indicate when the tone could no longer be heard. In a normal-hearing person or one with conductive pathology, the tone results in persistence of the tonal sensation indefinitely. In persons with end-organ pathology, however, the tonal sensation of a tone at 5 dB SL fades away after only 5–6 seconds of stimulation at that level. The duration of tonal sensation increases with increases in intensity (in 5-dB increments) until a level is reached which results in the persistence of a tonal sensation indefinitely. Figure 3 shows the intensity as a function of the length of tonal sensation at 2000 Hz. The level at which the persistence of a tonal sensation is attained is approximately 20–30 dB SL and is "the measure of the magnitude of the loss of sensitivity due to pathological adaptation" (Hood, 1955, p. 515). The loss of sensitivity was attributed to adaptation rather than fatigue for these reasons.

1. Immediate reapplication of the tone each time the tonal sensation faded away resulted in the restoration of loudness (on-effect) and sustained stimulation (not necessarily high-intensity stimulation) resulted in the disappearance of the tonal sensation (relapse).
2. The threshold elevation does not persist.

Hood (1955) also demonstrated the presence of adapta-

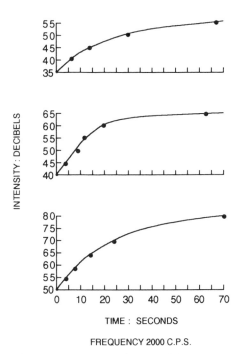

Figure 3 Intensity as a function of the time to inaudibility at 2000 Hz in three subjects with end-organ pathology. Reprinted from Hood (1955) with permission.

tion in cochlear-impaired subjects by the technique of threshold determination using interrupted as opposed to continuous tones. He found that the pure-tone threshold for interrupted tones is essentially similar to that for continuous tones in persons with normal-hearing or conductive hearing impairment. In persons with cochlear pathology such as Meniere's disease, the threshold for continuous tones is substantially higher than for interrupted tones. Thus, the pathological adaptation or relapse in subjects with end-organ pathology occurs so rapidly that no on-effect at all is initiated when the intensity is increased gradually in the manner described. Instead, relapse occurs during the increase in the intensity of the tone and the response of the end organs has reached a low level before the tone is heard. In contrast, "the short interrupted stimuli produce on-effects of high magnitude giving rise to a much lower threshold" (Hood, 1955, p. 518).

Jerger (1955) observed the phenomena of on-effect normalcy and relapse in subjects with acoustic trauma. He reported that when a 4000-Hz tone was presented to these subjects for 2 min at 10 dB SL with more intense but brief pips of the same frequency superimposed on the tone every 6 s, some subjects reported that the sustained tone faded away before it was terminated but the superimposed pips were easily heard, appearing to rise out of silence. Thus, the fading away of the sustained tone represented relapse whereas the ability to hear the pips after the sustained tone faded away represented on-effect normalcy.

Carhart (1957) cautioned against positing a cochlear site for relapse, observing that some normal-hearing persons

show abnormal auditory adaptation. The results of some animal experiments suggest that the site of auditory adaptation is the auditory nerve. Several investigators (Gisselson & Sorensen, 1959; Kiang & Peake, 1960; Ruben, Hudson, & Chiang, 1962) were unable to observe adaptation in the cochlear potentials of cats and guinea pigs. Marked adaptation has been observed in cases of eighth-nerve pathology (Flottorp, 1963; Gjaevenes & Söhoel, 1969; Johnson & House, 1964; Morales-Garcia & Hood, 1972; Owens, 1964a; Parker & Decker, 1971; Sorensen, 1962; Yantis, 1959). Thus, marked tone decay is consistent with the presence of eighth-nerve pathology. According to Morales-Garcia and Hood (1972), "the occasional presence of a marked tone decay in ears with cochlear lesions may be attributed to a subclinical loss in the integrity of certain elements of the auditory nerve (probably due to involvement of adjacent dendrites)" (p. 246). Harbert and Young (1964) proposed that lesions of the eighth nerve causing partial damage to the axons manifest marked tone decay. On the other hand, conditions such as nonprogressive congenital nerve deafness, in which a large proportion of fibers are nonfunctioning and the surviving fibers function normally, are not associated with marked tone decay. Harbert and Young referred to tone decay as slow adaptation since it is measured in seconds or minutes as opposed to fast adaptation, measured in milliseconds; the latter is evidenced when reduced amplitude continuous-tone Bekesy tracings are obtained.

A. PROCEDURE

1. CARHART THRESHOLD TONE-DECAY TEST
The threshold tone-decay test was developed in 1954 at Northwestern University and was described by Carhart in 1957. The procedure follows.

1. The subject raises his or her finger as soon as the tone is heard, keeping the finger raised for as long as the tone is heard.
2. The tone is presented at a level 10–15 dB below the threshold and then increased in intensity in 5-dB increments without interruption until the subject responds. This level is the starting level. The stopwatch is activated at the starting level.
3. If the subject hears the tone at the starting level for 1 min, the test is terminated. If the subject perceives the tone for less than 1 min, the intensity is increased gradually, without interruption, by 5 dB, the stopwatch reactivated, and a new minute of timing begun. This process continues until a level is reached at which the tone is heard for 1 min. A time-saving alternative proposed by Carhart was to terminate the test at an arbitrary level such as 30 dB SL.
4. The number of seconds the tone is heard at each intensity level is recorded.

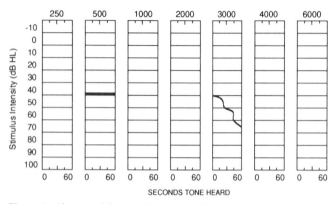

Figure 4 Chart used for graphing threshold tone decay with plots illustrating no decay at 500 Hz and appreciable decay at 4000 Hz. Reprinted from Carhart (1957) with permission.

5. Although the choice of frequencies at which the tone is administered is optional, Carhart suggested testing 500, 1000, 2000, and 4000 Hz, bilaterally.
6. The results are recorded on a chart such as that shown in Figure 4, on which the abscissa represents the number of seconds the tone is heard and the ordinate represents the intensity level. "The result of the test at a given frequency is plotted as a line connecting those points which represent the lengths of time during which successive presentation levels remain audible" (Carhart, 1957, p. 35).

The magnitude of the tone decay is obtained by subtracting the starting level from the level at which the test is terminated.

2. ROSENBERG TONE-DECAY TEST

Rosenberg (1969) developed a modification of the Carhart threshold tone-decay test. In this modification, the entire test takes only 1 min. The Rosenberg modification was developed because the Carhart threshold tone-decay procedure tended to become unwieldy and time-consuming when excessive tone-decay was present. The procedure follows.

1. The patient is instructed to raise his or finger as soon as the tone is heard and to lower it when the tone stops.
2. The tone is presented at threshold and the stopwatch activated.
3. Each time the tone is no longer heard and the patient lowers his or her hand, the intensity is increased quickly without interruption in 5-dB steps. This process continues for 60 s, at which time the tone is terminated.
4. The amount of tone decay is the difference between the level at which the test is terminated and the starting (threshold) level.
5. Rosenberg (1958) recommended administering the

tone-decay test at the lower and middle frequencies as well as at the higher frequencies.

Rosenberg (1958) classified 0–5 dB of tone decay as normal, 10–15 dB of tone decay as mild, 20–25 dB of tone decay as moderate, and 30 dB or more as marked tone decay. Rosenberg (1969) reported that mild to moderate tone decay was characteristic of pathology affecting the Organ of Corti whereas greater than 30 dB of tone decay was characteristic of retrocochlear pathology.

3. OTHER MODIFICATIONS OF THE CARHART THRESHOLD TONE-DECAY TEST

Sørensen (1962) developed another modification of the Carhart tone-decay test which differed from that test only by its requirement that the tone be heard for 90 rather than 60 s and its administration just at 2000 Hz. Yantis (1959) developed a procedure differing from the Carhart test only by a starting level of 5 dB SL relative to the pure-tone threshold rather than at threshold. Olsen and Noffsinger's (1974) modification followed the Carhart tone-decay procedure except that the starting level was 20 dB SL and no more than 10 dB of tone decay above the starting level could be measured, that is, the terminating level did not exceed 30 dB SL. Olsen and Noffsinger employed this starting level on the basis of Hood's (1955) finding that cochlear hearing-impaired persons can hear a tone presented at 20–30 dB SL indefinitely. The 30 dB SL termination level was selected on the basis of the finding that only 10 dB of tone decay beyond 20 SL need be measured before the result was consistent with retrocochlear pathology. The Olsen and Noffsinger (1974) procedure represents a screening device for measuring retrocochlear pathology. They reported that their procedure was easier for the patient to perform since the test was administered at a higher starting level than the other tone-decay tests, making the tone more audible.

4. HOOD TONE-DECAY TEST

In the Hood (1955) procedure, a tone is presented at 5 dB SL and the patient is asked to indicate when the tone is no longer heard. When the tone disappears, a rest period of 1 min is given and the procedure is repeated at a level that is 5 dB higher (10 dB SL). This procedure is continued until a level is reached which results in the persistence of a tonal sensation indefinitely. In normal-hearing persons or persons with conductive hearing loss, the tonal sensation persists indefinitely at 5 dB SL. In persons with end-organ pathology, the tonal sensation does not persist indefinitely until a level of 20–30 dB SL is reached.

a. Owens Modification

Owens (1964a) developed a modification of the Hood procedure. The Owens modification involved the following steps:

1. The subject was instructed to raise his or her hand upon hearing the tone and to lower the hand when the tone disappeared.
2. The tone is presented at 5 dB SL, and the timing is begun. If the tone is heard for 60 s, the test is terminated.
3. If the tone is not heard for a full 60 s at that level, a rest period of 20 s is given and the length of time the tone was heard is recorded. The 20-s rest period was chosen on the basis of Hood's (1950) finding that recovery from perstimulatory fatigue was most rapid within the first 10 s; flattening of the recovery curve occurs at about 20 s. Owens (1964a) felt that the shorter recovery period of 20 s rather than 1 min was clinically more feasible and would result in a shorter test.
4. The procedure in steps 1–3 is repeated at 10, 15, and 20 db SL, or until the tone is heard for 60 s, whichever occurs first. Only four intensity levels are administered because the reliability of additional levels is affected by boredom, fatigue, and discomfort at the higher intensity levels.

Table VIII shows the Owens classification of tone decay. Tone decay is classified as Type I if the tone is heard for a full 60 s at 5 dB SL. Type I is characteristic of normal-hearing persons or persons with cochlear pathology. Tone decay was classified as Type II if there is increasingly slower decay (the tone is heard for increasingly longer periods of time) with successive 5-dB increments. In Type IIA tone decay, the tone is heard for 60 s at 10 dB SL. In Type IIB tone decay, the tone is heard for 60 s at 15 dB SL. In Type IIC tone decay, the tone is heard for 60 s at 20 dB SL. In Type IID, the tone is never heard for a full 60 s although it is heard for increasing lengths of time with each successive 5-dB increment. In Type IIE tone decay, the tone is also never heard for a full 60 s, but is heard an average of 4–7 s longer with each successive 5-dB increment. Types IIA through IID are predominant in persons with cochlear pa-

thology. Type IIE is atypical, occurring in both cochlear and retrocochlear cases. Tone decay is classified as Type III if the tone is never heard for 60 s and there is very little or no change in the rate of decay with successive 5-dB increments; the tone is heard for essentially similar time periods at all four levels. Type III is predominant in persons with eighth-nerve pathology. Owens (1964a) recommended that at least two frequencies should be tested, preferably 500, 1000, and 2000 Hz.

b. Wiley and Lilly (1980) Modification

Wiley and Lilly (1980) modified the Hood procedure to allow a recovery period of 10 s rather than 1 min based on Bekesy's (1960) finding that the recovery period for a sustained tone with a duration of 2 min was 10 s. They also recommended that the procedure not be limited to four increments in intensity as proposed by Owens (1964a); the test should be continued in successive 5-dB increments until the tone is heard for 60 s or until the maximum output of the audiometer is reached because the temporal pattern of auditory adaptation may not be manifested entirely with only four presentation levels.

5. Suprathreshold Adaptation Test

Jerger and Jerger (1975b) hypothesized that, since abnormal tone decay is evidenced at the high intensity levels before being evidenced at the low intensity levels, the sensitivity (percentage of retrocochlear ears giving a positive test result) of the tone-decay test could be improved by administering it at a high intensity level. The procedure follows.

1. The test is administered at 110 dB SPL at 500, 1000, and 2000 Hz, which is approximately equivalent to 100 dB HL at 500 and 2000 Hz and 105 dB HL at 1000 Hz.
2. A broad-band noise of 90 dB SPL is presented to the nontest ear.
3. The patient is instructed to indicate when he or she hears the tone (raise hand) and when the tone is no longer heard (lower hand).
4. The tone (with masking noise in the opposite ear) is presented for a minute. If the tone is heard for the full 60 s, the test is scored as negative. If the tone is not heard for the full 60 s, the test is scored as positive for retrocochlear pathology and the length of time the tone was heard is recorded in the graph shown in Figure 5.
5. To ensure that the positive result is valid, the procedure is repeated with a pulsed tone. If the pulsed tone is heard for 60 s, then the positive test result with the continuous tone is valid. If the pulsed tone is not heard for 60 s, the positive result for the continuous tone is invalid.

Table VIII Examples of Tone-Decay Patterns Arbitrarily Chosen to Demonstrate the Variation in Those That Occurred[a]

Levels above threshold (dB)	Patterns of decay						
	I	II					III
		A	B	C	D	E	
5	60	25	7	12	15	5	14
10		60	34	26	23	14	16
15			60	40	30	18	12
20				60	39	21	14

[a] The numbers in the table represent seconds of time that the tone was heard. A twenty-second rest was given between 5-dB increments. Reprinted from Owens (1964a) with permission.

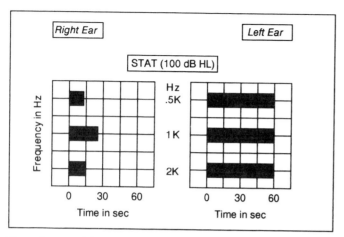

Figure 5 Plot of the time to inaudibility for each frequency in each ear using the STAT procedure. Reprinted from Jerger and Jerger (1981) with permission.

B. TONALITY VERSUS AUDIBILITY

Green (1963) found that when the instructions are modified so the patient signals one way when the tone loses tonality but retains audibility and signals another way when the tone loses audibility, more tone decay is measured for the former than latter instruction. Thus, the sensitivity of the test was improved when the patient responds to the tonality rather than the audibility of the tone. Pestalozza and Cioce (1962) observed that, during the tone-decay test, the tone lost its tonality, becoming like a "rustling noise" before fading into silence in some persons. Sørensen (1962) suggested that tone decay be measured for loss of pitch and the persistence of noise should be disregarded. Parker and Decker (1971) referred to the loss of tonality with preservation of audibility as tone perverson, that is, "subjective change of a pure-tone stimulus to an atonal sound" (p. 1). Harbert and Young (1964) observed that, in most persons, the tone fades into inaudibility without passing through a stage of tone perversion. In some persons, the tone loses its original tonal quality and begins to sound different in pitch and quality but still has a tonal quality, albeit a different one. Harbert and Young note that this diplacusis is commonly observed in cases of Meniere's disease. In other persons, the tone loses its tonal quality and becomes noiselike. Harbert and Young report that more tone decay is measured when the subject is instructed to respond only as long as the tone has a tonal quality than when the subject is instructed to respond as long as the tone is audible. Research substantiating the finding of increased sensitivity when subjects respond to tonality rather than audibility is lacking. In our experience, Green's modified instructions result in a greater frequency of positive tone-decay results in nonretrocochlear impaired ears, especially in the elderly.

Harbert and Young (1964) noted that

in some patients with severe partial damage to residual cochlear nerve fibers, the ability to appreciate the tonal

quality of pure tones may be lost or greatly impaired. A possible explanation for the loss of tonal quality is the fact that adaptation is greatest at the stimulated frequency. If there is adaptation for the stimulating frequency, the subject may become aware of the general turbulence produced by the traveling waves. This should result in the sensation of a broad-band noise. Rapid loss of tonality and failure to recognize tonality are considered indications of increasingly severe abnormal adaptation. In Meniere's and other hair cell lesions, there is a change in pitch, but this still has a tonal quality. (p. 59)

C. CLINICAL POPULATIONS

1. COCHLEAR-IMPAIRED EARS

Sørenson (1962), using his modification of the Carhart tone-decay test, reported that 97% of the 61 "typical" Meniere's-disease patients, 89% of the 36 "atypical" Meniere's-disease patients, 83% of the 6 acoustic-trauma cases, 100% of the 6 noise-induced cases, and 73% of the 11 head-trauma cases had negative tone-decay results (i.e., did not have excessive tone decay).

Owens (1964a), using the Owens tone-decay procedure, found that 89% of the 53 Meniere's-disease cases and 96% of the 28 cases with other cochlear pathology had Type I or Type IIA–E patterns (Type IIE occurred sporadically). He also reported that, at frequencies below 2000 Hz, tone decay was unlikely to occur when the hearing loss was less than 35 dB HL in patients with Meniere's disease. Tone decay was likely to occur at the high frequencies in Meniere's-disease cases. Of these patients, 60% had either no tone decay or tone decay at only one or two frequencies (high frequencies). Owens (1964a) also observed that the tone-decay phenomenon was independent of the loudness recruitment phenomenon.

Tillman (1969) reported that, with the Carhart tone-decay procedure, 96% of his 23 Meniere's disease patients had negative tone-decay results. Gjaevenes and Söhoel (1969) obtained similar findings for 94% of their 470 cochlear cases. Similary, Morales-Garcia and Hood (1972) reported that 96.5% of their 29 patients with Meniere's disease or noise-induced hearing loss had negative tone-decay results.

Olsen and Noffsinger (1974) compared the Carhart, Olsen–Noffsinger, and Rosenberg tone-decay procedures on a group of 40 patients with Meniere's disease, acoustic trauma, or presbycusis, and found that the Carhart and Olsen–Noffsinger procedures produced negative results in 88.5–90% whereas the Rosenberg procedure produced negative results in 95%.

Subsequent studies showed a reduced accuracy for the tone-decay test for the identification of cochlear pathology. Sanders, Josey, and Glasscock (1974), using the tone-decay procedure, found that the Carhart tone-decay test correctly identified 84% of their 83 cochlear-impaired cases. Olsen and Kurdziel (1976) found that the tone-decay results were negative in 82.5 and 85% for the Carhart and Olsen–Noffsinger procedures, respectively, in their 40 patients with Meniere's disease or acoustic trauma. On the other hand, Hall (1978) reported that the Carhart, Rosenberg, and Owens tone-decay tests yielded similar findings; negative results were obtained in approximately 88–90% of three different groups of approximately 205–283 cochlear cases.

2. Eighth-Nerve Pathology

Sørensen (1962) using the Sørensen modification of the Carhart threshold tone-decay test, reported that 100% of his 12 patients with cerebellopontine-angle tumors exhibited pronounced positive tone decay. Owens (1964a) obtained similar findings; 95% of his group of 19 cases of eighth-nerve pathology had a Type III pattern or Type IIE pattern at one or more frequencies. Four of the 19 cases exhibited Type IIA–D patterns along with the Type IIE and Type III patterns. Positive tone decay was present even when the test was administered at frequencies where the hearing was within normal limits. Abnormal tone-decay was usually present at several frequencies. Harbert and Young (1964) found excessive tone decay when subjects were instructed to respond to tonal quality rather than audibility in their 5 cases of eighth-nerve pathology. Gjaevenes and Söhoel (1969) found that 93% of their 14 cases of retrocochlear pathology had positive tone decay. Similarly, Tillman (1969) reported that, using the Carhart procedure, 89% of his 18 retrocochlear cases had pronounced tone decay.

Olsen and Kurdziel (1976) reported that both the Carhart and Olsen–Noffsinger procedures correctly identified 85% of their 20 cases with retrocochlear pathology. Olsen and Noffsinger (1974), who compared the Carhart, Olsen–Noffsinger, and Rosenberg tone-decay procedures, reported that positive tone decay was obtained in 95% of their 20 retrocochlear cases with the Carhart and Olsen–Noffsinger procedures and in only 65% with the Rosenberg procedure.

Lower accuracy rates were obtained for the tone-decay test in the later studies. For example, Sanders et al. (1974) reported that the Carhart procedure yielded a positive result in only 69% of their 26 ears. Hall (1978) reported that the Carhart, Rosenberg, and Owens tone-decay tests were similar in accuracy of correctly identifying eighth-nerve disorders; the procedures gave positive results in approximately 70–72% of three different groups of eighth-nerve cases with sample sizes ranging from 66 to 227. Josey (1987) reported that tone-decay testing revealed abnormal tone decay in only 64% of their 418 retrocochlear cases.

3. Normal-Hearing Persons

Morales-Garcia and Hood (1972) observed that tone decay was either absent or very minimal (i.e., no more than

5 dB at 500 and 1000 Hz and no more than 10–15 dB at 2000 and 4000 Hz) in persons with normal hearing-threshold levels. They also found that tone decay was frequency dependent, increasing as the stimulating frequency increased.

4. Conductive Pathology

Yantis (1959) reported that tone decay was absent in 3 patients with conductive pathology. Similarly, Sørensen (1962) reported the absence of tone decay in his group of 20 patients with conductive pathology.

5. Presbycusis

Goetzinger, Proud, and Dirks (1961) found that excessive adaptation was absent in their group of elderly persons. These findings were substantiated by Sørensen (1962). Gjaevenes and Söhoel (1969) reported that excessive adaptation was present in only 4% of their group of 606 presbycusic ears. On the other hand, Willeford (1960) reported that excessive tone decay was present in 3 of his 8 elderly cases. The discrepancies regarding the presence of tone decay in the elderly was attributed by Olsen and Noffsinger (1974) to differences in the particular tone-decay procedure employed.

D. RELIABILITY

Sung, Goetzinger, and Knox (1969) reported that the test–retest tone decay means using a modified Carhart threshold tone-decay test (in which the test was not terminated until the subject reported being able to hear the tone for 90 and 120 s) did not differ significantly at all frequencies evaluated (1000, 2000, and 4000 Hz) in their group of presbycusic ears, acoustic-trauma ears, and Meniere's-disease ears. The Pearson product-moment correlation coefficients were significant, ranging from 0.47 to 0.91 depending upon the test frequency, duration (90 or 120 s), and pathology (presbycusis, Meniere's disease, or noise-induced etiology). The standard error of measurement did not exceed 3 dB.

Jerger (1962a) reported that the reliability coefficients for the Carhart test at 1000 and 4000 Hz were 0.86 and 0.72, respectively. The standard error of measurement averaged approximately 5 dB over frequency for the Carhart procedure.

E. COMPARISON OF THE VARIOUS ADAPTATION PROCEDURES

Olsen and Noffsinger (1974) reported that the accuracy of the Carhart and Olsen–Noffsinger procedures in correctly identifying cochlear-impaired ears was similar and slightly worse than the Rosenberg procedure. Olsen and Kurdziel (1976) also found that the Carhart and Olsen–Noffsinger procedures were similar in accuracy in correctly identifying cochlear-impaired ears.

With respect to eighth-nerve pathology, Olsen and Noffsinger (1974) found the Carhart and Olsen–Noffsinger procedures to be identical in the proportion of retro-cochlear-impaired ears identified and markedly superior in accuracy to the Rosenberg procedure. Olsen and Noffsinger (1974) concluded that the 1-min limitation imposed by the Rosenberg test was time-saving but resulted in too great a sacrifice in the ability to detect retrocochlear pathology. Olsen and Kurdziel (1976) also reported that the Carhart and Olsen–Noffsinger procedures were essentially similar in the accuracy of correctly identifying eighth-nerve cases.

Parker and Decker (1971) compared the Owens and Car-hart tone-decay results in 50 cases with severe tone decay. They found that 9 cases with positive tone decay on the Carhart test showed the Owens Type IID or IIE pattern. In some cases, the rate of decay was slow initially, becoming rapid at intensities above those employed for the Owens test. Thus, the Carhart tone-decay test was superior to the Owens test.

In conclusion, the Carhart and Olsen–Noffsinger tone-decay tests are the most accurate of the tone-decay procedures. The latter procedure is shorter and therefore more clinically feasible than the former. The Owens tone-decay test is appropriate when the magnitude of the hearing loss and adaptation preclude the use of the Carhart and Olsen–Noffsinger procedures.

Turner, Shepard, and Frazer (1984), in their review of 170 papers published between 1968 and 1983, found that less than 150 ears had been evaluated with the STAT proce-dure whereas more than 1200 ears had been evaluated with the other protocols. Thus, too few studies have been done to judge the accuracy of the STAT test. The preliminary re-sults, however, indicate that the accuracy of the STAT test in correctly identifying retrocochlear ears as positive was substantially below that for the other tone-decay protocols (except for the STAT version done at 500–4000 Hz, for which there is only one study done on only 20 ears).

The increase in the false-negative rate for the tone-decay test from the early to the more recent studies probably reflects improved medical technology, for example, MRI or CAT scans, and increased awareness of retrocochlear pa-thology resulting in referral for audiologic follow-up at an earlier phase in the tumor growth. Because of its relatively high false-negative rate, the tone-decay test is not a good test for inclusion in the site-of-lesion battery.

F. TEMPORAL CHARACTERISTICS OF ADAPTATION

Owens (1964a) developed his tone-decay procedure on the basis of the observation that rapid decay was a distin-guishing feature of eighth-nerve pathology. Parker and Decker (1971) also reported that the rate of decay was important in the evaluation of tone decay. Olsen and Kurdziel (1976) recorded the rate of adaptation along with the magnitude of adaptation for the Carhart and Olsen–

Noffsinger procedures. The results revealed that the retro-cochlear ears, as a group, showed more rapid tone decay than the cochlear ears, as a group. Nevertheless, the few cochlear-impaired ears with excessive tone decay also showed rapid tone decay and the few retrocochlear ears without excessive tone decay failed to reveal rapid decay. Nevertheless, Olsen and Kurdziel (1976) recommended in-vestigating the rate as well as extent of tone decay.

Wiley and Lilly (1980) found that magnitude of adapta-tion using the Carhart and Rosenberg procedures failed to differentiate between the left ear with a surgically con-firmed eighth-nerve tumor and the right cochlear hearing-impaired ear. The rate of adaptation was assessed with the modified Hood procedure (10-s rather than 1-min rest pe-riod). They plotted the time to inaudibility in seconds as a function of sensation level. This plot revealed a rate-of-decay difference between the two ears. That is, for the retrocochlear ear, the longest time the tone was heard was 5 s. The right ear showed large times to inaudibility at all sensation levels. Wiley and Lilly (1980) noted that temporal information about auditory adaptation can be obtained using the Carhart procedure by recording the length of time the tone is heard at each intensity level. They also suggested that, if the Owens procedure is employed, the test should be continued beyond four increments until a complete descrip-tion of the auditory adaptation is obtained.

Silman, Gelfand, Lutolf, and Chun (1981) performed the Owens tone-decay test on a patient with a surgically con-firmed eighth-nerve tumor. The Owens tone-decay test was performed in this patient because the magnitude of the hearing loss (severe to profound in the pathological ear) precluded other tone-decay protocols. A Type III pattern was obtained in the pathological ear. They obtained infor-mation about the temporal characteristics of auditory ad-aptation by calculating the adaptation rate (dB/s) at each sensation level in the pathological ear. As the sensation level increased, the adaptation rate increased from 0.20 to 1.33 dB/s at 500 Hz and from 1.25 to 5.0 dB/s at 1000 Hz. They suggested that rate of adaptation was an important feature of tone decay, particularly when the hearing loss was severe or profound.

Future research is needed on the accuracy of the rate-of-adaptation measure in the cochlear and retrocochlear pop-ulations before this measure can be adopted clinically.

III. RECRUITMENT TESTS

A. ALTERNATE BINAURAL LOUDNESS BALANCE TEST

The earliest loudness recruitment test was the alternate binaural loudness balance (ABLB) test developed by Fowler (1936). The test involved the presentation of alternating tones between the two ears under earphones. The intensity of the tone in the hearing-impaired ear is varied until the loudness of that tone is judged by the subject to be equivalent to a tone at a constant intensity in the normal ear. This process of varying intensity is called a loudness balance. Loudness balances are done for various intensity levels in the normal-hearing ear. The results are then displayed on a laddergram. A laddergram contains parallel lines representing the two ears. Intensity in dB HL is represented on each of these lines. A horizontal line is drawn intersecting the parallel lines at the intensities where a loudness balance was achieved. Figure 6 illustrates a laddergram.

Fowler (1936) developed the ABLB test for the purpose of differentiating between conductive and sensorineural hearing losses. He concluded that persons with conductive hearing loss show no loudness recruitment whereas persons with sensorineural hearing loss manifest loudness recruitment. Loudness recruitment is the abnormally rapid growth of loudness with increases in intensity. Fowler (1939) and Lorente de Nó (1937) attributed the presence of recruitment to a neurologic mechanism. The results of subsequent research (Dix, Hallpike, & Hood, 1948; Hallpike & Hood, 1951, 1959; Jerger, 1961; Priede & Coles, 1974) show that loudness recruitment as measured by the Fowler ABLB method is characteristic of sensorineural hearing loss of cochlear etiology and absent in sensorineural hearing loss of neural etiology, normal-hearing ears, and conductive hearing loss. The ABLB test is a traditional tool employed in site-of-lesion testing to determine the locus of the sensorineural hearing impairment—auditory nerve or cochlea.

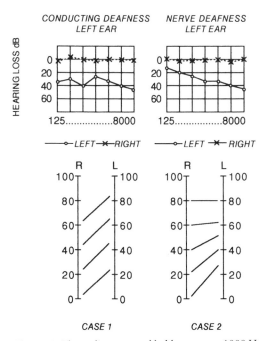

Figure 6 The audiograms and laddergrams at 1000 Hz for a person with conductive hearing loss (Case 1) and a person with cochlear pathology (Case 2). Recruitment is absent in Case 1 and complete in Case 2. Reprinted from Dix, Hallpike, and Hood (1948) with permission.

1. NATURE OF LOUDNESS RECRUITMENT

When the ABLB is performed on persons with unilateral conductive hearing loss and the data are plotted on a laddergram, the results indicate that a loudness balance at a particular frequency is attained at equal sensation levels in the two ears. Thus, if there is a tone of 60 dB SL relative to the pure-tone threshold in the normal-hearing ear, a loudness balance will occur at an equal sensation level (60 dB SL) in the hearing loss ear. In terms of dB HL, consider a person with a unilateral conductive hearing loss with a threshold of 30 dB HL at 1000 Hz in the hearing loss ear and a threshold of 0 dB HL at the same frequency in the normal-hearing ear. If a 1000-Hz stimulus is introduced to the normal-hearing ear at 20 dB HL, a loudness balance will occur at 50 dB HL in the hearing-loss ear, assuming that loudness balances are attained at equal SLs in the two ears in cases of conductive hearing loss. This example is illustrated in Case 1 of Figure 6. Similarly, if a 1000-Hz stimulus is introduced to the normal-hearing ear at 60 dB HL, then the intensity in the bad ear yielding a loudness balance will be 90 dB HL. Thus, "the loss of sensitivity or deafness of the affected ear, 30 dB at threshold, remains constant throughout the entire intensity range" (Dix *et al.*, 1948, p. 672).

The loudness of a tone grows abnormally rapidly in an ear with sensorineural hearing loss of cochlear etiology. That is, the sensitivity of the cochlear hearing-impaired ear is poorer than that of normal-hearing ears at intensities near threshold but is similar to that of normal-hearing ears at high intensities. Consider a person with a unilateral hearing loss of cochlear etiology with a threshold of 30 dB HL in the hearing-loss ear and 0 dB HL in the normal-hearing ear. The presentation of a 1000-Hz stimulus to the normal-hearing ear at 20 dB SL gave a loudness balance at only 10 dB SL in the hearing-impaired ear in Case 2 of Figure 6, since loudness grows more rapidly in the affected than normal ear. In terms of dB HL, the introduction of a tone at 80 dB HL in the normal-hearing ear will yield a loudness balance at the same level in the affected ear, as shown in Case 2. Thus, the loudness of an 80 dB SL tone in the normal-hearing ear is matched by that of a 50 dB SL tone in the hearing-impaired ear. "In other words, the deafness of the affected ear present at threshold disappears at higher intensities, and this in its simplest terms constitutes the phenomenon of loudness recruitment" (Dix *et al.*, 1948, p. 672).

Dix *et al.* (1948) reported that complete loudness recruitment was present in all of their 30 cases with Meniere's disease. Case 1 and Case 2 of Figure 7 have laddergrams reflecting complete recruitment. In complete loudness recruitment, there is a high intensity level in the normal-hearing ear at which a loudness balance is attained at equal dB HLs in the two ears. Over-recruitment, in which loudness grows faster in the affected than normal ear even at high intensities, was also present in some of these cases. In ears with over-recruitment, the affected ear seems more sensitive than the normal ear at high intensities. At high intensities, beyond that giving complete loudness recruitment, loudness balances will be achieved in which the intensity in dB HL in the affected ear is lower than that in the normal ear. Case 2 of Figure 7 is an illustration of over-recruitment.

The results of histological examination of the cochleas of the ears with Meniere's disease in the study by Dix *et al.* (1948) revealed changes in the Organ of Corti. The eighth-nerve fibers and cells of the spiral ganglion, on the other hand, were normal.

> The finding that the recruitment phenomenon is an unvarying occurrence in Meniere's disease, a disorder of the end-organ of hearing, appears to be related in an interesting way to the experimental work of Pumphrey and Gold (1948). According to Gold's theory based on this work, the microphonic potentials of the cochlea arise somewhere in Corti's organ and play a vital part in determining both its sensitivity and frequency selectivity. We should, therefore, certainly expect that a disorder of this microphonic mechanism, i.e. Corti's organ, would lead to deafness and to certain disorders of pitch sense, i.e., paracusis dysharmonica, well known to be characteristic of Meniere's disease. (Dix *et al.*, 1948, pp. 678–679)

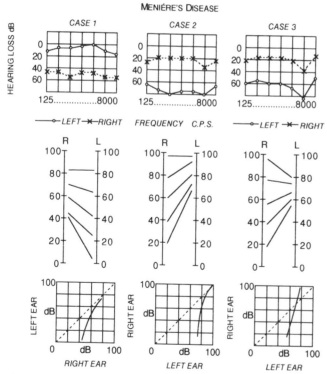

Figure 7 The audiograms, laddergrams, and Steinberg–Gardner plots for three cases with Meniere's disease. Complete recruitment is present in all the cases and over-recruitment is present in Case 3. Reprinted from Dix, Hallpike, and Hood (1948) with permission.

Dix *et al.* (1948) reported that loudness recruitment was completely absent in 14 of their 20 cases with eighth-nerve degeneration (neurofibroma and cerebellopontine angle lesions). In the remaining 6 cases, partial loudness recruitment was present. Partial loudness recruitment is abnormally rapid loudness growth in the affected ear with loudness balances at lower sensation levels in the affected than normal ear but without a loudness balance at equal dB HLs at some high intensity. The results of histological examination of the cochleas and eighth-nerves in these 20 cases revealed that the eighth-nerve lesion resulted in degeneration of cochlear fibers peripheral rather than central to the lesion. The effect of the lesion was to reduce substantially the number of cochlear fibers and cells of the spiral ganglion. Nevertheless, the Organ of Corti was unaffected by the lesion. Dix *et al.* (1948) concluded that loudness recruitment, present in cochlear pathology and absent in eighth-nerve pathology, resulted from disorders of the Organ of Corti.

Hallpike and Hood (1959) described the various loudness recruitment functions occurring in ears with Meniere's disease. They noted that three types of recruitment curves could occur. These three types of recruitment curves show hearing level in the normal ear as a function of the hearing level in the impaired ear for the various loudness balances; they are shown in Figure 8. In all three types, the loudness recruitment curve is linear to the point of complete recruitment. At higher intensities, the curve either follows the equal loudness line (Figure 8A) as in typical cases of moderate or worse hearing loss, continues past the equal loudness line with unchanging slope (Figure 8B) as in typical cases of mild hearing loss, or continues past the equal loudness line with a decrease in slope (Figure 8C).

Hood (1950) stated that the angle between the loudness recruitment curve and the abscissa in a Steinberg–Gardner plot exceeds 45° in recruiting ears. This angle is called the recruitment angle. Hood (1950) also reported that the size of the recruitment angle was directly related to the magnitude of the hearing loss. Figure 9 illustrates the relation of the recruitment angle to the degree of the hearing loss as seen on Steinberg–Gardner plots. This figure shows that mild hearing losses are associated with smaller recruitment angles than are more severe hearing losses.

Dix *et al.* (1948) offered the following explanation for the absence of loudness recruitment in cases of eighth-nerve lesions. Assuming that the lesion is evenly distributed, there is a specific fiber survival rate. Thus, if the fiber survival rate is 10 to 1 and if 1 bel excites 10 normal fibers, only one of the lesion fibers will be excited. A tenfold increase in intensity, i.e., a 2-bel stimulus, will result in the excitation of 100 normal fibers and only 10 lesion fibers. Therefore, an intensity in the affected ear which is 1 bel more than that in the normal ear is needed to excite the same number of fibers in the two ears. "This argument, therefore, leads us to expect that the sensitivity loss, or deafness, of the affected ear in a

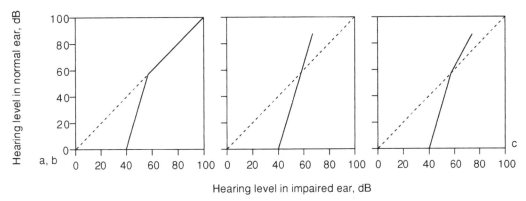

Figure 8 The various forms taken by loudness recruitment curves. Reprinted from Hood (1977) with permission.

case of diffuse degeneration of the VIII nerve, would be constant throughout the intensity range" (p. 685).

The presence of loudness recruitment in cases of end-organ pathology has been confirmed by several investigators (Coles & Priede, 1976; Dix & Hallpike, 1958; Hallpike, 1965; Jerger, 1961). Absence of loudness recruitment in eighth-nerve pathology also has been confirmed by several investigators (Dix & Hallpike, 1958; Hood, 1969; Jerger, 1961). Many cases with eighth-nerve pathology have derecruitment, in which the loudness growth with increases in intensity is slower than normal in the affected ear (loudness reversal). In derecruiting ears, loudness balances are attained at a higher sensation level in the affected

than in the normal ear. Case 3 in Figure 10 illustrates the loudness balance diagrams in a person with eighth-nerve pathology showing derecruitment. The other two cases in this figure show the loudness balance diagrams of two persons with eighth-nerve pathology demonstrating absence of recruitment.

Dix and Hallpike (1958) reported that loudness recruitment was present in 10% of their 69 cases of unilateral

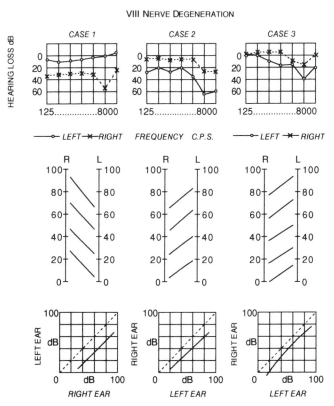

Figure 10 The audiograms, laddergrams, and Steinberg–Gardner plots for three cases with eighth-cranial-nerve pathology. Cases 1 and 2 demonstrate the absence of recruitment. Case 3 demonstrates derecruitment. Reprinted from Dix, Hallpike, and Hood (1948) with permission.

Figure 9 The loudness recruitment–amount of hearing loss relationship, showing two standard deviation limits of variation. From Hallpike and Hood (1959) with permission.

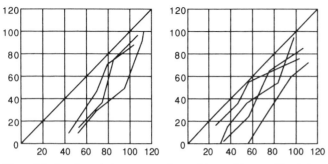

Figure 11 Loudness balance curves from subjects with nerve fiber lesions exhibiting loudness recruitment. Note irregularity of the curves. Reprinted from Hood (1969) with permission.

eighth-nerve pathology at one or more frequencies. They suggested that the presence of loudness recruitment in these cases was associated with interruption of the cochlear blood supply caused by tumor pressure upon the cochlear blood supply. These findings were supported by Simonton (1956) who found that, in several cases with loudness recruitment, the loudness recruitment disappeared after removal of the tumor. Further support came from Suga and Lindsay (1976), who conducted histological studies, the results of which revealed changes in the cochlea in some cases of eighth-nerve pathology. Hood (1969) noted that even when recruitment was present in eighth-nerve lesions, the recruitment curves were irregular rather than linear curves as seen in cases of cochlear pathology. Figure 11 shows the loudness recruitment curves in persons with eighth-nerve pathology who demonstrate recruitment.

2. AUDITORY ADAPTATION AND LOUDNESS RECRUITMENT

Hallpike and Hood (1951) conducted several experiments to evaluate the relation between loudness recruitment and auditory adaptation. In the first experiment, a simultaneous loudness balance was done with an intensity of 80 dB SL in the test ear. A balance was obtained when the varying-intensity tone in the control ear was 80 dB SL. A period of stimulation with a continuous tone in the test ear only then followed. Afterward, a simultaneous loudness balance was done again, with the test-ear intensity at 80 dB SL. In the repeat simultaneous loudness balance, loudness equality is attained at an intensity in the control ear that is less than 80 dB SL, depending upon the duration of the continuous stimulation between the initial and repeat loudness balances. If the test ear had a rest period, the final loudness balance was attained at a level in the control ear which more closely approximated that in the test ear; the longer the rest period, the closer the approximation in intensity of the tone in the control ear to that in the test ear. Figure 12 shows the relation between the duration of the recovery period in the test ear following the fatiguing tone to the intensity level in the control ear at which the loudness balance is obtained. The fatigue demonstrated by these experiments as evidenced by a decrease in the intensity of the tone needed to obtain loudness equality from the initial to the final loudness balance was termed perstimulatory fatigue since it was revealed during the actual application of the stimulus.

Hood (1955) reported that when the initial and final

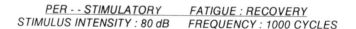

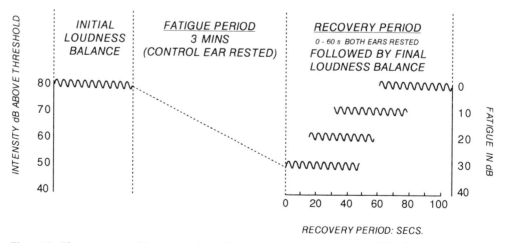

Figure 12 The time course of the recovery from adaptation (perstimulatory fatigue) following stimulation of the test ear at an intensity of 80 dB above threshold for three minutes at a frequency of 1000 Hz. Simultaneous loudness balances were carried out after both ears had been tested for varying periods. Each tracing represents a separate test. Reprinted from Hallpike and Hood (1951) with permission.

loudness balances involved alternate rather than simultaneous presentation of tones to the two ears, no adaptation (perstimulatory fatigue) was evidenced. Nevertheless, the alternating tone did not abolish adaptation resulting from the sustained tone to the test ear, as evidenced by the results of the following experiment. A simultaneous balance was followed by a fatiguing sustained tone in the test ear, then an alternate loudness balance, and then a simultaneous loudness balance. No loss of sensitivity was evidenced on the alternate loudness balance, although a loss of sensitivity was evidenced on the final simultaneous loudness balance. Thus, the response for the test ear was normal for alternating tones but relapsed to its adapted level when the sustained tone was applied.

Based on studies on the stretch receptor and the results of the experiments on alternate vs. simultaneous loudness balances following the application of a fatiguing tone, Hood (1955) concluded that the ability of the adapted cochlea to attain a loudness balance at equal intensities in the two ears when a fatiguing tone was followed by an alternating but not simultaneous loudness balance indicated the adapted cochlea's ability to initiate normal on-effects. Furthermore, the fact that loss of sensitivity (fatigue) in the test ear occurred only for the simultaneous loudness balance and not for the alternate loudness balance in the experiment in which a fatiguing tone was followed by an alternate and then a simultaneous loudness balance indicated that the adapted end organ can initiate normal on-effects but relapses with the reapplication of a sustained stimulus. Thus, when an alternate loudness balance procedure is employed, normal on-effects can be elicited whereas perstimulatory fatigues result when a simultaneous loudness balance is employed.

If a loudness balance test is done on a person with a recruiting unilateral hearing loss, the alternate loudness balance will show recruitment whereas recruitment may be absent with the simultaneous loudness procedure that causes relapse and subsequently the absence or even reversal of loudness recruitment. The recruiting ear behaves like an adapted end organ in that normal on-effects are obtained with short, interrupted stimuli and relapse is evidenced with sustained stimuli. If there is insufficient time between the application of successive stimuli to the same ear, the magnitude of the on-effect is reduced. In the case of the normal ear, a fatiguing tone is needed to bring the cochlea to the adapted state. In the case of the recruiting ear, the cochlea is already adapted. Hallpike and Hood (1951) suggested that

> if loudness recruitment as assessed by the alternate balance procedure depends on the capacity of diseased hair cells to initiate normal on-effects, then it follows that care should be taken to design the test procedure accordingly, i.e., with short, intermittent stimuli suitably spaced. It would, in fact, be possible to suggest as suit-

able values, 0.5 second for the stimulus duration and 1 second for the duration of the rest period. (p. 274)

Jerger and Harford (1960) supported the use of the alternate rather than the simultaneous loudness balance for reasons other than perstimulatory fatigue. They compared the ABLB with the simultaneous loudness balance procedure. In the case of the simultaneous loudness balance procedure, the responses represent median-plane localization responses. That is, the binaural intensity relations are manipulated until the phantom image is localized in the center of the head. Jerger and Harford demonstrated that there was a discrepancy between the ABLB and simultaneous loudness balance procedure in both recruiting and nonrecruiting ears. For example, in nonrecruiting ears, median-plane judgments were not accomplished at equal sensation levels with the simultaneous loudness balance procedure; loudness balances were attained at equal sensation levels in the nonrecruiting ears with the alternate loudness balance procedure. Therefore, simultaneous loudness balancing to achieve median-plane localization did not constitute a true loudness judgment. Therefore, Jerger and Harford (1960) recommended alternate rather than simultaneous loudness balancing.

3. Methodology
a. Hood versus Jerger
The discrepancy in the reports regarding the accuracy of the ABLB has been attributed by Hood (1969) to the different methodologies employed in the ABLB test administration. Jerger (1961), for example, reported that recruitment was present in only 75% of the ears with Meniere's disease and was absent in only 82% of the acoustic neuroma cases. Dix and Hallpike (1958), on the other hand, using the Hood method, reported that recruitment was present in 100% of their cases with Meniere's disease and absent in 90% of the retrocochlear-impaired ears. The Hood method follows.

1. The tones are manually alternated in order to adjust the pace of the test to the patient's abilities.
2. Initially, large intensity increments of 10 dB are employed in the bracketing procedure; the increment size is then progressively decreased to as small as 1 dB in cases with recruitment.
3. The ear receiving the louder sound is randomized rather than alternated so the patient cannot anticipate which ear will have the louder sound.
4. No more than 8 repetitions of a tone are given when there is a change of intensity in the impaired ear after which the patient must make a loudness judgment.
5. The ear receiving the initial stimulus is varied to avoid any precedence effects.
6. The interval between tones to the same ear is no less

than 1 s to maximize the magnitude of the on-effects. Hood (1969) suggested the use of a 1.5 s interval between successive stimuli to the same ear.

7. The duration should be sufficient to produce a tonal sensation. Hood (1969) suggested using a tonal duration of 0.3 sec.

8. Loudness balances are done at 20-dB increments up to 100 dB HL in the normal ear.

9. The fixed ear is the normal-hearing ear.

10. The varying-intensity ear is the impaired ear. The range of uncertainty regarding loudness judgments is reduced when the affected ear with enhanced loudness discrimination is the ear receiving the varying intensities.

11. The examiner adjusts the intensity using the method of limits procedure in the impaired ear until equality of loudness with the constant-intensity tone in the normal-hearing ear is attained. Hood (1969) suggested that it was preferable for the examiner rather than the patient to adjust the intensity since the examiner is able to perform checks on the reliability and validity of the patient's responses.

12. The results are displayed on a Steinberg–Gardner plot.

13. The hearing loss of the affected ear need not exceed 20 dB HL.

14. Recruitment is present if the angle between the loudness recruitment curve and the abscissa (intensity level in the impaired ear) exceeds 45°. Complete recruitment is present if the loudness-function curve and the equal-loudness line intersect at some point. No recruitment is present if the angle between the loudness function and the abscissa is equal to 45°. Over-recruitment is present if the loudness function continues past the point of intersection with the equal-loudness curve. Loudness reversal (derecruitment) is present when the angle between the loudness function and the abscissa is smaller than 45°.

The Jerger (1962b) method follows.

1. Tones alternate automatically.

2. Intensity increments of 2-dB are employed in the bracketing procedure.

3. The interval between tones to the same ear is 500 ms. Jerger and Jerger (1966) evaluated the critical off-times (COT) for obtaining pure-tone threshold levels in their patients with abnormal tone decay. They found that essentially no adaptation resulted when the COT exceeded 200 ms. Moreover, Dallos and Tillman (1966) and Tillman (1966) reported that the use of a 50% duty cycle with a 250 ms off-time in their patients with abnormal adaptation enabled complete recovery from the effects of adaptation.

4. The tonal duration is 500 ms (50% duty cycle).

5. The fixed-intensity ear is the affected ear.

6. The varying-intensity ear is the normal-hearing ear. Jerger (1962b) concluded that fewer levels at which loudness balancing is done are needed to obtain information about the presence or absence of recruitment when the fixed ear is the affected ear than when the fixed ear is the normal-hearing ear.

7. The patient varies the intensity using the method of adjustments in the normal-hearing ear to attain equality of loudness.

8. Loudness balances are accomplished with the intensity in the fixed ear at 20 and 40 dB SL relative to the bad-ear threshold.

9. The results are displayed on a laddergram.

10. The hearing loss in the affected ear must be at least 20 dB HL.

11. The maximum permissible total harmonic distortion at the maximum output of the audiometer should not exceed 1%.

12. If the loudness balances are made at equal sensation levels (± 10 dB), recruitment is absent. If there are one or more loudness balances made at equal intensity levels (± 10 dB), recruitment is complete. Partial recruitment occurs when the loudness balance falls between the two categories of no recruitment and complete recruitment.

Hood (1969) argued against the use of laddergrams and the Jerger criteria for interpretation, contending that the Jerger criteria would lead to misclassification of certain loudness functions. This point is illustrated in Figure 13, which shows some loudness-function curves. Curve C1 would be interpreted as showing incomplete recruitment by Hood's criteria and complete by Jerger's criteria. Curve D would be interpreted as showing partial recruitment by Hood's criteria but no recruitment by Jerger's criteria.

Priede and Coles (1974) and Coles and Priede (1976) support the use of the Hood technique rather than the Jerger technique with the exception of using the bad rather than the good ear as the fixed-intensity ear for the following reasons.

1. With the good ear fixed, variations in intensity level are made in the bad ear, which is subject to auditory distortion and also to loudness discomfort at the higher levels.

2. When test–retest loudness balances were done in 10 cochlear ears using 5-dB steps, the standard deviation was 3.9 dB for the Jerger ABLB test as opposed to 4.1 dB for the Hood ABLB test. Considering the actual slopes of the loudness functions, the standard deviation for the Jerger method corresponds in terms of accuracy for the measurement of the recruitment slope to a standard deviation of only 2.0 dB when the bad ear is the fixed ear. To achieve the same accuracy in slope of recruitment

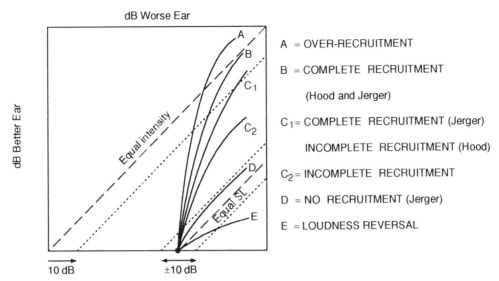

Figure 13 The loudness functions and interpretation of these curves according to the Hood and the Jerger criteria. Curve A shows over-recruitment. Curve B shows complete recruitment by both criteria. Curve C1 shows complete recruitment for the Jerger criteria and incomplete recruitment for the Hood criteria. Curve C2 shows incomplete recruitment. Curve D shows no recruitment (Jerger criteria). Curve E shows loudness reversal. Reprinted from Priede and Coles (1974) with permission.

as the Jerger bad-ear-fixed technique, smaller increments are required with the Hood good-ear-fixed technique. The loudness-function curves obtained by the Hood good-ear-fixed method corresponded with fewer of the recruitment functions measured in the same 19 patients by the acoustic-reflex threshold and loudness-discomfort level tests than the Jerger bad-ear-fixed method. Moreover, the Hood good-ear-fixed method yielded loudness functions that were 10 dB higher than those of the Jerger bad-ear-fixed method, indicating that the Hood method overestimated the degree of recruitment. Hood (1977) argued that Coles and Priede (1976) failed to give information on the hearing-levels of their subjects. Coles and Priede (1976) also suggested that there was a discrepancy between the high frequency of over-recruitment for the Hood ABLB test in Hallpike and Hood's (1959) study on 200 cases with Meniere's disease and the low frequency of over-recruitment for loudness-discomfort levels in the Hood and Poole (1966) study on patients with Meniere's disease.

Hood (1977) compared the loudness-discomfort levels and good-ear-fixed ABLB test results as follows. He considered the loudness-discomfort level test as a loudness balance at a high intensity (since it produces an equal sensation of loudness in the two ears) and plotted the loudness-discomfort level loudness-balance data along with the other loudness-balance data derived from the ABLB test in 400 ears. He then measured the discrepancy between the loudness-discomfort levels and the rest of the loudness-function curve. He found that the discrepancy was less than 3 dB in 81% and was less than 5 dB in 97%. Thus, he

concluded that Coles and Priede (1976) measured less recruitment with the bad-ear-fixed method than was actually present. Hood (1977) also contended that the frequency of over-recruitment with the ABLB method cannot be compared with that of the assumed over-recruitment using the loudness-discomfort level measurement since loudness discomfort does not necessarily occur at levels at which over-recruitment is present. Hood (1977) suggested that over-recruitment appears to be characteristic only of conditions involving impaired cochlear metabolic processes such as Meniere's disease. Thus, over-recruitment would be absent in ears with noise-induced hearing loss. Hood (1977) also concluded that over-recruitment was more likely to occur when the hearing loss was mild than when it was severe. Consequently, Hood (1977) contended that Coles and Priede's (1976) group with cochlear pathology might have included many ears with severe hearing losses, accounting for their failure to detect over-recruitment in their group of subjects. Hood (1977) argued that a comparison between the standard deviations of the good-ear-fixed method with those of the bad-ear-fixed method cannot be done when the increment size is 5 dB rather than less than or equal to 1 dB, as employed in the Hood method. Finally, Hood (1977) showed that if loudness balances with the bad ear fixed are obtained at 20 SL relative to the bad-ear threshold and at 120 dB HL, the loudness function in a recruiting ear will show less recruitment than the loudness function obtained using the Hood method.

Sanders (1979) recommended the following guidelines for interpretation of the ABLB results plotted on laddergrams when the bad ear is fixed. No recruitment is present if loudness balances occur at equal sensation levels

(± 10 dB). Partial recruitment is present if loudness balances occur at more than equal sensation levels (± 10 dB) but less than equal dB HLs (± 10 dB). Complete recruitment is present if there is a loudness balance at equal dB HLs (± 10 dB). Derecruitment is present if loudness balances are obtained at less than equal sensation levels (± 10 dB).

b. Miskolczy-Fodor

A modification of the ABLB test was proposed by Miskolczy-Fodor (1964). In this tracking method, the patient is instructed to press the button when the tone in the test ear becomes just noticeably louder than in the reference ear and to release the button of a hand-held switch when the tone in the test ear becomes just noticeably softer than in the reference ear. In the reference ear, a tone of gradually increasing (or decreasing) intensity (rate of 0.38 dB/s) is presented. In the test ear, manipulation of the button causes the intensity to increase or decrease more rapidly (rate of 2.5 dB/s). The midline of the loudness function tracked represents the equal-loudness level. The tones to the two ears can be at the same or different frequencies and either continuous or alternating. An advantage of this tracking method is that a complete continuous rather than discrete loudness function can be obtained. Also, the width of the tracked excursions represents the "limits of error for the respective individual judgment of equal loudness, and thus offers a basis of evaluating the subject's reliability" (Miskolczy-Fodor, 1964, p. 362).

Carver (1970) demonstrated that the Miskolczy-Fodor ABLB tracking method was not as reliable as the fixed ABLB test using the Jerger technique. The loudness curve obtained with the tracking method did not approximate the theoretically expected loudness function regardless of whether the intensity in the reference ear was ascending or descending, since a hysteresis effect was present. On the other hand, the loudness function obtained with the fixed method closely approximated the theoretically expected loudness function. Averaging of the tracking functions obtained with ascending and descending intensities resulted in cancellation of the hysteresis effect and close approximation of the theoretically expected loudness function but failed to improve reliability. Gelfand (1976) found that when the tracking ABLB test was applied to sensorineural hearing-impaired subjects, overshoot and undershoot artifacts were obtained, depending upon which ear received the reference tone.

c. Fritze

Fritze (1978) believed that the reference ear and the reference intensities for each loudness balance should be randomized. This randomization would reduce any bias resulting when only one ear is the reference ear. Fritze (1978) employed a computer to randomize the intensity levels and reference ear. Loudness balancing is performed by the subject using the method of adjustments. The computer plots

the equal-loudness data on a Steinberg–Gardner plot, the regression line, the angle of the regression line, and the deviation of the angle from 45°. Using the randomization procedure, 100% of the 14 ears were correctly identified as not having significant recruitment. The results of this computerized procedure with randomization of the reference ear and intensity were also compared with the poor-ear-fixed and the good-ear-fixed methods. Of the 26 patients with unilateral cochlear losses, 100% were identified with the randomization procedure, 88% were identified with the good-ear-fixed procedure, and 31% were identified with the bad-ear-fixed procedure. Further research is needed to substantiate Fritze's findings on normal and pathological ears. This procedure requires linkage of a computer with the audiometer but does not have a longer test administration time than the conventional procedures.

The Hood method is preferable to the Jerger method for the following reasons.

1. In cases with substantial hearing loss with a reduced dynamic range, the bad-ear-fixed method does not permit the obtaining of a sufficient number of loudness-balance data points.
2. Fritze (1978) showed, as mentioned earlier, that the good-ear-fixed method identified a higher percentage of patients with unilateral cochlear losses as having recruitment than the bad-ear-fixed method.

We recommend that, regardless of the method employed, the ABLB should be done only on unilateral hearing-loss cases in which the affected ear has a hearing loss of at least 40 dB HL at the test frequency. In our own clinical experience, children under the age of 13 years have difficulty performing loudness balances. We recommend that ABLB testing not be done in children less than 13 years of age.

4. CROSS-HEARING

Hood (1977) demonstrated that, when cross-hearing occurs during the ABLB test, for example, when a loudness balance is done between a completely deaf ear and a normal-hearing ear, the results of the loudness function curve reflect the responses of the normal-hearing ear. Figure 14 shows loudness-function curves in cases in which cross-hearing occurs during the ABLB test. Figure 14A illustrates no recruitment when an ABLB test is done between a completely deaf ear and a normal ear. If the possibility of cross-hearing exists in a case where the affected ear has a nonrecruiting hearing loss, the responses will be derived for the normal-hearing ear and the sensation level of the tone that has crossed over from the affected to the normal-hearing ear is greater than that in the affected ear. Therefore, the loudness-function curve will appear recruiting up to the point where it intersects with the cross-conduction curve (see Figure 14B). Thus, a spurious loudness recruitment curve will be obtained when the affected ear is nonrecruit-

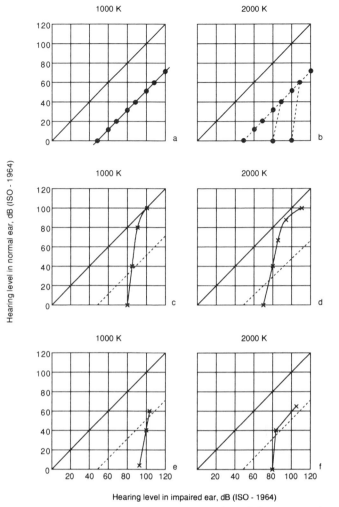

Hearing level in normal ear, dB (ISO - 1964)

Hearing level in impaired ear, dB (ISO - 1964)

Figure 14 Loudness balance curves. (a) Loudness balance curve due entirely to cross-conduction which would result from balancing a completely deaf ear against a normal ear, assuming an interaural attenuation of 50 dB. (b) Loudness balance curves due entirely to cross-conduction which would result in 2 cases of nonrecruiting deafness with hearing losses of 80 and 100 dB, respectively, assuming an interaural attenuation of 50 dB. (c, d) End organ lesion illustrating loudness recruitment which can be considered valid. (e, f) Actual example showing false recruitment in a case of confirmed eighth-cranial-nerve tumor. Reprinted from Hood (1977) with permission.

ing and there is cross-hearing during the ABLB. When loudness balancing is done between a recruiting hearing-loss ear and a normal-hearing ear, there is cross-hearing, and the resulting loudness-function curve shows loudness recruitment, that curve is derived from the affected—not the normal hearing—ear. Figures 14C and D illustrate this situation. For example, consider the loudness balance attained with 90 dB in the bad ear and 80 dB in the good ear in Figure 14C. If 90 dB is presented to the bad ear, the amount crossing over to the good ear is about 40 dB (assuming approximately 50 dB of interaural attenuation). Since 40 dB is less than the 80 dB required to attain a loudness

balance between the two ears, the impaired ear's responses to tones presented are not derived from the normal-hearing ear. The loudness-function curve therefore is a recruiting curve which continues to recruit beyond the cross-conduction curve.

To determine whether cross-hearing has affected the loudness-balance results, examine the loudness-function curve. If it is recruiting up to the cross-conduction curve and then follows the cross-conduction curve, the responses when tones are presented to the impaired ear are derived from the normal-hearing ear and a spurious recruiting curve is obtained. If the loudness-function curve continues to recruit beyond the cross-conduction curve, cross-hearing was not a factor and the recruiting curve is valid.

5. THEORIES OF LOUDNESS RECRUITMENT

One theory of loudness recruitment was proposed by Lorente de Nó (1937) in a discussion of a paper by Fowler. Lorente de Nó suggested that, if either the hair cells or cochlear fibers were affected, the near-threshold stimuli would appear weak in loudness. With high-intensity stimuli, however, the nonaffected hair cells or nerve fibers are maximally excited, resulting in the limiting number of impulses per second generated at the impaired ear. Consequently, both the impaired and normal-hearing ears would similarly perceive the loudness of a high-intensity tone. Although later studies indicate that recruitment is a phenomenon originating in the hair cells, this theory holds if the concept is restricted to hair-cell and not to nerve-fiber damage.

Another theory of loudness recruitment, which was proposed by Lurie (1940), ascribed a portion of the loudness growth to the outer hair cells and another portion to the inner hair cells. It was assumed that the outer hair cells responded to less intense stimuli whereas the inner hair cells responded only to more intense stimuli. If the outer hair cells were damaged, the pure-tone threshold would be elevated to the extent consistent with the hair-cell damage and perception of the loudness of faint tones would be impaired. With increases in intensity, the inner hair cells are excited, resulting in a loudness sensation which eventually equals that in the impaired ear. Thus, the recruitment seen in Meniere's disease could result from damage to the outer hair cells with selective sparing of the inner hair cells (Hallpike & Hood, 1959). The absence of recruitment would result from diffuse damage affecting both the inner and outer hair cells whereas derecruitment would result from damage primarily to the inner hair cells (Hallpike & Hood, 1959). This theory, however, does not account for overrecruitment. Moreover, Hallpike and Cairns (1938) did not find any histological evidence supporting the concept of the selective sparing of the inner hair cells in Meniere's disease. Hallpike and Hood (1959) also noted another failing of this theory. They suggested that if the loudness sensation of a high-intensity tone evoked by the inner hair cells in an ear with outer hair-cell damage is equal to that evoked in a normal-hearing ear, then the inner hair cells would have to account for a high porportion of the total action-potential activity. In order to do so, the inner hair cells either would have to be subserved by very large axons or many axons. This is not the case, that is, there are fewer inner than outer hair-cell axons and the axons subserving the inner hair cells are not particularly large. Nevertheless, this theory does account for the sudden abrupt angling of the loudness function in recruiting ears signaling the shift from excitation of the outer hair cells to excitation of the inner hair cells.

Another theory of loudness recruitment involves the summation principle (Simmons & Dixon, 1966). According to this theory, the loudness of a tone is related to the size of the area of the basilar membrane that is excited. The larger the area of the basilar membrane excited, the greater the number of nerve fibers activated, and the greater the loudness sensation. More intense sounds are presumed to excite larger areas of the basilar membrane than less intense sounds. Also, as intensity increases, the spread of energy along the basilar membrane is in a basilar direction. Hallpike and Hood (1959) noted that, if this theory held, the loss of a few receptors could affect the loudness response at low intensities. At high intensities, the contribution of these affected receptors to the loudness response would be minimal so a normal loudness sensation in the affected ear would occur for high-intensity stimuli. Hallpike and Hood (1959) noted that in some cases there was diffuse damage of the hair cells resulting in a hearing loss at all frequencies. Consequently, high-intensity stimuli would activate additional receptors which were already damaged, so the loudness response at high intensities as well as low intensities would be affected. As a result, a loudness loss would occur at all levels of the intensity scale. Hence, this theory would lead one to expect that recruitment would be absent in ears with Meniere's disease as well as in ears with eighth-nerve pathology. In support of this theory, Simmons and Dixon (1966) reported that in cases of steeply sloping unilateral hearing loss, the ABLB results show derecruitment at the frequency where no hearing loss exists in the two ears. This derecruitment resulted because, as the intensity increased, resulting in a spread of energy towards the basal end, high-frequency fibers could not be activated since they were already activated or missing, so loudness could not grow normally. Simmons and Dixon (1966) refer to this phenomenon as a summation deficit because increases in intensity result in a spread of energy along the basilar membrane to the basal end. Simmons and Dixon observed that rising sensorineural hearing-loss configurations almost always show recruitment regardless of the cause of the hearing loss, since increases in intensity cause activation of the undamaged high-frequency fibers.

Tonndorf (1980, 1981) proposed a "center-clipping"

theory of loudness recruitment. According to this theory, the cilia of the hair cells in the Organ of Corti lose their stiffness because of cochlear dysfunction, thereby becoming decoupled from the tectorial membrane. The decoupling occurs as the cilia pass through their center points as they move from side to side during the shearing action. At the moment of decoupling, there is an amplitude loss in the response waveform. This amplitude reduction has a fixed magnitude. As the intensity increases, the proportion of amplitude loss with respect to the total amplitude becomes smaller and smaller and eventually disappears.

Another model of recruitment states that a recruiting ear has an increased (steeper) slope of the curve describing the neural discharge rate as a function of intensity. Therefore, a small increase in intensity results in a larger than normal increase in the neural discharge rate and consequently an abnormally large change in loudness. Experimental support for this theory is provided by the animal studies of Henderson, Salvi, and Hamernik (1982).

Another theory of loudness recruitment (Evans, 1976; Kiang, Moxon, & Levine, 1970) is based on the rate at which nerve fibers are activated and the shape of the tuning curve—narrow at low intensities and broad at high intensities. In the normal ear, as the intensity increases, the number of nerve fibers activated per dB increases. The tuning curves in pathological ears are significantly wider than those in normal ears. Therefore, at a given intensity above the hearing threshold in a pathological ear, the number of nerve fibers activated per dB is greater than in a normal-hearing ear. The total number of fibers activated in pathological ears, however, is smaller than in normal ears because of the effect of the hearing impairment (the nerve fibers normally involved at low intensities are not activated). At high intensities, there is an approximately equal number of fibers activated in normal and recruiting ears. Experimental support for this theory comes from the study by Henderson *et al.* (1982). Salvi, Henderson, Hamernik, and Ahroon (1983), however, contended that, although this model is logical, some psychoacoustical data in the literature on loudness growth do not support this model.

In summary, many theories of loudness recruitment exist. Further research is needed before a single theory of loudness recruitment can be accepted which accounts for the phenomena of derecruitment and over-recruitment as well as complete recruitment.

6. ACCURACY

Several investigators conducted studies on the ABLB results in both cochlear and retrocochlear ears. Tillman (1969) found recruitment in 100% of his cochlear-impaired ears. Sanders *et al.* (1974) reported that recruitment was present in 85% of their 72 cochlear-impaired ears. Palva, Jauhiainen, Sjoblom, and Ylikoski (1978) found that only 73% of their 36 ears with Meniere's disease had recruitment. Thus, recruitment was not present in 27% of coch-lear ears in these studies.

Tillman (1969) reported that recruitment was absent when measured with the ABLB test in his group of 21 retrocochlear-impaired ears. Sanders *et al.* (1974) found that the ABLB test identified 67% of their 15 ears with retrocochlear pathology. Palva *et al.* (1978) obtained similar findings; the ABLB correctly showed a lack of recruitment in 65% of their group of 32 retrocochlear-impaired ears.

The variability in the accuracy of the ABLB test probably reflects the nature of the retrocochlear group. That is, retrocochlear ears with large tumors are more likely to have higher hit rates for the ABLB test than those with small tumors. This conclusion is supported by Johnson's (1977) finding that 72% of ears with large tumors were detected by the ABLB test whereas only 24% of ears with small tumors were detected by the ABLB test. The relatively low accuracy of the ABLB test in detection of retrocochlear pathology may also reflect the fact that acoustic tumors sometimes disrupt the cochlear blood supply, resulting in recruitment, as described earlier. This explanation, however, cannot account for the majority of retrocochlear cases with recruitment.

In summary, since the ABLB test has a low hit rate (percentage of retrocochlear ears identified by the test) and a moderately high false-positive rate (many cochlear ears do not show recruitment), can only be administered with certain (unilateral) losses, and some patients have difficulty performing loudness balances, it is not useful addition to the site-of-lesion battery.

B. MONAURAL LOUDNESS BALANCE TEST

The monaural loudness balance (MLB) test was developed to assess recruitment in cases with bilateral hearing impairment. In the MLB test, a loudness balance is done in one ear between a frequency at which the pure-tone threshold is normal and a frequency with a pure-tone hearing loss. The procedure for the MLB test is the same as that for the ABLB test except that two tones of different frequencies are presented to the same ear. One difficulty with the MLB is that tones of different frequency but of the same intensity are not necessarily perceived as equally loud. The results of the MLB need to be corrected according to the Fletcher and Munson equal-loudness contours (Denes & Naunton, 1950). The results are difficult to correct when the distance between the frequencies is large. Moreover, many patients find it difficult to do a loudness balance between tones heard in the same ear.

C. DIFFERENCE-LIMEN TESTS

The difference-limen tests of recruitment are based on the measurement of the rate of change in loudness as the inten-sity increases. The rate of change in loudness with increases in intensity is greater in recruiting than nonrecruiting ears. The change in intensity in dB which results in a just-barely-noticeable loudness change is termed the intensity difference limen (DL) for loudness. The presence or absence of recruitment is determined by measuring the intensity DL for loudness in the affected ear and comparing it to the DL in normal-hearing ears.

In Bekesy testing, the patient presses a button which changes the intensity in 2.5-dB steps when the sound is just barely heard and releases the button as soon as the sound becomes inaudible. This is done for tones varying in frequency from 100 to 10,000 Hz. The width of the tracking excursions on the graphic chart shows the intensity DL for loudness. From this record, the intensity DL for loudness can be measured and compared with that for normal-hearing ears to determine the presence or absence of recruitment. The problems with the excursion width of the Bekesy tracing as a measure of recruitment are the individual variability in the reaction time to respond to the change of loudness by pressing or releasing the button of the hand-held switch, a fatigue effect from listening to near-threshold tones (which affects the reliability of the tests), and the frequency dependency of the intensity DL at threshold (Denes & Naunton, 1950).

The Lüscher and Zwislocki (1948) recruitment test involves an amplitude-modulated tone. The size of the amplitude modulation which results in the perception of a loudness change is called the critical percentage modulation. The critical percentage modulation represents the intensity DL for loudness. If it is smaller than that in normal-hearing ears, recruitment is present; if it is the same size as that in normal-hearing ears, recruitment is absent. The test is done at 40 dB SL since the intensity DL in normal-hearing ears at this level is independent of frequency. Persons having a critical percentage modulation less than 8% were considered to have recruitment. Some problems with this test as a measure of recruitment include:

1. Persons with mild or nonsteeply sloping audiometric configurations obtained critical modulation percentages greater than 8% and some normal-hearing persons obtained critical modulation percentages less than 8% (Denes & Naunton, 1950).
2. Individual variability in judgment affected the reliability of the test (Denes & Naunton, 1950). Denes and Naunton (1950) suggested that the test may be measuring an intensity DL for quality rather than an intensity DL just for loudness.

Denes and Naunton (1950) developed another recruitment test based on the intensity DL for loudness. In this test, two tones of the same frequency are presented to an ear and the intensity of one of the tones is varied until a perception of a just-noticeable change in loudness results. This test was done at 4 and 44 dB SL. If the intensity DL increased or remained the same as the sensation level increased, recruitment was assumed to be present; if the intensity DL decreased as the sensation level increased, recruitment was assumed to be absent. Thus, the determination of recruitment was based on a relative rather than absolute measure of the intensity DL for loudness. Denes and Naunton (1950) contended that their DL recruitment test was more reliable than the Bekesy and Zwislocki test since comparison of intensity DLs obtained at the two levels resulted in elimination of the "effects of many of the individual and spurious variations in loudness judgments" (Denes & Naunton, 1950, p. 397).

Hirsh, Palva, and Goodman (1954) reported, however, that a modified version of the DL test did not differentiate between recruiting and nonrecruiting ears. Harris (1963) reported that the DL test had large intersubject variability, possibly associated with insufficient training of the subject taking the test. Thus, the difficulties in administering the test, which involves lengthy training of the subject, makes the DL test clinically infeasible as a test of recruitment. They also contended that the DL test for intensity was not a measure of recruitment. Further elaboration on this point is provided later in the section on the SISI test.

D. LOUDNESS-DISCOMFORT LEVEL TEST

Hood and Poole (1966) reported that patients with recruitment are intolerant of loud sounds. They proposed that the loudness discomfort level (LDL), the intensity level at which the patient first indicates a feeling of loudness discomfort, could be used as a test of recruitment. They found that the LDLs of patients with unilateral cochlear pathology and recruitment as indicated by the ABLB test were similar to those of normal-hearing persons. That is, the LDLs are obtained within the intensity range of 90–105 dB HL regardless of the degree of the hearing loss in normal-hearing and cochlear-impaired persons. The LDLs of patients with conductive and eighth-nerve disorders, however, are generally elevated to levels beyond 120 dB SPL. Therefore, the LDL test may be used to determine the presence or absence of loudness recruitment.

Kamm, Dirks, and Mickey (1978) found that a nonlinear relation exists between the magnitude of the hearing loss and the LDL. The LDLs in sensorineural hearing-impaired persons were increased with increases in hearing loss beyond 50 dB. They also found large intersubject variability so the LDL could not accurately be predicted from the magnitude of the hearing loss. Because of the dependence of the LDL upon the magnitude of the hearing loss beyond 50 dB HL and its large intersubject variability, the LDL test is not a clinically feasible measure of recruitment.

E. ACOUSTIC-REFLEX THRESHOLD

Recall from Chapter 3 that Metz (1946) reported that the acoustic-reflex threshold could be used as a test of loudness recruitment. He found that the acoustic-reflex thresholds of subjects with sensorineural hearing impairment were elicited at sensation levels markedly lower (<60 dB SL) than those of normal-hearing subjects. The conclusion that acoustic-reflex thresholds present at reduced sensation levels are indicative of loudness recruitment was based on the observation that the acoustic-reflex thresholds levels (in dB HL) of normal-hearing and cochlear hearing-impaired persons are similar.

Since the acoustic-reflex thresholds in ears with moderate or worse cochlear hearing impairment are not the same as those in normal-hearing hears, the basic premise of the Metz test with respect to loudness recruitment does not appear to hold. Hellman and Scharf (1984) contend, however, that there is a relation between the acoustic-reflex threshold and loudness. It remains a fact that the presence of acoustic-reflex thresholds at reduced sensation levels is consistent with cochlear pathology. On the other hand, the lack of reduced sensation levels for the acoustic-reflex threshold cannot be considered an indication that the ear is not cochlear-impaired (see Chapter 3).

IV. SHORT INCREMENT SENSITIVITY INDEX

Research interest on recruitment measurement by means of the intensity difference limen for loudness was stimulated by the need to develop a recruitment test that, unlike the ABLB, could be employed in persons with bilateral as well as unilateral hearing loss. The short increment sensitivity index (SISI) developed as an outgrowth of the intensity DL for loudness. The concept of the intensity DL for loudness was discussed earlier in this chapter in the section on the ABLB test. The intensity DL for loudness measure will be more fully explored in this section.

A. INTENSITY DIFFERENCE LIMEN FOR LOUDNESS

1. LÜSCHER–ZWISLOCKI METHOD

The test developed by Lüscher and Zwislocki (1948, 1949) was a modification of that developed by Riesz (1928). With Riesz's measure of the intensity DL, the subject's task was to determine whether an amplitude-modulated continuous tone was undulating (beating) or steady. Riesz (1928) employed a sinusoidal envelope for the continuous tone. The envelope of Riesz's stimulus is illustrated in Figure 15, which shows the waveform envelopes of the stimuli used in several investigations of the intensity DL

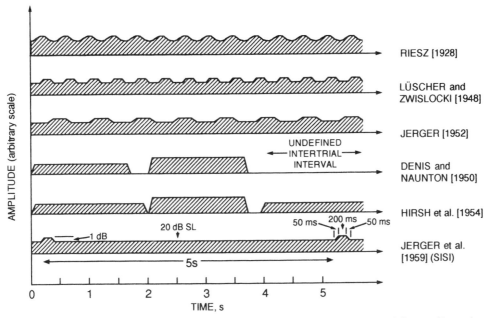

Figure 15 Envelopes of the stimuli used in several classical studies of intensity difference limens in normal-hearing and hearing-impaired listeners. Riesz (1928), Lüscher and Zwislocki (1948, 1949), Jerger (1952), and Jerger, Shedd, and Harford (1959) used amplitude modulation, whereas Denes and Naunton (1950) and Hirsh *et al.* (1954) used separate tone bursts differing in amplitude. The stimulus used for the SISI test, which is a continuous tone at 20 dB SL with a 1-dB increment presented every 5 s is shown at the bottom. The increment has a 200-ms steady state duration with a 50-ms linear transition so the total duration from beginning to end of the increment is 300 msec. Reprinted from Buus, Florentine, and Redden (1982a).

for loudness. Lüscher and Zwislocki (1948) used a tone that was amplitude modulated at a rate of 2/s. Each pulse had a trapezoidal rather than sinusoidal envelope with a rise–fall time of 80 ms as can be seen in Figure 15. The size of the amplitude modulations was expressed as a percentage of the mean intensity and was referred to as the percentage modulation. The intensity DL was the percentage modulation resulting in the perception of beating, also referred to as the critical percentage modulation. Lüscher and Zwislocki (1949) measured the critical percentage modulation at 40 dB SL since this is the level at which the intensity DL is independent of frequency. They found that recruiting ears had critical percentage modulations (intensity DLs) less than or equal to 8%. Nonrecruiting ears, on the other hand, had critical percentage modulations exceeding 8%. Lüscher (1951) reported that the IDLs were reduced in ears with cochlear impairment, normal in ears with retrocochlear pathology, and increased in ears with functional hearing loss. Neuberger (1950) reported that all of his 14 patients with unilateral recruiting losses (as evidenced by the results of ABLB testing) had reduced intensity DLs using the Lüscher–Zwislocki (1949) technique. König (1962) obtained similar findings.

Jerger (1952) changed the presentation level for the Lüscher–Zwislocki test from 40 to 15 dB SL, since the

literature shows that the intensity DL was most affected between 10 and 30 dB SL (Doerfler, 1948) in impaired ears. Jerger also employed a stimulus with a slightly different envelope (see Figure 15) and an ascending instead of a descending presentation approach. Jerger (1952) found that all of his 53 patients with reduced intensity DLs had nonconductive hearing impairments. Some of these patients with reduced intensity DLs received ABLB testing which revealed the presence of recruitment. Most of the patients with enlarged intensity DLs had functional hearing loss and most with normal intensity DLs had conductive hearing loss or presbycusis. The overlap in categories was reduced when the relative measure of the intensity DL was evaluated by comparing the intensity DLs at 10 and 40 dB SL (Jerger, 1953). Denes and Naunton (1950) had also employed a relative measure of the intensity DL but their comparison levels were 4 and 44 dB SL.

Several investigators (Lidén & Nilsson, 1950; Lund-Iversen, 1952; Zöllner & Hallbrock, 1952a,b) obtained intensity DL findings which contradicted those reported by Lüscher and Zwislocki (1949), Lüscher (1951), Neuberger (1950), and Jerger (1952, 1953). For example, Lidén and Nilsson (1950) found larger intersubject variability and overlap in the intensity DLs between normal-hearing and hearing-impaired persons. Lund-Iverson (1952) failed to obtain agreement between the results of the ABLB test and the Lüscher–Zwislocki intensity DL test in his group of 81 patients. Zöllner and Hallbrock (1952a,b) reported that their cochlear-impaired patients had intensity DLs larger than those reported by Lüscher and Zwislocki (1949) and Lüscher (1951). Zöllner and Hallbrock (1952a,b) found that nonauditory factors such as a person's occupation could affect the intensity DL; musicians, for example, had smaller intensity DLs than other normal-hearing listeners.

Lüscher (1951) modified the intensity DL test to employ a presentation level of at least 80 dB HL; levels above 80 dB HL which represented at least 15–20 dB SL were employed in persons with hearing-loss magnitudes exceeding 60 dB HL. The rationale underlying this modification was twofold. Recruitment is present at this level and the intensity DL at this level is small (4–6%) in normal-hearing persons, indicating that the task of making loudness judgments was simplified. Complete recruitment was assumed to be present if a hearing-impaired person obtained an intensity DL of 4–6% at this presentation level. Larger values implied the presence of partial recruitment and still larger values implied the absence of recruitment. König (1962) supported the use of this modified Lüscher–Zwislocki test.

Several problems affected the clinical utility of the amplitude-modulation approach to measurement of the intensity DL. Lüscher and Zwislocki (1949) acknowledged that the critical percentage modulation could exceed 8% in recruiting ears if the hearing loss was mild (i.e., less than 30 dB HL) or if the audiometric configuration was insufficiently steep. They also observed that normal-hearing listeners could obtain intensity DLs less than 8% with practice. Denes and Naunton (1950) contended that individual differences in judgment influenced the intensity DL and that the intensity DL actually was a DL for quality rather than for loudness. Jerger, Shedd, and Harford (1959) criticized the amplitude-modulation intensity DL test since the task of judging when the tone was just perceptibly beating was difficult for the patient and the tester was often forced to make a subjective judgment of the patient's responses, which were not always straightforward.

2. DENES–NAUNTON METHOD

Denes and Naunton (1950) used a technique to measure the intensity DL that differed from the amplitude-modulation technique. Their technique is often referred to as the "memory method" of measuring the intensity DL. Denes and Naunton's (1950) technique involved the sequential presentation of two tones at the same frequency to the same ear. This is illustrated in Figure 15. The intensity of the second tone was varied until the patient reported that it was just noticeably louder than the first tone. Then the intensity of the second tone was varied until the patient reported that it was just noticeably softer than the first tone.

The intensity DL derived with this method in fact represents twice the intensity DL, since two increments of loudness, from less to equally loud and from equally loud to louder are measured. Since the slope of the loudness curve is greater for recruiting than nonrecruiting ears, the intensity DL should be smaller in recruiting than nonrecruiting ears. Denes and Naunton (1950) reported that there was a large overlap in the intensity DLs of their normal-hearing and recruiting ears. They attributed this overlap to intersubject variability in loudness judgment, attention level, and so forth. To eliminate these effects, Denes and Naunton made the intensity DL test a relative rather than an absolute one. The intensity DLs were compared at two presentation levels: 4 and 44 dB SL. If the intensity DL decreased with increasing sensation level, the ear was assumed to be nonrecruiting. If the intensity DL increased or remained unchanged with increasing sensation level, the ear was assumed to be recruiting. Denes and Naunton proposed that the intensity DL in recruiting ears would increase or remain the same as intensity increased since the loudness growth is most rapid near threshold. They found that only 3 of their 43 recruiting ears (as defined by the results of ABLB tests) did not show increasing or unchanging intensity DLs as the sensation level increased. The results for 2 of these 3 cases were attributed to crosshearing.

The amplitude-modulation approach resulted in intensity DLs that differed in size from those measured using the memory approach. For example, Hirsh et al. (1954), using a modification of the memory approach (see Figure 15 for a description of the stimuli), reported essentially equivalent intensity DLs for their normal-hearing and hearing-impaired ears. Also, the intensity DL obtained with the memory method was essentially frequency independent (Floretine, 1981; Jesteadt, Wier, & Green, 1977; Penner, Leshowitz, Cudahy, & Ricard, 1974) rather than frequency dependent as demonstrated with the amplitude-modulation approach (Riesz, 1928). Harris (1963) compared the intensity DL using the memory method with that using the amplitude-modulation method in a patient with a unilateral hearing loss and reported that the intensity DL in the impaired ear compared with the normal ear was reduced with the former method and equivalent with the latter method.

3. BEKESY

Some researchers have contended that the excursion size of the Bekesy sweep-frequency audiogram represents the intensity DL. (Further details about Bekesy testing will be given later in this chapter.) Therefore, when recruitment is present, the excursion size (intensity DL) is narrowed. When recruitment is absent, the excursion size (intensity DL) remains unchanged. Denes and Naunton (1950) reported that the excursion size was an inaccurate measure of intensity DL because of the considerable intersubject variability in the response time, that is, the time to respond to loudness change by pressing on the button controlling the intensity. The intersubject variability in response time was attributed to differences in sense of rhythm and the fatigue effect of listening to near-threshold sounds. Hirsh *et al.* (1954) contended that the excursion size reflected moment-to-moment variability in the threshold. Harbert, Young, and Weiss (1969) reported that the correlation between excursion size of the continuous tone and recruitment was not "close." "Reduced amplitude therefore represents a defect in the ability to continue to hear a sound decreasing from threshold. We consider this a manifestation of rapid adaptation which takes place in milliseconds" (Harbert *et al.*, 1969, p. 441).

4. Intensity DL as a Measure of Recruitment

Hirsh *et al.* (1954) contended that the intensity DL was not a measure of recruitment. They contended that the fact that a particular intensity change resulting in a greater change in loudness sensation for a recruiting than a nonrecruiting ear did not necessarily indicate that a particular intensity change was more readily detected by a recruiting than a nonrecruiting ear. They also stated that the assumption underlying the concept that recruitment was related to the intensity DL was erroneous. That is, Fechner's law, which states that the number of just-noticeable-difference (jnd) levels increases as loudness increases, does not hold. Furthermore, the fact that loudness increases more rapidly at low than high frequencies implies that the intensity DL should be reduced at low frequencies. The results of research, however, indicate that the intensity DL obtained with the amplitude-modulation method is larger at low than at mid and high frequencies (Riesz, 1928) and the intensity DL obtained with the memory method is frequency independent (Dimmick & Olson, 1941). Also, the fact that loudness growth is most rapid around threshold implies that the intensity DL should be smallest at the low intensities. Research using the amplitude-modulation approach however, shows that the intensity DL is in fact reduced at high intensities and increased at low intensities in both recruiting and nonrecruiting ears (Neuberger, 1950).

Another line of evidence against the concept of intensity DL as a measure of recruitment comes from the finding that the intensity DL obtained with the memory method fails to differentiate among normal-hearing, nonrecruiting hearing-impaired, and recruiting hearing-impaired ears (Hirsh *et al.*, 1954).

Lastly, several researchers found that the intensity DL did not decrease as the signal-to-noise ratio decreased, regardless of the technique used to measure the intensity DL. A decrease in the intensity DL with decreases in signal-to-noise ratio would have reflected a recruitment-like phenomenon similar to that seen when there is incomplete masking of a pure tone with a noise (L'amore & Rodenburg, 1980).

B. DESCRIPTION OF THE SISI TEST

Jerger *et al.* (1959) asserted that the crucial issue regarding the significance of the intensity DL was not whether it was related to loudness recruitment. Rather, the issue was whether the ability to hear small changes in sound intensity was a predictor of cochlear impairment. Jerger *et al.* (1959) noted that hypersensitivity to small changes in intensity may be unrelated to the intensity DL.

> For example, it may be that behavior simulating abnormally acute differential sensitivity will arise only through the use of a test methodology involving relatively sustained stimulation. At the same time, the patient's intensity difference limen might be entirely normal when defined by a methodology not involving sustained stimulation (e.g., the method of constant stimulus differences. (Jerger *et al.*, 1959, p. 83)

Guided by the principle that persons with cochlear impairment might demonstrate hypersensitivity to small intensity increments superimposed on a sustained rather than an interrupted tone, Jerger *et al.* (1959) developed the SISI test. They simplified the task of determining loudness change by requiring the patient merely to indicate whenever increments were heard rather than to indicate when a tone began to wobble with the amplitude-modulation technique of measuring the intensity DL. To simplify the decision of when the increments were heard, they employed a stimulus with a temporal pattern similar to that employed in the quantal psychophysical method (see Figure 15). The test stimulus had a rise–fall time of 50 ms and had a total duration of 300 ms. Each increment was 1 dB, superimposed upon a continuous tone at 5-s intervals. The test presentation level was 20 dB SL. The patient was instructed to indicate whenever he or she was certain there was a little jump in loudness and not to respond if he or she was uncertain whether or not there was a little jump in loudness. A test run consisted of 28 increments. The first 5 increments were 5 dB in size, serving to familiarize the patient with the task. Then the run of 20 1-dB increments was given. To prevent false-positive and false-negative responses, 3 increments were inserted between the 5th and 6th, 10th and 11th, and 15th and 16th increments. The size of the interspersed increment depended upon the nature of the previous responses. If the patient responded to 2 or fewer of the previous 5 increments, the sixth increment was increased to 5 dB. If the patient responded to 3 or more of the previous 5 increments, the sixth increment was decreased to 0 dB. Responses to these interspersed items were not scored.

The short increment sensitivity index was derived from the responses to the 20 1-dB increments and was expressed as a percentage, with each response equivalent to a score of 5%. Jerger *et al.* (1959) suggested representing the scores on a "SISI-gram." Figure 16 illustrates a SISI-gram. On a SISI-gram, the "O" represents the right-ear score, the "X" represents the left-ear score, and the shaded area between 0 and 10% represents the range of scores for normal-hearing ears. Jerger (1961) considered scores between 60 and 100% to be positive, that is, indicative of cochlear pathology, scores between 20 and 55% to be questionable, and scores between 0 and 15% to be consistent with conductive or retrocochlear pathology.

1. EFFECTS OF PATHOLOGY

Jerger *et al.* (1959) presented their findings for the SISI test administered at 1000 and 4000 Hz to 75 patients with various types of hearing loss. They found that none of their 21 patients with conductive pathology obtained a SISI score exceeding 15% at either test frequency. None of their 9 patients with acoustic trauma had SISI scores exceeding

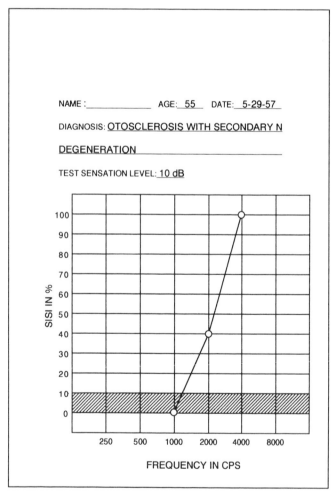

Figure 16 SISI-gram of a patient with otosclerosis accompanied by secondary sensorineural loss. Modified from Jerger, Shedd, and Harford (1959).

40% at 1000 Hz where the hearing was normal, although all had scores exceeding 70% at 4000 Hz, the region of greatest hearing loss. All of their 8 patients with Meniere's disease had scores exceeding 65% at both frequencies. In their 34 presbycusic patients, the SISI scores were more variable, ranging from 0 to 100%. Thus, high SISI scores traditionally are associated with cochlear pathology and low SISI scores are associated with normal-hearing, conductive, and retrocochlear-impaired ears.

2. CRITERIA FOR SCORING

The following various criteria for a negative score have been used: (a) 0–15%, (b) 0–20%, (c) 0–25%, (d) 0–30%, and (e) 0–35%. The following various criteria for a questionable score have been used: (a) 20–55%, (b) 35–55%, (c) 35–60%, (d) 25–55%, (e) 40–70%, and (f) 25–75%. The following various criteria for a positive score have been used: (a) 60–100%, (b) 65–100%, (c) 70–100%, (d) 75–100%, and (e) 80–100%. Pennington and Martin (1972) reported that most audiologists consider positive SISI scores to be between 80 and 100%. Buus, Florentine, and Redden (1982a) suggested that a SISI score falling between 80 and 100% not be considered a positive score unless the patient has been given sufficient pre-test practice. Since most SISI scores fall at the extreme ends of the range, it appears that defining a score as positive if it exceeds 55% (as recommended by Jerger, 1961) rather than 80% would probably not decrease the number of ears identified as retrocochlear impaired. Similarly, defining a SISI score as negative if it falls below 35 rather than 20% probably would not increase the number of cochlear-impaired ears misidentified as retrocochlear impaired.

3. RELATION OF PRESENTATION LEVEL TO THE SISI SCORE

Young and Harbert (1967) reported that the SISI scores of 5 trained, normal-hearing listeners exceeded 60% at dB SPLs greater than or equal to 45 at frequencies between 250 and 4000 Hz. Their distribution of SISI scores were similar across all frequencies. These findings were substantiated by the study of Harbert *et al.* (1969) except that high scores near 100% were obtained at intensities greater than or equal to 60 dB SPL in their group of 33 naive normal-hearing listeners. Their distribution of SISI scores in the affected and unaffected ears of unilateral cochlear-impaired subjects, presbycusic subjects, and congenital sensorineural hearing-impaired subjects showed a pattern similar to that of the trained normal-hearing subjects. That is, the SISI score exceeded 65% at intensities greater than or equal to 60 dB SPL. The SISI scores of unaffected ears of the unilateral hearing-impaired subjects differed from those of the trained normal-hearing subjects only in the intensity range between 45 and 60 dB SPL, suggesting that SISI scores in this intensity range may be affected by practice, motivation level, and intersubject variability. Differences in the SISI scores between the cochlear-impaired and normal-hearing ears are observed only when the SISI scores are plotted as a function of intensity in dB SL. When the data are plotted in dB SL, the SISI scores in cochlear-impaired ears are positive regardless of the sensation level whereas positive scores in normal-hearing ears are obtained only at sensation levels exceeding 20 dB.

The results of Young and Harbert (1967) indicate that the pattern of distribution of SISI scores from conductive-impaired ears when the air–bone gap is subtracted from the presentation level in dB SPL is similar to that for normal-hearing ears. That is, positive SISI scores are obtained whenever the presentation level entering the cochlea exceeds 60 dB SPL. Negative SISI scores are obtained in retrocochlear-impaired ears regardless of the presentation level.

Harbert *et al.* (1969) reported that the SISI scores of 17 patients with mild cochlear hearing loss were similar to those of normal-hearing persons when the data were plotted as a function of dB SL. That is, negative SISI scores were obtained in the hearing-impaired ear when the presentation level was less than or equal to 20 dB. Positive SISI scores were obtained in these affected ears, however, when the carrier tone was presented at levels exceeding 55 dB SPL. Consequently, ears with cochlear hearing impairment may give negative SISI scores if the presentation level does not exceed 20 dB SL and the hearing loss is mild since, in these cases, the dB SPL reaching the cochlea would not reach 60 dB. Similar findings were obtained by other investigators (Bartholomeus & Swisher, 1971; Harford, 1967; Owens, 1965a; Swisher, Stephens, & Doehring, 1966).

4. Reliability

Jerger *et al.* (1959) investigated the SISI scores of a patient on whom the SISI test had been administered in the right ear at 1000 and 4000 Hz a total of 8 times over a period of 10 months by 3 different testers. The diagnosis for the right ear was otitis media with secondary nerve degeneration. The loss at 1000 Hz was primarily conductive whereas the loss at 4000 Hz had a sensorineural as well as a conductive component. At 1000 Hz, over the 8 sessions the SISI scores ranged from 0 to 5%. At 4000 Hz, over the 8 sessions the SISI scores ranged from 65 to 95%.

Jerger (1962a) obtained test–retest scores in 27 patients. Test–retest reliability was poor at 250 Hz ($r = 0.10$), moderately high at 1000 Hz ($r = 0.72$), and high at 4000 Hz ($r = 0.88$). The poor reliability at 2000 Hz was spurious since the total range of scores at that frequency was restricted. Thus, test–retest reliability of the SISI test was good at the mid to high frequencies.

Jerger *et al.* (1959) investigated the split-half reliability of the SISI test. The analysis was based on 129 SISI records.

The Spearman–Brown correlation coefficients were 0.72, 0.95, and 0.96 at 250, 1000, and 4000 Hz, respectively. Thus, the correlation was moderately high at 250 Hz and very high at 1000 and 4000 Hz. Jerger *et al.* concluded that the 20-item SISI test had sufficiently good internal consistency. These findings were substantiated by Griffing and Tuck in their analysis of 300 SISI records.

Griffing and Tuck (1963) reported that a small practice effect was present. They also reported that the test–retest reliability was only slightly diminished when the number of increments was reduced from 20 to 10. On the other hand, Fulton and Spradlin (1972) found a significant practice effect, particularly when the first SISI score was questionable. Findings contrary to those reported by Fulton and Spradlin (1972) were obtained by Fournier and Jirsa (1976), who reported the absence of an order effect for frequency.

5. Modifications

a. High-Level SISI

Thompson (1963) suggested administering the SISI test at a presentation level of 75 dB HL. He reasoned that, at this level, normal-hearing, conductive-impaired, and cochlear-impaired subjects would obtain positive scores whereas only retrocochlear-impaired ears would obtain negative SISI scores. This rationale was confirmed by the results of SISI testing on 2 patients with a unilateral hearing loss due to suspected acoustic neuroma. Koch, Bartels, and Rupp (1969) observed that the SISI scores of normal-hearing and cochlear-impaired subjects increased as the carrier-tone level increased beyond 20 dB SL whereas those of their 5 patients with retrocochlear pathology remained low as the carrier-tone level increased. Cooper and Owen (1976) recommended a minimum presentation level of 90 dB HL. In cases where the hearing loss was greater than or equal to 70 dB, Cooper and Owen recommended a 20 dB SL presentation level—lower, if 20 dB SL exceeded audiometric limits.

Sanders, Josey, and Glasscock (1978) recommended a presentation level of 75 dB HL as proposed by Thompson (1963) since this level adequately separated retrocochlear- from cochlear-impaired ears. They recommended against higher levels since they found that these levels resulted in positive SISI scores in patients with retrocochlear pathology. Young and Harbert (1967) recommended administering the SISI test at 70 dB SPL or more if required for audibility. They concluded that a positive score at this level indicates that the ear is responding like a normal-hearing ear; a negative score indicates the presence of abnormal adaptation.

b. Increment Size

Harbert *et al.* (1969) suggested using an increment size of 1.5 dB on the basis of the findings by Weiss, Harbert, and Wilpezeski (1967) that the minimum increment that can be detected in normal-hearing and recruiting ears fell in the range of 0.5 to 1.5 dB and the minimum increment that could be detected in abnormally adapting ears exceeded 1.5 dB.

Hanley and Utting (1965) attempted to determine which SISI increment size (0.50, 0.75, and 1.00 dB) resulted in a SISI score equal to or exceeding 60% in no greater than 5% of the normal-hearing population. They administered the SISI test using 3 different increment sizes to 48 normal-hearing adults at the conventional presentation level of 20 dB SL. They reported that 33% of the subjects who received the 1-dB increments, 4% of the subjects who received the 0.75-dB increments, and 0% of the subjects who received the 0.50-dB increments obtained SISI scores equal to or exceeding 60%. It still remained questionable whether the use of the 0.75- or 0.50-dB increments was sufficiently large to allow patients with cochlear involvement to obtain positive SISI scores. Therefore, Hanley and Utting administered the SISI test using the 0.75- and 0.50-dB increments at 4000 Hz to 11 patients with cochlear pathology who had obtained a score of at least 70% on the standard SISI test with the 1-dB increment. They found that only 1 of the 11 patients obtained a score below 70% for the 0.75-dB increment but 4 of the 11 obtained scores below 70% for the 0.50-dB increment. They also reported that the average SISI score for the 11 sensorineural hearing-impaired subjects was significantly higher with the 1-dB than with the 0.75-dB increment, although all subjects obtained scores well above 60% for both increment sizes. In conclusion, Hanley and Utting recommended the use of the 0.75-dB increment to separate cochlear-impaired from retrocochlear-impaired ears. Nevertheless, Hanley and Utting's results should be viewed with caution. A comparison of the SISI scores obtained with the 1-dB increment in Hanley and Utting's normal-hearing subjects with those obtained in Jerger's (1962b) normal-hearing subjects reveals that the mean scores were significantly different (10% in the Jerger study as opposed to 42% in the Hanley and Utting study). Hanley and Utting could not account for the discrepant findings.

Sanders and Simpson (1966) evaluated the SISI scores using a 0.75- and a 1.00-dB increment in 24 normal-hearing listeners and 9 cochlear-impaired listeners. Their mean of 19.4% for the 1-dB increment in the normal-hearing listeners was similar to Jerger's (1962b) mean of 10%. All 9 of their cochlear-impaired patients receiving the 1-dB increment but only 7 of these 9 receiving the 0.75-dB increment obtained scores exceeding 60%. Furthermore, only 1 of their 24 subjects with normal hearing who received the 1.00-dB increment obtained a score exceeding 60%. Therefore, Sanders and Simpson (1966) concluded, contrary to Hanley and Utting, that the 1.00-dB increment was preferable to the 0.75-dB increment.

Owens (1965a) reported that a substantial number of his retrocochlear-impaired ears could hear 2- and 3-dB increments. Thus, his findings argue against the presentation of increments larger than 1 dB to retrocochlear-impaired persons as suggested by Young and Harbert (1967).

6. DECAY OF THE CARRIER TONE

Owens (1965a) reported that some patients commented that the carrier tone faded away and the increments appeared to arise out of silence during the SISI test. Hughes (1968) reported that their 11 patients with Meniere's disease, 4 patients with vascular disease, and 3 patients with eighth-nerve pathology had positive SISI scores despite having tone decay greater than or equal to 20 dB at all frequencies tested, as evidenced by the modified Rosenberg tone-decay test (presentation level of 5 rather than 0 dB SL). Thus, despite the fading of the carrier tone, high SISI scores were obtained, even in the case of retrocochlear pathology. Hughes (1968) concluded that the validity of the SISI test was not compromised by the fading of the carrier tone to inaudibility. Bartholomeus and Swisher (1971) reported that the SISI scores of subjects with no tone decay at all are higher than those of subjects having some nonsignificant (5–20 dB) tone decay when the two groups are equated for hearing loss. Buus, Florentine, and Redden (1982b) suggested asking the patient what was heard before reporting the obtained SISI score.

7. CONTRALATERAL MASKING

Blegvad (1969) evaluated the effect of masking with a broad-band noise at 80 dB SPL on the SISI scores of the affected ears of 32 patients with unilateral losses of predominantly cochlear origin. His data show that, although masking did not alter the total number of positive scores, it caused a few negative scores to fall in the questionable range. The masking resulted in dramatic improvement in SISI in a few of the subjects. Shimizu (1969) reported that, although all of his 12 subjects with normal hearing or conductive impairment obtained negative scores without contralateral masking, 7 obtained positive scores with contralateral masking using a broad-band noise at 40 dB SL. Swisher, Dudley, and Doehring (1969) used contralateral sawtooth and broad-band noise masking in listeners with normal hearing. The masking improved the ability to hear 1-dB increments only when the carrier tone exceeded 38 dB SPL. Below 38 dB SPL, masking did not have an effect on differential intensity discrimination. Blegvad and Terkildsen (1967) reported that the mean SISI score improved from 22 to 46% when contralateral masking with a broad-band noise of 70 dB SPL was employed. The improvement in SISI scores with contralateral masking is supported by the finding of Osterhammel, Terkildsen, and Arndal (1970), who showed that the evoked cortical response increased significantly when contralateral masking with an 80 dB SPL broad-band noise was employed.

Perhaps the increase in SISI score is related to the release-from-masking phenomenon. That is, internal noise such as blood rushing may sometimes mask out the increment. Consequently, when noise is added to the contralateral ear, it is then perceived as spatially separate from the increments, which can then be heard. If this hypothesis holds, then the release-of-masking phenomenon should occur in normal-hearing persons and improvement of SISI scores should result from contralateral masking in normal-hearing persons but not in diagnostic groups such as presbycusics, in whom the masking-level difference has been reported to be reduced.

Buus *et al.* (1982b) suggested a midline position between that advocated by Studebaker (1973) on the one hand, who asserted that contralateral masking usually is unnecessary, and Priede and Coles (1974) and Martin (1978) on the other hand, who suggested the use of contralateral masking during SISI testing whenever the possibility of cross-hearing existed. Buus *et al.* (1982b) took into account (a) the finding that negative SISI scores are obtained in normal-hearing and cochlear-impaired listeners at levels below 35–45 dB SPL, and (b) the finding that normal-hearing and cochlear-impaired ears obtain high SISI scores above approximately 45–60 dB SPL. Therefore, Buus *et al.* (1982b) suggested using contralateral masking only when the level of crossover into the nontest ear exceeds 30 dB SPL, provided that the bone-conduction threshold is below the crossover level of the SISI carrier tone. That is, masking of the contralateral ear should be employed whenever the SISI presentation level minus the interaural attenuation (IA − 40 dB) exceeds 30 dB, provided that the bone-conduction threshold is less than 30 dB in the nontest ear at the test frequency. Bearing in mind the fact that contralateral masking can increase the SISI score and the finding by Young and Wenner (1968) that very low SISI scores are obtained at signal-to-noise ratios of + 10 dB or less, Buus *et al.* (1982) suggested the following formula for the minimum effective masking level for the SISI test.

$$EM_{SISI} = HL_{SISI} - (IA + 10 \text{ dB}) + ABG_{nte}$$

where EM is the minimum effective masking level, HL is the presentation level, and ABG is the air–bone gap in the nontest ear. Buus *et al.* (1982b) suggested that the amount of masking in ears with severe hearing impairment can be reduced by reducing the presentation level to 10 dB SL, since research shows that cochlear-impaired persons obtain high SISI scores even at a sensation level of 10 dB.

8. Nature of Auditory Function

The results of SISI testing employing an increment superimposed on the carrier tone (modification of the amplitude-modulation intensity DL method) differ from the results of testing with the tonebursts (intensity DL using the memory method). Buus *et al.* (1982b) suggested that the former technique requires the ability to detect the onset of an intensity increase whereas the latter requires a comparison of the loudness of one tone with that of another tone. Buus *et al.* (1982b) based their conclusion on the results of studies by Harris (1963), Nelson, Eruklar, and Bryan (1966), and Evans and Whitfield (1965). Harris (1963) found that intensity discrimination improved as the rise-time of the modulation decreased. Nelson *et al.* (1966) reported that some neurons in the inferior colliculus respond to the onset of the intensity increase. Evans and Whitfield reported that some neurons in the cortex respond to the onset of an intensity increase. Buus *et al.* (1982b) suggested that detection of onset of an increase in intensity is not the sole mechanism underlying detection of increments superimposed upon a carrier tone, since duration has a marked effect on the intensity DL that is even greater than the effect of rise–fall time as shown by Harris (1963).

Buus *et al.* (1982b) proposed another mechanism for the detection of SISI increments on the basis of the study by Eggermont and Odenthal (1974). Eggermont and Odenthal reported that the input–output function of the action potential has two components, a slowly rising section followed by a rapidly rising section. Buus *et al.* (1982b) hypothesized that the slowly rising component was consistent with low SISI scores whereas the sharply rising component was consistent with high SISI scores. Buus *et al.* (1982b) stated that Swisher (1966) hypothesized that low SISI scores reflect the participation of the outer hair cells and high SISI scores reflect the participation of the inner hair cells. Buus *et al.* (1982b) asserted that Swisher's hypothesis is untenable in light of the fact that temporal-bone studies of patients with Meniere's disease, who usually obtain high SISI scores, indicate that both the inner and outer hair cells generally appear unaffected (Schuknecht, 1974).

9. Pediatric Population

Fulton and Spradlin (1974) employed a modification of the SISI test in severely retarded children ranging in age from 10 to 19 years. The increment size was 1.25 dB, with a duration of 357 ms, and an interstimulus interval of 14 s, provided no responses were given during the interstimulus interval. The children were rewarded with candy when appropriate responses were made. One subject, who was given both the standard and modified SISI procedures, obtained similar SISI scores for both versions of the test. Fulton and Spradlin (1974) concluded that the modified SISI yielded results essentially similar to those for the standard SISI in difficult-to-test children.

Owens (1979) suggested that the SISI test could be successfully employed in children without mental impairment who are as young as 6–7 years if play responses were employed. Mártony (1974) reported that the intensity DL obtained with the memory method decreased markedly with age, and plateaued at about 11 years of age in a group of 26 severely hearing-impaired and 23 normal-hearing subjects. On the other hand, Fior (1972) reported the lack of a developmental effect on the intensity DL obtained with the amplitude-modulation technique in 70 normal-hearing subjects ranging in age from 3 to 13 years. The studies by Fior (1972) and Mártony (1974) also differed with respect to presentation level. Because the issue of developmental effects has not been settled, Buus *et al.* (1982a) suggested interpreting the SISI scores cautiously in children 11 years of age or younger.

10. ACCURACY

Buus *et al.* (1982a) evaluated the results of 12 SISI studies between 1959 and 1977 on normal-hearing and pathological ears. The SISI scores were characterized as low (−), questionable (?), or high (+) (as defined by each investigator) for patients with normal hearing, conductive pathology, retrocochlear pathology, Meniere's disease, acoustic trauma, presbycusis, and undefined cochlear pathology. Across the twelve studies, the results indicate that approximately 7% of the normal hearing, 8% of the conductive impaired, and 31% of the retrocochlear impaired obtained positive scores; approximately 16% of the Meniere's or hydrops group, 14% of the acoustic trauma group, 21% of the presbycusis group, and 16% of the undefined cochlear group obtained negative scores. The percentage of questionable scores did not exceed 9% for any group. Inspection of the data reported by Buus *et al.* revealed that

1. When positive scores do occur in normal-hearing ears, they occur primarily at 4000 Hz.
2. The SISI scores of conductive-impaired, normal-hearing, and retrocochlear-impaired ears are similar.
3. The SISI score is strikingly frequency dependent in cochlear hearing-impaired ears. That is, negative scores are obtained in many of the cochlear-impaired subjects at 250–1000 Hz, with the largest number seen at 250 Hz. This frequency dependency indicates that the SISI score is related to the magnitude of the hearing loss. For example, most patients with acoustic trauma obtain low scores at 250–1000 Hz where the hearing is normal whereas the majority obtain high scores at the high frequencies—the region of the hearing loss. This finding is consistent with Jerger's (1973) statement that "cochlear signals are usually evident only at frequencies above 1000 Hz. The SISI score, for example, will usually be quite low (0–20%) at 250 and 500 Hz, questionable (40–60%) at 1000 Hz, and very high (80–100%) at 2000, 3000, and 4000 Hz" (p. 81).
4. Most SISI scores fall into the negative or positive category and very few fall into the questionable category.

As shown by the findings of Buus *et al.* (1982a) and other investigators, the SISI test is a poor detector of retro-cochlear pathology. For example, Brand and Rosenberg (1963) reported that the SISI scores of their retrocochlear-impaired ears ranged from 0–100%. Shapiro and Naunton (1967) reported that 2 of their 3 patients with retrocochlear pathology had preoperative SISI scores exceeding 70%. Hughes (1968) found that all of his 3 subjects with surgically-confirmed eighth-nerve tumors obtained scores exceeding 80% at all frequencies tested, despite the fact that they had tone decay exceeding 25 dB at these frequencies.

Buus *et al.* (1982a) suggested that some patients with retrocochlear pathology may also have cochlear impairments resulting from interruptions in cochlear blood supply caused by the pressure of the tumor on the internal auditory artery (Benitez, Lopez-Rios, & Novon, 1967; Perez de Moura, 1967) or alterations in the chemical composition of the intracochlear fluids (Perez de Moura, 1967). This hypothesis was discussed earlier in this chapter in relation to the ABLB test and represents an extension of the hypothesis by Dix and Hallpike (1958). In cases where there is cochlear involvement secondary to the acoustic tumor, the SISI scores could be positive. Nevertheless, this explanation can account for only some of the retrocochlear ears with high SISI scores.

Very few studies have been done on the accuracy of the modified SISI test (high presentation level). Turner *et al.* (1984) reported that the modified SISI test, on average, based on a total of 5 studies and 286 ears, yielded negative scores in 69% of retrocochlear-impaired ears and positive SISI scores in 90% of cochlear-impaired ears.

11. PREDICTIVE VALUE

According to L'amoré and Rodenburg (1980), the predictive value of the SISI test is the probability that a positive SISI score represents a cochlear-impaired ear. This probability is dependent upon the prevalence rate of cochlear and retrocochlear pathology. L'amoré and Rodenburg suggested that the prevalence of cochlear impairment was the probability that a cochlear impairment (Co+) was present [i.e., Pr(Co+)]. When considering only the population of sensorineural hearing-impaired ears, the prevalence of noncochlear impairment (Co−) is equivalent to the probability of retrocochlear (RE) impairments [i.e., Pr(Co−) which is the same as Pr(RE)].

The sensitivity of the SISI test is defined as the probability of a positive score (T+) given that the impairment is cochlear [Pr(T+/Co+). The specificity of the SISI test is the probability that the SISI score is negative (T−) given that the impairment is noncochlear or retrocochlear [Pr(T−/Co−) or Pr(T−/RE). The predictive value of the SISI test with respect to cochlear impairment is the probability that the hearing impairment is cochlear given a positive score, that is, Pr(Co+/T+). L'amoré and Rodenburg (1980) used Bayes's theorem to yield the following formula for the predictive value of the SISI test with respect to cochlear impairment:

$$Pr(CO+/T+) = \frac{Pr(T+/Co+) \times Pr(Co+)}{[Pr(T+/Co+) \times Pr(Co+)] + [Pr(T+/RE) \times Pr(RE)]}$$

Similarly, the predictive value of the SISI test with respect to retrocochlear impairment is the probability that a hearing impairment is retrocochlear given a negative score. Again, using Bayes's theorem, the predictive value of the SISI test with respect to retrocochlear impairment is represented by the formula

$$Pr(Re/T-) = \frac{Pr(T-/RE) \times Pr(RE)}{[Pr(T-/RE) \times Pr(RE)] + [Pr(T-/Co+) \times Pr(Co+)]}$$

Based on previous research findings indicating that approximately 60% of cochlear ears demonstrate positive SISI scores, the probability of a positive SISI score given a cochlear impairment is set as $Pr(T+/Co+) = 0.60$. Similarly, previous research indicates that approximately 55% of patients with retrocochlear pathology obtain negative scores. Hence, the probability of a negative score given a retrocochlear impairment is set as $Pr(T-/RE) = 0.55$. Therefore, the probability of a positive score given a retrocochlear impairment is set as $Pr(T+/RE) = 0.45$. L'amoré and Rodenburg assumed that 80% of sensorineural hearing-impaired ears in the population are cochlear-impaired and the remaining 20% are retrocochlear-impaired. Thus, the prevalence of cochlear-impaired ears or the probability of a cochlear impairment given a sensorineural hearing impairment is $Pr(Co+) = 0.80$. Similarly, the prevalence of retrocochlear impairment or the probability of a retrocochlear impairment given a sensorineural hearing loss is $Pr(RE) = 0.20$. Substituting the values of 0.80, 0.55, 0.60, 0.20, and 0.45 into the formula for the predictive value of a positive result yields the moderately predictive value of 0.84 for the SISI test with respect to cochlear pathology.

The probability of a negative score given a cochlear impairment is defined as $Pr(T-/Co+)$ and represents $1 - Pr(T+/Co+) = 1 - 0.60 = 0.40$. Substituting the values of 0.55, 0.84, 0.20, and 0.80 into the formula yields a low predictive value of 0.26 for the SISI test with respect to retrocochlear pathology. In summary, 84% of the time the positive SISI score represents a cochlear-impaired ear whereas only 26% of the time a negative SISI score represents a retrocochlear-impaired ear. These predictive values were obtained by eliminating questionable results, that is, considering only positive and negative results.

Buus *et al.* (1982a) employed similar formulas for the predictive value of the SISI test. That is, the predictive value of the SISI test with respect to cochlear impairment was given by the formula

$$Pr(Co+/T+) = \frac{Pr(T+/Co+) \times Pr(Co+)}{[Pr(T+/Co+) \times Pr(Co+)] + [Pr(T+/Co-) \times Pr(Co-)]}$$

where $Pr(T+/Co+)$ is the probability of a high SISI score given a cochlear impairment (Co+), $Pr(T+/Co-)$ is the probability of a high SISI score given a noncochlear (retrocochlear) impairment, $Pr(Co-)$ is the prevalence rate of noncochlear (retrocochlear) impairment in the population.

Buus *et al.* (1982a) used the following formula to derive the predictive value of the SISI test with respect to retrocochlear impairment:

$$Pr(Re+/T-) = \frac{Pr(T-/RE+) \times Pr(RE+)}{[Pr(T-/RE+) \times Pr(RE-)] + [Pr(T-/Co+) \times Pr(Co+)]}$$

where $Pr(RE+/T-)$ is the probability for a retrocochlear impairment given a negative SISI score, $Pr(T-/Re+)$ is the probability of a negative score given a retrocochlear impairment, and $Pr(T-/Co+)$ is the probability of a low SISI score given a cochlear impairment.

Buus *et al.* (1982a) took the value of 0.77 rather than the 0.60 used by L'amoré and Rodenburg (1980) for the probability of a positive SISI score given a cochlear impairment and the value of 0.60 rather than the 0.55 used by L'amoré and Rodenburg (1980) for the probability of a negative SISI score given a retrocochlear impairment, based on their review of 12 SISI studies. Buus *et al.* (1982a) also did not disregard the questionable scores as L'amoré and Rodenburg (1980) did. Therefore, $Pr(T+/RE+)$ did not equal $1 - Pr(T-/RE+)$ and $Pr(T-/Co+)$ did not equal $1 - Pr(T+/Co+)$. $Pr(T+/Re+)$ and $Pr(T-/Co+)$ were set at the values of 0.31 and 0.15, respectively, based on their review of 12 SISI studies. Assuming the same prevalence rates for cochlear and retrocochlear pathology as employed by L'amoré and Rodenburg (1980), Buus *et al.* (1982a) derived a predictive value of 0.91 for the SISI test with respect to cochlear pathology and a predictive value of 0.48 for the SISI test with respect to retrocochlear pathology. In summary, 91% of the time a positive SISI score represents a cochlear-impaired ear whereas 48% of the time a negative SISI score represents a retrocochlear-impairment. These predictive values are higher than those reported by L'amoré and Rodenburg (1980).

The percentage of retrocochlear-impaired ears detected with the SISI test is too low (approximately 60% as reported by Buus *et al.*, 1982a) to warrant the use of this test as a tool in the site-of-lesion battery or as a screening tool for the detection of retrocochlear pathology in persons who appear to be at low risk for retrocochlear pathology. Many patients require extensive training to perform the SISI test. Also, the tone-decay test detects more retrocochlear-impaired ears than the SISI test.

V. BEKESY TESTING

Bekesy audiometry, first described by Bekesy (1947) is a technique whereby the subject tracks his or her own hearing threshold levels. The signal, which is changing in intensity, is presented through one of the earphones and the subject presses the button on a hand-held switch whenever the signal is heard, thereby causing the signal intensity to decrease at a rate of 2.5 dB/sec in steps of 0.25 dB (an essentially stepless change). The subject releases the button as soon as the signal disappears, thereby causing the signal intensity to increase at the same rate. A broad-band noise or narrow-band noise is presented to the ear contralateral to the test ear whenever the possibility of cross-hearing exists. Because a graphic-level recorder is connected to the audiometer, a graphic representation of the subject's tracking behavior can be obtained. The signal is either continuous or pulsed [200 ms on-time with a 50% duty cycle: on-time/ (on-time + off-time)] and fixed in frequency or changing in frequency (sweep frequency). When a sweep-frequency Bekesy audiogram is obtained, the direction of the frequency change can be forward (low to high frequencies) or backward (high to low frequencies), usually over the range of about 100 to 10,000 Hz (the range on most currently available Bekesy audiometers). (The backward sweep is also referred to as the reverse sweep.) The graphic representation of the tracking behavior is referred to as the Bekesy tracing or the Bekesy audiogram.

Several investigators have studied the relation between the Bekesy audiogram and pure-tone thresholds obtained by conventional audiometry (Burns & Hinchcliffe, 1957; Corso, 1956, 1957; Erlandsson, Hakanson, Ivarsson, & Nilsson, 1979; Harris, 1979; Reger, 1952; Rodda, 1956). Researchers have attempted to specify whether the midpoints, peaks, or troughs of the excursion correspond to the pure-tone threshold. The results show that the variations in stimulus and recording parameters account for the differences between studies. The results also show good correspondence between the pulsed-tone tracings and the pure-tone thresholds in normal-hearing and hearing-impaired ears. Differences between the Bekesy tracings and the conventional pure-tone thresholds result, at least in part, from differences in psychophysical procedure: conventional pure-tone audiometry is based on the method of limits whereas Bekesy tracking is based on the method of limits and of adjustments and the adaptive procedure (Gelfand, 1981). In general, the midpoint of the excursion is considered the best estimate of the pure-tone threshold.

Bekesy (1947) reported that Bekesy tracings revealed reduced amplitude in the excursion width in patients with hearing impairment and loudness recruitment. He suggested that the tracing amplitude represents the first just-noticeable difference (jnd) in loudness. He also proposed that the reduction in amplitude was an indirect measure of

loudness recruitment. The jnd for loudness or the intensity DL for loudness was discussed earlier in Sections III,C and IV,A,3 of this chapter. The concept of reduced amplitude in relation to loudness recruitment will be addressed more fully later on in this chapter.

Lundborg (1952) and others reported that the amplitude of the Bekesy tracing represented a tool for differential diagnosis of the auditory site of lesion. Lundborg (1952) found that reduced amplitude (2–3 dB) was associated with ears having cochlear pathology; ears with retrocochlear pathology did not demonstrate reduced amplitude. No drift of the continuous-tone tracing occurred in the retrocochlear-impaired ears. Reger and Kos (1952), on the other hand, reported that the continuous tone tracing drifted downward substantially in persons with retrocochlear pathology. Differences between the studies result from differences in attenuator; Lundborg used a Bekesy audiometer in which the intensity varied in 2.0 rather than 0.25-dB steps, leading to a pulsed rather than a continuous signal whereas Reger and Kos used an essentially stepless (0.25-dB steps) attenuator. Jerger (1960) found considerable overlap among the various pathologic groups on measures such as the width of the continuous tracing in dB, the number of threshold crossings per quarter octave, the difference between the continuous and interrupted tracing widths, and the difference between the continuous and interrupted tracing midpoints.

A. BEKESY TYPES

Jerger (1960) evaluated the accuracy of Bekesy audiograms in determining auditory site of lesion in 434 subjects, based on the relation between the continuous (C) and interrupted (I) tracings. The rate of intensity change was 2.5 dB/s and the rate of frequency change was 1 octave/min between 100 and 10,000 Hz. The attenuator step was 0.25 dB. The interruption rate for the pulsed tones was 2.5 ips (interruptions per second). Fixed-frequency as well as sweep-frequency tracings were obtained. For the fixed-frequency tracing, the subject tracked threshold over a 3-min period. The interrupted tracing was obtained before the continuous tracing. Blue and red inks were used for the interrupted and continuous tracings, respectively. The instructions for the interrupted tracing were:

When I put these earphones on, you are going to hear a beeping sound in your ear. As long as you don't do anything the sound will keep getting louder. But you can make it fade away by holding down this switch. When you let up on this switch the sound will get louder again. Now, here is what I want you to do. Listen very carefully, and, as soon as you hear the beeping sound, hold this switch down until you can't hear it anymore. As soon as the beeping sound is gone, let up on the switch until it comes back. Then, as soon as you hear it again, hold the switch down until it goes away again, and so forth. The idea is to keep going back and forth from where you can just hear the beeping sound to where you can just not hear it anymore. Never let the sound get very loud and never let it stay away too long. Hold this switch down as soon as you hear the sound, and then let it up as soon as the sound is gone. (Jerger, 1960, p. 277)

For the continuous tracings, the instructions were

Now we are going to do the same thing again, but this time the sound will be steady instead of beeping on and off. Your job is still the same. Hold the switch down as soon as you hear the steady sound and let it up as soon as the steady sound goes away. (Jerger, 1960, p. 277)

On the basis of the relation between the continuous and interrupted tracings, Jerger (1960) classified the Bekesy audiogram as Type I, Type II, Type III, or Type IV. Figures 17 and 18 illustrate these Bekesy types for fixed- and sweep-frequency tracings. The sweep-frequency Bekesy audiogram was classified as Type I if the interrupted and continuous tracings interwove. The width of the Type I tracings was 10 dB on average although it varied between 3 and 20 dB. These features also characterized fixed-frequency Type I Bekesy audiograms. In sweep-frequency Type II Bekesy audiograms, the C tracing dropped below the I tracing between 500 and 1000 Hz. Jerger (1962b) indicated that

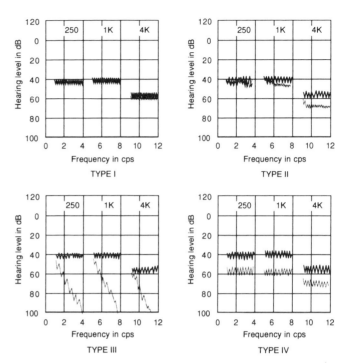

Figure 18 The four types of fixed-frequency Bekesy tracings. Dark is interrupted; light, continuous. Reprinted from Jerger (1960) with permission.

the C tracing ran parallel to the I tracing after the separation and the gap between the C and I tracings usually did not exceed 20 dB. After the C tracing dropped away from the I tracing, the amplitude of the C tracing narrowed to about 3–5 dB. This narrowing of the excursion amplitude was considered a classical sign of loudness recruitment. In the fixed-frequency Type II Bekesy audiogram, the C tracing dropped below the I tracing within the first 60 s and then stabilized. The C–I gap ranged from 5–20 dB, becoming constant after the first minute. The gap appeared only at frequencies above 500 to 1000 Hz. In the sweep-frequency Type III Bekesy audiogram, the C tracing dropped rapidly below the I tracing. The separation began between 100 and 500 Hz. In the fixed-frequency Type III Bekesy audiogram, the C tracing immediately broke away from the I tracing and descended to the audiometric limits. The width of the Type III continuous tracing was usually normal. The sweep-frequency Type IV Bekesy audiogram resembled the sweep-frequency Type II Bekesy audiogram except that the C tracing separated from the I tracing below 500 Hz rather than between 500 and 1000 Hz and the width of the C tracing did not necessarily become narrowed after the separation. Also, the C tracing sometimes rejoined the I tracing after the separation. These features also characterized the fixed-frequency Type IV Bekesy audiograms. Jerger (1962b) reported that the C–I gap was larger in Type IV than Type II fixed- and sweep-frequency Bekesy audiograms.

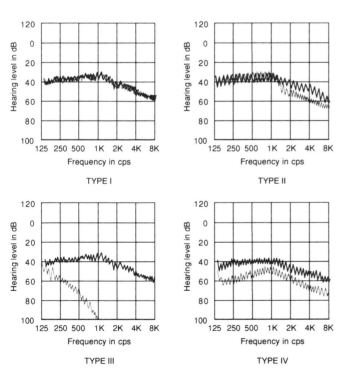

Figure 17 The four types of conventional Bekesy audiograms. Dark represents threshold tracing for a periodically interrupted tone; light for a continuous tone. Reprinted from Jerger (1960) with permission.

Some Bekesy audiograms, such as those with excessive tracing widths (e.g., 30–40 dB), cannot be classified into one of these four types. Some tracings may be contaminated by the presence of tinnitus. According to Jerger (1960), the obtaining of unclassifiable tracings indicates that the Bekesy audiogram is invalid for that patient. Questionable Bekesy audiograms may also result from slow reaction time, patient confusion regarding the task, or attentional or motivational factors.

1. INTERPRETATION

Jerger (1960) reported that 100% of his normal-hearing ears had Type I Bekesy audiograms. Of his conductive hearing-impaired ears, 94% had Type I Bekesy audiograms. Of his cochlear hearing-impaired ears, 76% had Type II Bekesy audiograms and most of the remainder had Type I Bekesy audiograms. Of his presbycusic ears, 34% had Type II Bekesy audiograms and 55% had Type I Bekesy audiograms. Of the acoustic-neuroma ears, 60% had Type III Bekesy audiograms and 40% had Type IV audiograms. Of the ears with unknown sensorineural hearing loss, 61% had Type II tracings, 28% had Type I tracings, and 6% had Type IV tracings. Of the mixed hearing-loss ears, 77% were characterized by Type II tracings, 15% were characterized by Type I tracings, and 8% were characterized by Type IV tracings. Of the ears with sudden onset of hearing loss, 63% had Type III tracings, 25% had Type IV tracings, 6% had Type I tracings, and 6% had Type II tracings. Thus, a Type I Bekesy audiogram is characteristic of normal-hearing and conductive hearing-impaired ears. A Type II Bekesy audiogram is characteristic of cochlear hearing-impaired ears, although many cochlear-impaired ears show Type I Bekesy audiograms, particularly at the low frequencies, and some cochlear-impaired ears show Type IV Bekesy audiograms. Retrocochlear pathology is associated predominantly with Type III and occasionally with Type IV Bekesy audiograms.

Owens (1964b) hypothesized that, in cases of combined eighth-nerve and cochlear involvement secondary to interruption of the cochlear blood supply because of pressure from the eighth-nerve lesion, a Type I or II Bekesy audiogram is likely to be present. This hypothesis was offered by Dix and Hallpike (1958) for the ABLB test in cases of retrocochlear pathology with recruitment (see Section III of this chapter). Dix and Hallpike's explanation has also been invoked in cases of retrocochlear pathology with nonsignificant tone decay and in cases of retrocochlear pathology with positive SISI scores (see Section III of this chapter). Again, as mentioned earlier, this explanation can account for only some cases of retrocochlear pathology with cochlear signs (in this case, Type I or II Bekesy audiograms).

Bekesy audiometry has been found to be clinically feasible in children as young as 7 years of age (Price & Falck, 1963; Stark, 1965).

2. MODIFICATIONS OF CRITERIA

Owens (1964b) suggested the omission of Type IV Bekesy audiograms and the broadening of the definition of Type II Bekesy audiograms so that Type II applied to those Bekesy audiograms in which the C tracing separated from the I tracing anywhere along the frequency range and then ran parallel to the I tracing with a separation of 4–26 dB or rejoined the I tracing.

Johnson and House (1964) suggested that the classification of a Bekesy audiogram as Type II or IV be dependent upon the size of the C–I gap. That is, a Bekesy audiogram is classified as Type II if the C–I gap is less than or equal to 25 dB and as Type IV if the C–I gap is greater than 25 dB. Hughes, Winegar, and Crabtree (1967) also supported differentiating between Types II and IV Bekesy audiograms on the basis of the C–I gap; the Bekesy audiogram was Type II if the C–I gap did not exceed 20 dB and was Type IV if the C–I gap exceeded 20 dB.

Hopkinson (1966) noted that it was generally more difficult to classify Types II and IV than to classify Types I and II Bekesy audiograms. Hopkinson offered three suggestions to improve interpretation of Type II and IV Bekesy audiograms:

1. Broader interpretation of the problem identified by a Type IV.
2. Interpretation of Types II and IV based on fixed-frequency tracings.
3. For tracings confounded by a combination of characteristics of different types, the use of descriptive terms giving details regarding "degree of separation" and "width of swing" rather than a specific classification. (Hopkinson, 1966, p. 80)

With respect to the first suggestion, Hopkinson suggests classifying a difficult Bekesy audiogram as an "equivocal" Type II, III, or IV audiogram and then explaining significant features such as the size of the C–I gap or the width of the tracing and why the Bekesy audiogram was considered equivocal. Stark (1968) also supported giving an operational description of the tracing.

Ehrlich (1971) noted, similar to Hopkinson (1966), that differentiation between Types II and IV was often difficult. Ehrlich evaluated 68 fixed-frequency Bekesy audiograms. The following aspects of the Bekesy audiograms were evaluated: (a) the C–I gap, (b) the amplitude of the C tracing (number of threshold crossings in 1 inch), (c) the ratio of the C amplitude to the I amplitude, (d) the rate of decay (C–I gap divided by 60), and (e) the pattern of decay of the C tracing. Figure 19 shows the four patterns of decay of the C tracing which were present in these 68 Bekesy tracings with patterns suggestive of retrocochlear lesions from patients with cochlear or retrocochlear lesions. Ehrlich calculated the probabilities of identifying cochlear or retrocochlear

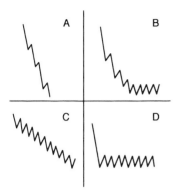

Figure 19 Patterns of decay. Reprinted from Ehrlich (1971) with permission.

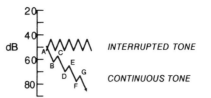

Figure 21 Example of a Type III Bekesy tracing showing a steady downward shift in which the patient hears the tone from time to time. Reprinted from Owens (1965b) with permission.

pathology on the basis of these various Bekesy tracing measures. She found that a large C–I gap size (>26 dB), fast rate of decay (>0.49 dB/s), and type A pattern of decay (see Figure 19) were highly indicative of retrocochlear pathology at all frequencies. A reduced amplitude of the C tracing (>8 excursions per inch) was highly predictive of cochlear pathology only at the low frequencies. Ehrlich (1971) recommended describing the probability that the Bekesy audiogram represents cochlear or retrocochlear pathology based on tracing measures such as the C–I gap size, amplitude of the C tracing, and so forth rather than classifying the tracings as Type I–V.

We suggest that the Jerger classification be employed with the modification proposed by Johnson and House (1964) with respect to the differentiation of Type II from Type IV on the basis of whether or not the C–I gap size exceeds 25 dB.

3. Mechanism Underlying the Pattern of the C Tracing

Owens (1965b) provided explanations for the C patterns in the various Bekesy types. Figures 20, 21, and 22 show the various C patterns for which Owens gave explanations. In one form of the Type III Bekesy pattern (see Figure 20), the C tracing plummets to the limits of the audiometer. The C tone is never heard because it decays at a rate that is faster than the 2.5 dB/s rate in increase of signal intensity induced when the button of the hand-held switch is released. Thus,

the C tracing proceeds nearly straight down to the limits of the audiometer.

In another form of the Type III Bekesy audiogram (see Figure 21), the rate of tone decay is slower than the 2.5 dB/s rate in intensity increase induced by releasing the button of the hand-held switch. Thus, at some point, the intensity increase will overcome the tone decay from point A to point B and result in the perception of an audible tone at point B. When the patient presses the button of the hand-held switch, the intensity decrease combined with the phenomenon of tone decay will cause the tone to become inaudible very rapidly (points B to C). Again, at point C the patient releases the button and, at some point, the intensity increase again overcomes the tone decay. (The tone decay is occurring at the same rate regardless of the intensity of the tone.) Thus, the tone is once again heard at point D. This sequence continues until the tracing reaches the limit of the audiometer.

A type II tracing occurs when the rate of tone decay decreases as the intensity of the signal increases. In Figure 22 it can be seen that, as a result of tone decay, the tone is not heard until the intensity increase overcomes the tone decay at point B. At point B, the button is pressed and the intensity decrease combined with the tone decay causes the tone to become inaudible rapidly. At the point of inaudibility (C), the button of the hand-held switch is again released and the intensity of the tone increases. Now less time is required for the intensity increase to overcome the tone decay (point D) since the tone decay is inversely proportional to the intensity level. Therefore, the distance C–D is shorter than the distance A–B. When the tone is heard at

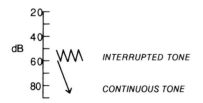

Figure 20 Example of a plummeting Type III Bekesy tracing. Reprinted from Owens (1965b) with permission.

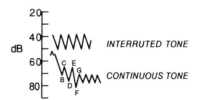

Figure 22 Example of a Type II Bekesy tracing showing the slight downward shift, noticeable narrowing, and stabilization (equilibrium). Reprinted from Owens (1965b) with permission.

point D, the button is pressed, the intensity again decreases, but the tone becomes inaudible more slowly than before, so D–E is longer than B–C. Similarly, E–F is shorter than C–D and F–G is longer than D–E, and so forth until equilibrium is reached.

B. VARIABLES AFFECTING BEKESY AUDIOGRAMS

1. FIXED VERSUS SWEEP-FREQUENCY

Owens (1964b) evaluated fixed- and sweep-frequency Bekesy tracings. He observed that, whenever adaptation was present in the fixed-frequency tracing, it was also present in the same frequency region in the sweep-frequency tracing. Similarly, reduced amplitude of the C tracing in cochlear ears was present in both sweep- and fixed-frequency tracings. Nevertheless, fixed-frequencies usually displayed greater adaptation, as evidenced by the C–I gap size, than the sweep-frequencies. Owens (1964b) concluded that the fixed-frequency tracings were more accurate than the sweep-frequency tracings. Moreover, the fixed-frequency tracings were more useful in cases of severe hearing impairment. These findings were substantiated by several investigators (Bilger, 1965; Jerger & Jerger, 1966; Katinsky & Toglia, 1968). Hopkinson (1966) suggested that fixed-frequency Bekesy audiograms were less confusing for the patient since they did not require the patient to become adjusted to rapidly changing frequencies.

2. STARTING INTENSITY

Rosenblith and Miller (1949) found that, when the starting direction of intensity was high to low, slightly better pulsed-tone thresholds were obtained than when the starting direction of intensity was low to high. The opposite effect was found for the continuous tracing. Harbert and Young (1968) reported that equivalent thresholds resulted for the I tracing in normal-hearing and cochlear-impaired ears regardless of whether the starting level was high with an initially decreasing intensity or low with an initially increasing intensity. For the continuous tracing, as the starting level increased, the elevation in threshold increased in normal-hearing and pathological ears.

3. MASKING

a. Contralateral

Blegvad (1968) obtained sweep- and fixed-frequency C and I tracings in 31 patients with unilateral cochlear hearing impairment. Patients were selected such that the interaural differences in hearing threshold levels were not sufficient to result in cross-hearing. While the tracings were obtained in the test ear, a broad-band noise of 80 dB SPL was introduced into the contralateral ear. The introduction of the masking resulted in increased hearing thresholds (on average), particularly for the C tracings. This effect was also

observed in normal-hearing listeners at 1000 and 4000 Hz (Blegvad, 1967). The average size of the threshold shift in their cochlear-impaired subjects was 1–4.5 dB for the fixed-frequency I tracings and 5–8.5 dB for the fixed-frequency C tracings. The masking also resulted in an increase in the C–I gap of approximately 3 dB on average in the fixed-frequency Bekesy tracings. A similar increase in the C–I gap as a result of the masking was also obtained in the sweep-frequency tracings. The masking also resulted in slightly decreased (about 1 dB) mean tracing amplitudes (taken as the average of the amplitudes for the first and second minutes). The decrease, however, was statistically significant for the 250 and 1000 Hz but not the 4000 Hz fixed-frequency C and I tracings, and for the sweep-frequency C but not I tracings. Using Jerger's (1960, 1962b) criteria for classifying Bekesy audiograms, Blegvad (1968) found that contralateral masking resulted in a shift of some of the Type I to Type II Bekesy audiograms, Type II to Type IV Bekesy audiograms, and Type I to Type IV Bekesy audiograms. Similar findings were obtained by Dirks and Norris (1966) and Grimes and Feldman (1969).

Hughes and Johnson (1978) suggested that such effects could be the result of central masking, interaural interference, or distraction of the subject.

b. Ipsilateral

Several researchers (Collins & Menzel, 1965; Small & Minifie, 1961; Young, 1968) have shown that the tracking amplitude of I and C tracings is essentially unaffected by the presence of ipsilateral masking with broad-band or narrow-band noise. The I thresholds, however, are elevated by the presence of ipsilateral noise (broad-band and narrow-band); this effect is enhanced in patients with retrocochlear pathology (Harbert & Young, 1965).

4. INSTRUCTIONS

The findings of Pollack (1948), Sørensen (1962), and Owens (1965b) on the effect of instructions on conventional pure-tone threshold assesssment or tone-decay testing indicates that Bekesy tracings may be affected by the instructions given to the patient. That is, requiring the patient to listen for any sound or for a tonal signal may result in different Bekesy tracings. At the conclusion of Bekesy testing, the audiologist should inquire about the kind of sound the patient heard. If the patient indicates that the response was to a noise, interpretation should be made cautiously.

C. MODIFICATIONS OF THE BEKESY TECHNIQUE

1. CRITICAL OFF-TIME

Harbert and Young (1962) reported that the threshold for the I tracing in a patient with injury to the seventh and eighth nerves increased as the off-time decreased. Jerger and

Jerger (1966) attempted to sensitize the Bekesy test to the presence of retrocochlear pathology by varying the off-time of the I tones between 20 and 500 ms (the on-time was kept constant). They employed this modification with 6 patients having retrocochlear pathology. They found that the critical off-time (breakpoint in the curve showing threshold as a function of off-time) was increased and the amount of threshold elevation caused by decreases in off-time was increased in the impaired ear compared with the normal-hearing ear of these patients. Dallos and Tillman (1966) obtained similar findings.

2. BRIEF-TONE AUDIOMETRY

Hughes (1946) was the first to show that, as the stimulus duration decreased, the pure-tone threshold increased. Garner and Miller (1947) showed that this effect, referred to as temporal integration or summation, occurs for stimulus durations below 200 ms. A number of procedures such as the classical methods of limits and of adjustments as well as Bekesy tracking have been employed in brief-tone audiometry.

Sanders, Josey, and Kemker (1971) obtained brief-tone audiometry data for normal-hearing, cochlear-impaired, and retrocochlear-impaired subjects. They found that the slopes of the temporal-integration functions were similar to those of normal-hearing subjects and were steeper than those for the cochlear-impaired subjects. Thus, brief-tone audiometry differentiated between retrocochlear-impaired and cochlear-impaired ears but not between retrocochlear-impaired and normal-hearing ears. These findings were not substantiated by other investigators. Olsen, Rose, and Noffsinger (1979) reported that, although the median temporal-integration slopes were shallower for the cochlear- than the retrocochlear-impaired and the normal-hearing, there was substantial overlap in the temporal integration functions among normal-hearing, cochlear-impaired, and retrocochlear-impaired ears. Pedersen (1976) and Stephens (1976) obtained findings similar to those reported by Olsen et al. (1979). Olsen (1987) concluded that recent studies in the clinical utility of brief-tone audiometry are lacking because of the large intersubject variability in the temporal-integration functions, the large overlap in the results for normal-hearing and cochlear-impaired ears, and the low sensitivity of brief-tone audiometry to retrocochlear pathology.

3. FORWARD–BACKWARD SWEEP TRACINGS

Palva, Karja, and Palva (1970) evaluated the forward and backward sweep C tracings in a large sample (231 ears). Pulsed backward and forward I tracings were also obtained if there was abnormal separation between the forward and backward sweep-frequency C tracings. A forward–backward discrepancy was considered to be present if there was a separation between the forward and backward trac-ings of more than 10 dB over at least one octave. A forward–backward discrepancy (in which the reverse tracing showed poorer hearing threshold levels than the forward tracing) occurred more frequently in ears with brainstem, brain base, and cerebellar lesions than in normal-hearing or cochlear-impaired ears. Also, forward–backward discrepancies were more frequently identified with the C than I tracings.

Young and Harbert (1971) obtained the forward and backward C and I sweep tracings in a small group of patients. Forward C and I fixed-frequency tracings were also obtained. The results revealed that the amplitude of the I and C tracings was independent of the sweep direction. The sweep direction, however, affected the C–I gap. That is, when there was more abnormal adaptation in the high than low frequencies (as indicated by the results of tone-decay testing), then the backward sweep tracing showed greater C–I gaps than the forward sweep. Similarly, if there was more abnormal adaptation in the low than high frequencies, then the forward sweep showed greater C–I gaps than the backward sweep. When there was no abnormal adaptation or the amount of abnormal adaptation was similar across frequencies, then no discrepancy between the forward and backward tracings resulted.

Jerger et al. (1972) evaluated the forward and backward sweep-frequency I and C tracings in 185 subjects with various auditory disorders. The forward I tracing was first obtained followed by the forward C tracing and then the backward C tracing. The frequency sweep encompassed the range between 200 and 8000 Hz. Jerger et al. then applied Palva et al.'s (1970) criteria for the presence of a forward–backward discrepancy to their normal-hearing group. The application of Palva et al.'s (1970) criteria resulted in the presence of a forward–backward discrepancy in 7% of the ears. To reduce this rate, Jerger et al. developed more stringent criteria for the presence of a forward–backward discrepancy: separation of more than 10 dB over at least 2 octaves (not necessarily adjacent), a 30-dB or greater separation over at least one octave, or a 50-dB or greater separation over at least half an octave. None of their normal-hearing ears had forward–backward discrepancies as defined by these more stringent criteria.

Jerger et al. (1972) reported that many of their retrocochlear ears had a forward–backward discrepancy. In cases where the forward tracing revealed a Type III Bekesy audiogram, a mirroring pattern of discrepancy often occurred. Figure 23 illustrates this mirroring pattern of discrepancy. This was not the only pattern of discrepancy that occurred. Therefore, duration of stimulation was not the sole mechanism underlying the discrepancy pattern. Generally, but not consistently, the backward sweep revealed greater hearing threshold levels than the forward sweep. It was the magnitude rather than the direction of the discrepancy which had diagnostic utility. Jerger et al. also found

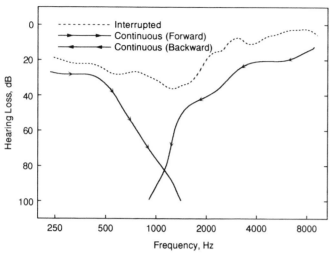

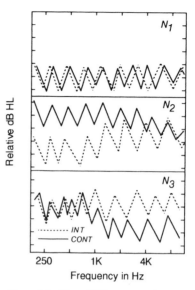

Figure 23 Three Bekesy tracings (interrupted, continuous-forward, and continuous-backward) on right ear of patient 1. Audiometric findings were consistent with eighth cranial nerve disorder. Type III Bekesy audiogram is associated with mirroring of forward and backward continuous tracings. Reprinted from Jerger, Jerger, and Mauldin (1972) with permission.

Figure 24 Three BCL patterns characterizing patients with normal sensitivity or peripheral hearing impairment. These patterns, labeled N_1, N_2, and N_3, are reported as negative BCL results. Reprinted from Jerger and Jerger (1974b) with permission.

that the forward–backward discrepancy was present in ears with functional hearing loss as well as ears with retrocochlear pathology. (See Chapter 4 for a detailed discussion of functional hearing loss.) Figure 23 shows the interrupted and continuous forward tracings and continuous backward tracing for an ear with retrocochlear pathology.

Rose, Kurdziel, Olsen, and Noffsinger (1975) evaluated the forward–backward sweep-frequency tracings and fixed-frequency tracings in 18 patients with surgically-confirmed retrocochlear pathology. The forward–backward tracings revealed more adaptation than the fixed-frequency tracings in 56% of the cases. When the criterion of 20 dB of adaptation was employed to detect retrocochlear pathology, the hit rates for the forward–backward tracings and fixed-frequency tracings were essentially similar. For this reason, and because fixed-frequency tracings required less administration time than forward–backward tracings, Rose *et al.* concluded that fixed-frequency tracings were preferable to forward–backward tracings in site-of-lesion testing.

4. Bekesy Comfortable Loudness Tracings

Jerger and Jerger (1974b) proposed that since eighth-nerve signs appear to be manifested first at suprathreshold levels and then at threshold levels, tests which evaluate auditory performance at suprathreshold levels should be more sensitive to retrocochlear disorders than those at threshold levels. Therefore, they developed a modification of the Bekesy test which required the patient to track the signals at a comfortable loudness level instead of at threshold. The comfortable loudness level was tracked for I and C signals.

Jerger and Jerger (1974b) obtained the Bekesy Comfortable Loudness (BCL) tracings in 164 ears with various pathologies. Based on their inspection of the tracings, they developed 6 BCL types: three negative and three positive types. Figures 24 and 25 show the BCL tracings for the negative and positive types. The BCL tracing was classified as N_1 if the C and I tracings interwove. The BCL tracing was classified as N_2 if the C tracing ran above the I tracing by

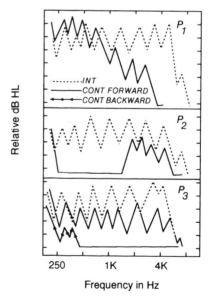

Figure 25 Three BCL patterns characterizing patients with eighth-cranial-nerve lesions or brain stem disorders. These patterns, labeled P_1, P_2, and P_3, are reported as positive BCL results. Reprinted from Jerger and Jerger (1974b) with permission.

more than 10 dB for at least 2 adjacent octaves or by more than 5 dB for at least 3 adjacent octaves. The BCL tracing was classified as N_3 if the C tracing separated from the I tracing at some point and then ran below and parallel to the I tracing. The N_1, N_2, and N_3 Types are consistent with normal hearing, conductive pathology, or cochlear pathology.

The BCL tracing was classified as Type P_1 if the C tracing broke away from the I tracing and then descended to the audiometric limits. The BCL tracing was classified as Type P_2 if the C interwove with or was parallel to the I tracing at the high frequencies and ran substantially below the I tracing at the low to mid frequencies. The BCL tracing was classified as Type P_3 if the forward I and C tracings interwove but there was a substantial discrepancy between the forward and backward C tracings. The P_1, P_2, and P_3 Types are consistent with retrocochlear pathology.

D. RELATIONS AMONG BEKESY TRACINGS, AUDITORY ADAPTATION AND LOUDNESS RECRUITMENT

Hallpike and Hood (1951) and Dix and Hood (1953) observed that the recruiting ear demonstrates "perstimulatory fatigue" as evidenced by the drift downward in threshold tracking for C tones. The size of the drift was as large as 15 dB. Reger and Kos (1952) observed that patients with cochlear hearing impairment demonstrated only a slight downward drift in the C threshold tracing when compared with a patient with retrocochlear pathology who demonstrated a drift of 30 dB (at the output level of the audiometer) within 2 min. This drift was termed the "temporary threshold shift" (TTS). Yantis (1959) also observed drifts downward in the C threshold tracing of his patients with retrocochlear pathology. The drift appeared to be associated with retrocochlear rather than cochlear pathology.

Owens (1965b) observed that a Type I Bekesy occurred when loudness recruitment was present but tone decay was absent; Type II Bekesy occurred when both loudness recruitment and tone decay were present; Type III occurred when tone decay was present and loudness recruitment was absent.

Jerger, Carhart, and Lassman (1958) suggested that auditory adaptation after sustained stimulation at threshold was present in ears with cochlear and retrocochlear pathology. In retrocochlear-impaired ears, however, the magnitude of the adaptation was substantially greater than in cochlear-impaired ears. Therefore, ears with retrocochlear pathology evidence greater drifts in the C threshold tracing than ears with cochlear pathology. Jerger et al. (1958) observed that no auditory adaptation or drift in tracking is observed for I threshold tracings in either retrocochlear or cochlear-impaired ears.

The topic of narrowed excursions in the C tracings in subjects with cochlear pathology has been a subject of controversy in the literature. Bekesy (1947), as mentioned in the beginning of this section, attributed the reduced amplitude to loudness recruitment. Denes and Naunton (1950), as mentioned in Section III, contended that the reduced Bekesy amplitude was not a measure of recruitment; rather, the reduced width reflected intersubject variability in reaction time, fatigue effects from listening to near-threshold tones, and the frequency dependence of the intensity DL at threshold. Hirsh et al. (1954) suggested that the tracing amplitude reflected moment-to-moment variability in absolute auditory threshold. Owens (1965b) proposed that the reduced excursion width "reflects the interplay of tone decay and abnormal loudness growth; seemingly, there is a moderately rapid buildup of loudness on the one side and a rapid decrease in loudness (from combined tone decay and audiometer attenuation) on the other" (p. 56). Harbert and Young (1964) hypothesized that the reduced amplitude reflected a rapid adaptation process occurring in milliseconds.

It is apparent that the reduced amplitude of the Bekesy excursion is not a measure of recruitment. Nevertheless, the presence of reduced amplitude of the C tracing is consistent with cochlear pathology.

E. HIT AND FALSE-ALARM RATES

1. CONVENTIONAL BEKESY AUDIOMETRY

Tillman (1969) reported a hit rate (presence of Types III or IV Bekesy audiograms) of 70% for his group of 23 cases with eighth-nerve pathology. Sanders et al. (1974) obtained a hit rate of only 52% for their group of 27 cases with retrocochlear pathology. Johnson (1973) found that conventional Bekesy audiometry detected 60% of their 321 ears with retrocochlear pathology. Palva et al. (1978) obtained a hit rate of only 15% for their 32 tumor cases. A recent study by Antonelli, Bellotto, and Grandori (1987) revealed positive Bekesy findings in 62.5% of their 25 acoustic-neuroma cases.

Several researchers have suggested that tumor size affects the Bekesy pattern (Jerger & Waller, 1962; Johnson, 1968; Shapiro & Naunton, 1967). Johnson (1977) reported that Type III or IV Bekesy patterns were seen in 72% of their cases with large eighth-nerve tumors but only 39% of their cases with small tumors.

Tillman (1969) had a false-alarm rate of 0% for conventional Bekesy testing in his 23 patients with Meniere's disease. Sanders et al. (1974) had a false-alarm rate of 7% for their group of 61 cochlear-impaired cases. Johnson (1977) reported positive Bekesy results in 17% of their group of 89 cochlear-impaired ears. Palva et al. (1978) found a false-alarm rate of 23%. Antonelli et al. (1987) reported that 13% of their group of 56 cochlear-impaired ears had positive Bekesy results.

2. FORWARD–BACKWARD BEKESY TESTING

For the forward–backward measure, Jerger *et al.* (1972) found a hit rate of 78% using the Jerger *et al.*(1972) criteria as opposed to 83% using the Palva *et al.* (1970) criteria in their group of 23 retrocochlear-impaired ears. Palva *et al.* (1978) found a forward–backward discrepancy in 63% of their 32 acoustic-neuroma cases; only 15% had positive results on conventional audiometry testing. Karjalainen, Karja, Sorri, and Plava (1984) reported that the hit rate for the forward–backward measure using the Plava *et al.* (1970) criteria was 62% for their group of 21 patients with eighth-nerve tumors; the hit rate for conventional Bekesy audiometry was only 38%. Thus, Karjalainen *et al.* (1984) found that the forward–backward measure was more sensitive than conventional Bekesy audiometry to retrocochlear pathology.

For the forward–backward measure, Jerger *et al.* (1972) reported a false-alarm rate of 1% using the Jerger *et al.* (1972) criteria as opposed to 5% using the Palva *et al.* (1970) criteria. Jerger *et al.* (1972) concluded that their criteria were associated with a lower false-positive rate but slightly higher false-negative rate than the Palva *et al.* (1970) criteria. Palva *et al.* (1978) found a false-alarm rate of 4% for the forward–backward measure in their group of 36 ears with Meniere's disease; on conventional Bekesy testing, 23% obtained positive results. Karjalainen *et al.* (1984) found that only 2% of their 107 cochlear cases had a forward–backward discrepancy.

3. BEKESY COMFORTABLE LOUDNESS

For the BCL measure, Jerger and Jerger (1974b) reported that a P pattern was obtained in approximately 69% of their 16 cases with retrocochlear pathology including those with intra-axial brainstem pathology. The P_1 pattern was present in 37.5%, the P_2 pattern was present in 12.5%, and the P_3 pattern was present in approximately 19%. In approximately 19%, the BCL pattern could not be classified. In approximately 12.5%, N patterns were obtained.

Jerger and Jerger (1974b) reported that a P_1 pattern was obtained in 2% of their 148 ears with normal hearing-threshold levels, conductive hearing impairment, or cochlear hearing impairment. In 8% of these 148 cases, the BCL tracings could not be classified since the sounds never became too loud or even comfortably loud. The remaining 90% demonstrated N patterns; the N_1 Type was the most prevalent and the N_3 pattern was the least prevalent.

Jerger and Jerger (1974b) also compared BCL testing with conventional Bekesy audiometry in 10 patients with retrocochlear pathology, including those with intra-axial brainstem pathology. They reported that BCL testing detected 9 of the 10 patients whereas conventional Bekesy audiometry detected only 6 of these 10 patients. Jerger and Jerger (1974b) concluded that BCL testing was more sensitive than conventional Bekesy testing to the presence of retrocochlear pathology.

Turner *et al.* (1984) reviewed 170 papers on site-of-lesion testing published between 1968 and 1983. They found that the average hit rate for BCL testing was 85% and the average false-alarm rate for BCL testing was 8%. But these averages were based on a total of only 3 studies with a total of 40 retrocochlear-impaired ears and 119 cochlear-impaired ears. Although further research is needed to assess the clinical utility of BCL testing with respect to differential diagnosis, it is likely that the trend observed for the other site-of-lesion tests relating to decreased sensitivity over time would also apply to the BCL because of the improvements in medical technology leading to detection of the tumor at an earlier stage of development and hence earlier referral for audiologic follow-up.

In conclusion, the more recent studies show that conventional Bekesy audiometry and forward–backward Bekesy testing detect less than 70% of retrocochlear-impaired ears. Few studies have been done on BCL tesing. Nevertheless, as mentioned earlier, it is unlikely that BCL testing is associated with high hit rates based on the trend of reduced hit rates over time. Also, Jerger and Jerger (1974b) reported that the BCL patterns could not be classified in a large number of their patients—19% of their retrocochlear cases and 8% of their cochlear cases. Based on these findings, Bekesy testing (conventional and modified) does not appear to be a strong diagnostic or screening tool for site-of-lesion testing. Moreover, Owens (1964b) concluded that Bekesy audiometry was limited in cases of severe hearing impairment with large C–I gaps; in such cases, the C tracing may not stabilize until beyond the limits of the audiometer and accurate classification is thereby precluded.

Further research is needed to explore methods for increasing the sensitivity of the Bekesy test. For example, since the literature shows a relation between adaptation rate and the rate in change of intensity during Bekesy audiometry, the effect of attenuation rates less than the patient's adaptation rate on the Bekesy audiogram in pathological ears needs to be investigated.

VI. MASKING FOR SUPRATHRESHOLD TONAL TESTS

The suprathreshold tonal tests such as the tone-decay, SISI, and Bekesy Comfortable Loudness tests often must be done with masking in the ear contralateral to the test ear to prevent cross-hearing of the test signal by the nontest ear. Masking of the nontest ear is required whenever the presentation level minus the interaural attenuation for air-conduction (40 dB) equals or exceeds the air- or bone-conduction threshold in the nontest ear. Narrow-band noise is used as the masker (broad-band noise for sweep-frequency Bekesy testing) for the suprathreshold tonal tests.

A. INITIAL MASKING

Initial masking (IM) for suprathreshold tonal testing can be derived using the formula

$$IM = A_{nt} + MEM$$

where A_{nt} is the air-conduction threshold of the nontest ear at the test frequency and MEM is minimum effective masking for pure-tone testing. (See Chapter 1 for the procedure to obtain MEM for pure-tone testing.)

B. OVERMASKING

Overmasking during suprathreshold tonal testing may occur if the following holds:

$$ML_{nt} \geq B_t + IA$$

where ML_{nt} is the masking level in the nontest ear, B_t is the bone-conduction threshold of the test ear at the test frequency, and IA is the interaural attenuation for air-conduction testing.

C. MAXIMUM MASKING

The maximum amount of masking noise that one can confidently introduce into the nontest ear without resulting in overmasking of the test ear during suprathreshold tonal testing can be derived from the formula

$$MM = B_t + IA - 5\ dB$$

where MM is maximum masking, B_t is the bone-conduction threshold of the test ear at the test frequency, and IA is the interaural attenuation for air-conduction testing (40 dB).

REFERENCES

Anderson, H., Barr, B., & Wedenberg, E. (1969). Intra-aural reflexes in retrocochlear lesions. In C. Hamberger & J. Wersall (eds.), *Nobel symposium 10: Disorders of the skull base region*, pp. 49–55. Stockholm: Almqvist and Wiksell.

Antonelli, A. R., Bellotto, R., & Grandori, F. (1987). Audiologic diagnosis of central versus eighth nerve and cochlear hearing impairment. *Audiology, 26*, 209–226.

Bartholomeus, B., & Swisher, L. (1971). Tone decay and SISI scores. *Arch. Otolaryngol., 93*, 451–455.

Bauch, C. D., Olsen, W. O., & Harner, S. G. (1983). Audiologic results for matched pairs of tumor and non-tumor patients. Paper presented at the Annual Convention of the American Speech–Language–Hearing Association, Cincinnati, Ohio.

Beattie, R. C., & Raffin, M. J. M. (1985). Reliability of threshold, slope, and PB max for monosyllabic words. *J. Speech Hear. Dis., 50*, 166–177.

Beattie, R. C., & Warren, V. G. (1983). Relationships among speech threshold, loudness discomfort, comfortable loudness, and PB max in the elderly hearing impaired. *Am. J. Otol., 3*, 353–358.

Bekesy, G. v. (1947). A new audiometer. *Acta Otolaryngol., 35*, 411–422.

Bekesy, G. v. (1960). *Experiments in hearing.* New York: McGraw-Hill.

Benitez, J., Lopez-Rios, G., & Novon, V. (1967). Bilateral acoustic neuromas; a human temporal bone study. *Arch. Otolaryngol., 86*, 51–57.

Bess, F. H. (1983). Clinical assessment of speech recognition. In D. F. Konkle & W. F. Rintelmann (eds.), *Principles of speech audiometry*, pp. 127–201. Baltimore: University Park Press.

Bess, F. H., Josey, A. F., & Humes, L. E. (1979). Performance intensity functions in cochlear and eighth nerve disorders. *Am. J. Otol., 1*, 27–31.

Bess, F. H., Josey, A. F., Glasscock, M. E., & Wilson, L. K. (1984). Audiologic manifestations in bilateral acoustic tumors (von Recklinghausen's disease). *J. Speech Hear. Dis., 49*, 177–182.

Bilger, R. C. (1965). Some parameters of fixed-frequency Bekesy audiometry. *J. Speech Hear. Res., 8*, 85–95.

Blegvad, B. (1966). The SISI test in normal listeners. An investigation with non-commercial equipment. *Acta Otolaryngol., 62*, 201–212.

Blegvad, B. (1967). Contralateral masking and Bekesy audiometry in normal listeners. *Acta Otolaryngol., 64*, 157–165.

Blegvad, B. (1968). Bekesy audiometry and clinical masking. *Acta Otolaryngol., 64*, 229–240.

Blegvad, B. (1969). Differential intensity sensitivity and clinical masking. *Acta Otolaryngol., 67*, 428–434.

Blegvad, B., & Terkildsen, K. (1967). Contralateral masking and the SISI-test in normal listeners. *Acta Otolaryngol., 63*, 557–563.

Brand, S., & Rosenberg, P. (1963). Problems in auditory evaluation for neurosurgical diagnosis. *J. Speech Hear. Dis., 28*, 355–361.

Brandy, W. T. (1966). Reliability of voice tests of speech discrimination. *J. Speech Hear. Res., 9*, 451–465.

Burns, W., & Hinchcliffe, R. (1957). Comparison of the auditory threshold as measured by individual pure tone and by Bekesy audiometry. *J. Accoust. Soc. Am., 29*, 1274–1277.

Buus, S., Florentine, M., & Redden, R. B. (1982a). The SISI test: A review. Part I. *Audiology, 21*, 273–293.

Buus, S., Florentine, M., & Redden, R. B. (1982b). The SISI test: A review. Part II. *Audiology, 21*, 365–385.

Carhart, R. (1957). Clinical determination of abnormal auditory adaptation. *Arch. Otolaryngol., 65*, 32–39.

Carver, W. F. (1970). The reliability and precision of a modification of the ABLB test. *Ann. Otol. Rhinol. Laryngol., 79*, 398–411.

Causey, G. D., Hermanson, C. L., Hood, L. J., & Bowling, L. S. (1983). A comparative evaluation of the Maryland NU-6 auditory test. *J. Speech Hear. Dis., 48*, 62–69.

Clemis, J. D., & Carver, W. F. (1967). Discrimination scores for speech in Meniere's disease. *Arch. Otolaryngol., 86*, 614–168.

Coles, R. R. A., & Priede, V. M. (1976). Factors influencing the choice of fixed-level ear in the ABLB test. *Audiology, 15*, 465–479.

Collins, J., & Menzel, O. J. (1965). The relation between intensity difference limen and Bekesy threshold tracings (Abstract). *Asha, 7*, 428 (1965).

Cooper, J. C., Jr., & Owen, J. H. (1976). In defense of SISI's. The short increment sensitivity index. *Arch. Otolaryngol., 102*, 396–399.

Corso, J. F. (1956). Effects of testing methods on hearing thresholds. *Arch. Otolaryngol., 63*, 78–91.

Corso, J. F. (1957). Additional variables on the Bekesy-type audiometer. *Arch. Otolaryngol., 66*, 719–728.

Dallos, P. J., & Tillman, T. W. (1966). The effects of parameter variations in Bekesy audiometry in a patient with acoustic neurinoma. *J. Speech Hear. Res., 9*, 557–572.

Denes, P., & Naunton, R. F. (1950). The clinical detection of auditory recruitment. *J. Laryngol. Otol., 65*, 375–398.

Dewey, G. (1923). *Relative frequency of English speech sounds.* Cambridge: Harvard University Press.

Dimmick, F. L., & Olsen, R. M. (1941). The intensity difference limen in audition. *J. Acoust. Soc. Am., 12,* 517–525.

Dirks, D. D., & Morgan, D. E. (1983). Measures of discomfort and most comfortable loudness. In D. F. Konkle & W. F. Rintelmann (eds.), *Principles of speech audiometry,* pp. 285–319. Baltimore: University Park Press.

Dirks, D. D., & Norris, J. D. (1966). Shifts in auditory thresholds produced by ipsilateral and contralateral maskers at low intensity levels. *J. Acoust. Soc. Am., 40,* 12–19.

Dirks, D. D., Kamm, C., Bower, D., & Betsworth, A. (1977). Use of performance-intensity functions for diagnosis. *J. Speech Hear. Dis., 42,* 408–415.

Dix, M. R., & Hallpike, C. S. (1958). The otoneurological diagnosis of tumours of the VIII nerve. *Proc. R. Soc. Med., 51,* 689–897.

Dix, M. R., & Hood, J. D. (1953). Modern developments in pure-tone audiometry and their application to the clinical diagnosis of end-organ deafness. *J. Laryngol. Otolaryngol., 67,* 343–357.

Dix, M. R., Hallpike, C. S., & Hood, J. D. (1948). Observations upon the loudness recruitment phenomenon, with especial reference to the differential diagnosis of disorders of the internal ear and VIII nerve. *Proc. R. Soc. Med., 41,* 516–526.

Doerfler, L. G. (1948). *Differential sensitivity to intensity in perceptually deafened ears.* Ph.D. Thesis. Evanston, Illinois: Northwestern University.

Dubno, J. R., & Dirks, D. D. (1983). Suggestions for optimizing reliability with the synthetic sentence identification test. *J. Speech Hear. Dis., 48,* 98–102.

Egan, J. P. (1948). Articulation testing methods. *Laryngoscope, 58,* 955–991.

Eggermont, J. J., & Odenthal, D. W. (1974). Action potentials and summating potentials in the normal human cochlea. *Acta. Otolaryngol. Suppl., 316.*

Ehrlich, C. H. (1971). Analysis of selected fixed-frequency Bekesy tracings. *Arch. Otolaryngol., 93,* 12–24.

Elpern, B. S. (1960). Differences in difficulty among the CID W-22 auditory tests. *Laryngoscope, 70,* 1560–1565.

Erlandsson, B., Hakanson, H., Ivarsson, A., & Nilsson, P. (1979). Comparison of the hearing threshold measured by manual pure tone and by self-recording (Bekesy) audiometry. *Audiology, 18,* 414–429.

Evans, E. F. (1976). Temporary sensorineural hearing loss and VIII nerve changes. In D. Henderson, R. P. Hamernik, D. S. Dosanji, & J. Mills (eds.), *Effects of noise on hearing,* pp. 79–92. New York: Raven Press.

Evans, E., & Whitfield, I. (1965). Classification of unit responses in the auditory cortex of the unanesthetized and unrestrained cat. *J. Physiol., 171,* 476–493.

Fior, R. (1972). Physiological maturation of auditory function between 3 and 13 years of age. *Audiology, 11,* 317–321.

Florentine, M. (1981). Intensity discrimination as a function of level and frequency and its relation to high-frequency hearing. *J. Acoust. Soc. Am., 70,* S87.

Flottorp, G. (1963). Pathological fatigue in part of the hearing nerve only. *Acta. Otolaryngol., 50,* 438–450.

Fournier, M. S., & Jirsa, R. E. (1976). Lack of reliability of the SISI procedure for determining inner ear threshold. *J. Am. Aud. Soc., 1,* 206–208.

Fowler, E. P. (1936). A method for the early detection of otosclerosis: A study of sounds well above threshold. *Arch. Otolaryngol., 24,* 731–741.

Fowler, E. P. (ed.) (1939). *Medicine of the ear.* New York: Nelson.

French, N. R., Carter, C. W., & Koenig, W. (1930). The words and sounds of telephone conversations. *Bell Syst. Tech. J., 9,* 290–324.

Fritze, W. (1978). A computer-controlled binaural balance test. *Acta Otolaryngol., 86,* 89–92.

Fulton, R., & Spradlin, J. (1972). Effects of practice on SISI scores with normally-hearing subjects. *J. Speech Hear. Res., 15,* 127–224.

Fulton, R. T., & Spradlin, J. E. (1974). The short-increment sensitivity index. In R. T. Fulton (ed.), *Auditory stimulus-response control,* pp. 53–64. Baltimore: University Park Press.

Gang, R. P. (1976). The effects of age on the diagnostic utility of the rollover phenomenon. *J. Speech Hear. Dis., 41,* 63–69.

Garner, W. R., & Miller, G. A. (1947). The masked threshold of pure tones as a function of duration. *J. Exp. Psychol., 37,* 293–303.

Gates, G. A. (1976). Interpretation of diagnostic tests for acoustic neuroma: A self instructional package. Chicago: American Academy of Ophthalmology and Otolaryngology.

Gelfand, S. A. (1976). The tracking ABLB in clinical recruitment testing. *J. Aud. Res., 16,* 34–41.

Gelfand, S. A. (1981). *Hearing: An introduction to psychological and physiological acoustics.* New York: Marcel Dekker.

Gisselsson, L., & Sorensen, H. (1959). Auditory adaptation and fatigue in cochlear potentials. *Arch. Otolaryngol., 50,* 391–405.

Gjaevenes, K., & Söhoel, T. H. (1969). The tone decay test. *Acta Otolaryngol., 68,* 33–42.

Goetzinger, C. P., Proud, G., & Dirks, D. (1961). A clinical study of hearing in advanced age. *Arch. Otolaryngol., 61,* 810–820.

Gradenigo, G. (1893). On the clinical signs of the affections of the auditory nerve. Translated by S. E. Alle. *Arch. Otol., 22,* 213–215.

Green, D. S. (1963). The modified tone decay test (MTDT) as a screening procedure for eighth nerve lesions. *J. Speech Hear. Dis., 28,* 31–36.

Griffing, T., & Tuck, G. (1963). Split-half reliability of the SISI. *J. Aud. Res., 3,* 159–164.

Grimes, C. T., & Feldman, A. S. (1969). Comparative Bekesy typing with broad and modulated narrow-band noise. *J. Speech Hear. Res., 12,* 840–846.

Hagerman, B. (1976). Reliability in the determination of speech discrimination. *Scand. Audiol., 5,* 219–228.

Hall, J. (1978). Diagnostic audiometry in sensorineural loss: A critical survey. Paper presented at the Annual Convention of the American Speech-Language-Hearing Association, San Francisco, California.

Hallpike, C. S. (1965). Clinical otoneurology and its contributions to theory and practice. *Proc. R. Soc. Med., 58,* 185–196.

Hallpike, C. S., & Cairns, H. (1938). Observations on the pathology of Meniere's syndrome. *J. Laryngol., 53,* 625–655.

Hallpike, C. S., & Hood, J. D. (1951). Some recent work on auditory adaptation and its relationship to the loudness recruitment phenomenon. *J. Acoust. Soc. Am., 23,* 270–274.

Hallpike, C. S., & Hood, J. D. (1959). Observations upon the neurological mechanism of loudness recruitment. *Acta Otolaryngol., 50,* 472–486.

Hanley, C., & Utting, J. (1965). An examination of the normal hearer's response to the SISI. *J. Speech Hear. Dis., 30,* 58–65.

Harbert, F., & Young, I. M. (1962). Threshold auditory adaptation. *J. Aud. Res., 2,* 229–246.

Harbert, F., & Young, I. M. (1964). Threshold auditory adaptation measured by the tone decay test and Bekesy audiometry. *Ann. Otol. Rhinol. Laryngol., 73,* 48–60.

Harbert, F., & Young, I. M. (1965). Spread of masking in ears showing abnormal adaptation and conductive deafness. *Acta Otolaryngol., 60,* 49–58.

Harbert, F., & Young, I. M. (1968). Clinical application of Bekesy audiometry. *Laryngoscope, 78,* 487–497.

Harbert, F., Young, I., & Weiss, B. (1969). Clinical application of the intensity difference limen. *Acta Otolaryngol., 67,* 435–443.

Harford, E. (1967). Clinical application and significance of the SISI test. In A. B. Graham (ed.), *Sensorineural hearing processes and disorders,* pp. 223–233. Boston: Little, Brown.

Harris, D. A. (1979). Microprocessor versus self-recording audiometry. *J. Aud. Res., 19,* 137–150.

Harris, J. D. (1963). Loudness discrimination. *J. Speech Hear. Res. Monogr. Suppl., 11,* 24–32.

Harrison, R. (1962). *Audiological manifestations in Meniere's disease.* Unpublished Ph.D. thesis. Chicago, Illinois: Northwestern University.

Hellman, R., and Scharf, B. (1984). Acoustic reflex and loudness. In S. Silman (ed.), *The acoustic reflex: Basic principles and clinical applications,* pp. 469–516. New York: Academic Press.

Henderson, D., Salvi, R. J., & Hamernik, R. P. (1982). Neurological basis of the symptoms of noise induced hearing loss. In P. Alberti (ed.), *Personal hearing protection in industry,* pp. 103–124. New York: Raven Press.

Hirsh, I. J., Davis, H., Silverman, S. R., Reynolds, E. G., Eldert, F., & Benson, R. W. (1952). Development of materials for speech audiometry. *J. Speech Hear. Dis., 17,* 321–337.

Hirsh, I. J., Palva, T., & Goodman, A. (1954). Difference limen and recruitment. *Arch. Otolaryngol., 60,* 525–540.

Hodgson, W. R. (1967). Audiologic report of a patient with left hemispherectomy. *J. Speech Hear. Dis., 32,* 38–45.

Hood, J. D. (1950). Studies in auditory fatigue and adaptation. *Acta Otolaryngol. Suppl., 92,* 1–57.

Hood, J. D. (1955). Auditory fatigue and adaptation in the differential diagnosis of end-organ disease. *Ann Otol. Rhinol. Laryngol., 64,* 507–518.

Hood, J. D. (1969). Basic audiological requirements in neuro-otology. *J. Laryngol. Otol., 83,* 695–711.

Hood, J. D. (1977). Loudness balance procedures for the measurement of recruitment. *Audiology, 16,* 215–228.

Hood, J. D., & Poole, J. P. (1966). Tolerable limit of loudness: Its clinical and physiological significance. *J. Acoust. Soc. Am., 40,* 47–53.

Hood, J. D., & Poole, J. P. (1971). Speech audiometry in conductive and sensorineural hearing loss. *Sound, 5,* 30–38.

Hood, J. D. & Poole, J. P. (1980). Influence of the speaker and other factors affecting speech intelligibility. *Audiology, 19,* 434–455.

Hopkinson, N. T. (1966). Modifications of the four types of Bekesy audiograms. *J. Speech Hear. Dis., 31,* 79–82.

Hughes, J. W. (1946). The threshold of audition for short periods of stimulation. *Proc. R. Soc. Lond., B133,* 486–490.

Hughes, R. (1968). Atypical responses to the SISI. *Ann. Otol. Rhinol. Laryngol., 77,* 332–337.

Hughes, R. L., & Johnson, E. W. (1978). Bekesy audiometry. In J. Katz (ed.), *Handbook of clinical audiology,* pp. 201–217. 2d ed., Baltimore: Williams & Wilkins.

Hughes, R. L., Winegar, W. J., & Crabtree, J. A. (1967). Bekesy audiometry: Type II versus type IV patterns. *Arch. Otolaryngol., 86,* 424–430.

Jerger, J. (1952). A difference limen test and its diagnostic significance. *Laryngoscope, 62,* 1316–1332.

Jerger, J. (1953). DL difference test. *Arch. Otolaryngol., 57,* 490–500.

Jerger, J. F. (1955). Differential intensity sensitivity in the ear with loudness recruitment. *J. Speech Hear. Dis., 20,* 183–191.

Jerger, J. (1960). Bekesy audiometry in analysis of auditory disorders. *J. Speech Hear. Res., 3,* 275–287.

Jerger, J. (1961). Recruitment and allied phenomena in differential diagnosis. *J. Aud. Res., 2,* 145–151.

Jerger, J. (1962a). Comparative evaluation of some auditory measures. *J. Speech Hear. Res., 5,* 3–17.

Jerger, J. (1962b). Hearing tests in otologic diagnosis. *Asha, 4,* 139–145.

Jerger, J. (1973). Diagnostic audiometry. In J. Jerger (ed.), *Modern developments in audiology, 2nd ed.,* pp. 75–115. New York: Academic Press.

Jerger, J. F., & Harford, E. R. (1960). Alternate and simultaneous binaural balancing of pure tones. *J. Speech Hear. Res., 3,* 15–30.

Jerger, J. F., & Jerger, S. (1966). Critical off-time in VIIIth nerve disorders. *J. Speech Hear. Res., 9,* 573–583.

Jerger, J. F., & Jerger, S. (1971). Diagnostic significance of PB word functions. *Arch. Otolaryngol., 93,* 573–580.

Jerger, J. F., & Jerger, S. W. (1974a). Auditory findings in brainstem disorders. *Arch. Otolaryngol., 99,* 342–349.

Jerger, J., & Jerger, S. (1974b). Diagnostic value of Bekesy comfortable loudness tracings. *Arch. Otolaryngol., 99,* 351–360.

Jerger, J. F., & Jerger, S. (1975a). Clinical validity of central auditory tests. *Scand. Audiol., 4,* 147–163.

Jerger, J., & Jerger, S. (1975b). A simplified tone decay test. *Arch. Otolaryngol., 101,* 403–407.

Jerger, J., & Jerger, S. (1976). Comment on "The effects of age on the diagnostic utility of the rollover phenomenon." *J. Speech Hear. Dis., 41,* 556–557.

Jerger, J., & Thelin, J. (1968). Effects of electroacoustic characteristics of hearing aids on speech understanding. *Bull. Prosthetics Res., 10,* 159–197.

Jerger, J., Carhart, R., & Lassman, J. (1958). Clinical observations of an excessive threshold adaptation. *Arch. Otolaryngol., 68,* 617–623.

Jerger, J., Shedd, J., & Harford, E. (1959). On the detection of extremely small changes in sound intensity. *Arch. Otolaryngol., 69,* 200–211.

Jerger, J., Speaks, C., & Trammell, J. (1968). A new approach to speech audiometry. *J. Speech Hear. Dis., 33,* 318–328.

Jerger, J., Jerger, S., & Mauldin, L. (1972). The forward–backward discrepancy in Bekesy audiometry. *Arch. Otolaryngol., 72,* 400–406.

Jerger, J., & Waller, J. (1962). Some observations on masking and on the progression of auditory signs in acoustic neuroma. *J. Speech Hear. Dis., 27,* 140–143.

Jerger, S. & Jerger, J. (1981). *Auditory disorders: A manual for clinical evaluation.* Boston: Little, Brown.

Jerger, S., & Jerger, J. (1983). Evaluation of diagnostic audiometric tests. *Audiology, 22,* 144–161.

Jesteadt, W., Wier, C., & Green, D. (1977). Intensity discrimination as a function of frequency and sensation level. *J. Acoust. Soc. Am., 61,* 169–177.

Jewett, D., & Williston, J. (1971). Auditory-evoked far fields averaged from the scalp of humans. *Brain, 94,* 681–696.

Johnson, E. W. (1968). Auditory findings in 268 cases of acoustic neuromas. *Arch. Otolaryngol., 88,* 598–603.

Johnson, E. W. (1973). Clinical application of special hearing tests. *Arch. Otolaryngol., 97,* 92–96.

Johnson, E. W. (1977). Auditory test results in 500 cases of acoustic neuroma. *Arch. Otolaryngol., 103,* 152–158.

Johnson, E. W., & House, W. F. (1964). Auditory findings in 53 cases of acoustic neuromas. *Arch. Otolaryngol., 80,* 667–677.

Josey, A. F. (1987). Audiologic manifestations of tumors of the eighth nerve. *Ear Hear., 4, Suppl.,* 19S–21S.

Kamm, C., Dirks, D. D., & Mickey, M. R. (1978). Effect of sensorineural hearing loss on loudness discomfort level and most comfortable loudness judgments. *J. Speech Hear. Res., 21,* 668–681.

Kamm, C., Carterett, E. C., Morgan, D. E., & Dirks, D. D. (1980). Tutorial: Use of digitized speech materials in audiological research. *J. Speech Hear. Res., 23,* 709–721.

Karjalainen, S., Karja, J., Sorri, M., & Palva, A. (1984). Reverse frequency-sweep audiometry in patients with retrocochlear and cochlear deafness. *Audiology, 23,* 53–58.

Katinsky, S. E., & Toglia, J. V. (1968). Audiologic and vestibular manifestations of meningiomas of the cerebellopontine angle. *J. Speech Hear. Dis., 33,* 351–360.

Kiang, N. Y., & Peak, W. T. (1960). Components of electrical responses recorded from the cochlea. *Ann. Otol. Rhinol. Laryngol., 69,* 448–458.

Kiang, N. Y. S., Moxon, E. C., & Levine, R. A. (1970). Auditory-nerve activity in cats with normal and abnormal cochleas. In G. W. Wolstenholme & J. Knight (eds.), *Sensorineural hearing loss.* London: Churchill. pp. 94–101.

Koch, L. J., Bartels, D., & Rupp, R. R. (1969). The use of a "modified" short increment sensitivity index in assessing site of auditory lesion. Paper presented at the Annual Convention of the American Speech and Hearing Association, Chicago, Illinois.

König, E. (1962). Difference limen for intensity. *Int. Audiol., 1,* 198–202.

Kos, C. (1955). Auditory function as related to the complaint of dizziness. *Laryngoscope, 65,* 711–721.

Kreul, E. J., Bell, D. W., & Nixon, J. C. (1969). Factors affecting speech discrimination test difficulty. *J. Speech Hear. Res., 12,* 281–287.

L'amoré, P. J. J., & Rodenburg, M. (1980). Significance of the SISI test and its relation to recruitment. *Audiology, 19,* 75–85.

Lehiste, I., & Peterson, G. E. (1959). Linguistic considerations in the study of speech intelligibility. *J. Acoust. Soc. Am., 31,* 280–286.

Lidén, G., & Nilsson, G. (1950). Differential audiometry. *Acta Otolaryngol., 38,* 521–527.

Lorente de Nó, R. (1937). Discussion of paper by Fowler. *Trans. Amer. Otol. Soc., 27,* 219–220.

Loven, F. C., & Hawkins, D. B. (1983). Interlist equivalency of the CID W-22 word lists presented in quiet and in noise. *Ear Hear., 4,* 91–97.

Lund-Iversen, L. (1952). An investigation on the difference limen determined by the method of Lüscher and Zwislocki in normal hearing and in various forms of deafness. *Acta Otolaryngol., 42,* 219–224.

Lundborg, T. (1952). Diagnostic problems concerning auditory problems. *Acta Otolaryngol. Suppl., 99,* 1–110.

Lurie, M. H. (1940). Studies of acquired and inherited deafness in animals. *J. Acoust. Soc. Am., 11,* 420–426.

Lüscher, E. (1951). The difference limen of intensity variations of pure tones and its diagnostic significance. *J. Laryngol. Otol., 65,* 486–510.

Lüscher, E., & Zwislocki, J. (1948). Eine einfache Methode zur monauralen Bestimmung des Lautstärkeausgleiches. *Arch. Ohr.-Nas.-Kehl. Heilk., 155,* 323.

Lüscher, E., & Zwislocki, J. (1949). A simple method for indirect monaural determination of the recruitment phenomenon (difference limen in intensity in different types of deafness). *Acta Otolaryngol. Suppl., 78,* 156–172.

McNamee, J. (1960). An investigation of the use of CID Auditory Test W-22 with children. M.S. Thesis. Columbus, Ohio: Ohio State University.

Martin, F. (1978). The SISI test. In J. Katz (ed.), *Handbook of clinical audiology,* 2d ed., pp. 179–187. Baltimore: Williams & Wilkins.

Martin, F. N., & Mussell, S. A. (1979). The influence of pauses in the competing signal on synthetic sentence identification scores. *J. Speech Hear. Dis., 44,* 282–292.

Mártony, J. (1974). Some psychoacoustic tests with hearing-impaired children. *STL-OPSR, 2/3,* 72–89.

Mencher, G. R., Clark, T. D., & Rupp, R. R. (1970). The difference limen for intensity and central auditory pathway. *J. Aud. Res., 10,* 372–377.

Metz, O. (1946). The acoustic impedance measured on normal and pathological ears. *Acta Otolaryngol. Suppl., 63,* 1–254.

Meyer, D. H., & Mishler, E. T. (1985). Rollover measurements with the Auditec NU-6 word lists. *J. Speech Hear. Dis., 50,* 356–360.

Miller, M. H. (1985). The integration of audiologic findings. In J. Katz (ed.), *Handbook of clinical audiology,* 3d ed., pp. 259–272. Baltimore: Williams & Wilkins.

Miskolczy-Fodor, F. (1964). Automatically recorded loudness balance testing. *Arch. Otolaryngol., 79,* 355–365.

Morales-Garcia, C., & Hood, J. D. (1972). Tone-decay test in neuro-otological diagnosis. *Arch. Otolaryngol., 96,* 231–247.

Nelson, P., Eruklar, S., & Bryan, S. (1966). Responses of units of the inferior colliculus to time varying acoustic stimuli, *J. Neurophysiol., 29,* 834–860.

Neuberger, F. (1950). Untersuchengen über den qualitativen Zusammenhang der Unterschieds-Schwelle fur Tonintensitätsänderungen und dem Lautstärkeausgleich. *Mschr. Ohrenheilk. Lar.-Rhinol., 84,* 169–182.

Noffsinger, D. (1982). Clinical applications of selected binaural effects. *Scand. Audiol. Suppl., 15,* 157–165.

Noffsinger, D. W., Olsen, W. O., Carhart, R., Hart, C. W., & Sahgal, V. (1972). Auditory and vestibular aberrations in multiple sclerosis. *Acta Otolaryngol., 303, Suppl.,* 1–63.

Olsen, W. O. (1987). Brief tone audiometry: A review. *Ear Hear. Suppl., 8,* 13S–18S.

Olsen, W. O., & Kurdziel, S. A. (1976). Extent and rate of tone decay for cochlear and for VIIIth nerve lesion patients. Paper presented at the Annual Convention of the American Speech and Hearing Association, Houston, Texas.

Olsen, W., & Matkin, N. (1979). Speech audiometry. In W. F. Rintelmann (ed.), *Hearing assessment,* pp. 133–206. Baltimore: University Park Press.

Olsen, W. O., & Noffsinger, D. (1974). Comparison of one new and three old tests of auditory adaptation. *Arch. Otolaryngol., 96,* 231–247.

Olsen, W. O., Noffsinger, D., & Kurdziel, S. (1975). Speech discrimination in quiet and in white noise by patients with peripheral and central lesions. *Acta Otolaryngol., 80,* 375–382.

Olsen, W. O., Rose, D. E., & Noffsinger, D. (1979). Brief-tone audiometry with normal, cochlear, and eighth nerve tumor patients. *Arch. Otolaryngol., 99,* 185–189.

Osterhammel, P., Terkildsen, K., & Arndal, P. (1970). Evoked responses to SISI stimuli. Contralateral masking effects. *Acta Otolaryngol. Suppl., 263,* 245–247.

Owens, E. (1964a). Tone decay in VIIIth nerve and cochlear lesions. *J. Speech Hear. Dis., 29,* 14–22.

Owens, E. (1964b). Bekesy tracings and site of lesion. *J. Speech Hear. Dis., 29,* 456–468.

Owens, E. (1965a). The SISI test and VIIIth nerve versus cochlear involvement. *J. Speech Hear. Dis., 30,* 252–269.

Owens, E., (1965b). Bekesy tracings, tone decay, and loudness recruitment. *J. Speech Hear. Dis., 30,* 50–57.

Owens, E. (1979). Differential intensity discrimination. In W. F. Rintelmann (ed.), *Hearing assessment,* pp. 235–260. Baltimore: University Park Press.

Palva, T., Karja, J., & Palva, A. (1970). Forward vs reversed Bekesy tracings. *Arch. Otolaryngol., 91,* 449–452.

Palva, T., Jauhiainen, C., Sjoblom, J., & Ylikoski, J. (1978). Diagnosis and surgery of acoustic tumors. *Acta Otolaryngol., 86,* 233–240.

Parker, W., & Decker, R. L. (1971). Detection of abnormal auditory threshold adaptation. *Arch. Otolaryngol., 94,* 1–7.

Pedersen, C. B. (1976). Brief-tone audiometry. *Scand. Audiol., 5,* 27–33.

Penner, M. J., Leshowitz, B., Cudahy, E., & Ricard, R. (1974). Intensity discrimination for pursled sinusoids of various frequencies. *Percept. Psychophys., 15,* 568–570.

Pennington, C. D., & Martin, F. D. (1972). Current trends in audiometric practices. Part II. Auditory tests for site of lesion. *Asha, 14,* 199–203.

Penrod, J. (1979). Talker effects on word discrimination scores of adults with sensorineural hearing impairment. *J. Speech Hear. Dis., 44,* 340–349.

Perez de Moura, L. (1967). Inner ear pathology in acoustic neurinomas. *J. Speech Hear. Dis., 32,* 29–35.

Pestalozza, G., & Cioce, C. (1962). Measuring auditory adaptation. *Laryngoscope, 72,* 240–259.

Peterson, G. E., & Lehiste, I. (1962). I. Revised CNC lists for auditory tests. *J. Speech Hear. Dis., 27,* 62–69.

Pollack, I. (1948). The atonal interval. *J. Acoust. Soc. Am., 20,* 146–149.

Posner, J., & Ventry, I. M. (1977). Relationships between comfortable loudness levels for speech and speech discrimination in sensorineural hearing loss. *J. Speech Hear. Dis., 42,* 370–375.

Pratt, L., & Egan, J. (1968). SISI test in preoperative mixed loss patients. *Laryngoscope, 78,* 1965–1970.

Price, L. L., & Falck, V. T. (1963). Bekesy audiometry with children. *J. Speech Hear. Res., 6,* 129–133.

Priede, V. M., & Coles, R. R. A. (1974). Interpretation of loudness recruitment tests—Some new concepts and criteria. *J. Laryngol. Otol., 88,* 641–662.

Pumphrey, R. J., & Gold, T. (1948). *Proc. R. Soc., 41,* 183–187.

Raffin, M. J. M., & Schafer, D. (1980). Application of a probability model based on the binomial distribution to speech discrimination scores. *J. Speech Hear. Res., 23,* 570–575.

Reger, S. N. (1951). A clinical and research version of the Bekesy audiometer. *Laryngoscope, 62,* 1333–1351.

Reger, S. N., & Kos, C. M. (1952). Clinical measurements and implications of recruitment. *Ann. Otol. Rhinol. Laryngol., 61,* 810–823.

Riesz, R. (1928). Differential sensitivity of the ear for pure-tones. *Physiol. Rev., 31,* 867–875.

Rintelmann, W. F., Schumaier, D. R., Jetty, A. J., Burchfield, S. A., Beasley, D. S., Mosher, N. A., Mosher, R. A., & Penley, E. D. (1974). Six experiments on speech discrimination utilizing CNC monosyllables *J. Aud. Res. Suppl., 2,* 1–30.

Rodda, M. (1956). The consistency of audiometric testing. *Ann. Otorhinolaryngol., 74,* 673–676.

Rose, D. E., Kurdziel, S., Olsen, W. O., & Noffsinger, D. (1975). Bekesy test results in patients with eighth nerve lesions. *Arch. Otolaryngol., 101,* 573–575.

Rosenberg, P. E. (1969). *Tone decay.* Maico Audiological Library Series VIII, Rep. 6.

Rosenblith, W. A., & Miller, G. A. (1949). The threshold for continuous and interrupted tones (Abstract). *J. Acoust. Soc. Am., 22,* 674.

Ross, M., & Huntington, D. A. (1962). Concerning the reliability and equivalence of the CID W-22 auditory tests. *J. Aud. Res., 2,* 220–228.

Ruben, R. J., Hudson, W., & Chiang, A. (1962). Anatomical and physiological effects of chronic section of the eighth nerve in cat. *Acta Otolaryngol., 55,* 473–484.

Runge, C. A., & Hosford-Dunn, H. (1985). Word recognition performance with modified CID W-22 word lists. *J. Speech Hear. Res., 28,* 353–362.

Salvi, R. J., Henderson, D., Hamernik, R., & Ahroon, W. A. (1983). Survey paper: Neural correlates of sensorineural hearing loss. *Ear Hear., 4,* 115–129.

Sanders, J. (1965). Labyrinthine otosclerosis. *Arch. Otolaryngol., 81,* 553–565.

Sanders, J. W. (1979). Recruitment. In W. F. Rintelmann (ed.), *Hearing assessment,* pp. 261–280. Baltimore: University Park Press.

Sanders, J. W. (1984). Diagnostic audiology. In J. L. Northern (ed.), *Hearing disorders,* pp. 25–39. Boston: Little, Brown.

Sanders, J., & Simpson, M. (1966). The effect of increment size on short increment sensitivity scores. *J. Speech Hear. Res., 9,* 297–304.

Sanders, J. W., Josey, A. F., & Kemker, F. J. (1971). Brief-tone audiometry in patients with VIIIth nerve tumor. *J. Speech Hear. Res., 14,* 172–178.

Sanders, J. W., Josey, A. F., & Glasscock, M. E. (1974). Audiologic evaluation in cochlear and eighth-nerve disorders. *Arch. Otolaryngol., 100,* 283–293.

Sanders, J. W., Josey, A. F., & Glasscock, M. D. (1978). The SISI at high intensity in eighth nerve ears. Paper presented at the Annual Convention of the American Speech-Language-Hearing Association, San Francisco, California.

Sanderson-Leepa, M. E., & Rintelmann, W. F. (1976). Articulation function and test-retest performance of normal-learning children on three speech discrimination test: WIPI, PBK 50, and NU auditory Test No. 6. *J. Speech Hear. Dis., 41,* 503–519.

Schubert, K. (1944). Hörermüdung und Hördauer. *Hals-Nas.-Ohrenheilk., 51,* 19–74.

Schuknecht, H. (1974). *Pathology of the ear,* pp. 388–403. Cambridge: Harvard University Press.

Schuknecht, H. F., & Woellner, R. C. (1955). An experimental and clinical study of deafness from lesions of the the cochlear nerve. *J. Laryngol., 69,* 75–97.

Shapiro, I., & Naunton, R. (1967). Audiologic evaluation of acoustic neurinomas. *J. Speech Hear. Dis., 32,* 29–35.

Shimizu, H. (1969). Influence of contralateral noise stimulation on tone decay and SISI tests. *Laryngoscope, 79,* 2155–2164.

Silman, S., Gelfand, S. A., Lutolf, J., & Chun, T. H. (1981). Letters to the editor: A response to Wiley and Lilly. *J. Speech Hear. Dis., 46,* 217.

Simmons, F. B., & Dixon, R. F. (1966). Clinical implications of loudness balancing. *Arch. Otolaryngol., 83,* 449–454.

Simonton, K. M. (1956). End-organ deafness: Diagnosis and significance. *Arch. Otolaryngol., 63,* 262–269.

Small, A. M., Jr., & Minifie, F. A. (1961). Intensive differential sensitivity and masked threshold. *J. Speech Hear. Res., 4,* 164–171.

Sohmer, H., & Feinmesser, M. (1970). Cochlear and cortical audiometry conveniently recorded in the same subject. *Israel J. Med. Sci., 6,* 219–223.

Sorensen, H. (1962). Clinical application of continuous threshold recordings. *Acta Otolaryngol., 54,* 403–422.

Speaks, C. (1967). Intelligibility of filtered synthetic sentences. *J. Speech Hear. Res., 19,* 289–298.

Speaks, C., & Jerger, J. (1965). Method for measurement of speech identification. *J. Speech Hear. Res., 8,* 185–194.

Speaks, C., Jerger, J., & Jerger, S. (1966). Performance-intensity characteristics of synthetic sentences. *J. Speech Hear. Res., 9,* 305–312.

Stark, E. W. (1968). Bekesy audiometry. *Maico Audiol. Lib., 6,* 5–8.

Starr, A., & Achor, L. (1975). Auditory brain stem responses in neurological disease. *Arch. Neurol., 32,* 761–768.

Stephens, S. D. G. (1976). Auditory temporal summation in patients with central nervous system lesions. In S. D. G. Stephens (ed.), *Disorders of auditory function, II.,* pp. 231–243. London: Academic Press.

Studebaker, G. (1973). Auditory masking. In J. Jerger (ed.), *Modern developments in audiology,* 2d ed., pp. 117–154. New York: Academic Press.

Suga, F., & Lindsay, J. R. (1976). Inner ear degeneration in acoustic neuromata. *Ann. Otol. Rhinol. Laryngol., 85,* 343–358.

Sung, S. S., Goetzinger, C. P., & Knox, A. W. (1969). The sensitivity and reliability of three tone-decay tests. *J. Aud. Res., 9,* 167–177.

Swisher, L. P. (1966). Response to intensity change in cochlear pathology. *Laryngoscope, 76,* 1706–1713.

Swisher, L. P. (1967). Auditory intensity discrimination in patients with temporal lobe damage. *Cortex, 3,* 179–193.

Swisher, L., Stephens, M., & Doehring, D. (1966). The effects of hearing level and normal variability on sensitivity to intensity change. *J. Aud. Res., 6,* 249–259.

Swisher, L. P., Dudley, J. G., & Doehring, D. G. (1969). Influence of contralateral noise on auditory intensity discrimination. *J. Acoust. Soc. Am., 45,* 1532–1536.

Thompson, G. A. (1963). Modified SISI technique for selected cases with suspected acoustic neuroma. *J. Speech Hear. Dis., 28,* 299–302.

Thorndike, E. L. (1932). *A teacher's word book of the twenty thousand words found most frequently and widely in general reading for children and young people.* New Uork: Teachers College, Columbia University.

Thorndike, E. L., & Lorge, I. (1944). *The teacher's word book of 30,000 words.* New York: Columbia University Press.

Thornton, A. R., & Raffin, M. J. M. (1978). Speech-discrimination scores modeled as a binomial variable. *J. Speech Hear. Res., 21,* 507–518.

Tillman, T. W. (1966). Audiologic diagnosis of acoustic tumors. *Arch. Otolaryngol., 83,* 574–581.

Tillman, T. W. (1969). Special hearing tests in otoneurologic diagnosis. *Arch. Otolaryngol., 89,* 52–56.

Tillman, T. W., & Carhart, R. (1966). An expanded test for speech discrimination utilizing CNC monosyllabic words (Northwestern University Test No. 6). Technical Report, SAM-TR-66-55 USAF School of Aerospace Medicine, Aerospace Medical Division (AFSC), Brooks Air Force Base, Texas.

Tillman, T. W., & Olsen, W. O. (1973). Speech audiometry. In J. Jerger (ed.), *Modern developments in audiology*, 2d ed., pp. 37–74. New York: Academic Press.

Tillman, T. W., Carhart, R., & Wilber, L. (1963). A test for speech discrimination composed of CNC monosyllabic words (Northwestern University Auditory Test No. 4). Technical Report, SAM-TDR-62-135 USAF School of Aerospace Medicine, Aerospace Medical Division (AFSC), Brooks Air Force Base, Texas.

Tonndorf, J. (1980). Special hearing tests in otoneurological diagnosis. *Arch. Otolaryngol., 89,* 25–30.

Tonndorf, J. (1981). Stereociliary dysfunction, a cause of sensory hearing loss, recruitment, poor speech discrimination and tinnitus. *Acta Otolaryngol., 91,* 469–480.

Turner, R. G., Shepard, N. T., & Frazer, G. J. (1984). Clinical performance of audiological and related diagnostic tests. *Ear Hear., 5,* 187–194.

Walsh, T. E., & Goodman, A. (1955). Speech discrimination in central auditory lesions. *Laryngoscope, 65,* 1–8.

Ward, W. D. (1970). Cited by Green, D. S. (1978) Tone decay. In J. Katz (ed.), *Handbook of clinical audiology*, 2d ed., pp. 188–200. Baltimore: Williams & Wilkins.

Weiss, B. G., Harbert, F., & Wilpezeski, C. R. (1967). Suprathreshold intensity discrimination. Paper presented at the Annual Convention of the American Speech and Hearing Association, Chicago, Illinois.

Wiley, T. L., & Lilly, D. J. (1980). Temporal characteristics of auditory adaptation: A case report. *J. Speech Hear. Dis., 45,* 209–215.

Willeford, J. A. (1960). *The association of abnormalities in auditory adaptation to other auditory phenomena.* Ph.D. Thesis. Evanston: Illinois: Northwestern University.

Wilson, R. H., & Margolis, R. H. (1983). Measurements of auditory thresholds for speech stimuli. In D. F. Konkle & W. F. Rintelmann (eds.), *Principles of speech audiometry*, pp. 79–126. Baltimore: University Park Press.

Wilson, R. H., Coley, K. E., Hanel, J. L., & Browning, K. M. (1976). Northwestern University Test No. 6: Normative and comparative intelligibility functions. *J. Am. Aud. Soc., 5,* 221–228.

Yantis, P. Q. (1959). Clinical application of temporary threshold shift. *Arch. Otolaryngol., 70,* 779–787.

Yantis, P., & Decker, R. (1964). On the short increment sensitivity index (SISI test). *J. Speech Hear. Dis., 29,* 231–246.

Young, I. M. (1968). Effects of ipsilateral masking on Bekesy amplitude. *J. Aud. Res., 8,* 357–365.

Young, I. M., & Harbert, F. (1967). Significance of the SISI test. *J. Aud. Res., 7,* 303–311.

Young, I. M., & Harbert, F. (1971). Forward and backward sweep responses in Bekesy audiometry. *Ann. Otol. Rhinol. Laryngol., 80,* 612–617.

Young, I., & Wenner, C. (1968). Effects of masking noise on the SISI test. *J. Aud. Res., 8,* 331–337.

Zöllner, F., & Hallbrock, K. (1952a). Erfahrungen mit überschwelligen Hörmessungen. I. *Z. Lar. Rhinol. Otol., 31,* 245–358.

Zöllner, F., & Hallbrock, K. (1952b). Erfahrungen mit überschwelligen Hörmessungen. II. *Z. Lar. Rhinol Otol., 31,* 309–322.

CHAPTER 6

CENTRAL AUDITORY SPEECH TESTS

An interference with the central auditory nervous system (CANS) from the cochlear nuclei to the auditory cortex in the temporal lobe including the interhemispheric pathways (see Chapter 2) may result in central auditory dysfunction. Interference can result from a lesion directly or indirectly affecting the CANS. Such lesions may be space-occupying neoplasms, degenerative diseases, infections, vascular disorders, congenital neurologic deficits, or acquired neurologic deficits such as that resulting from head trauma. Central auditory dysfunction can also result from minimal lesions of the CANS which cannot be detected by sophisticated radiologic and neurologic techniques.

Central auditory testing has been employed (a) to detect and localize the site of a central auditory lesion, (b) to identify children with central auditory processing disorders who demonstrate learning or communication problems, (c) to quantify and describe the deficit in central auditory processing in order to determine the nature of remediation, (d) to assess the benefits of educational and medical including surgical remediation on central auditory function, (e) to determine ear dominance and hemispheric specialization for various types of auditory stimuli, and (f) to examine the effects of maturation on central auditory processing. The primary focus of this chapter is on central auditory testing for the purposes of detecting and localizing the site of a central auditory lesion, and for assessing central auditory function to monitor or determine remediation.

In the subsequent sections, diagnostic application of each audiologic test with respect to identification and localization of central auditory dysfunction will be discussed. This section will focus on the diagnostic application of central auditory speech tests with respect to central auditory dysfunction.

Interest in the use of special speech tests for the assessment of central auditory dysfunction grew after clinical case studies revealed that the pure-tone thresholds and monosyllabic PB-word recognition scores were essentially normal in hemispherectomized patients (Goldstein, 1961; Goldstein, Goodman, & King, 1956; Hodgson, 1967). The failure of pure-tone threshold tests to identify central audi-

tory dysfunction is related to the decreasing importance of frequency and intensity analysis at increasingly rostral levels of the auditory pathway and the intrinsic redundancy of the CANS. The failure of conventional speech-recognition threshold and monosyllabic PB-word tests to identify central auditory dysfunction is related to the concept of intrinsic and extrinsic redundancy.

Intrinsic CANS redundancy is based on the multiplicity of neural pathways, centers, and decussations; interrelatedness of these pathways, centers, and decussations; and bilateral representation of the auditory system. Extrinsic redundancy stems from aspects of the auditory signal such as the frequency range, sound duration, context in which the message is given, rhythm, and the individual's familiarity with the semantic, syntactic, and phonologic rules of language. Extrinsic redundancy is inherent in the speech message and enables the message to be perceived even when parts of the message are degraded or absent. Intrinsic redundancy is reduced by CANS lesions but the effect of this reduction on performance on conventional speech-recognition tests is not apparent unless the lesion affects a significant proportion of the neurons and nuclei in the CANS. Extrinsic redundancy of speech can be reduced by various means of degradation such as filtering, time alteration, or noise. Since pure-tone signals have fewer parameters than speech signals, the extrinsic redundancy of pure-tones is more difficult to reduce than that of speech.

The principles of "subtlety" and "bottleneck" also apply when investigating central auditory function (Jerger, 1960a). The former principle states that the subtlety of the auditory signs of central auditory dysfunction increases as the level of the lesion becomes more rostral. Thus, at peripheral levels, a lesion may be detected by simple tests such as the audiogram. At central levels, however, the lesion can be detected only by more complex tests such as distorted speech tests. According to the bottleneck principle, a complex signal such as speech encounters neural congestion at the junction of the eighth nerve and brainstem; lesions at these sites have a very deleterious effect on speech-recognition scores whereas lesions more peripheral or central to these sites have less deleterious effects on speech-recognition scores.

The development of specialized (degraded) speech tests for assessment of central auditory dysfunction was based on the concept that the central auditory dysfunction is manifested by taxing the CANS through reduction in extrinsic redundancy. Central auditory tests based on the principle of reduction of extrinsic redundancy include the monaural and dichotic speech tests. Since extra-axial brainstem disorders behave like eighth-nerve disorders, this section will concentrate on the use of central auditory speech tests for detection of intra-axial brainstem and cortical lesions.

I. MONAURAL LOW-REDUNDANCY SPEECH TESTS

Monaural presentation involves the presentation of one message to a single ear at a time. In monaural speech tests, the extrinsic redundancy is reduced by filtering and by time alteration such as compression or interruption.

A. LOW-PASS FILTERED

Bocca, Calearo, and Cassinari (1954) and Bocca, Calearo, Cassinari, and Migliavacca (1955) obtained performance-intensity functions for low-pass filtered (cutoff frequency of 500 Hz) lists of PB words in persons with temporal-lobe tumors with normal-hearing threshold levels. They found a contralateral-ear effect (i.e., scores were poorer in the ear contralateral to the side of the temporal-lobe lesion) that was absent (or reduced) when the lists were presented without frequency distortion. Similar findings were obtained by Goldstein et al. (1956), using the Rush Hughes poor-quality (presumably frequency distorted) recordings of PB words, and Jerger (1960a,b,1964), using low-pass filtered PAL PB-50 word lists.

Lynn and Gilroy (1972, 1975, 1976, 1977) have conducted several investigations on the effects of various central auditory lesions on low-pass filtered speech scores. For example, Lynn and Gilroy (1977) obtained the scores for low-pass filtered NU-6 monosyllabic PB words (cutoff-frequency of 500 Hz with a rejection rate of 34 dB/octave) presented at 60 dB SL relative to the PTA or SRT in a group of 11 patients with surgically confirmed right temporal-lobe tumors and 11 patients with left temporal-lobe tumors. The contralateral-ear effect was present in the right and left temporal-lobe tumor cases, with an average interaural difference of approximately 16% for the right temporal-lobe cases and approximately 12% for the left temporal-lobe cases. Lynn and Gilroy (1977) found that, in their group of 35 patients with temporal-lobe tumors, 74% had contralateral-ear effects, 3% had ipsilateral-ear effects, and 24% had normal scores on the low-pass filtered speech test.

Studies (Lynn & Gilroy, 1977; Musiek, Wilson, & Pinheiro, 1979) have revealed that the scores for both ears for low-pass filtered speech are generally unaffected by lesions of the interhemispheric pathways (corpus callosum). In a recent study, Baran, Musiek, and Reeves (1986) reported that post-surgical scores on the low-pass filtered speech test did not differ significantly from the preoperative scores in a group of 8 patients who underwent anterior section of the corpus callosum. Lynn and Gilroy (1977) found that, in a group of 38 patients with parietal-lobe tumors affecting the interhemispheric auditory pathways, 74% had normal scores, 22% had abnormal scores in the left ear, and 4% had abnormal scores in the right ear.

Consistent findings on low-pass filtered speech tests have not been obtained for brainstem lesions. Ipsilateral, contralateral, and bilateral ear effects have been reported in persons with brainstem lesions (Calearo & Antonelli, 1968; Lynn & Gilroy, 1977). According to Lynn and Gilroy (1977), the diffuse nature of many brainstem lesions affects the correlation between locus of the tumor and the ear affected on the low-pass filtered speech test. The level of the lesion in the central nervous system and magnitude of the lesion also affect the correlation between locus of the tumor and the ear affected (Rintelmann, 1985).

The low-pass filtered speech test in the Willeford battery has a cutoff frequency of 500 Hz with a rejection rate of 18 dB/octave and uses Michigan consonant-nucleus-consonant (CNC) words. The presentation level is 50 dB SL relative to the PTA or SRT.

Because of the limited normative data available for the Willeford (CNC) and Lynn and Gilroy (NU-6) low-pass filtered speech test, lack of standardized procedure and tape, and the variety of cutoff frequencies available on commercial recordings of the filtered speech tests, each clinic should establish its own normative data.

B. TIME COMPRESSED

Early investigations of time-compressed speech employed fast playback of the tape recorder. A drawback of the fast playback procedure was the concomitant shifts in spectrum of the recorded signal (Beasley & Freeman, 1977). The chop–splice procedure was then developed by Garvey (1953a,b), which corrected for the problem of frequency shifts associated with temporal alteration of the signal by manually cutting portions from the recording and then splicing back the remaining sections of the tape. This procedure, however, was tedious and awkward. Fairbanks, Everitt, and Jaeger (1954) developed a procedure for time compression which avoided the problems associated with the playback and chop–splice procedure. Fairbanks et al. (1954) used an electromechanical time compressor/expander which electromechanically deleted samples and electromechanically spliced the remaining samples yielding a recording that is some percentage compressed or expanded relative to the original recording. The Springer Information Rate Changer was an electromechanical device similar to the Fairbanks device except that the discard interval had a limited range of variability. The Lee (1972) Varispeech device, a modification of the Fairbanks instrument, contains a small tape recorder and minicomputer and is the one most widely used currently for time-compressed speech. A drawback of both the Fairbanks and Lee devices was that the sampling was random so samples discarded could be within as well as between linguistic sections. More sophisticated devices based on digital computers and speech synthesizers which allow for selectivity in removal of specific sections are available but these devices are extremely expensive and are not employed clinically.

Calearo and Lazzaroni (1957) found that contralateral-ear effects were present in temporal-lobe tumor cases for time-compressed speech. Nevertheless, the contralateral-ear effects for time-compressed speech were not as pronounced as those for frequency-distorted speech. Calearo and Lazzaroni (1957) also reported that decreased suprathreshold speech-recognition scores for time-compressed speech were present for diffuse disorders of the central auditory nervous system and for brainstem pathology. Similar findings were obtained by deQuiros (1964).

Calearo and Antonelli (1968) reported that 14 of 23 cases with brainstem pathology had reduced scores on time-compressed speech tests, generally on one ear.

Kurdziel, Noffsinger, and Olsen (1976) obtained scores for 0, 40, and 60% time compression of NU-6 monosyllables for 15 patients with diffuse central nervous system lesions (e.g., cerebral vascular accident cases) and 16 patients with discrete anterior temporal-lobe lesions. Contralateral-ear effects were present in the diffuse-lesion group but not the discrete temporal-lobe lesion group. The contralateral-ear effects were enhanced at the highest compression rate (60%). Thus, the time-compressed speech is sensitive to diffuse hemispheric but not discrete anterior temporal-lobe lesions. Beck and Mueller (1983) observed only slight contralateral-ear effects in patients with discrete brain injury resulting from head injury.

Studies of the effects of time compression on speech recognition in normal-hearing elderly listeners enabled the investigation of the effects of diffuse central nervous system dysfunction. Sticht and Gray (1969) investigated the effects of time compression of CID W-22 word lists on the suprathreshold speech-recognition scores of young and old normal-hearing adults. Their results showed that older adults had more errors with time-compressed speech than younger adults at all degrees of time compression investigated. Konkle, Beasley, and Bess (1977), who also used time-compressed W-22 word lists, obtained similar findings. The results indicate that time-compressed speech may

help differentiate between peripheral and central auditory dysfunction in the elderly.

Beasley and his colleagues (1972a,b) have collected extensive normative data for several rates of time compression and several sensation levels of presentation of NU-6 word lists using the Zemlin modification of the Fairbanks et al. (1954) procedure. Normative data were also obtained by deChicchis, Orchik, and Tecca (1981) for the Auditec uncompressed recordings of the NU-6 and W-22 word lists compressed using the Varispeech II time compressor/expander. The scores reported by deChicchis et al. (1981) for the NU-6 word lists were significantly poorer than those reported by the Beasley et al. (1972a,b) norms. Beattie (1986) obtained normative performance-intensity functions for the Auditec CID W-22 recordings with 30 and 60% time compression.

A 30 and 60% time-compressed version of the NU-6 Form A tape was made commercially available by Auditec of St. Louis in 1978. Compression was obtained using the Varispeech II device. Grimes, Mueller, and Williams (1984) collected data on normal-hearing and sensorineural hearing-impaired persons for the four randomizations of the Auditec 60% time-compressed NU-6 Form A lists presented at 32 dB SL relative to the SRT. Interlist equivalency was present only for lists I and IV in the sensorineural group and for lists I, II, and IV in the normal-hearing group. In the normal-hearing group, the score reflecting two standard deviations below the mean of 73.2% was approximately 58% (across lists I, II, and IV). Grimes et al. suggested that interaural differences in time-compressed scores of at least 20% can be considered significant in normal-hearing listeners. Grimes et al. (1984) also reported the presence of significant learning effects which were larger in the normal-hearing group. Nevertheless, significant learning effects were not manifested between the first and second presentation. Grimes et al. (1984) concluded that the learning effect was clinically insignificant because not more than two lists are generally presented to a patient.

Beasley et al. (1972b) also reported significant list differences in their recording of the NU-6 test. Riensche, Konkle, and Beasley (1976), who investigated interlist equivalency for the Beasley recording of the NU-6 Form A time-compressed lists while controlling for the order effect, reported a smaller interlist differences than reported by Beasley et al. (1972b) for Form B of the same recording.

II. DICHOTIC SPEECH TESTS

Dichotic testing refers to stimulation of both ears with different stimuli. That is, the signals presented to the left ear differ from the signals presented simultaneously to the right ear.

A. MODEL FOR CONTRALATERAL AND IPSILATERAL EAR EFFECTS

Kimura (1961a,b), using a dichotic digits test, found that patients with unilateral anterior temporal lobe resections made more errors in identifying digits presented to the ear contralateral to the resection and that patients with left temporal-lobe damage had poorer contralateral-ear scores than patients with right temporal-lobe damage. Sparks and Geschwind (1968) reported that an ipsilateral-ear effect emerged from dichotic testing in patients with lesions involving the interhemispheric auditory pathway (corpus callosum).

Speaks (1975) proposed a model to account for the contralateral- and ipsilateral-ear effects. His model is a modification of the one proposed by Sparks, Goodglass, and Nickel (1970). The model is based on the premise that the contralateral pathways are more numerous or stronger than the ipsilateral pathways. During monotic listening, either the contralateral and/or the ipsilateral pathway enable recognition of the stimulus. The model assumes that during dichotic listening, the ipsilateral pathways are suppressed so only the contralateral pathways contribute to recognition. Figure 1 illustrates the mechanism underlying the ear effect obtained in a normal-hearing, non-brain-damaged person for a dichotic speech test. This figure shows that the signal for the left ear is routed contralaterally to the right temporal lobe where acoustic analysis (probably feature detection) and possibly preliminary linguistic analysis of the speech signal occurs. The signal is then routed from the

right to the left hemisphere (which is usually dominant for language) for further linguistic analysis. As the signal is routed between hemispheres, it undergoes slight degradation so the left ear (dichotic) score is slightly reduced. The signal (speech) presented to the right ear is routed contralaterally to the left hemisphere for both acoustic and in-depth linguistic analysis. Since the signal does not need to be transmitted across hemispheres, there is no degradation of the signal presented to the right ear. Therefore, the dichotic score for the right ear is superior to that for the left ear. This slight right-ear superiority is known as the right-ear advantage. If the dominant hemisphere for language is the right rather than the left hemisphere, then a slight left-ear advantage is obtained for a normal-hearing, non-brain-damaged person during dichotic speech tests. The right-ear advantage is difficult to demonstrate using monotic speech materials. It is revealed during dichotic speech testing since dichotic tests sufficiently tax the auditory system enabling the manifestation of subtle effects.

Figure 2 illustrates the mechanism underlying the increased right-ear advantage in persons with damage to the right temporal lobe. The left-ear signal is routed contralaterally to the right lobe where it is degraded because of the damage in that lobe. The signal is then transmitted to the left temporal lobe, undergoing further degradation in the transmission between hemispheres. This results in a left-ear score which is reduced more than it is in normal-hearing non-brain-damaged listeners. The right-ear score is unaffected since the right-ear signal is routed contralaterally to the intact, left, language-dominant hemisphere for both

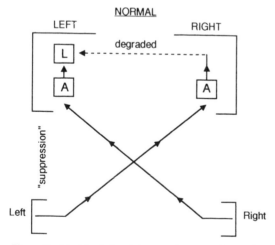

Figure 1 Model of the right-ear advantage during dichotic testing in normal persons. The linguistic area of the temporal lobe is represented as L and the area of the temporal lobe responsible for preliminary acoustic analysis is represented as A. The diagonal, solid lines from the two ears represent the contralateral pathways. The ipsilateral pathways are not shown because of suppression during dichotic testing. The horizontal dashed line between the temporal lobes represents the interhemispheric pathways. Reprinted from Speaks (1975) with permission.

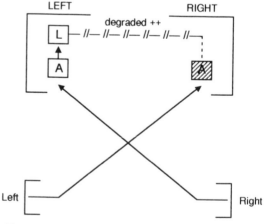

Figure 2 Model of ear effects in persons with damage to the right temporal lobe. The linguistic area of the temporal lobe is represented as L and the area of the temporal lobe responsible for preliminary acoustic analysis is represented as A. The diagonal, solid lines from the two ears represent the contralateral pathways. The ipsilateral pathways are not shown because of suppression during dichotic testing. The symbols connecting the right and left temporal lobes represent the interhemispheric pathways. Reprinted from Speaks (1975) with permission.

acoustic and linguistic analysis. Thus, a larger-than-normal right-ear advantage resulting from good right-ear scores and poorer-than-normal left-ear scores is expected on dichotic speech tests in persons with a right temporal-lobe lesion. In other words, a significant contralateral-ear effect is observed in right-hemisphere lesions, that is, the score for the ear opposite to the side of the lesion is reduced compared to that for the ear on the same side as the lesion.

Figure 3 shows the mechanism underlying the left-ear advantage in persons with damage in the left temporal lobe confined to the area involving acoustic analysis. The right-ear signal is routed directly to the impaired left temporal lobe where it is degraded by the lesion. The left-ear signal is routed to the intact right temporal lobe for acoustic analysis and then to the intact linguistic area of the left temporal lobe for linguistic analysis. During the interhemispheric transmission there is a slight degradation in the signal. Thus, the score for the left ear is only slightly reduced and is similar to that for the left ear of non-brain-damaged persons. The right-ear signal is routed to the left temporal lobe for acoustic and linguistic processing where it is degraded by the lesion in the acoustic area. Therefore, the right-ear score is depressed compared with the right-ear score for non-brain-damaged listeners. The slightly degraded left-ear score and significantly degraded right-ear score yields a left-ear advantage or contralateral-ear effect in cases with damage in the left hemisphere involving the acoustic area.

Figure 4 shows the mechanism underlying the left-ear advantage in persons with damage to the linguistic and auditory areas of the left temporal lobe. The right-ear signal

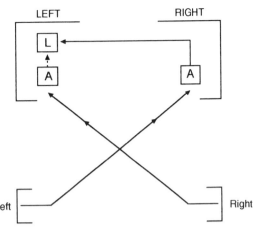

Figure 4 Model of ear effects in persons with damage to the linguistic area and area responsible for preliminary acoustic analysis in the left temporal lobe. The linguistic area of the temporal lobe is represented as L and the area of the temporal lobe responsible for preliminary acoustic analysis is represented as A. The diagonal, solid lines from the two ears are the contralateral pathways. The ipsilateral pathways are not shown since they are suppressed during dichotic testing. The solid horizontal line between temporal lobes represents the interhemispheric pathways. Reprinted from Speaks (1975) with permission.

is routed contralaterally to the damaged left temporal lobe where it is severely degraded because both the auditory and linguistic areas are affected. The left-ear signal is routed to the intact right hemisphere for acoustic processing and then is routed to the left hemisphere for linguistic processing. The left-ear score is degraded slightly by the interhemispheric transmission and is also degraded by the lesion in the left hemisphere. The degradation in the right-ear score is greater than that in the left-ear score (which receives normal acoustic processing in the right hemisphere) yielding a left-ear advantage or contralateral-ear effect.

Figure 5 shows the mechanism underlying the ipsilateral-ear effect in persons with damage in the left hemisphere involving the terminal callosal fibers. The left-ear signal is first routed to the right hemisphere for acoustic processing and then is routed to the left hemisphere for linguistic processing. Since the interhemispheric pathway is impaired, the left-ear signal is severely degraded by the interhemispheric transmission. The right-ear signal is routed to the intact left hemisphere for acoustic and linguistic processing. The degraded left-ear score and normal right-ear score yields a right-ear advantage or ipsilateral-ear effect (because the depression in manifested in the ear ipsilateral to the side of the lesion).

Sparks *et al.* (1970) reported that 4 of his 20 patients with right hemisphere damage failed to yield the expected contralateral-ear effect. Speaks, Rubens, Podraza, and Kuhl (1973) reported that one of their patients with deep supra-Sylvian lesions involving the terminal callosal fibers failed to show the ipsilateral-ear effect. Since the dichotic speech

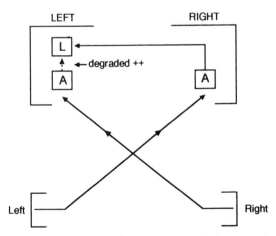

Figure 3 Model of ear effects in persons with damage to the left temporal lobe confined to the area responsible for preliminary acoustic analysis. The linguistic area of the temporal lobe is represented as L and the area of the temporal lobe responsible for preliminary acoustic analysis is represented as A. The diagonal, solid lines from the two ears represent the contralateral pathways. The ipsilateral pathways are not shown since they are suppressed during dichotic testing. The horizontal solid line between the temporal lobes represents the interhemispheric pathways. Reprinted from Speaks (1975) with permission.

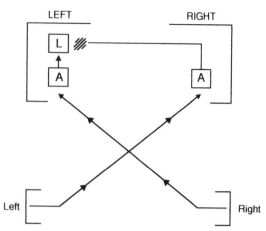

Figure 5 Model of ear effects in persons with damage in the left hemisphere involving the terminal callosal fibers. The linguistic area of the temporal lobe is represented as L and the area of the temporal lobe responsible for preliminary acoustic analysis is represented as A. The diagonal, solid lines from the two ears represent the contralateral pathways. The ipsilateral pathways are not shown since they are suppressed during dichotic testing. The horizontal solid line between the two hemispheres represents the interhemispheric pathways. The area with small diagonal lines at the left end of the solid horizontal line represents the damaged part of the interhemispheric pathways. Reprinted from Speaks (1975) with permission.

tests do not always yield the expected results even in populations with well-defined lesions, Speaks (1975) suggested that determination of the side of lesion be based on neurologic rather than dichotic listening tests. Instead, Speaks (1975) suggested that dichotic listening results be used to answer the question of whether there was impaired auditory processing of speech. Nevertheless, Speaks (1975) contended that in cases of left-hemisphere lesions involving the callosal fibers, it is not always possible to differentiate between an ipsilateral-ear effect and a normal (but larger than average) right-ear advantage. The presence of aphasia has a confounding effect on the production of contralateral- and ipsilateral-ear effects.

Because dichotic speech tests do not always yield the expected contralateral- or ipsilateral-ear effect, some investigators refer to the ear with the more depressed score as the "weak" ear and the ear with the higher score as the "strong ear."

Recently, the model to account for dichotic speech-test results developed by Sparks *et al.* (1970) with the minor modifications by Speaks (1975) has been questioned (Efron, 1985). Efron (1985) contended that symmetrical hearing-threshold levels do not rule out asymmetry in suprathreshold measures such as loudness recruitment, frequency discrimination, or gap-detection threshold, or asymmetry in subcortical function. Efron (1985) also contended that earphone reversal between blocks of trials does not ensure completely sufficient counterbalancing; earphone reversal

also does not counterbalance for interaural differences in ear-canal resonance. Efron (1985) also contended that the use of the hemispheric specialization model to account for the dichotic speech-test results is weakened by the fact that although nearly all right-handed people are left-hemisphere dominant, only about 50% of normal subjects actually show right-ear advantages on dichotic speech tests. According to Efron (1985), the hemispheric-specialization model is further weakened by the fact that ear effects can be elicited with nonspeech as well as speech stimuli. Efron (1985) proposed that some of the ear effects may result from efferent (feedback) pathways from the cortex to subcortical structures rather than from degradation of the signal during interhemispheric transmission from the nondominant to the dominant hemisphere. Although Efron's arguments are cogent, further research is needed to clarify the issue of the mechanism underlying the observed ear effects on dichotic-listening tests.

B. DIGITS

In the early 1960s, Kimura carried out several investigations of the deficits associated with temporal-lobe lesions using the Broadbent (1954) technique. In the Broadbent (1954) technique, two different digits are presented simultaneously to the two ears through earphones, one digit to each ear. Typically, three pairs of digits are presented sequentially. After the six digits are presented (three to each ear in a pair-wise fashion), the patient is asked to report all the numbers heard in any order.

Kimura (1961b) demonstrated that, on the dichotic-digits test, unilateral temporal lobectomy resulted in impaired digit recognition in the ear contralateral to the side of the lobectomy. Kimura (1961b) also observed that overall efficiency (total number of digits reported from both ears) was impaired by left but not right temporal lobectomy. Kimura (1961b) also observed that, regardless of the side of the lobectomy, the preoperative dichotic-digits score was higher for the right than for the left ear. This right-ear superiority was also observed in normal subjects (Kimura, 1961a). Kimura (1961a,b) concluded that the contralateral pathways were stronger or more numerous than the ipsilateral pathways and that the left temporal lobe was more important than the right temporal lobe in speech-recognition ability.

Sparks *et al.* (1970) reported that 17 of their 20 patients with right-hemisphere lesions and 13 of their 28 patients with left-hemisphere lesions demonstrated contralateral-ear effects on the dichotic-digits test. Ipsilateral-ear effects, however, were observed in 1 of the 20 patients with right-hemisphere lesions and 15 of the 28 patients with left-hemisphere lesions. According to Sparks *et al.* (1970), the ipsilateral-ear effects occurred in cases where the lesion was deep and involved the callosal fibers from the right hemisphere, yielding reduced left-ear scores similar to those observed in patients with right-hemisphere lesions.

Baran *et al.* (1986) administered the Musiek (1983a) version of the dichotic-digits test to 7 patients with anterior sections of the corpus callosum. Baran *et al.* (1986) reported that the average preoperative score was 66.3% for the left ear and 86.3% for the right ear; the average postoperative score was 67.4% for the left ear and 83.3% in the right ear. Thus, a left-ear deficit was demonstrated preoperatively and postoperatively and the scores did not change in either ear, on average, following anterior sections of the corpus callosum. Baran *et al.* (1986) concluded that the lack of change following anterior sections of the corpus callosum compared with results in patients with complete commissurotomies supports the hypothesis that the majority of the auditory fibers transverse the posterior rather than the anterior half of the corpus callosum.

Musiek (1983a) developed a modified dichotic-digits test which differed from Kimura's test in that two instead of three pairs of digits are delivered pair-wise (two digits presented simultaneously to the two ears, one to each ear). The presentation level was 50 dB SL relative to the SRT. Forty pairs of digits are delivered. The patient is instructed to report the digits heard in any order (free recall). Musiek's dichotic-digits test is commercially available from his laboratory.

Musiek (1983b) administered the dichotic-digits test to 30 patients with surgically, radiologically, and/or neurologically diagnosed intracranial lesions. Of the 30, 18 had hemispheric (cortical) lesions (11 right-hemisphere damage, 4 left-hemisphere damage, and 3 bilateral-hemisphere damage) and 12 had brainstem lesions (3 right-brainstem damage, 4 left-brainstem damage, and 5 diffuse or undetermined). The cutoff dichotic-digits score for each ear defining normal performance was 90%. (The mean left-ear score in a group of normal-hearing subjects between 15 and 46 years of age was 96.5% for the left ear and 97.8% for the right ear with a standard deviation of 1.7% for the left ear and 2.9% for the right ear.) Only 18 of the 30 subjects had normal hearing-threshold levels. The results revealed that 83% of the hemispheric-lesion cases and 75% of the brainstem-lesion cases had an abnormal dichotic-digits score in one or both ears. Thus, the dichotic-digits test was slightly more sensitive to hemispheric lesions than to brainstem lesions. Of the 15 patients with hemispheric lesions confined to one hemisphere, approximately 87% had abnormal contralateral-ear scores and 40% had abnormal ipsilateral-ear scores. Of the 13 hemispheric-lesion patients with abnormal dichotic-digits scores in the ipsilateral and/ or contralateral ear, 85% had a greater contralateral than ipsilateral deficit. Of the 7 patients with unilateral brainstem lesions, approximately 57% had abnormal contralateral-ear scores and approximately 86% had abnormal ipsilateral-ear scores. Of the 6 brainstem-lesion patients

with abnormal dichotic-digits scores on the ipsilateral and/ or contralateral ear, 83% had greater ipsilateral than contralateral deficits.

Musiek (1983b) concluded that the failure to demonstrate the contralateral-ear effect in all of the unilateral hemispheric-lesion cases reflected an indirect effect of the lesion on the interhemispheric pathways. The obtaining of ipsilateral rather than contralateral effects in the brainstem cases conflicted with the finding by Jerger and Jerger (1975) that intra-axial brainstem lesions show contralateral effects. Nevertheless, ipsilateral as well as contralateral effects in intra-axial brainstem-lesion cases have been reported by Lynn and Gilroy (1977). According to Musiek (1983b), the anatomical position, magnitude and type of lesion within the brainstem affect the production of ipsilateral vs. contralateral effects on the dichotic-digits test. Musiek (1983b) also hypothesized that other factors which could have yielded ipsilateral-ear effects in the brainstem-lesion cases included

> pathologic effects associated with the primary lesion, but not in the same anatomical region; complex pathophysiologic processes which interact in ways that cannot be measured accurately by present tests; and an inability to interpret present tests in a broad enough manner to understand the meaning of unique or unusual results. (p. 322)

Musiek (1983b) noted that although the brainstem-lesion group differed from the hemispheric-lesion group in the nature of the ear effect (ipsilateral vs. contralateral), only the production of a depressed score in one or both ears rather than the nature of the ear effect has clinical utility since an ear effect can be defined as ipsilateral or contralateral only after the laterality of the lesion has been neurologically and/or surgically confirmed.

Collard, Lesser, Luders, Dinner, Morris, Hahn, and Rothner (1986) administered the Musiek (1983a) version of the dichotic-digits test to 14 patients with left temporal lobectomies and 12 patients with right temporal lobectomies, all of whom had normal hearing-threshold levels. Collard *et al.* (1986) scored the results in terms of decreased score in the ipsilateral ear from presurgery to postsurgery, decreased score in the contralateral ear from presurgery to postsurgery, decreased total-correct score (number of digits reported correctly in the ipsilateral ear combined with the number of digits reported correctly in the contralateral ear) from presurgery to postsurgery, and decreased double-correct score (number of digits correct when both ears correctly report a digit pair) from presurgery to postsurgery. Statistical testing revealed the lack of a statistically significant decrease from presurgery to postsurgery on all of these dichotic-digit measures. The findings by Collard *et al.* (1986) do not support the results by Kimura (1961b) and Musiek (1983b) and others. Factors which may contribute to the discrepancy include etiology of the lesion, anatomical position, and magnitude of the lesion. Further research is needed to resolve the discrepancy relating to the dichotic-digits test results in the brain-damaged population.

C. CONSONANT–VOWEL NONSENSE SYLLABLES

Berlin and his colleagues introduced the use of consonant–vowel (CV) nonsense syllables for the purpose of central auditory nervous system assessment in the early 1970s. The CV stimuli consisted of the following syllables: /pa/, /ta/, /ka/, /ba/, /da/, and /ga/. Alignment of the syllables under the simultaneous condition is accomplished by computer and is accurate within 2.5 msec. Under the simultaneous condition, 30 pairs of dichotic CVs are presented. Under the time-staggered condition, two CV syllables are presented, one to each ear, aligned so that one ear receives the syllable a fixed number of milliseconds before the other, that is, onsets were delayed at asynchronies of 30, 60, 90, and 120 ms with 30 pairs in each condition for both right and left ears. The amplitude of the vowel segments are within 2.5 dB of a recorded 1000-Hz calibration tone. Stimulus duration is 310 ms for each CV (320 for /pa/), the inter-stimulus interval is 6 s, and signal-to-noise ratio is at least +30 dB. The CV nonsense syllables are available from the Kresge Hearing Research Laboratory of the South, Louisiana State Medical Center.

Various presentation levels have been employed such as 55 dB SL (Collard *et al.*, 1986), most comfortable listening level (Jacobson, Deppe, & Murray, 1983), 78 dB SPL (Olsen, 1983), 75 dB SPL (Bingea & Raffin, 1986; Lowe, Cullen, Berlin, Thompson, & Willett, 1970), and 80 dB SPL (Berlin, Cullen, Hughes, Berlin, Lowe-Bell, & Thompson, 1975b). Before dichotic testing, the 15 CV nonsense syllables are presented monaurally to familiarize the patient with the stimuli and to ensure correct identification of the test items (Olsen, 1983; Rintelmann & Lynn, 1983).

1. SIMULTANEOUS

Several studies have shown that, in normal subjects, the right-ear score is usually between 70 and 80% and the left-ear score is usually between 58 and 70% (Berlin, Lowe-Bell, Cullen, Thompson, & Stafford, 1972a; Berlin, Lowe-Bell, Cullen, Thompson, & Loovis, 1973; Cullen, Thompson, Samson, & Hughes, 1973; Hannah, 1971; Lowe, 1970; Thompson, Stafford, Cullen, Hughes, Lowe-Bell, & Berlin, 1972). Thus, there is usually a right-ear advantage for the simultaneous presentation of dichotic CVs. When the syllables were presented monaurally, 96–100% scores were obtained. Therefore, dichotic presen-

tation resulted in poorer recognition than monaural presentation.

Berlin and his colleagues observed that, when simultaneous dichotic CVs were presented to 3 temporal lobectomy patients (2 left and 1 right) shortly after the operation (Berlin, Lowe-Bell, Jannetta, & Kline, 1972b) and 3 years postoperatively (Berlin *et al.* (1975b), a marked contralateral-ear effect (performance near chance levels) was present, with the ipsilateral ear performing better than normal in the right temporal lobectomy cases but poorer than normal in left temporal lobectomy cases. Berlin *et al.* (1975b) also reported that, in their group of 4 patients with hemispherectomy (3 right and 1 left), a marked contralateral-ear effect (performance near chance levels) was found. The hemispherectomy patients differed from the temporal lobectomy patients in that the ipsilateral-ear score was essentially 100% in the right hemispherectomy cases and about 84% for the left hemispherectomy (on average); for both right and left hemispherectomy cases, the ipsilateral-ear score was better than in normal subjects. Berlin *et al.* (1975b) concluded that, in the hemispherectomy cases, the CV syllable presented to the contralateral ear did not interfere with recognition of the CV syllable in the ipsilateral ear. Figure 6 summarizes these findings. Berlin *et al.* (1975b) concluded that, since the left temporal lobectomy cases had poorer than normal ipsilateral-ear scores, some "acoustic-level suppression" occurred. Since the hemispherectomy cases had excellent scores in the ipsilateral ear, they " have neither phonetic nor acoustic competition between the channels."

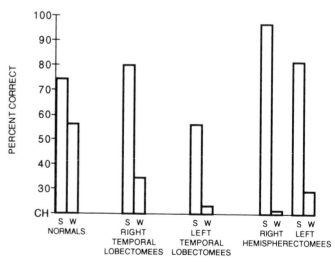

Figure 6 Average performance of normal subjects and patients on dichotic stop-consonant-vowel test. S, Strong ear; W, weak ear. In patients, the weak ear is contralateral to the side of the lesions. In normals, the weak ear is the left ear. Reprinted from Cullen, Berlin, Hughes, Thompson, & Samson (1975) with permission.

Olsen (1983) presented the dichotic CV test under the simultaneous condition to 50 normal subjects and 67 anterior temporal lobectomy patients (33 right temporal lobe and 34 left temporal lobe). The temporal lobectomies were performed to control medically intractable seizures. The mean scores for the normal group were 69.3% for the right ear and 59.2% for the left ear; the ranges were 47–93% for the right ear and 43–77% for the left ear. This large range shows the large intersubject variability in scores for the dichotic CV test. The presurgical and postsurgical scores fell within the normal range for the right and left temporal-lobe groups.

Olsen (1983) considered scores below 66% for the right ear and below 60% for the left ear as abnormal, since these were the lowest scores obtained in the normal group. Tables I and II show the number of patients in each pattern of results (averaged across the simultaneous and two lag conditions) presurgically and postsurgically for the right temporal-lobe group and left temporal-lobe group, respectively. As can be seen in Table I, the pattern reflecting normal right- and left-ear dichotic CV scores was the most frequently occurring one in the right temporal-lobe group. The next most frequently occurring pattern in the right temporal-lobe group was the one reflecting decreased dichotic CV performance in the left ear (contralateral-ear effect). Table I also reveals that ipsilateral- and bilateral-ear effects were also present in the right temporal-lobe group. Similar to the right temporal-lobe group, the most frequently occurring pattern of results for the left temporal-lobe group was normal dichotic CV scores for the right and left ears as shown in Table II. Table II also shows that ipsilateral-ear effects occurred with approximately the same frequency as contralateral-ear effects in the left temporal-lobe group. This finding supports Speaks' (1980) contention that ear-effects cannot be used to identify the side of the CANS lesion. In summary, approximately 42% of all the temporal-lobe patients obtained normal dichotic CV scores for both ears presurgically and postsurgically. Thus, the dichotic CV test identified approximately 58% of

Table I Patterns of Results in Terms of Normal and Abnormal Performance for Dichotic CV Test Materials[a] for 33 Right Temporal-Lobe Seizure Patients[b]

Pattern of results	Presurgery (N)	Postsurgery (N)
R normal L normal	14	18
R normal L abnormal	9	11
R abnormal L normal	5	1
R abnormal L abnormal	5	3

[a] Averaged across three test conditions.
[b] Reprinted from Olsen (1983) with permission.

Table II Patterns of Test Results in Terms of Normal and Abnormal Performance for Dichotic Test Materials[a] for 34 Left Temporal-Lobe Seizure Patients[b]

Pattern of results	Presurgery (N)	Postsurgery (N)
R normal L normal	14	10
R normal L abnormal	7	8
R abnormal L normal	7	10
R abnormal L abnormal	6	6

[a] Averaged across three test conditions.
[b] Reprinted from Olsen (1983) with permission.

the group, a sensitivity rate that is near chance levels. Olsen (1983) also found that in more than 60% of the right and left temporal-lobe groups, the presurgical dichotic pattern of results was the same as the postsurgical pattern. The lack of change in dichotic CV score from the presurgical to the postsurgical condition led Olsen (1983) to conclude that removal of the anterior portion of the temporal lobe did not depress dichotic CV performance in the majority of the patients.

Collard *et al.* (1986) administered the simultaneous dichotic CV test preoperatively and postoperatively to 30 patients with temporal-lobe lesions from medically intractable seizures. The results revealed a significant mean score change (+7.7%) from the preoperative to the postoperative condition for the ipsilateral but not the contralateral ear. Thus, the postoperative dichotic CV score was slightly improved in comparison with the preoperative dichotic CV score and a contralateral-ear deficit was not observed, on average, either preoperatively or postoperatively. The contralateral-ear deficit (i.e., normal in the ipsilateral ear with a deficit in the contralateral ear or a deficit bilaterally which is worse in the contralateral ear) was present in 27% of the left temporal-lobe group preoperatively and postoperatively. In the right temporal-lobe group, the contralateral-ear deficit was present in 25% preoperatively and in 50% postoperatively. The findings by Collard *et al.* (1986) show that temporal lobectomy did not have an adverse effect on dichotic CV scores and did not yield the expected contralateral-ear deficit in the majority of the cases.

2. TIME-STAGGERED

In normal listeners, the results of time-staggered dichotic (30–90 ms) CV tests reveal that the scores are better for the lagging than for the leading ear, that is, for the ear receiving the second syllable (Berlin *et al.*, 1973; Studdert-Kennedy, Shankweiler, & Schulman, 1970). This was called the "lag effect." Therefore, when the right ear leads, the right-ear advantage is overcome, resulting in a left-ear advantage. Conversely, when the left ear leads, the right-ear advantage is increased compared with that obtained under simultaneous dichotic CV conditions. The presence of a lag effect indicates that processing of the lead syllable is disrupted by the lag syllable. At onset asynchronies exceeding 90 ms, the score for the lead syllable becomes equal to that for the lag syllable, indicating that the lag syllable no longer disrupts the processing of the lead syllable (Berlin *et al.*, 1973; Porter, 1975).

Berlin *et al.* (1972b) reported that in their 4 cases with left or right temporal lobectomy, no lag effect was present, that is, the contralateral-ear effect occurred at all time-staggered conditions (30–90 ms). These findings persisted even after a 3-year follow-up (Berlin *et al.*, 1975b). Berlin *et al.* (1975a) found that the lag effect was also absent in patients with hemispherectomy. The hemispherectomy patients differed from the temporal lobectomy patients in that the ipsilateral ear outperformed normal ears, approaching 100%.

Olsen (1983) administered the time-staggered CV test under conditions of the left-ear lagging by 90 ms or the right-ear lagging by 90 ms in 50 normal subjects and 67 temporal-lobe lesion patients. In the normal subjects, the mean scores for the left-ear lag condition were 86.3% for the right ear and 79.3% for the left ear; the range was 63–100% for the right ear and 56–100% for the left ear. For the right-ear lag condition, the mean scores were 87.7% for the right ear and 79.2% for the left ear. Thus, the expected lag effect, present in the right-ear lag condition (90 ms), was not observed under the left-ear lag condition (90 ms) in the normal subjects, on average. In the right temporal-lobe lesion group, the mean data revealed that, as expected, the lag effect was absent and the contralateral-ear deficit was present under the right- and left-ear lag conditions, presurgically and postsurgically. In the left temporal-lobe lesion group, contrary to what was expected, the mean data reveal the presence of an ipsilateral rather than contralateral-ear deficit under both lag conditions, both presurgically and postsurgically. The finding of a contralateral-ear deficit, on average, for the right temporal-lobe lesion group supports the findings by Berlin *et al.* (1972b, 1975a) but the absence of a contralateral-ear deficit, on average, for the left temporal-lobe lesion group conflicts with the results of Berlin *et al.* (1972, 1975b). Olsen (1983) also reported that, under the right-ear and left-ear lag conditions, the postsurgical dichotic CV scores for both ears in the postsurgical condition were not decreased in comparison with the presurgical scores; this lack of decrease from the preoperative to postoperative condition was also observed under the simultaneous dichotic CV condition. Olsen (1983) concluded that anterior temporal lobectomy does not disrupt the time-staggered dichotic CV test or simultaneous dichotic CV test performance. Olsen (1983) further concluded that the obtaining of ipsilateral-ear as well as contralateral-ear deficits precluded the use of ear effects to determine the side of the CANS lesion.

Berlin, Cullen, Berlin, Tobey, and Mouney (1975a) administered the simultaneous dichotic CV test to a patient with a brainstem lesion in the region of the medial geniculate bodies. At the first evaluation (January, 1975), the left-ear dichotic score was reduced to below 10% whereas the right-ear score was at essentially normal levels. At the second evaluation (May, 1975), after chemotherapy and radiation therapy, the left-ear score improved to nearly 40% and the right-ear score increased to approach 90%.

Bingea and Raffin (1986) investigated dichotic CV scores under the 0, 30, 60, 90, and 120 ms delay conditions (right and left lag) in a group of 30 young adults ranging in age from 19 to 70 years who showed (a) a score of at least 25 out of 30 when the CVs were administered monaurally, (b) hearing-threshold levels not exceeding 20 dB HL, (c) air–bone gaps not exceeding 10 dB, (d) interaural pure-tone thresholds not exceeding 10 dB, (e) spondee-recognition thresholds within 10 dB of the 3-frequency pure-tone average, (f) NU-6 speech-recognition scores of at least 92% in quiet and at least 60% at a 0 dB signal-to-noise ratio, (g) NU-6 speech-recognition score with contralateral competing message (message-to-competition ratio of -10 dB) of at least 92%, (h) absent tone decay at 500 and 2000 Hz, (i) normal simultaneous binaural median-plane localization at 500 Hz, (j) masking-level differences not less than 7 dB at 500 Hz, (k) normal tympanometric peak pressures, (l) contralateral acoustic-reflex thresholds present between 70 and 100 dB HL at 500 and 1000 Hz, (m) ipsilateral acoustic-reflex thresholds present between 70 and 105 db SPL at 500 and 1000 Hz, and (n) negative acoustic-reflex decay at 500 Hz. Subjects responded using a multiple-choice answer form. The intensity level was equivalent to that of a 1000-Hz calibration tone of 75 dB SPL. Single-ear and double-correct scores were obtained for each subject in each condition. The mean single-ear and double-correct scores were also obtained in each condition. The binomial model (Thornton & Raffin, 1978) was also applied to determine whether there was a significant ear advantage (left-ear arc-sine transformed score differs significantly from the right-ear arc-sine transformed score) and whether there was a significant difference in arc-sine transformed single-ear or double-correct score between onset time asynchronies using the 99th percentile critical difference limits. Thirty items were presented in each condition.

Bingea and Raffin (1986) reported that analysis of the single-ear mean data revealed that the right-ear score was superior to the left-ear score in both right-lag and left-lag conditions at all onset-time asynchronies. Analysis of variance revealed the absence of a significant lag effect for the group. Large intersubject variability in single-ear correct scores was evidenced by the large ranges for both ears at all onset-time asynchronies as shown in Figure 7. The ranges were substantially greater for the double-correct scores

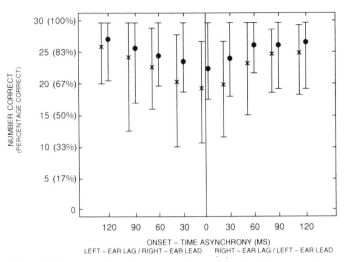

Figure 7 Single ear dichotic means and ranges for 30 subjects as a function of interchannel onset time asynchrony and lag. Circles represent right ear means; Xs represent left ear means. The vertical lines associated with each symbol subtend the range of scores obtained for each ear condition. Reprinted from Bingea and Raffin (1986) with permission.

than for the single-ear scores at each onset-time asynchrony. Significant (with respect to the binomial model) left-ear advantages under the left-lag condition were obtained by 0% at the 120 ms condition, 0% at the 30 ms condition, 3% at the 90 ms condition, and 3% at the 60 ms condition. Significant (with respect to the binomial model) right-ear advantages under simultaneous and right-lag conditions were obtained by only 27% at the 0 ms condition, 37% at the 30 ms condition, 10% at the 60 msec condition, 13% at the 90 msec condition, and 3% at the 120 ms condition. Thus, the vast majority of subjects did not demonstrate the expected (significant) ear advantage. Also, although the mean data revealed a right-ear advantage at simultaneity, the individual data revealed that most subjects did not show a right-ear advantage. The frequency of occur-

rence of significant differences (with respect to the binomial model) in single-ear and double-correct scores between onset-time a synchronies was greatest when the onset-time asynchrony was at least 90 msec. The percentage of subjects with significant differences between onset-time asynchronies never exceeded 57% for any comparison of two onset-time asynchrony conditions. Thus, most subjects did not reveal significant differences between onset-time asynchronies. Since the frequency of occurrence of difference between onset-time asynchronies was greatest when the onsets differed by at least 90 ms and the lag effect was most prevalent at 30–90 ms, Bingea and Raffin (1986) recommended that the 0 and 90 ms right- and left-lag conditions were sufficient for clinical use. Table III shows the percentage of cases with significant differences in single-ear or double-correct scores between onset-time asynchronies.

Bingea and Raffin (1986) suggested that ear advantage be calculated by determining whether the right-ear score is significantly different (according to the binomial model) than the left ear score rather than by calculating the ear differences or absolute ear indexes. They also concluded that it is inaccurate to say that a dichotic score for an ear from a CANS-lesion patient is better than normal because the score is higher than the normal group's mean; the score for an ear from a CANS-lesion patient has to be considered within the context of the range of normal scores. Bingea and Raffin (1986) recommend that future research on dichotic-test results in patients with lesions analyze ear effects (contralateral, ipsilateral, lag) and presurgical and postsurgical comparisons based on the binomial model rather than by using mean scores.

D. STAGGERED SPONDAIC WORDS

The staggered spondaic word (SSW) dichotic test was developed by Katz (1962, 1968). For each test item, two spondaic words are presented with staggered onset, one to each ear, such that there are three separate sequential events. The first

Table III Number of Subjects out of 30 Who Demonstrated Significant Differences between Onset Time Asynchronies for at Least One Ear (Right or Left) for Single-Ear Scores and Double-Correct Scores[a]

	120 ms		90 ms		60 ms		0 ms	
	SE[b]	DC[c]	SE	DC	SE	DC	SE	DC
90 msec	3(10%)	6(20%)						
60 msec	6(20%)	6(20%)	3(10%)	2(7%)				
30 msec	15(50%)	18(60%)	8(27%)	10(33%)	2(7%)	4(13%)		
0 msec	11(37%)	17(57%)	10(33%)	12(40%)	4(13%)	5(17%)	2(7%)	1(3%)

[a] Reprinted from Bingea and Raffin (1986) with permission. A binomial model, incorporating arc-sine transformed scores, was used to determine the significance of differences between scores. Significance is $p < 0.01$. Onset time asynchronies are 120, 90, 60, 30, or 0 m.
[b] SE, single-ear.
[c] DC, double-correct.

half of the first spondaic word (the half-word is a monosyllabic word) is presented in isolation to one ear followed by the second half of the first spondaic word (monosyllabic word) to the same ear simultaneously with the first half of the second spondaic word (monosyllabic word) in the other ear, followed by the second half of the second spondaic word (monosyllabic) word in that ear. The first event with the monosyllable in the first ear is a noncompeting event; the second event with different monosyllables in each ear is the competing event; the third event with a monosyllable in the second ear is also a noncompeting event. For example, if the first item is "upstairs, downtown," then "up" is delivered to the first ear (e.g., the right ear), followed by "stairs" to the right ear simultaneously with "down" to the second (left) ear, followed by "town" to the left ear. The spondaic words are familiar words. When the noncompeting segments of each item are combined, they also form familiar, spondaic words. In this example, combination of the noncompeting segments yields "uptown."

1. PROCEDURE

The latest recording of the SSW, the version EE, does not have the problems of poor acoustic quality, noise, and poor alignment of the competing portions associated with the earlier recording (SSW-EC) of the test (Johnson & Sherman, 1980). Nevertheless, most investigations use version EC since normative data have been obtained with this version. The SSW (version EC) is commercially available from Precision Acoustics (Vancouver, Washington). There are 40 items; each item consists of two spondaic words, one to each ear. Half of the items are presented so that the first monosyllable arrives at the right ear and the other half of the items are presented so that the first monosyllable arrives at the left ear. Error scores (omissions, substitutions, or distortions) are obtained for the right noncompeting (RNC), right competing (RC), left competing (LC), and left noncompeting (LNC) conditions, the right and left ears, and the total test. In the example given previously, if the first monosyllable is presented to the right ear, then "up" is RNC, "stairs" is RC, "down" is LC, and "town" is LNC. Response biases, ear and order effects, and reversals may also be assessed.

The SSW test is presented at 50 dB SL relative to the three-frequency pure-tone average in normal-hearing persons, at SLs below 50 but no lower than 25 in cases with tolerance problems, or at 30 dB SL (provided this level is at least 50 dB HL) in cases with conductive hearing impairment of at least 20 dB. Doyle (1981) found that presentation levels as low as 20 dB SL could be employed successfully in normal-hearing persons. Flynn, Danhauer, Gerber, Goller, & Arnst (1984) found that the SSW can be presented to persons with cochlear hearing impairment at presentation levels as low as 30 dB SL. The patient is instructed to repeat all of the words heard.

2. SCORING

Figures 8, 9, and 10 illustrate a sample SSW scoring form. Errors are noted by drawing a dash through the word that was omitted or repeated incorrectly and, if a substitution was given, writing the substitution (linquistic or nonlinguistic) above the dashed line. Omission or addition of a plural or possessive "s" is not considered an error. If the order of the words was incorrectly repeated, the order is noted by writing numbers below the words to represent the order in which the words were repeated. An item is considered a reversal (R is circled in the reversal column) if the order of the words is repeated incorrectly and not more than one omission or substitution is obtained. If the first item is right-ear first, then a line is drawn through "Left First" in Figure 10; if the first item is left-ear first, then a line is drawn through "Right First" in Figure 9.

The eight cardinal numbers are obtained by totaling the errors at the bottom of columns A, B, C, D, E, F, G, and H (all competing and noncompeting conditions for the right and left ears for right-ear first and left-ear first items). The "SUM" rows in Figures 9 and 10 represent the total errors for these columns for the first 20 and second 20 items. The "TOTAL" row in Figure 10 yields the total errors for these columns for all the items; the numbers in the "TOTAL" row represent the 8 cardinal numbers.

In the "COMBINED TOTALS" box (see Figure 10), the total errors for the RNC, RC, LC, and LNC conditions are recorded. The total number of errors for these conditions by entering the number of errors for columns A–D (or E–H, depending on which ear is first) in the first row and for columns E–H (or A–D, depending on which ear is first) in the second row of the "COMBINED TOTALS" box. Addition of the numbers in each column in the "COMBINED TOTALS" box yields the total number of errors for the RNC, RC, LC, and LNC conditions. These four numbers are then transferred to the first row of the "R-SSW" box in Figure 8 and multiplied by 2.5 to yield the raw SSW percentage error (R-SSW % error) scores (third row of the R-SSW box in Figure 8) for each of the RNC, RC, LC, and LNC conditions. The right-ear (RE) R-SSW percentage error score (in the R-SSW box in Figure 8) is obtained by averaging the RNC and RC percentage error scores from row 3 of the R-SSW box in Figure 8. The left-ear (LE) R-SSW percentage error score is obtained by averaging the LC and LNC percentage error scores from row 3 of the R-SSW box in Figure 8. The total (T) R-SSW percentage error score is obtained by averaging the right-ear and left-ear R-SSW percentage error scores in the R-SSW box in Figure 8. Fractions are rounded off to the nearest even number. In summary, 7 R-SSW percentage error scores are derived from the errors in columns A-H: 4 condition scores (RNC, RC, LC, LNC), 2 ear scores (RE and LE), and 1 total score (T). These scores can be plotted on the graph shown in Figure 8.

STANDARD SSW TEST-LIST EC

Name _____ Date _____ REF LEF

AGE _____ Sex: M F   Handed: R L A   Tester _____

1. R-SSW — Enter totals from page 3

CONDITION	RNC	RC	LC	LNC
Total Errors				
Multiplier	x	x	x	x
R-SSW %Error				
EAR	RE		LE	
R-SSW %Error				
TOTAL		T		
R-SSW % Error				

3. A - SSW — Enter least biased errors from page 3

CONDITION	RNC	RC	LC	LNC
Least Biased Errors				
Multiplier	x	x	x	x
Least Biased % Errors				
-WDS % Error	–	–	–	–
A-SSW % Error				
EAR	RE		LE	
A-SSW % Error				
TOTAL		T		
A-SSW % Error				

PERCENT ERROR graph: 100, 75, 50, 25, 0, (-25)
RIGHT NC C   LEFT C NC
X=R-SSW
O=C-SSW
A=A-SSW

2. C-SSW — Enter R-SSW % error

CONDITION	RNC	RC	LC	LNC
R-SSW % Error				
-WDS % Error	–	–	–	–
C-SSW % Error				
EAR	RE		LE	
C-SSW % Error				
TOTAL		T		
C-SSW % Error				

SSW SUMMARY
Score

Response Bias

Reversals ____ SIG NS
Sig-Order ____/____ H/L L/H
Sig-Ear ____/____ L/H H/L
Type A LC RC
Other: _____

COMMENTS: _____

AUDIOMETRIC SUMMARY

	3-FREQ SP AVG	SRT	WDS	SSW HL
RE				
LE				

PRECISION ACOUSTICS
411 N.E. 87th Avenue, Suite B
Vancouver, WA 98664
(206) 892-9367

Multipliers

#ITEMS	R-SSW	A-SSW
20 ___	5 ___	10 ___
25 ___	4 ___	8 ___
30 ___	3.3 ___	6.7 ___
40 ___	2.5 ___	5 ___
If other: ___		
( )	___	___

TEC ANALYSIS

	C-SSW Total	Ear	Cond.	A-SSW Total	Ear	Cond.
#						
CAT						
	Combined TEC			Combined TEC		

© *JACK KATZ, Ph.D.* 1970, 1977, 1985

Figure 8 Page 1 of the SSW test form. Reprinted with permission from Jack Katz.

PAGE 2

PRACTICE ITEMS

a.	air	plane	wet	paint
c.	north	west	stair	way

b.	cow	boy	white	bread
d.	oat	meal	flash	light

Left First	L-NC (A)	L-C (B)	R-C (C)	R-NC (D)	Rev	WRONG
Right First	R-NC	R-C	L-C	L-NC		
1.	up	stairs	down	town	R	
3.	day	light	lunch	time	R	
5.	corn	bread	oat	meal	R	
7.	flood	gate	flash	light	R	
9.	meat	sauce	base	ball	R	
11.	house	fly	wood	work	R	
13.	sun	day	shoe	shine	R	
15.	back	door	play	ground	R	
17.	snow	white	foot	ball	R	
19.	blue	jay	black	bird	R	
SUM						

	R-NC (E)	R-C (F)	L-C (G)	L-NC (H)	Rev	WRONG
	L-NC	L-C	R-C	R-NC		
2.	out	side	in	law	R	
4.	wash	tub	black	board	R	
6.	bed	spread	mush	room	R	
8.	sea	shore	out	side	R	
10.	black	board	air	mail	R	
12.	green	bean	home	land	R	
14.	white	walls	dog	house	R	
16.	school	boy	church	bell	R	
18.	band	saw	first	aid	R	
20.	ice	land	sweet	cream	R	
SUM						

COMMENTS: _____

_____

_____

_____

_____

Figure 9 Page 2 of the SSW test form. In this example, item 1 begins in the right ear. Reprinted with permission from Jack Katz.

PAGE 3

	(A)	(B)	(C)	(D)	Rev	WRONG		(E)	(F)	(G)	(H)	Rev	WRONG
21.	hair	net	tooth	brush	R		22.	fruit	juice	cup	cake	R	
23.	ash	tray	tin	can	R		24.	nite	light	yard	stick	R	
25.	key	chain	suit	case	R		26.	play	ground	bat	boy	R	
27.	corn	starch	soap	flakes	R		28.	birth	day	first	place	R	
29.	day	break	lamp	light	R		30.	door	knob	cow	bell	R	
31.	bird	cage	crow's	nest	R		32.	week	end	work	day	R	
33.	book	shelf	drug	store	R		34.	wood	work	beach	craft	R	
35.	hand	ball	milk	shake	R		36.	fish	net	sky	line	R	
37.	for	give	milk	man	R		38.	sheep	skin	bull	dog	R	
39.	race	horse	street	car	R		40.	green	house	string	bean	R	
SUM Page 3							SUM Page 3						
SUM Page 2							SUM Page 2						
TOTAL	(CARDINAL NUMBERS)						TOTAL	(CARDINAL NUMBERS)					
Left First	L-NC (A)	L-C (B)	R-C (C)	R-NC (D)				R-NC (E)	R-C (F)	L-C (G)	L-NC (H)		
Right First	R-NC	R-C	L-C	L-NC				L-NC	L-C	R-C	R-NC		

EAR EFFECT		
Total Errors	REF	LEF
☐ Sig. ☐ N. Sig.		

REVERSALS
TOTAL =

ORDER EFFECT			
1	2	3	4
(A+E)	(B+F)	(C+G)	(D+H)
TOTAL		TOTAL	
1st SPONDEE		2nd SPONDEE	
☐ Sig		☐ N. Sig	

COMBINED TOTALS				
	RNC	RC	LC	LNC
(A) - (D) or (E) - (H)				
(H) - (E) or (D) - (A)				
GRAND TOTALS				

Enter these figures on Page 1

Figure 10 Page 3 of the SSW test form. In this example, item 1 begins in the right ear. Reprinted with permission from Jack Katz.

According to Katz (1968), one can account for the effect of a peripheral hearing impairment on the SSW results by subtracting the suprathreshold speech-recognition error score (for W-22s) from each of the R-SSW percentage error condition scores to obtain the corrected SSW (C-SSW) percentage error scores. The "C-SSW" box is shown in Figure 8. The C-SSW RE, LE, and T percentage error scores in the C-SSW box in Figure 8 are calculated from the C-SSW condition error scores the same way that the R-SSW RE, LE, and T percentage error scores were calculated from the R-SSW condition percentage error scores. The C-SSW percentage error condition scores can also be plotted on the graph in Figure 8.

Arnst and Doyle (1983) evaluated the C-SSW scores in 92 adult males with bilaterally symmetrical cochlear hearing impairment with a negative history of central nervous system impairment. The Pearson Product Moment Correlation between the R-SSW and the percentage error on the W-22 monosyllabic PB-word recognition test was high ($r = 0.80$). The Pearson Product Moment Correlation between the C-SSW and percentage error on the W-22 monosyllabic PB-word recognition test was very low and insignificant ($r = 0.13$, $p < 0.05$). Arnst and Doyle (1983) concluded that the C-SSW procedure "appears to neutralize the R-SSW/WDS relationship when cochlear dysfunction is present. The net effect is to reduce the influence of a peripheral distortion on SSW results" (p. 245). They also reported that the C-SSW scores for the subjects having 3-frequency pure-tone averages greater than 50 dB were poorer by 10–15% on average than those for the subjects having 3-frequency pure-tone averages less than 40 dB. Therefore, cochlear hearing impairment having a magnitude greater than 50 dB may shift the C-SSW score to a more abnormal performance category. Arnst and Doyle (1983) concluded that the C-SSW results must be interpreted cautiously in persons with 3-frequency pure-tone averages greater than 50 dB HL. Jacobson *et al.* (1983) contended that modification of the R-SSW score to take into account the speech-recognition error score has not been justified.

An order effect, a type of response bias, represents a tendency to have more errors on the first than the second spondaic word or vice-versa. To determine whether the order effect is present, performance on the first spondaic word is compared with the performance on the second spondaic word. In the "ORDER EFFECT" box in Figure 10, column 1 is the sum of the errors for columns A and E, column 2 is the sum of the errors for columns B and F, column 3 is the sum of the errors for columns C and G, and column 4 is the sum of the errors for columns D and H (assuming the right-ear was first on the odd-numbered items). The number of errors on the first spondaic word is the total of the number of errors in columns 1 and 2 in the "ORDER EFFECT" box in Figure 10. The number of errors on the second spondaic word is the total of the number

of errors in columns 3 and 4 in the "ORDER EFFECT" box in Figure 10. A difference of at least 5 between the errors on the first spondaic word and the errors on the second spondaic word is considered significant. The number of errors on the first spondaic word is reported before that on the second spondaic word. For example, Order 7/10 means that 7 errors were obtained on the first spondaic word and 10 errors were obtained on the second spondaic word. if significantly fewer errors (by at least 5) are made on the second than on the first spondaic word, then the general classification is Order high/low (O H/L). Conversely, if significantly (by at least 5) fewer errors are made on the first than on the second spondaic word, the general classification is O L/H.

An ear effect, a type of response bias, represents a tendency to make more errors on items when the right-ear is first than when the left ear is first or vice versa. The number of errors on right-ear first items is compared with that for left-ear first items. In the "EAR EFFECT" box in Figure 10, the right-ear first errors represent the sum of the errors on columns A through D and the left-ear first errors represent the sum of the errors for columns E through H (when the right ear is first on the odd-numbered items). A difference of 5 between right-ear first errors and left-ear first errors is considered significant. The number of errors on right-ear first items is reported before that for left-ear items. For example, Ear 9/8 indicates that 9 errors were made on items for which the right ear was first and 8 errors were made on items for which the left ear was first. If significantly (by at least 5) fewer errors are made when the right ear was first than when the left ear was first, then the general classification would be Ear low/high (E L/H). If significantly fewer errors were made when the left ear was first than when the right ear was first, the general classification would be E H/L.

A reversal, another type of response bias, occurs when an item is repeated in the incorrect sequence and no more than one omission or substitution was made. Two or more reversals are considered to be significant.

Type A and B patterns are also response biases. Type A pattern is considered to be present if any of the 8 cardinal numbers is at least twice as large as each of the other 7 cardinal numbers and is larger than the next largest number by at least 3. The Type B pattern is a specific form of the Type A pattern in that the large number occurs in column C or G.

When highly positive C-SSW scores are obtained and response biases are present, then the adjusted (A-SSW) scores can be obtained. The A-SSW score is obtained by lowering the C-SSW score by the magnitude of the response bias.

Analysis of the total, ear, and condition C-SSW or A-SSW scores (TEC analysis) can be done to determine the category (overcorrected, normal, mild, moderate, and severe) associated with each of these scores. A combined category is obtained based on the category associated with the total score, the category associated with the most positive of the ear and condition scores, and the most negative of the ear and condition scores. The results of this analysis are entered in the right-hand boxes at the bottom of Figure 8.

Further details regarding the scoring of the SSW can be obtained from Brunt (1978), Katz (1984), and Lukas and Genchur-Lukas (1985).

3. INTERPRETATION

According to Katz (1984), a moderate or severe combined TEC category in persons between 11 and 60 years of age may be associated with disorders of the auditory reception area (Heschl's gyrus) located in the posterior superior portion of the temporal lobe in the hemisphere contralateral to the side (ear) with the peak errors. The presence of posterior response biases (E H/L or O L/H effects) lend additional support to the interpretation of auditory reception area dysfunction in the case of a moderate or severe combined TEC category.

A moderate or severe combined TEC category is also observed in cases with high (upper) brainstem pathology or interhemispheric pathway (corpus callosum) dysfunction (Katz, 1984). In cases with interhemispheric pathway dysfunction, the peak errors occur in the ear opposite the hemisphere nondominant for language. Katz (1984) stated that a normal or mild combined TEC category is associated with nonauditory reception area involvement (the brain exclusive of the auditory reception area), provided there was known brain dysfunction.

According to Katz (1984), an overcorrected combined TEC category is associated with sensorineural hearing impairment (of cochlear, eighth nerve, or low brainstem origin). A normal combined TEC category is associated with cochlear hearing impairment, nonauditory reception area dysfunction (if there is a known brain disorder), or an intact peripheral and central system. A mild combined TEC category is consistent with cochlear hearing impairment and/or a nonauditory reception area disorder. The presence of "anterior" response biases (E L/H, O H/L, reversals) along with a normal or mild combined TEC category is associated with dysfunction of the front or anterior nonauditory reception region of the brain. The finding of posterior response biases (E H/L or O L/H) with a normal or mild combined TEC category suggests dysfunction near but not in the auditory reception area.

Lukas and Genchur-Lukas (1985) reported that the Type A pattern has been observed in a variety of disorders at a variety of anatomical sites. The Type B pattern is considered rare.

Although Katz and his associates developed this model of interpretation of combined TEC categories, many recent investigators have not used this model. In several recent investigations, interpretation was based on the SSW scores in the competing conditions, and R-SSW scores outside the normal range were considered consistent with dysfunction of the auditory brainstem or cortical regions (Baran et al., 1986; Lynn & Gilroy, 1977; Musiek, 1983b, Olsen, 1983).

4. PATHOLOGIC GROUPS

Musiek (1983b) reported that the mean R-SSW scores (based on list EC) in a group of 32 normal subjects between 15 and 46 years of age was 98.0% for the left ear and 98.7% for the right ear; the standard deviations were 3.1 and 2.7% for the left and right ears, respectively. Based on these results, Musiek (1983b) established 90% as the lower limit of the normal range. Lynn and Gilroy (1977) reported that the mean R-SSW scores (based on list EC) for a group of 20 normal-hearing persons were 98.8 and 98.7% in the noncompeting conditions for the right and left ears, respectively, and were 97.3 and 96.4% in the competing conditions for the right and left ears, respectively. The ranges for the noncompeting conditions were 95–100% and 94–100% for the right and left ears, respectively; the range for the right and left competing conditions was 90–100%. The standard deviation for the noncompeting condition was 1.8% for the right ear and 2.0% for the left ear; for the competing condition, the standard deviation was 2.2% for the right ear and 3.8% for the left ear.

Lynn and Gilroy (1977) reported that the hit rate for the SSW test under the competing condition was 91% (abnormal contralateral-ear scores in 85% and abnormal ipsilateral-ear scores in 6%) for their group of 35 patients with right or left temporal-lobe lesion; in the noncompeting condition, the hit rate was 56% (abnormal contralateral-ear scores in 53% and abnormal ipsilateral-ear scores in 3%).

Musiek (1983b) found a hit rate of 78% for his group of 18 patients with hemispheric lesions and a hit rate of 58% for his group of 12 patients with brainstem lesions. (The R-SSW in the competing condition was considered abnormal if it was below the lower limit of the normal range in the normal group.) Thus, the sensitivity of the SSW test was greater for hemispheric than for brainstem lesions. Further analysis on 15 patients with hemispheric lesions confined to one side revealed that 80% had contralateral R-SSW scores below the normal cutoff and approximately 26% had ipsilateral R-SSW scores below the normal cutoff. Of the 12 hemispheric patients with abnormal scores in the ipsilateral and/or contralateral ear, approximately 92% had poorer scores in the contralateral than ipsilateral ear. Further analysis on the results from 7 patients with brainstem lesions limited to one side revealed that 28.5% had contralateral R-SSW scores below the normal cutoff and approximately 71% had ipsilateral R-SSW scores below the normal cutoff. Of the 5 patients with unilateral brainstem lesions with abnormal scores on the ipsilateral and/or contralateral ear, 100% had poorer scores in the ipsilateral than contralateral ear. These results showed that laterality effects were striking for the brainstem-lesion and hemispheric-lesion groups when abnormal scores are obtained. Nevertheless, the facts that the R-SSW scores do not reliably distinguish between hemispheric and brainstem groups and contralateral effects generally are obtained for the former group whereas ipsilateral effects generally are obtained for the latter group indicate that the SSW test cannot be used to determine laterality.

Olsen (1983) reported that only 6% of 33 patients with right temporal-lobe disorders had R-SSW scores in one or both competing conditions below the normal cutoff of 90% established by Lynn and Gilroy (1972), presurgically. Similar findings were obtained following anterior right temporal lobectomy. Of their 34 patients with left temporal lobe seizure, only approximately 3% obtained R-SSW scores in one or both competing conditions below the normal cutoff presurgically; postsurgically, only approximately 9% obtained R-SSW scores in one or both competing conditions below the normal cutoff.

Collard et al. (1986) reported that contralateral-ear deficits (only for the contralateral ear or for both ears but contralateral worse than ipsilateral) on the competing conditions of the SSW were present preoperatively in 13% of their patients and postoperatively in 0% of their 15 patients with left temporal-lobe lesions who underwent unilateral anterior temporal lobectomy; ipsilateral deficits (only for the ipsilateral ear or for both but with ipsilateral worse than contralateral) on the competing conditions of the SSW were present preoperatively in 20% of their patients and postoperatively in 0% of these 15 patients. Contralateral-ear deficits in the competing conditions of the SSW were present preoperatively in 33% and postoperatively in 33% of their 15 patients with right temporal-lobe lesions who underwent anterior right temporal lobectomy; ipsilateral-ear deficits were absent preoperatively and postoperatively in these patients. Thus, ipsilateral and contralateral effects were distributed similarly in the left temporal-lobe lesion group but contralateral effects predominated over ipsilateral effects in the right temporal-lobe lesion group. Collard et al. (1986) also reported that the mean SSW score for the whole group of 30 patients with temporal-lobe lesions in the ipsilateral but not contralateral ear changed significantly (an average of +4.8%) from the preoperative to the postoperative condition in the direction of improvement. Because of the relatively small number of ears with contralateral or ipsilateral deficits, Collard et al. (1986) concluded that temporal-lobe lesions with epileptogenic foci and unilateral anterior temporal lobectomy do not have an adverse effect on SSW performance.

Jacobson et al. (1983) investigated the sensitivity of the SSW test based on the R-SSW error scores in each of the competing and noncompeting conditions in 20 subjects with confirmed multiple sclerosis. Jacobson et al. (1983) found that only 2 subjects (10%) obtained abnormal SSW scores (one was classified as mildly abnormal and one was classified as moderately abnormal). Jacobson et al. (1983) concluded that the SSW was not an effective audiologic tool for detection of demyelinating diseases.

The widely varing reports of sensitivity for the SSW test may reflect the sample differences from varying etiology, site of the lesion, and magnitude of the lesion. In the report by Musiek (1983b), subjects had epileptic focus lesions, vascular insults, and space-occupying lesions. In the Olsen (1983) and Collard et al. (1986) reports, the subjects had epileptic focus lesions. Further large-sample studies are needed to determine the effect of brainstem and temporal-lobe lesions on the SSW test results. The SSW test remains one of the few central speech tests which is relatively unaffected by cochlear hearing impairment (when the C-SSW score is evaluated).

Studies on the SSW in the elderly show an increase in SSW error scores with age and an increase in variability (Amerman & Parnell, 1980; Arnst, 1982).

E. COMPETING SENTENCES

Willeford (1968) developed the dichotic competing sentences test involving simple natural sentences. In this test, the primary sentence is presented to one ear at 35 dB SL relative to the PTA (or SRT in normal-hearing persons) and the competing sentence is presented to the opposite ear at 50 dB SL. The message-to-competition ratio is −15 dB, indicating that the intensity of the competition is greater than that of the test sentences by 15 dB. Ten pairs of sentences are presented with the primary sentences to the right ear and the competing sentences to the left ear. Another ten pairs of sentences are presented with the primary sentences to the left ear and the competing sentences to the right ear. The sentences average 6–7 words in length. The competing sentence has a content similar to that of the primary sentence. The patient's task is to repeat the primary sentences and ignore the louder, competing sentences. All of the sentences are first presented monaurally to ensure that the patient can repeat the sentences (Lynn and Gilroy, 1975). Then five practice dichotic pairs of sentences are given before the test sentences to familiarize the patient with the task. The competing sentence pairs are shown in Table IV. The onsets and offsets of the sentences are approximately but not precisely aligned since recognition of the primary sentence involved active processes of larger than individual word components (Willeford, 1977). The Competing Sentences Test is commercially available from Auditec of St. Louis.

As noted by Musiek and Baran (1987), scoring procedures are not standardized and there is an element of subjectivity in the scoring procedure leading to variability among clinicians in interpretation of the results. Musiek (1983b) scored the competing sentences test as follows.

Table IV Competing Sentence Test Items[a]

1. It was a long ride by car. I thought we would never get there.	16. That movie was on TV. I saw it when it was a play.
2. He went to the South on his vacation. I get two weeks off in the summer.	17. I saw lots of different kinds of animals. There are lions and tigers in the zoo.
3. He read the whole book in one week. I think they made the book into a movie.	18. It is dangerous to swim there. He likes to swim the backstroke.
4. I put the letter in the mail box. You must write to her more often.	19. He is only resting. I had to take a nap.
5. He drank all of the milk. I like my coffee black.	20. I had a wonderful Christmas. He's off for Easter week.
6. He watched the cartoon on TV. I like the Bugs Bunny cartoon.	21. I think hide and seek is a lot of fun. The children played tag for a long time.
7. He was very late to class yesterday. I went to the cafeteria at noon.	22. They went to the zoo Sunday. I was able to go to the park.
8. The airplane flew very low. The jet took off smoothly.	23. My sister is older than I am. Your uncle is not over there.
9. I have the best teacher in school. He was a student here before me.	24. There is a color television over there. I think I hear a radio playing.
10. I saw the funny clown. The circus was very good.	25. He's too old to play with toys. I like to run my model train.
11. This is a long freight train. The caboose is always last.	26. There was fried chicken for dinner. I had a sandwich for lunch.
12. I don't like to go to school either. Recess is my favorite time.	27. Dessert was a chocolate sundae. I put strawberries on my ice cream.
13. My car is very fast. Put gas in the tank.	28. Mother made pancakes for breakfast. I like maple syrup on my waffles.
14. They say candy is bad for your teeth. I do not like to eat dinner alone.	29. Nobody is at home. They won't answer the phone.
15. Put a bandage on that cut. That cut may get infected.	30. It's raining very hard. There's a lot of snow on the ground.

[a] Reprinted from Auditec of St. Louis with permission. Items are pairs of primary and competing sentences.

1. A score of 10% was assigned if the meaning and content of the sentence was correctly communicated; a verbatim response was not necessary to obtain the score of 10%.
2. If the meaning/content was not completely correct, a score of 2.5%, 5%, or 7.5% was assigned according to the magnitude of the loss of content.

Lynn and Gilroy (1975) reported that normal-hearing subjects always obtain scores of 100% on the Competing Sentences Test. Similarly, they observed mean scores of 100% for the right and left ears for their group of 20 normal subjects in a later report (Lynn & Gilroy, 1977). Musiek (1983b) obtained mean scores of 97.9% and 97.8% fot the right and left ears, respectively, in his group of 31 normal-hearing subjects between 15 and 46 years of age. The standard deviations were 4.5 and 3.4% for the

right and left ears, respectively. The range was 80–100% for the right and for the left ear.

Lynn and Gilroy (1975) administered the Competing Sentences Test to 10 patients with posterior temporal-lobe tumors. The mean scores were 84.0% for the ipsilateral ear and 33.0% for the contralateral ear. The range was 0–100% for both ears. These results show slight deficit in the ipsilateral ear with a greater deficit in the contralateral ear. In a later study (Lynn & Gilroy, 1977) on 11 patients with right temporal-lobe tumors, the mean score was 100% for the ipsilateral ear and approximately 64% for the contralateral ear; the mean contralateral-ear score was significantly different from the ipsilateral-ear score. The mean score was 100% for the ipsilateral ear and approximately 52% for the contralateral ear in their group of 11 patients with left temporal-lobe tumors; the mean contralateral-ear score was significantly different from that for the ipsilateral ear. Lynn and Gilroy (1977) also reported that the hit rate was 63% (57% in the contralateral ear and 6% in the ipsilateral ear) for their group of 35 patients with right or left temporal-lobe lesions.

Lynn and Gilroy (1975) reported that the mean score for the ipsilateral and contralateral ears in a group of 10 patients with temporal-lobe rumors in the anterior inferior regions were similar to those in normal-hearing subjects. Thus, the Competing Sentences Test was not sensitive to antero-inferior temporal-lobe tumors. With respect to patients with brainstem lesions, Lynn and Gilroy (1977) reported that inconsistent findings were obtained on the Competing Sentences Test; normal findings, ipsilateral-ear effects, contralateral-ear effects, and bilateral-ear effects have been observed in these cases.

Lynn and Gilroy (1975) reported that, in their group of 12 patients with deep parietal-lobe tumors involving the corpus callosum, the mean right-ear score was 88.8% and the mean left-ear score was 62.2% with a range of 0–100% for both ears; these results revealed a slight deficit in the right ear and the expected left-ear deficit (ear ipsilateral to the hemisphere dominant for language) in cases with involvement of the interhemispheric pathways. In a later study on 14 patients with deep right parietal-lobe tumors and 10 patients with deep left parietal-lobe tumors, Lynn and Gilroy (1977) obtained similar findings. The mean right-ear score was 100% for the right parietal-lobe group and approximately 94% for the left parietal-lobe group; the mean left-ear score was approximately 56 and 58% for the right and left parietal-lobe groups, respectively. Lynn and Gilroy (1977) also reported that the hit rate of the test was 52% (48% in the left ear and 4% in the right ear) for their group of 28 patients with deep right or left parietal-lobe tumors involving the interhemispheric pathways. Musiek, Kibbe, and Baran (1984) reported a marked left-ear deficit for the Competing Sentences Test following total commisurotomy. The left-ear deficit following anterior sectioning of the corpus callosum was less marked (Baran *et al.*, 1986).

Musiek (1983b) investigated the sensitivity of the Competing Sentences Test in a group of 18 patients with hemispheric lesions and 12 patients with brainstem lesions. Their findings were similar to those reported by Lynn and Gilroy (1977). Musiek (1983b) reported a hit rate (abnormal score in one or both ears) in 56% of the hemispheric-lesion group and 50% of the brainstem group. These results show that the sensitivity of the test is approximately at chance levels for both the hemispheric and brainstem lesion groups and the test does not differentiate between brainstem and hemispheric lesions. Of the 15 patients with hemispheric lesions limited to one hemisphere, 60% had abnormal contralateral-ear scores and approximately 27% had abnormal ipsilateral-ear scores. Of the 9 patients with abnormal scores in the contralateral and/or ipsilateral ears, approximately 78% had deficits greater in

the contralateral than ipsilateral ear. Of the 7 patients with brainstem lesions limited to one side, 28.5% had abnormal contralateral-ear scores and approximately 71% had abnormal ipsilateral-ear scores. Of the unilateral brainstem-lesion patients with abnormal scores in the ipsilateral and/or contralateral ear, 100% had greater deficits in the ipsilateral than contralateral ear. Although the laterality effects are more striking for the brainstem-lesion than the hemispheric-lesion groups, the fact that hemispheric-lesion cases cannot be differentiated from brainstem-lesion cases and contralateral-ear effects predominate for the hemispheric lesion cases whereas ipsilateral-ear effects predominate for the brainstem lesion cases, laterality cannot be determined on the basis of this test. Musiek (1983b) also reported that in their 3 patients with bilateral hemispheric lesions, 1 had normal scores bilaterally and 2 had abnormal scores in only one ear.

F. BINAURAL FUSION

Matzker (1959) developed a binaural test in which German two-syllable PB words were filtered through a low-pass band (500–800 Hz) in one ear and a high-pass band (1815–2500 Hz) in the other ear. The high-pass band was presented simultaneously with the low-pass band. Normal subjects are able to fuse the high-pass band and low-pass band and recognize the word. That is, they integrate the information at the two ears (summate binaurally). When only one of the bands (high- or low-pass) is presented to an ear, normal subjects cannot recognize the word. This test is considered a special case of dichotic speech tests since different but complementary stimuli are presented simultaneously to the two ears. Matzker's procedure involved first dichotic presentation, then diotic presentation (which did not require binaural summation or fusion), followed again by dichotic presentation. In normal-hearing subjects, performance in the dichotic mode is essentially equivalent to performance in the diotic mode. Matzker hypothesized that patients with brainstem pathology, particularly lower brainstem pathology, would perform poorly on the dichotic mode of the binaural-fusion test; that is, they would be unable to fuse the high-and low-pass bands of information.

Linden (1964) developed a Swedish version of the Matzker binaural-fusion test based on Swedish spondaic words. His low-pass band was from 560 to 715 Hz and his high-pass band was from 1800 to 2200 Hz. Linden hypothesized that patients with various central pathologies would obtain binaural-fusion test scores in the dichotic mode lower than those when high-and low-pass bands were presented simultaneously to one ear. The results did not bear out his hypothesis. Linden concluded that his modification of the binaural-fusion test was not useful for the detection of central auditory pathology.

In Ivey's (1969) version of the binaural-fusion test, the low-pass band extended from 500 to 700 Hz and the high-pass band extended from 1900 to 2100 Hz. The rejection rate of the filter was 36 dB per octave. Two lists of 20 children's spondaic words were presented with the low-pass band at 25 dB SL relative to the 500-Hz pure-tone threshold and the high-pass band at 25 dB SL relative to the 2000-Hz threshold. The first list was given with the low-pass band to one ear and the high-pass band to the other ear. With the second list, the ears receiving the high- and low-pass bands were reversed. Each item was assigned a value of 5%. Arbitrarily, the binaural-fusion score is attributed to the ear in which the low-pass band is presented. Ivey (1969) administered the binaural fusion test to a group of normal-hearing listeners. The mean score for list 1 was higher than that for list 2 (93.8% and 86.0%, respectively).

Willeford (1977) modified the Ivey (1969) version of the binaural-fusion test, using the presentation of 30 rather than 25 dB SL (higher sensation levels if low scores are obtained at 30 dB SL). Willeford (1977), as noted by Lukas and Gendeur-Lukas (1985), recommended that a 10% correction factor be added to scores obtained for list 2. Monaural recognition is first obtained for each frequency band for each ear. Then the binaural-fusion recognition scores are obtained with one list presented such that the right ear receives the low-frequency band and the other list presented such that the left ear receives the low-frequency band. Willeford (1977) reported that the mean binaural-fusion score for his group of 20 normal adults was 89% with a range of 75–100%. According to Lynn and Gilroy (1975), normal binaural-fusion scores usually surpass the highest monaural single-band score by at least 50%.

Lynn and Gilroy (1972) reported that performance on the binaural-fusion test was abnormal in some of their patients with temporal-lobe tumors. Nevertheless, in some cases there was evidence of secondary brainstem compression. In a later study on 4 patients with posterior temporal-lobe tumors, Lynn and Gilroy (1975) reported that abnormal binaural-fusion test scores were obtained in 1 patient and questionable binaural-fusion test scores were obtained in another patient. Lynn and Gilroy (1975) also observed that the binaural-fusion test results were abnormal in only 1 of their 6 patients with antero-inferior temporal-lobe tumors, 0 of their 5 patients with superficial parietal-lobe tumors, and 1 of their 8 patients with deep parietal-lobe tumors (with a questionable score in another patient). These results suggest that the binaural-fusion test is not sensitive to temporal-lobe or parietal-lobe tumors.

In the Smith and Resnick (1972) version of the binaural-fusion test, monosyllables (CNC) were employed. The low-frequency band was 360–890 Hz and the high-frequency band was 1750–2220 Hz. The test was presented under three conditions; (a) dichotic with the low-pass band to one

ear and the high-pass band to the opposite ear, (b) diotic with high- and low-pass bands presented binaurally, and (c) the same dichotic condition as in (a) except that the ears receiving the low- and high-pass bands were reversed. Smith and Resnick (1972) found that performance on the binaural-fusion test was similar across the three conditions in subjects with normal hearing-threshold levels, bilateral sensorineural hearing impairment, and temporal-lobe pathology. In all 4 of their subjects with brainstem pathology, performance in at least one of the two dichotic conditions was reduced compared with that in the diotic condition. Smith and Resnick's (1972) findings suggested that the binaural-fusion test could be used to detect brainstem pathology. Palva and Jokinen (1975) reported that poor binaural-fusion test scores (with good scores when the low- and high-pass bands were presented monaurally) occurred frequently in patients with brainstem lesions of vascular or traumatic etiology. On the other hand, Lynn and Gilroy (1977) did not observe consistent findings or patterns on the binaural-fusion test in patients with brainstem lesions. Also, Musiek and Geurkink (1982), who used the Willeford (1977) version of the binaural-fusion test, reported that only 30% of their 10 patients with brainstem lesions demonstrated abnormal binaural-fusion test scores. These later reports suggest that the binaural-fusion test has a low sensitivity to brainstem lesions, contrary to what was originally theorized. Large-sample studies on the binaural-fusion test are required before this test can be used clinically to detect brainstem dysfunction.

The binaural-fusion test tape can be obtained from Auditec of St. Louis.

III. OTHER SPEECH TESTS

A. SYNTHETIC SENTENCE IDENTIFICATION TEST

The Synthetic Sentence Identification SSI test was developed by Speaks and Jerger (1965) who constructed a diagnostic speech test based on sentence rather than word stimuli in order to investigate the relation between the temporal characteristics of the message and speech-recognition ability. The SSI is a closed-set test and contains sentence stimuli controlled for length, vocabulary, syntax, and word familiarity. Synthetic (artificial) sentences were used to overcome the problems of sentence recognition through identification of a key word, and construction of equivalent lists of sentences.

Speaks and Jerger (1965) employed Miller and Selfridge's (1950) procedure to construct the synthetic sentences. In the first-order approximations of sentences, each word of the sentence is selected at random from the Thorndike and Lorge (1944) listing. In the second-order approximations of sentences, the first word in the sentence is randomly selected from the Thorndike and Lorge (1944) listing of the 1000 most common words and then an individual gives the next word that could logically follow the first word. Another individual then gives the third word that could logically follow the second word without having knowledge of the first word. This process continues with each individual supplying a word based on knowledge of only one word until the sentence is completed. When constructing a third-order approximation, the first word pair is chosen randomly from the second-order sentences. Then an individual gives a word that could logically follow the word pair. The next individual gives a word that could logically follow the second and third words. This process continues with each individual supplying a word based on knowledge of two words until the sentence is constructed. Jerger, Speaks, and Trammel (1968) developed 10 third-order approximations of sentences. This list of third-order synthetic sentences is shown in Table V. The patient is given a placard with the list of 10 sentences and is asked to identify the number of the sentences that was heard.

Since many hearing-impaired as well as normal-hearing listeners obtained scores of 100% at high intensities, the test was made more difficult by adding a competing message—the narrative story of Davy Crockett. (Jerger *et al.*, 1968). The talker who presented the synthetic sentences was the same one who presented the competing message.

The competing message can be presented ipsilaterally (SSI–ICM) or contralaterally (SSI–CCM). The SSI-ICM test is presented at +10, 0, −10, and −20 dB message-to-competition ratios (MCR). The SSI–CCM test is presented at 0, −20, and −40 dB message-to-competition ratios. The intensity of the speech is 40 dB SL at all MCRs. The test is used in normal-hearing persons with symmetrical audiometric configurations. According to Jerger *et al.* (1968) and Keith (1977), normal-hearing persons obtain scores of 90–100% at all MCRs for the SSI–CCM test. Jerger (1970) reported that for the SSI–ICM test, the mean scores were 100% at +10 MCR, 94% at 0 MCR, 80% at −10 MCR, and 55% at −20 MCR; the range between one standard

deviation above the mean and one standard deviation below the mean was 0% at +10 MCR, 85–100% at 0 MCR, 70–92% at −10 MCR, and 45–65% at −20 MCR. Keith (1977) obtained similar findings for the SSI–ICM in his group of 20 normal-hearing listeners. Figure 11 shows the forms used for recording the SSI–ICM and SSI–CCM results. The crossed-hatched area in the SSI–ICM form shows the range (one standard deviation above and below the mean) in normal-hearing listeners. The SSI–ICM and SSI–CCM tapes are commercially available from Auditec of St. Louis.

PATHOLOGIC AND ELDERLY GROUPS

Jerger and Jerger (1974) reported on the SSI–ICM and SSI–CCM results in a group of 11 patients with intra-axial brainstem tumors having pure-tone averages not exceeding 38 dB in either ear. All of the patients exhibited reduced SSI–ICM scores bilaterally or in the contralateral ear. Even when the SSI scores were poor bilaterally, the score for the contralateral ear was poorer than for the ipsilateral ear. The SSI–CCM scores were either normal bilaterally or were slightly reduced (not below 70%) in the contralateral ear.

Jerger and Jerger (1975) administered the SSI–ICM and SSI–CCM tests to a group of 10 patients with intra-axial brainstem lesions and 6 patients with temporal-lobe lesions. When scores on the SSI–ICM were averaged across MCRs, the mean score of the brainstem group showed a deficit of

Table V List of Third-Order Synthetic Sentences Used in the SSI Test[a]

1. Small boat with a picture has become
2. Built the government with the force almost
3. Go change your car color is red
4. Forward march said the boy had a
5. March around without a care in your
6. Your neighbor who said business is better
7. Battle cry and be better than ever
8. Down by the time is real enough
9. Agree with him only to find out
10. Women view men with green paper should

[a] Reprinted from Jerger, Speaks, and Trammel (1968) with permission.

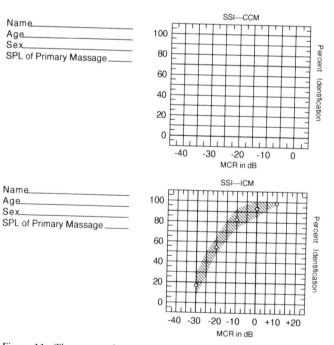

Figure 11 The top graph represents the SSI–CCM form and the bottom graph represents the SSI–ICM form. The cross-hatched area represents the range from one standard deviation below to one standard deviation above the mean. The circles represent the means in normal-hearing subjects. Modified from Keith (1977).

approximately 40% in the contralateral ear and the temporal-lobe group had a deficit of approximately 30% on the ipsilateral ear and 40% on the contralateral ear. When performance on the SSI–CCM was averaged across all MCRs, the brainstem group obtained a mean score within normal limits, and the mean score of the temporal-lobe group showed a deficit on the contralateral ear of approximately 20%. Based on these and previous findings, Jerger and Jerger (1975) concluded that, for the brainstem group, poor scores are obtained on the SSI–ICM on the contralateral ear and good scores on the SSI–CCM are obtained bilaterally. Some brainstem patients may show SSI–ICM deficits bilaterally and/or a slight SSI–CCM deficit contralaterally. Jerger and Jerger (1975) also concluded that, for the temporal-lobe group, poor scores are obtained on the SSI–ICM bilaterally and on the SSI–CCM contralaterally. Some temporal-lobe patients have SSI–ICM deficits only in the contralateral ear or normal SSI–ICM scores. In summary, the brainstem patients do more poorly on the SSI–ICM than on the SSI–CCM whereas the temporal-lobe patients do more poorly on the SSI–CCM than on the SSI–ICM. Figure 12 shows the expected SSI–ICM and SSI–CCM results in patients with eighth-nerve tumors, brainstem lesions, and temporal-lobe lesions.

Antonelli, Bellotto, and Grandori (1987) administered the SSI–ICM and SSI–CCM to a group of 12 patients with intra-axial lesions and a group of 10 patients with temporal-lobe lesions. Scores on the Italian version of the SSI–ICM were considered abnormal if the average of the

scores at MCRs of 0, −10, and −20 dB was below 70%. Scores on the Italian version of the SSI–CCM were considered abnormal if average of the scores at MCRs of 0, −20, and −40 dB was below 100%. Antonelli *et al.* (1987) reported poor ICM scores in 75% of the brainstem group and poor SSI–CCM scores in 80% of their temporal-lobe group. Nonetheless, 16.7% of their brainstem group also obtained poor SSI–CCM scores.

Jacobson *et al.* (1983) evaluated the SSI–ICM and SSI–CCM test results in 20 patients with multiple sclerosis. All had multiple sites of involvement in the central nervous system as indicated by neurologic findings but varied with respect to the particular sites involved (spinal cord, brainstem, cerebellar, cerebral, ocular). Nearly all had normal hearing-threshold levels. The SSI–ICM was reduced unilaterally or bilaterally in 25% of their cases at one or more MCRs. All had normal scores on the SSI–CCM. These findings conflicted with those obtained by Russolo and Poli (1983) who reported that 55% of their patients with multiple sclerosis showed deficits on the SSI–ICM and 50% showed deficits on the SSI–CCM. Jerger, Oliver, Chmiel, and Rivera (1986) reported that 50% of their 62 patients with multiple sclerosis obtained abnormal scores on the SSI–ICM test (unilateral deficits in 19% and bilateral deficits in 31%). These studies indicate that the SSI–ICM and SSI–CCM tests do not have a high sensitivity to the presence of multiple sclerosis and whether the deficit is in the SSI–ICM or SSI–CCM scores may depend upon the particular regions of the central nervous system affected by the disease and upon the extent of the involvement.

Orchik and Burgess (1977) administered the SSI–ICM test at five MCRs to four groups of normal-hearing patients aged 10–12 years, 20–29 years, 40–49 years, and 60 years or more. They found that the SSI–ICM scores were decreased in the two older groups compared with the two younger groups. Jerger and Hayes (1977) found that the SSI–ICM maximum scores at 0 dB MCR decreased with age in subjects between 10 and 89 years of age although the PB_{max} scores remained relatively unchanged with age. Jerger and Hayes (1977) concluded that comparison of the PB_{max} and SSI–ICM maximum scores could grossly indicated the extent to which an auditory deficit was peripheral or central. Similar findings were obtained by Shirinian and Arnst (1982).

Otto and McCandless (1982) investigated the SSI–ICM performance intensity function at 0 dB MCR in 30 elderly and 30 young subjects with relatively matched mild-to-moderate sensorineural hearing impairment. Excessive rollover was present in 30%. Stach, Jerger, and Fleming (1985) reported on the performance-intensity function for the SSI–ICM at 0 dB MCR in an elderly patient on four occasions over a 9-year period. Over this period, the peripheral sensitivity changed minimally. The SSI scores, however, changed over this period. Rollover increased first, followed by a

N VIII TUMOR – RIGHT	
SSI – RIGHT **ICM** Poor Score **CCM** Poor Score	**SSI – LEFT** **ICM** Good Score **CCM** Good Score

BRAIN STEM LESION – RIGHT	
SSI – RIGHT **ICM** Good or Poor Score **CCM** Good Score	**SSI – LEFT** **ICM** Poor Score **CCM** Good Score

TEMPORAL LOBE LESION – RIGHT	
SSI – RIGHT **ICM** Good or Poor Score **CCM** Good Score	**SSI – LEFT** **ICM** Poor Score **CCM** Poor Score

Figure 12 Characteristic SSI results on patients with eighth nerve, brainstem, and temporal-lobe lesions. Reprinted from Keith (1977) with permission.

decline in the maximum SSI score. Stach *et al.* (1985) suggested that the SSI decline paralleled changes in central auditory function with age. These findings suggest that SSI–ICM and SSI–CCM tests should not be used to detect central auditory dysfunction of etiology other than aging in the elderly since aging can produce deterioration in the SSI scores.

B. RAPIDLY ALTERNATING SPEECH PERCEPTION TEST

Bocca and Calearo (1963) developed a swinging speech test following the method of Cherry and Taylor (1954). In the swinging speech test, the message alternates periodically between ears so that each ear receives half of the message. Recognition of the entire message occurs only if the information to the two ears is fused or resynthesized. Figure 13 illustrates the poor recognition in each ear alone with complete recognition when the two ears receive the complementary segments.

Bocca and Calearo (1963) found that performance on the rapidly alternating speech perception (RASP) test was unaffected by pathology of the auditory cortex. Since RASP performance was affected by some cases of diffuse cerebral pathology and many cases of brainstem pathology, they suggested that the RASP test was dependent upon the integrity of the central auditory nervous system at the level of the brainstem.

Lynn and Gilroy (1975) developed their own English language version of the Bocca and Calearo swinging speech test. The stimuli alternated every 300 ms. Normative data collected in their laboratory revealed monaural scores ranging from 0–10% and binaural scores from 95–100%. In a later study based on 18 normal adults, Lynn and Gilroy (1977) obtained mean monaural scores of 7.2 and 3.9% for the right and left ears, respectively, with standard deviations of 9.0 and 5.1% for the right and left ears, respectively; in the binaural condition, the mean score was 97.2% and the standard deviation was 7.4%. The Willeford (1977) version of the RASP test differed from the Lynn and Gilroy (1975) version essentially with respect to the stimulus items. The presentation level is 30 dB SL relative to the pure-tone average. Some investigators have recommended

the use of 40 dB SL relative to the SRT (Tobin, 1985) or 50 dB SL relative to the SRT or PTA (Musiek & Geurkink, 1982; Pinheiro, 1978). The procedure involves first presenting the sentences monaurally to each ear (with a score for each ear) and then presenting the sentences in the alternating mode with the two ears receiving the complementary segments. Twenty sentences are presented, each sentence having an assigned value of 5%. The sentences used in the RASP are shown in Table VI. In the alternating mode, 10 sentences are presented so that the right ear receives the first segment and 10 sentences are presented so that the left ear receives the first segment. Willeford (1977) reported that the mean scores for the RASP in a group of 20 normal adults was 99% with a range of 90–100%.

Lynn and Gilroy (1977) reported that the RASP mean score was 100% in their group of 11 patients with right temporal-lobe tumors, approximately 80% for their group of 11 patients with left temporal-lobe tumors, approximately 92% for their group of 14 patients with right parietal-lobe tumors, approximately 92% for their group of 10 patients with left parietal-lobe tumors, approximately 38% for their group of 6 patients with low pons cerebello-pontine-angle lesions, and approximately 84% for their group of 9 patients with upper brainstem lesions. These results show that the poorest RASP scores were obtained in patients with low brainstem lesions. Musiek and Geurkink (1982) reported abnormal scores on the RASP test in only 50% of their 10 patients with brainstem lesions. Antonelli *et al.* (1987) obtained findings similar to those of Musiek

Table VI Sentences from the Rapidly Alternating Speech Perception Test[a]

SENTENCE BEGINS_____ TRACK	
L	1. The children came home late from school.
L	2. He likes to play and splash in the water.
R	3. She is mad because the television was broken.
R	4. It rained very much for hours.
R	5. The wind almost blew the roof off.
L	6. What time did you get in yesterday?
L	7. The school room was very large.
R	8. I took a picture of her with my camera.
L	9. What is your favorite television program?
R	10. Where have you been all day?
L	11. The telephone rang for a real long time.
L	12. How did you put that together again?
R	13. They went to the park to play games.
L	14. Let the dog in at the back door.
R	15. Answer the telephone as soon as it rings.
R	16. Please turn the radio up louder.
L	17. Are you going to the office this morning?
L	18. That window is very dirty.
R	19. His father is on the police force.
R	20. I had bacon and eggs for breakfast.

[a] Reprinted with permission from Auditec of St. Louis.

BINAURAL RESYNTHESIS

RAPIDLY ALTERNATING SPEECH PERCEPTION

RE: I'   EE YO   GH AF   L CH

LE: LL S   U RI T   TER UN

BIN: I'LL SEE YOU RIGHT AFTER LUNCH

Figure 13 Binaural resynthesis sample from the Rapidly Alternating Speech Perception Test. Reprinted from Lynn and Gilroy (1975) with permission.

and Geurkink (1982). Antonelli *et al.* (1987) reported that approximately 56% of their 16 cases with intra-axial brainstem lesions had abnormal alternating speech test scores whereas only approximately 6% of their 16 cases with temporal-lobe lesions had abnormal alternating speech scores.

According to Tobin (1985), the RASP and binaural-fusion tests do not necessarily assess the same aspect of binaural interaction function; the former test involves "integration of segments over time" (p. 164) whereas the latter is a "spectral function" (p. 164).

The RASP tape is commercially available from Auditec of St. Louis.

C. MASKING LEVEL DIFFERENCE TEST

Binaural advantages in detection of signals in masking noise have been investigated in various clinical populations. These binaural advantages are also known as binaural release from masking, masking level differences (MLDs), or binaural unmasking. The mechanism for extraction of the signal from a background of noise is believed to be analysis of interaural phase (time) differences (Durlach & Colburn, 1978).

Consider the case of a person who has a noise (N) and a signal (S) such as speech presented to one ear. This condition, which reflects monotic presentation of the signal and noise, has been represented in the literature as SmNm. The condition in which the signal is presented to one ear but the noise is presented to both ears with a 180° interaural phase difference is represented as SmNπ. The condition in which the signal is presented to one ear but the noise is presented to both ears with a 0° interaural phase difference is represented as SmNo. The condition in which the signal is presented to both ears with a 0° interaural phase difference and the noise is presented to both ears with a 0° interaural phase difference is represented as SoNo. The condition in which the signal is presented to both ears with a 180° interaural phase difference and the noise is presented to both ears with a 0° interaural phase difference is represented as SπNo. The condition in which the signal is presented to both ears with a 0° interaural phase difference and the noise is presented to both ears with a 180° interaural phase difference is represented as SoNπ. The condition in which the signal is presented to both ears with a 180° interaural phase difference and the noise is presented to both ears with a 180° phase difference is represented as SπNπ.

Figure 14 illustrates some of these experimental conditions. The SoNo condition is homophasic since the noise and signals are in phase. The SoNπ, SπNo, and SπNπ are antiphasic conditions since the noises and/or the signals are out of phase.

According to Diercks and Jeffress (1962), the SmNm, SoNo, and SπNπ produce the poorest thresholds. The

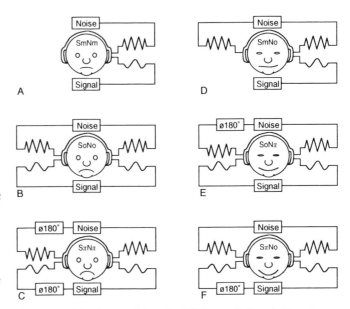

Figure 14 Stimulus conditions for MLD test. S, Signal; N, noise; m, monaural; o, in phase at two ears; π 180° out of phase at two ears. Reprinted from Olsen and Noffsinger (1976) with permission.

SoNπ and SπNo produce the best thresholds. This situation is illustrated by the magnitude of the smile or frown in Figure 14. In normal-hearing persons, the threshold for a signal in the SmNo or SmNπ condition is better than that in the SmNm condition. Also, the threshold for a signal in the SoNπ or SπNo condition is better than that in the SoNo condition. These improvements reflect release from masking. The MLD can be obtained by subtracting the threshold level for the signal in the SmNo or SmNπ condition from the threshold level for the signal in the SmNm condition. The MLD can also be obtained by subtracting the threshold level for the signal in the SoNπ or SπNo condition from the threshold level for the signal in the SoNo condition.

The MLD for speech is most commonly measured by obtaining the spondee recognition threshold in the SoNo condition (reference condition) and SoNπ or SπNo condition. The size of the MLD is defined as the difference between the SRT in the homophasic condition and that in the antiphasic (SπNo or SoNπ) condition. The intensity of the broad-band noise is usually presented at 80 dB SPL (Lynn, Gilroy, Taylor, & Leiser, 1981; Olsen & Noffsinger, 1976; Olsen, Noffsinger, & Carhart, 1976). Some two-channel audiometers (e.g., GSI-10) have a network that allows phase reversal of either the noise or test signal. Adaptors with the mixer and phase shift capability are commercially available for use with two-channel audiometer and can be purchased from some companies.

1. NORMATIVE DATA
Olsen and Noffsinger (1976) obtained mean spondee MLDs of 7.3 dB for the SπNo antiphasic condition and

6.9 dB for the SoNπ antiphasic condition when the reference condition was SoNo in their group of 12 normal-hearing subjects. Olsen et al. (1976) obtained a mean spondee MLD of 8.3 and 6.9 dB for the SπNo and SoNπ conditions, respectively, in their group of 50 normal-hearing subjects. Since only 6% obtained spondee MLDs less than or equal to 5 dB for the SπNo condition and less than or equal to 3 dB for the SoNπ condition, the cutoff MLD for normalcy below which the MLD was abnormally reduced was 5 dB for the former condition and 3 dB for the latter condition. Lynn et al. (1981) reported that the mean MLD in their group of normal-hearing subjects was 12.2 dB for the SπNo antiphasic condition and 10.2 dB for the SoNπ antiphasic condition; the standard deviation was 1.1 dB for both antiphasic conditions and the range was 10–14 dB for the SπNo antiphasic condition and 8–12 dB for the SoNπ antiphasic condition.

2. PATHOLOGIC GROUPS

Cullen and Thompson (1974) reported that the MLD score (% Michigan CNC words correct in SoNπ or SπNo condition minus % Michigan CNC words correct in the SoNo condition) in 4 patients with anterior temporal-lobe lesions involving the superior gyrus fell in the range defining one standard deviation above and below the mean in normal-hearing listeners. Cullen and Thompson (1974) concluded that an intact auditory association was not essential for release of masking to occur. They also concluded that the release from masking phenomenon was probably mediated at subthalamic levels. Lynn et al. (1981) reported that the mean MLD detection threshold in their group of 12 patients with cerebral lesions did not differ significantly from that of the normal subjects for both SπNo and SoNπ antiphasic conditions. Olsen et al. (1976) reported that abnormally small spondee MLDs were obtained in only 5% of their 20 patients with cortical lesions for the SπNo antiphasic condition and 0% of these patients for the SoNπ antiphasic condition. Olsen et al. (1976) concluded that the MLD was mediated at subcortical levels. Noffsinger (1982) reported that the spondee MLD (SoNo - SπNo) was abnormally small (less than 6 dB) in only 9% of their 67 cases with temporal-lobe lesions. The results of these investigations on the MLD in temporal-lobe lesions show that the MLD is generally unaffected by cortical lesions.

Olsen and Noffsinger (1976) reported that 58% of their 12 patients with multiple sclerosis and other pathologies of the midbrain and/or brainstem region had abnormlly small spondee MLDs of less than 6 dB for the SπNo antiphasic condition and/or less than 4 dB in the SoNπ antiphasic condition. They concluded that the MLD was often impaired by central-nervous system pathologies associated with multiple sclerosis or other midbrain and/or brainstem lesions. Noffsinger (1982) reported that 52% of their 114 patients with brainstem lesions and normal-hearing sensi-

tivity had spondee MLDs (SoNo minus SπNo) that were abnormally reduced (<6 dB). Noffsinger (1982) concluded that abnormally reduced MLDs in persons with normal hearing-thresholds signaled the presence of brainstem pathology. Lynn et al. (1981) reported that the mean MLDs for the speech-detection threshold did not differ significantly among the normal, cerebral, and upper pons/midbrain/thalamic groups. The mean MLD was significantly reduced in the pontomedullary group compared with the normal, cerebral, and upper pons/midbrain/thalamic groups. Lynn et al. (1981) concluded that the pontomedullary region of the brainstem (lower brainstem) mediates that MLD phenomenon and suggested that the region of the superior olivary nuclei was a likely site for mediation of the MLD since it was the most caudal anatomical site in the brainstem where there was integration of information from the two ears. The hypothesis of Lynn et al. (1981) was substantiated by the findings of Noffsinger, Martinez, and Schaefer (1982). Noffsinger et al. (1982) found that abnormally small MLDs and abnormally elevated or absent acoustic-reflex thresholds occurred in patients with brainstem lesions when abnormalities in the brainstem auditory-evoked potentials began with wave I, II, or III but normal MLDs and acoustic-reflex thresholds occurred in patients with brainstem lesions when abnormalities in the brainstem auditory-evoked potentials began with wave IV or V. Since waves I and II probably arise from the eighth cranial nerve, and the primary contribution to wave III is the superior olivary complex according to Britt and Rossi (1980) and Rossi and Britt (1980) or the cochlear nuclei according to Moller, Jannetta, and Moller (1981), Noffsinger et al. (1982) proposed that cochlear nuclei and/or the superior olivary complex may be responsible for the binaural interaction processes involved in the MLD phenomenon. Since abnormally reduced spondee MLDs occur in patient with eighth-nerve tumors even when there is normal-hearing sensitivity and symmetrical audiometric configurations (Noffsinger, 1982; Olsen et al., 1976), the presence of a reduced MLD in persons with bilateral normal-hearing thresholds and symmetrical audiometric configurations does not differentiate between eighth nerve and brainstem sites of lesion. The spondee MLD is associated with a higher sensitivity than the 500-Hz MLD to brainstem pathology (Olsen & Noffsinger, 1976; Noffsinger, 1982). Nevertheless, since the hit rate for the spondee MLD appears not to be substantially higher than chance, the spondee MLD test does not appear to hold great promise as a clinical tool for the detection of brainstem dysfunction in normal-hearing persons.

Several studies have shown reduced speech MLDs in patients with multiple sclerosis (Hannley, Jerger, & Rivera, 1983; Olsen & Noffsinger, 1976; Olsen et al., 1976). Hannley et al. (1983) reported a hit rate of 75% for their 20 patients with confirmed multiple sclerosis (75% of whom had normal-hearing sensitivity). Olsen *et al.* (1976), on the other hand, reported that the spondee MLD hit rate was 58% for the SπNo antiphasic condition and 41% for the SoNπ antiphasic condition in their group of 100 patients with multiple sclerosis and normal-hearing sensitivity. Olsen *et al.* (1976) hypothesized that reduced MLDs and normal hearing sensitivity in patients with multiple sclerosis indicated brainstem and/or midbrain lesions. The findings of Lynn, Gilroy, Taylor and Leiser (1981) MLDs in low brainstem but not midbrain lesions and Noffsinger *et al.* (1982) showing abnormal MLDs in patients with brainstem lesions when the abnormalities in the brainstem auditory-evoked potentials commenced with waves I, II, or III but not IV or V suggest that the reduced MLDs in patients with multiple sclerosis reflect dysfunction at the low brainstem rather than the midbrain.

IV. EFFECT OF PERIPHERAL HEARING IMPAIRMENT

Luterman, Welsh, and Melrose (1966) administered a speeded CID W-22 speech test to 10 normal-hearing young males and 18 young adult males with sensorineural hearing impairment. The hearing-impaired subjects had greater mean error scores than the normal-hearing subjects at all rates of time alteration. Sticht and Gray (1969) administered the time-compressed CID-22 test at 36, 46, and 59% rates of compression to a group of 7 young normal-hearing subjects, 7 young sensorineural hearing-impaired subjects, 7 elderly normal-hearing subjects, and 7 elderly sensorineural hearing-impaired subjects. The mean time-compressed scores revealed that the young hearing-impaired listeners obtained poorer scores than the young normal-hearing subjects and the elderly hearing-impaired subjects obtained poorer scores than the elderly normal-hearing subjects at all compression ratios. Korsan-Bengtsen (1973) found that patients with acquired sensorineural hearing impairment had reduced scores on a temporally interrupted speech test. Kurdziel, Rintelmann, and Beasley (1975) reported reduced scores on the time-compressed CNC monosyllables at all compression ratios in their hearing-impaired subjects. Grimes *et al.* (1984) administered the Auditec of St. Louis recording of the 60% time-compressed NU-6 test (lists I–IV) to 28 normal-hearing adults (19–37 years of age) and 28 subjects (25–59 years of age) with sensorineural hearing-impairment assumed to be secondary to noise exposure. The hearing-impaired subjects had varying magnitudes of hearing impairment in the mid to high frequencies. The sensorineural group obtained mean scores 35–40% below those of the normal group on all of the NU-6 lists. Significant differences among the mean scores were obtained between lists I and II, I and III, II and IV, and III and IV, indicating a lack of interlist equivalency in the hearing-impaired group. Speaks (1980) examined the issue of the effect of peripheral hearing impairment on temporally interrupted speech scores in 10 patients with bilateral sensorineural, bilateral mixed, or unilateral sensorineural hearing impairment and on time-compressed speech scores in 11 patients with bilateral sensorineural, bilateral mixed, bilateral conductive, or unilateral sensorineural hearing impairment. All of the subjects had 100% scores for the uninterrupted and uncompressed sentences. The results revealed substantial ear-difference scores for the temporally interrupted sentences. Abnormal ear-difference scores were obtained in 2–6 of the 11 patients, depending upon the compression rate and intensity. Speaks (1980) concluded that the results of time-compressed and temporally altered speech tests must be interpreted cautiously in persons with peripheral hearing impairment. The results of these studies suggest that peripheral hearing impairment has a deleterious affect on performance on time-compressed speech tests. The presence of sensorineural hearing impairment could confound interpretation of decreased scores since one cannot distinguish between the effects of peripheral hearing impairment or central auditory impairment.

Lynn & Gilroy (1977) reported that peripheral sensorineural hearing impairment could result in decreased low-pass filtered-speech scores, RASP scores, and dichotic speech scores. Lynn and Gilroy (1977) disagreed with Katz's statement that the PB speech-recognition score could be subtracted from the SSW score to yield an SSW score free of the effect of peripheral hearing impairment. According to Lynn and Gilroy (1977), there is no way to identify the peripheral as opposed to the central components of the PB speech-recognition score in persons with combined peripheral sensorineural hearing impairment and central auditory dysfunction. In some cases with symmetrical audiometric configuration and asymmetrical speech-recognition scores, the PB speech-recognition score may result entirely from the central auditory lesion and and not reflect the peripheral sensorineural hearing-impairment at all. Lynn and Gilroy (1977) concluded that, when abnormal central auditory test scores are obtained in persons with peripheral hearing impairment, the clinician should state that the status of the central auditory system cannot be accurately assessed. Cafarelli, Nodar, Collard, and Larkins (1977) reported that large intersubject and intrasubject variability in SSW scores were obtained in their group of hearing-impaired subjects. Arnst (1982) reported that the C-SSW score did not necessarily compensate for peripheral hearing impairment since 24% of the hearing-impaired subjects had C-SSW scores in the moderate or severe categories. Arnst (1982) concluded that the C-SSW scores should be interpreted cautiously in persons with pure-tone averages exceeding 40 dB HL.

Miltenberger, Dawson, and Raica (1978) evaluated the results of a central auditory test battery on 70 subjects with peripheral sensorineural hearing impairment of varying magnitude and slope. The central auditory test battery consisted of the competing-sentences test, the filtered-speech test, the binaural-fusion test, and the RASP. The results revealed that abnormal scores were obtained by 17% on the competing-sentences test, 24% on the binaural-fusion test, 21% on the RASP test, and 61% on the filtered-speech test. Abnormal scores on one or more of the central auditory tests were obtained by 77%. Miltenberger *et al.* (1978) concluded that the results of central auditory tests in persons with peripheral sensorineural hearing impairment must be interpreted cautiously.

Roeser, Johns, and Price (1976) reported that their group of hearing-impaired subjects obtained significantly poorer scores than the normal-hearing subjects on the dichotic digits test and the dichotic CV nonsense syllables test. Also, substantial ear-differences were obtained in the hearing-impaired subjects, particularly for the dichotic digits test. Speaks (1980) found that, although a patient with a unilateral sloping sensorineural hearing impairment obtained small ear-difference scores on the monotic performance-intensity functions for CVs, these small differences could account for the significant dichotic ear differences and substantial variation in dichotic ear advantage across intensities. In another patient with asymmetrical sensorineural hearing impairment and equal monotic performance-intensity functions for the CVs, the dichotic ear advantage varied across intensities, suggesting that symmetrical monotic CV scores cannot assure that the dichotic CV scores are unaffected by peripheral hearing impairment.

Olsen and Noffsinger (1976) reported that the MLD for spondees were reduced when the MLD was based on comparison of the SoNo with the SπNo or SoNπ conditions in 58% of the group of 12 patients with noise-induced hearing impairment and 100% of the group of 12 patients with Meniere's disease. Similar findings were obtained by Olsen *et al.* (1976). Olsen *et al.* (1976) found abnormally reduced MLDs for spondees in 50% of a group of 10 patients with unilateral conductive hearing impairment, 32% of a group of 50 patients with noise-induced sensorineural hearing impairment, 85% of the group of 20 patients with unilateral Meniere's disease, and 50% of the group of 20 patients with presbycusis when the MLD was based on the SoNo homophasic and SπNo antiphasic conditions. Bocca and Antonelli (1976) reported, based on mean data, that the masking-level difference for the sentence detection threshold was reduced in patients with asymmetrical conductive hearing impairment, presbycusis, unilateral sudden deafness, and Meniere's disease. The greatest reduction in MLD was observed in the poor ear of Meniere's disease cases. The mean MLD for the presbycusic group was only slightly reduced compared with that for the normal group. Reduced MLDs were obtained despite the fact that the signal intensity was set at the level producing a sound image

at the center of the head. The mean MLD for the group of symmetrical conductive hearing impairment was similar to that for the normal group. Bocca and Antonelli (1976) concluded that "hearing asymmetry—of any type—seems to produce unfavorable conditions for full binaural cooperation, not compensated by even complete intensity or loudness balancing between ears" (p. 486). Large intersubject variability in MLD was present in all of the groups. Noffsinger (1982) reported that abnormally reduced MLDs for spondees were obtained in 52% of the group of 54 patients with unilateral conductive hearing-impairment and 60% of the group of 200 patients with unilateral or bilateral cochlear hearing impairment. Noffsinger (1982) also reported that when the interaural signal and noise levels were adjusted by loudness balancing to achieve equal loudness at the two ears to subgroups of the conductive and sensorineural groups, the percentage of conductive hearing-impaired patients with reduced MLDs (for the 500-Hz pure tone) was decreased markedly and the percentage of unilateral cochlear hearing-impaired patients with reduced MLDs was only slightly reduced. Noffsinger (1982) concluded that the adjusted procedure increased the MLD (for tones) in patients with conductive but not sensorineural hearing impairment. Noffsinger (1982) also evaluated the MLD for the 500-Hz tone in two subgroups of Meniere's disease patients: one subgroup had an interaural threshold difference (at 500 Hz) of less than 15 dB and the other subgroup had an interaural threshold difference equal to or larger than 15 dB. The results revealed that the percentage of Meniere's-disease patients with abnormally reduced 500-Hz MLDs was similar for the small and larger interaural threshold groups. Therefore, interaural threshold difference at 500 Hz was not the primary factor producing small 500-Hz MLDs in Meniere's disease patients. These previously mentioned studies show that the MLD is abnormally reduced in persons with peripheral hearing impairment and in many presbycusic persons.

Based on the results of the previously mentioned investigations on the effects of peripheral hearing impairment on the central auditory speech tests, the clinician cannot straightforwardly interpret the central auditory test results unless there is normal hearing sensitivity bilaterally and symmetrical audiometric configurations. We suggest that central auditory testing be done only if normal hearing sensitivity is present bilaterally and the audiometric configuration is symmetrical (within 10 dB). Recently, the dichotic sentence identification test was developed for use with hearing-impaired adults (Fifer, Jerger, Berlin, Tobey, & Campbell, 1983). Further research on the DSI test in patients with peripheral hearing loss and on the sensitivity of this test in persons with central auditory dysfunction is needed before a recommendation can be made regarding the utilization of this test in the hearing-impaired population at risk for central auditory dysfunction.

V. ASSESSMENT OF CENTRAL AUDITORY PROCESSING DISORDERS IN THE PEDIATRIC POPULATION

Increasingly, in recent years, audiologists are seeing children for evaluation of suspected central auditory processing disorders. These children, who have been identified as learning disabled (or as having minimal brain dysfunction) or who exhibit abnormal auditory behavior, are generally referred by speech–language pathologists, learning-disabilities specialists, or special educators. Children with central auditory processing disorders exhibit abnormal scores on central auditory tests, unremarkable neurologic findings, at least normal intelligence, and normal peripheral hearing sensitivity. Signs of children with central auditory processing disorders include innattentiveness or short attention span, behavior like a hearing-impaired child despite normal peripheral hearing sensitivity; difficulty hearing in noise; difficulty understanding verbal directions; reversals in reading, writing, or repeating verbal information; frequent requests to repeat the message; hypoactivity or hyperactivity or high distractibility because of frustration resulting from lack of comprehension or fatigue in attempting to comprehend a message; poor memory for auditory information; and so forth (Musiek & Geurkink, 1980; Willeford, 1985). Although certain auditory and language skills interact in a complex manner, the precise nature of that interaction and the extent to which a central auditory processing disorder contributes to or is responsible for a language disorder remains unknown (Willeford, 1985). Nevertheless, children with central auditory processing disorders may or may not also exhibit a language disorder (Willeford, 1985; Willeford & Billger, 1978).

Normative data for the Willeford filtered-speech test, competing-sentences test, binaural-fusion test, and rapidly alternating speech perception test in children are shown in Tables VII, VIII, IX, and X, respectively. Table VII reveals improvement in score on the filtered-speech test with age (maturation effect), small interaural differences in scores at all ages, and a wide range in scores at all age levels consistent with large intersubject variability. Table VIII reveals improvement in the weak-ear competing-sentences score with age (maturation effect). The strong-ear competing sentences score is high even at age 5. The large range of scores in the weak ear through 9 years of age shows the large intersubject variability in the weak-ear competing-sentences score in children. A maturation effect is also seen for the binaural-fusion test, as shown in Table IX. Table X reveals that the rapidly alternating speech test scores in children as young as 5 years of age are similar to those in adults. The lack of a maturation effect on the rapidly alternating speech test indicates that this test is an easy one for children.

Willeford (1977) administered the competing-sentences test, the filtered-speech test, the binaural-fusion test, and the rapidly alternating speech test to 7 patients with learning disabilities or with academic performance at levels below expectations. Willeford (1977) reported abnormally reduced scores on one or more of these tests in each of the children.

The binaural-fusion test is considered to be a test of binaural integration which examines the ability to combine acoustic information presented simultaneously to the two ears. Martin and Clark (1977) employed the WIPI stimuli in their version of the binaural-fusion test administered to normal and language-learning-disabled children. They

Table VII Willeford Filtered-Speech Test Norms[a]

| | | | | Years of age | | | | |
	5	6	7	8	9	10	Adults[b]	Average 6–10
N	[c]	40	40	40	40	40	20	200
Mean								
LE	—	60.6	64.7	65.8	68.2	71.2	87.6	66.1
RE	—	60.9	64.6	65.7	67.9	72.7	87.4	66.4
Average ear difference[d]	—	5.4	6.3	6.7	5.4	5.3	0.2	5.8
SD								
LE	—	9.8	8.8	7.9	9.4	6.2	6.3	8.4
RE	—	9.7	7.5	8.4	9.2	6.2	5.7	8.2
Range								
LE	—	42/84	52/86	52/86	56/92	66/84	74/98	42/92
RE	—	44/82	52/86	56/92	56/92	64/82	74/98	44/92

[a] Modified from Willeford (1985).
[b] College students aged 18–29 years (Ivey, 1969).
[c] Insufficient at present.
[d] Only 18 of the 200 subjects had ear differences which exceeded 10%. The greatest difference in any subject was 16%.

Table VIII Norms for Willeford Competing-Sentences Test[a]

	Years of age						
	5	6	7	8	9	10	5–10
N	25	40	40	40	40	40	225
Expected result							
Weak ear	20	60	70	80	90	100	70
Strong ear[b]	90/100	90/100	100	100	100	100	100
Mean							
Weak ear	24.8	59.5	67.8	83.0	93.0	98.4	71.6
Strong ear	94.0	96.5	97.5	98.0	98.8	99.2	95.9
SD							
Weak ear	35.9	33.2	31.2	22.2	9.8	3.6	22.7
Strong ear	4.4	4.0	3.6	3.2	2.6	2.6	3.5
Range							
Weak ear	0/80	0/100	0/100	10/100	70/100	90/100	0/100
Strong ear	90/100	90/100	90/100	90/100	90/100	90/100	90/100

[a] Modified from Willeford (1985). Data are unilateral responses.
[b] Strong ears were predominantly right ears. Left ears were the strong ears in only 13 of the 225 subjects.

found that 50% of the learning-disabled subjects were detected with the binaural-fusion test. On the other hand, Harris (1963) found the binaural-fusion test to be ineffective in distinguishing between normal-hearing children and brain-damaged or reading-disabled children. Roush and Tait (1984) obtained similar findings to those obtained by Harris (1963). Willeford and Billger (1978) found that slightly more than half of the group of 150 learning-disabled children (64%) had abnormal binaural-fusion test scores. Ferre and Wilber (1986) reported that approximately 86% of their group of 13 learning-disabled children with presumed auditory impairment and 24% of their group of 13 learning-disabled children with presumed normal auditory skills had abnormal scores on the NU-CHIPS binaural-fusion test (low-pass band in the left ear).

Willeford (1985) reported that although none of 4 children with suspected auditory function obtained abnormal scores on a time-compressed WIPI test, the scores of 3 of the 4 children fell below age-mean scores as established by Maki, Beasley, and Orchik (1973). Willeford (1985) also noted, however, that he had also seen children with suspected central auditory processing disorder who obtained abnormal scores on only the time-compressed speech test. Manning, Johnston, and Beasley (1977) observed that children suspected of having central auditory processing dysfunction performed similarly on a time-compressed speech test at the 30% compression ratio as normal children but obtained poorer scores than normal at the 0 and 60% compression ratios. Ferre and Wilber (1986) reported that 68% of their 13 learning-disabled children with presumed auditory impairment and 68% of the 13 learning-disabled children with presumed normal auditory skills had abnormal scores on the NU-CHIPS 60% time-compressed speech test.

Martin and Clark (1977) reported that the low-pass filtered WIPI test failed to discriminate between the group of normal children and the group of language-learning-disabled children. Farrer and Keith (1981) observed that there was little overlap between the group of normal children and the group of auditory-learning-disabled children on the low-pass filtered PB-kindergarten word test when the cutoff frequency was 1000 Hz; clear separation between the groups was not obtained at cutoff frequencies of 500 or 750 Hz. Willeford and Billger (1978) reported that only

Table IX Willeford Binaural-Fusion Test Norms[a]

Age	N (ears)	Mean scores	Range	Norm
5	10	74	55–95	55–95
6	18	75	60–95	60–95
7	18	76	65–90	65–90
8	18	83	70–100	70–100
9	18	86	70–100	70–100
Adult	20	89	75–100	75–100

[a] Reprinted from Willeford (1977) with permission.

Table X Norms for the Willeford Rapidly Alternating Speech Perception Test[a]

Age	N (ears)	Mean scores	Range	Norm
5	20	99	90–100	
6	20	99	90–100	
7	20	99	90–100	80–100
8	20	98	80–90	
9	20	99	90–100	
Adult	20	99	90–100	

[a] Reprinted from Willeford (1977) with permission.

57% of their 150 learning-disabled children obtained abnormal filtered-speech test scores. Ferre and Wilber (1986) reported that abnormal performance on the low-pass filtered NU-CHIPS test was obtained in approximately 92% of the 13 learning-disabled children with presumed auditory impairment and approximately 24% of the 13 learning-disabled children with presumed normal auditory skills.

The competing-sentences test is a test of binaural separation which examines the ability to attend to acoustic information presented to one ear while suppressing the acoustic information presented simultaneously to the other ear. Willeford (1985) administered the competing-sentences test to a group of 9 learning-disabled children 5 to 7 years of age. He reported that 5 of 9 learning-disabled children did not obtain strong-ear scores within the normal range for the 5–7 year age levels. Weak-ear scores below the normal range for the 5–7 year age levels were also obtained by 5 of the 9 learning-disabled children. An abnormal weak-ear and/or strong-ear test score was obtained in 6 of the 9 children. Of the 8 learning-disabled children between 9 and 15 years of age, 6 had weak-ear and/or strong-ear scores on the competing-sentence test below the normal range for the 9–15 year age levels. Willeford and Billger (1978) reported that 48% of their 150 learning-disabled children obtained abnormal competing-sentences scores.

The weakest test for detecting central auditory processing disorders appears to be the rapidly alternating speech perception test (Willeford and Billger, 1978). Willeford and Billger (1978) found that only 18% of their group of 150 learning-disabled children obtained abnormal scores on this test.

The discrepancies among investigators on the results for a given central auditory test on learning-disabled children and the variability in scores among the various central auditory tests for a given learning-disabled child suggest that children with central auditory processing disorders are a heterogeneous population (Willeford, 1985). It appears, therefore, that a battery of central auditory tests rather than a single central auditory test may maximize detection of central auditory processing disorder. The limitations of test batteries, however, will be discussed in Chapter 9.

An intriguing approach to determining whether the basis of a central auditory processing disorder has a linguistic or an auditory basis was recently presented by Jerger, Johnson, and Loiselle (1988). They administered the Pediatric Speech Intelligibility (PSI) test to a group of 5 children with surgically and/or radiologically confirmed nonauditory CNS lesions, 10 children with surgically and/or radiologically confirmed intra-axial brainstem lesions, 4 children with surgically and/or radiologically confirmed temporal-lobe lesions, and 7 children with suspected central auditory processing disorders (identified by their school teachers as having abnormal auditory behavior). The results revealed that 6 of the 7 patients with suspected central auditory processing disorders had a PSI pattern similar to that obtained in the temporal-lobe group (i.e., the PSI–CCM scores were worse than the PSI–ICM scores). Since abnormal findings were obtained for the PSI–CCM but not the PSI–ICM, the investigators suggested that the central auditory processing disorders was auditory rather than linguistic in nature. The finding of an auditory-specific basis suggests that an auditory skills remediation program rather than a linguistic remediation program would be appropriate in children with central auditory processing disorders. Further research is needed to substantiate the Jerger *et al.* (1988) finding of an auditory-specific basis for central auditory processing disorders.

Other tests have also been employed to detect central auditory processing dysfunction in children. For example, Cherry (1980) developed a test of selective auditory attention abilities. Using the selective auditory attention test, normative data were obtained on 321 children between the ages of 4 and 8 years. The results indicated that children scoring below the 25th percentile are at risk for learning disabilities (Cherry, 1980). Cherry and Kruger (1983) found that 7-year-old learning-disabled children obtained lower mean scores than their 7-year-old normal counterparts on the test of selective auditory attention abilities. Similar findings were obtained for their 8-year-old learning-disabled and normal groups. Further research is necessary on this test to determine the clinical feasibility of this test as a screening tool for the detection of central auditory processing disorders in children. The test is commercially available from Auditec of St. Louis. Another promising test for the detection of central auditory processing disorders is the pediatric speech intelligibility (PSI) test developed by Jerger (1980) and Jerger, Jerger, and Abrams (1983) which was developed for use with children between 3 and 6 years of age. The PSI test is a modified version of the SSI test using picture stimuli representing words and actions within the vocabulary of children 3–6 years of age. Other tests for the detection of central auditory processing disorders have been developed but it is beyond the scope of this chapter to discuss these tests.

REFERENCES

Amerman, J. D., & Parnell, M. M. (1980). The staggered spondaic word test: A normative investigation of older adults. *Ear Hear., 1,* 42–45.

Antonelli, A. R., Bellotto, R., & Grandori, F. (1987) Audiologic diagnosis of central versus eighth nerve and cochlear auditory impairment. *Audiology, 26,* 209–226.

Arnst, D. J. (1982). Staggered spondaic word test performance in a group of older adults: A preliminary report. *Ear Hear., 3,* 118–123.

Arnst, D. J., & Doyle, P. C. (1983). Verification of the corrected staggered spondaic word (SSW) score in adults with cochlear hearing loss. *Ear. Hear., 4,* 243–246.

Baran, J. A., Musiek, F. E., & Reeves, A. G. (1986). Central auditory function following anterior sectioning of the corpus callosum. *Ear Hear.*, 7, 359–362.

Beasley, D. S., & Freeman, B. A. (1977). Time-altered speech as a measure of central auditory processing. In R. W. Keith (ed.), *Central auditory dysfunction*, pp. 129–176. New York: Grune & Stratton.

Beasley, D., Forman, B., & Rintelmann, W. (1972a). Perception of time-compressed CNC monosyllables by normal listeners. *J. Aud. Res.*, 12, 71–75.

Beasley, D. S., Schwimmer, S., & Rintelmann, W. F. (1972b). Intelligibility of time-compressed CNC monosyllables. *J. Speech Hear. Res.*, 15, 340–350.

Beattie, R. C. (1986). Normal intelligibility functions for Auditec CID W-22 test at 30% and 60% time compression. *Am. J. Otolaryngol.*, 7, 60–64.

Beck, W. G., & Mueller, H. G. (1983). Time-compressed speech recognition of a brain-injured population. Paper presented at the Annual Convention of the American Speech-Language-Hearing Association, Cincinnati, Ohio.

Berlin, C. I., Lowe-Bell, S. S., Cullen, J. K., Jr., Thompson, C. L., & Stafford, M. R. (1972a). Is speech special? Perhaps the temporal lobectomy patient can tell us. *J. Acoust. Soc. Am.*, 52, 702–705.

Berlin, C. I., Lowe-Bell, S. S., Jannetta, P. J., & Kline, D. G. (1972b). Central auditory deficits of temporal lobectomy. *Arch. Otolaryngol.*, 96, 4–10.

Berlin, C. I., Lowe-Bell, S. S., Cullen, J. K., Jr., Thompson, C. L., & Loovis, C. F. (1973). dichotic speech perception: An interpretation of right-ear advantage and temporal offset effects. *J. Acoust. Soc. Am.*, 53, 699–709.

Berlin, C. I., Cullen, J. K., Jr., Berlin, H., Tobey, E., & Mouney, D. (1975a). Dichotic listening in a patient with a presumed lesion in the region of the medial geniculate bodies. Paper presented at the 90th meeting of the Acoustical Society of America, San Francisco.

Berlin, C. I., Cullen, J. K., Jr., Hughes, L. F., Berlin, H. L., Lowe-Bell, S. S., & Thompson, C. L. (1975b). Acoustic variables in dichotic listening. In M. D. Sullivan (ed.), *Proceedings of a symposium on central auditory processing disorders*, pp. 36–46. Omaha: University of Nebraska Medical Center.

Bingea, R. L., & Raffin, M. J. M. (1986). Normal performance variability on a dichotic CV test across nine onset-time-asynchrony conditions. *Ear Hear.*, 7, 246–255.

Bocca, E., & Antonelli, A. (1976). Masking level difference: Another tool for the evaluation of peripheral and cortical defects. *Audiol.*, 15, 480–487.

Bocca, E., & Calearo, C. (1963). Central hearing processes. In J. Jerger (ed.), *Modern developments in audiology*, pp. 337–370. New York: Academic Press.

Bocca, E., Calearo, C., & Cassinari, V. (1954). A new method for testing hearing in temporal lobe tumors. *Acta Otolaryngol.*, 44, 219–221.

Bocca, E., Calearo, C., Cassinari, V., & Migliavacca, F. (1955). Testing "cortical" hearing in temporal lobe tumors. *Acta Otolaryngol.*, 42, 289–304.

Britt, R. H., & Rossi, G. T. (1980). Neural generators of brainstem auditory evoked responses. I. Lesion studies. *Neurosco. Abstr.*, 6, 594.

Broadbent, D. E. (1954). The role of auditory localization of attention and memory span. *J. Exp. Psychol.*, 47, 191–196.

Brunt, M. A. (1978). The staggered spondaic word test. In J. Katz (ed.), *Handbook of clinical audiology*, pp. 262–275. Second edition. Baltimore: Williams & Wilkins.

Cafarelli, D. L., Nodar, R. H., Collard, M., & Larkins, D. A. (1977). SSW test results by patients with Meniere's disease. Paper presented at the Annual Convention of the American Speech–Language–Hearing Association, Chicago, Illinois.

Calearo, C., & Antonelli, A. R. (1968). Audiometric findings in brainstem lesions. *Acta Otolaryngol.*, 66, 305–319.

Calearo, C., & Lazzaroni, A. (1957). Speech intelligibility in relation to the speed of the message. *Laryngoscope*, 67, 410–419.

Cherry, E. C., & Taylor, W. K. (1954). Some further experiments upon the recognition of speech, with one and with two ears. *J. Acoust. Soc. Am.*, 26, 554–559.

Cherry, R. S. (1980). *Selective auditory attention test (SAAT)* St. Louis: Auditec of St. Louis.

Cherry, R. S., & Kruger, B. (1983). Selective auditory attention abilities of learning disabled and normal achieving children. *J. Learn. Dis.*, 16, 202–205.

Collard, M. E., Lesser, R. P., Luders, H., Dinner, D. S., Morris, H. M., Hahn, J. F., & Rothner, A. D. (1986). *Ear Hear.*, 7, 363–369.

Cullen, J. K., & Thompson, C. L. (1974). Masking release for speech in subjects with temporal lobe resection. *Arch. Otolaryngol.*, 100, 113–116.

Cullen, J. K., Berlin, C. I., Hughes, L., Thompson, C. L., & Samson, D. (1975). Speech information flow: A model. In M. D. Sullivan (Ed.), *Central auditory processing disorders*, pp. 108–127. Omaha: University of Nebraska Medical Center.

Cullen, J. K., Jr., Thompson, C. L., Samson, D. S., & Hughes, L. R. (1973). The effects of monaural and binaural masking on a dichotic speech task. Paper presented at the Annual Convention of the American Speech and Hearing Association, Detroit, Michigan.

deChicchis, A., Orchik, D. S., & Tecca, J. (1981). The effect of word list and talker variation on word recognition scores using time-altered speech. *J. Speech Hear. Dis.*, 45, 213–216.

deQuiros, J. (1964). *Accelerated speech audiometry, An examination of test results*. Translated by J. Tonndorf. Chicago: Beltone Institute of Hearing Research.

Diercks, K. J., & Jeffress, L. A. (1962). Interaural phase and the absolute thresholds for tone. *J. Acoust. Soc. Am.*, 34, 981–984.

Doyle, P. C. (1981). Performance–intensity functions for a normal hearing population on the staggered spondaic word test. Paper presented at the 29th Annual Convention of the California Speech–Language–Hearing Association, San Francisco.

Durlach, N. I., & Colburn H. S. (1978). Binaural phenomena. In E. C. Carterette & M. F. Friedman (eds.), *Handbook of perception*, Vol. 4, pp. 365–366. Orlando, Florida: Academic Press.

Efron, R. (1985). The central auditory system and issues related to hemispheric specialization. In M. L. Pinheiro & F. E. Musiek (eds.), *Assessment of central auditory dysfunction: Foundations and clinical correlates*, pp. 143–154. Baltimore: Williams & Wilkins.

Fairbanks, G., Everitt, W. L, & Jaeger, R. P. (1954). Methods for time or frequency compression–expansion of speech. *Transact. I.R.E.-P.G.A.*, AU-2, 7–12.

Farrer, S., & Keith, R. (1981). Filtered word testing in the assessment of children's central auditory abilities. *Ear Hear.*, 2, 267–269.

Ferre, J. M., & Wilber, L. A. (1986). Normal and learning disabled children's central auditory processing skills: An experimental test battery. *Ear Hear.*, 7, 336–343.

Fifer, R. C., Jerger, J. F., Berlin, C. I., Tobey, E. A., & Campbell, J. C. (1983). Development of a dichotic sentence identification test for hearing-impaired adults. *Ear Hear.*, 4, 300–305.

Flynn, P. A., Danhauer, J. L., Gerber, S. E., Goller, M. C., & Arnst, D. J. (1984). SSW test performance-intensity functions for hearing-impaired adults. *Ear Hear.*, 5, 346–348.

Garvey, W. D. (1953a). The intelligibility of abbreviated speech patterns. *Q. J. Speech*, 39, 296–306.

Garvey, W. D. (1953b). The intelligibility of speeded speech. *J. Exp. Psychol.*, 45, 102–108.

Goldstein, R. (1961). Hearing and speech follow-up after left hemispherectomy. *J. Speech Hear. Dis.*, 26, 126–129.

Goldstein, R., Goodman, A. C., & King, R. B. (1956). Hearing and speech in infantile hemiplegia before and after left hemispherectomy. *Neurol.*, 6, 869–875.

Grimes, A. M., Mueller, H. G., & Williams, D. L. (1984). Clinical considerations in the use of time-compressed speech. *Ear Hear., 5*, 114–117.

Hannah, J. E. (1971). Phonetic and temporal titration of the dichotic right ear effect. Unpublished Ph. D. Thesis. New Orleans: Louisiana State University.

Hannley, M., Jerger, J. F., & Rivera, V. M. (1983). Relationships among auditory brain stem responses, masking level differences, and the acoustic reflex in multiple sclerosis. *Audiology, 22*, 20–33.

Harris, R. (1963). Central auditory functions in children. *Percept. Motor Skills, 16*, 207–214.

Hodgson, W. (1967). Audiological report of a patient with left hemispherectomy. *J. Speech Hear. Dis., 32*, 39–45.

Ivey, R. G. (1969). Tests of CNS function. Unpublished M. S. Thesis. Fort Collins: Colorado State University.

Jacobson, J. T., Deppe, U., & Murray, T. J. (1983). Dichotic paradigms in multiple sclerosis. *Ear Hear., 4*, 311–318.

Jerger, J. (1960a). Observations on auditory behavior in lesions of the central auditory pathways. *Arch. Otolaryngol, 71*, 797–806.

Jerger, J. (1960b). Audiological manifestations of lesions in the auditory nervous system. *Laryngoscope, 70*, 417–425.

Jerger, J. F. (1964). Auditory test for disorders of the central auditory mechanisms. In W. Fields & B. Alford (eds.), *Neurological aspects of auditory and vestibular disorders*, pp. 77–93. Springfield, Illinois: Charles C. Thomas.

Jerger, J. (1970). Diagnostic significance of SSI test procedures: Retrocochlear site. In C. Rojskjaer (ed.), *Speech audiometry*, pp. 163–175. Odense, Denmark: Second Danavox Symposium.

Jerger, J., & Hayes, D. (1977). Diagnostic speech audiometry. *Arch Otolaryngol., 103*, 216–222.

Jerger, J. F., & Jerger, S. W. (1974). Auditory findings in brainstem disorders. *Arch. Otolaryngol., 99*, 342–349.

Jerger, J., & Jerger, S. (1975). Clinical validity of central auditory tests. *Scand. Audiol., 4*, 147–163.

Jerger, J., Speaks, C., & Trammel, J. (1968). A new approach to speech audiometry. *J. Speech Hear. Dis., 33*, 318–328.

Jerger, J. F., Oliver, T. A., Chmiel, R. A., & Rivera, V. M. (1986). Patterns of auditory abnormality in multiple sclerosis. *Audiology, 25*, 193–209.

Jerger, S. W. (1980). Evaluation of central auditory function in Children. In R. W. Keith (ed.), *Central auditory and language disorders in children*, pp. 30–60. Houston: College-Hill Press.

Jerger, S. W., Jerger, J. R., & Abrams, S. (1983). Speech audiometry in young children. *Ear Hear., 4*, 56–66.

Jerger, S., Johnson, K., & Loiselle, L. (1988). Pediatric central auditory dysfunction: Comparison of children with confirmed lesions versus suspected processing disorders. *Am. J. Otol. Suppl., 9*, 63–71.

Johnson, D. W., & Sherman, R. E. (1980). The new SSW test (List EE) and the CES test. *Audiol. Hear. Ed., 6*, 5–8.

Katz, J. (1962). The use of staggered spondaic words for assessing the integrity of the central auditory system. *J. Aud. Res., 2*, 327–337.

Katz, J. (1968). The SSW test—An interim report. *J. Speech Hear. Dis., 33*, 132–146.

Katz, J. (1984). Staggered spondaic word test. In H. Kaplan, V. S. Gladstone, & J. Katz (eds.), *Site of lesion testing: Audiometric testing*, Vol. 2, pp. 253–325. Baltimore: University Park Press.

Keith, R. W. (1977). Synthetic sentence identification. In R. W. Keith (ed.), *Central auditory dysfunction*, pp. 73–102. New York: Grune & Stratton.

Kimura, D. (1961a). Cerebral dominance and the perception of verbal stimuli. *Can. J. Psychol., 15*, 166–171.

Kimura, D. (1961b). Some effects of temporal lobe damage on auditory perception. *Can. J. Psychol., 15*, 157–165.

Konkle, D., Beasley, D., & Bess, F. (1977). Intelligibility of time-altered speech in relation to chronological aging. *J. Speech Hear. Res., 20*, 108–115.

Korsan-Bengtsen, M. (1973). Distorted speech audiometry: A methodological and clinical study. *Acta Otolaryngol. Suppl., 310*, 7–75.

Kurdziel, S., Rintelmann, W. F., & Beasley, D. (1975). Performance of noise-induced hearing impaired listeners on time-compressed CNC monosyllables. *J. Am. Audiol. Soc., 1*, 54–60.

Kurdziel, S., Noffsinger, D., & Olsen, W. (1976). Performance by cortical lesion patients on 40 and 60% time-compressed materials. *J. Am. Audiol. Soc., 2*, 3–7.

Lee, F. F. (1972). Time compression and expansion of speech by the sampling method. *J. Audiol. Engineer. Soc., 20*, 738–742.

Linden, A. (1964). Distorted speech and binaural speech resynthesis test. *Acta Otolaryngol., 58*, 32–48.

Lowe, S. S. (1970). Perception of dichotic and monotic simultaneous and time-staggered syllables. Unpublished Ph. D. Thesis. New Orleans: Louisiana State University.

Lowe, S. S., Cullen, J. K., Jr., Berlin, C. I., Thompson, C. L., & Willett, M. E. (1970). Perception of simultaneous dichotic and monotic monosyllables. *J. Speech Hear. Res., 13*, 812–822.

Lukas, R. A., & Genchur-Lukas, J. (1985). Spondaic word tests. In J. Katz (ed.), *Handbook of clinical audiology*, 3d ed., pp. 383–403. Baltimore: Williams & Wilkins.

Luterman, D. M., Welsh, O. L., & Melrose, J. (1966). Responses of aged males to time-altered speech stimuli. *J. Speech Hear. Res., 9*, 226–230.

Lynn, G. W., & Gilroy, J. (1972). Neuro-audiological abnormalities in patients with temporal lobe tumors. *J. Neurol. Sci., 17*, 167–184.

Lynn, G. E., & Gilroy, J. (1975). Effects of brain lesions on the perception of monotic and dichotic speech stimuli. In M. Sullivan (ed.), *Central auditory processing disorders: Proceedings of a conference*, pp. 47–83. Omaha: University of Nebraska Medical Center.

Lynn, G. E., & Gilroy, J. (1976). Central aspects of audition. In J. L. Northern (ed.), *Hearing disorders*, pp. 102–116. Boston: Little, Brown.

Lynn, G. E., & Gilroy, J. (1977). Evaluation of central auditory dysfunction in patients with neurological disorders. In R. W. Keith (ed.), *Central auditory dysfunction*, pp. 177–222. New York: Grune & Stratton.

Lynn, G. E., Gilroy, J., Taylor, P. C., & Leiser, R. P. (1981). Binaural masking-level differences in neurological disorders. *Arch. Otolaryngol., 107*, 357–362.

Maki, J., Beasley, D., & Orchik, D. (1973). Children's perception of time-compressed speech using two measures of speech discrimination. Paper presented at the Annual Convention of the American Speech and Hearing Association.

Manning, W., Johnston, K., & Beasley, D. (1977). The performance of children with auditory perceptual disorders on a time-compressed speech discrimination measure. *J. Speech Hear. Dis., 42*, 77–84.

Martin, F. N., & Clark, J. G. (1977). Audiologic detection of auditory processing disorders in children. *J. Am. Aud. Soc., 3*, 140–146.

Matzker, J. (1959). Two methods for the assessment of central auditory functions in cases of brain disease. *Ann. Otol. Rhinol. Laryngol., 68*, 115–1197.

Miller, G. A., & Selfridge, J. A. (1950). Verbal context and recall of meaningful material. *Am. J. Psychol., 53*, 176–185.

Miltenberger, G. E., Dawson, G. J., & Raica, A. N. (1978). Central auditory testing with peripheral hearing loss. *Arch. Otolaryngol., 104*, 11–15.

Moller, A. R., Jannetta, P. J., & Moller, M. B. (1981). Neural generators of brainstem evoked potentials: Results from human intracranial recordings. *Ann. Otol. Rhinol. Laryngol., 90*, 591–596.

Musiek, F. E. (1983a). Assessment of central auditory dysfunction: The dichotic digit test revisited. *Ear. Hear., 4*, 79–83.

Musiek, F. E. (1983b). Results of three dichotic speech tests on subjects with intracranial lesions. *Ear. Hear., 4*, 318–323.

Musiek, F. E., & Baran, J. A. (1987). Central auditory assessment: Thirty years of challenge and change. *Ear Hear. Suppl., 8*, 228–358.

Musiek, F. E., & Gurkink, N. A. (1980). Auditory perceptual problems in children: Considerations for the otolaryngologist and audiologist. *Laryngoscope, 90,* 962–971.

Musiek, F. E., & Geurkink, N. A. (1982). Auditory brainstem response and central auditory test findings for patients with brainstem lesions: A preliminary report. *Laryngoscope, 92,* 891–900.

Musiek, F. E., Wilson, D. H., & Pinheiro, M. L. (1979). Audiological manifestations in split-brain patients. *J. Am. Audiol. Soc., 5,* 25–29.

Musiek, F. E., Kibbe, K., & Baran, J. A. (1984). Neuroaudiological results from split-brain patients. *Sem. Hear., 5,* 219–229.

Noffsinger, D. (1982). Clinical application of selected binaural effects. *Scand. Audiol. Suppl., 15,* 157–165.

Noffsinger, D., Martinez, C. D., & Schaefer, A. B. (1982). Auditory brainstem responses and masking level differences from persons with brainstem lesions. *Scand. Audiol. Suppl., 15,* 81–93.

Olsen, W. O. (1983). Dichotic test results for normal subjects and for temporal lobectomy patients. *Ear Hear., 4,* 324–330.

Olsen, W. O., & Noffsinger, D. (1976). Masking level differences for cochlear and brain stem lesions. *Ann. Otol. Rhinol. Laryngol., 85,* 820–825.

Olsen, W. O., Noffsinger, D., & Carhart, R. (1976). Masking level differences encountered in clinical populations. *Audiology, 15,* 287–301.

Orchik, D., & Burgess, J. (1977). Synthetic sentence identification as a function of the age of the listener. *J. Am. Audiol. Soc., 3,* 42–46.

Otto, W. C., & McCandless, G. A. (1982). Aging and auditory site of lesion. *Ear Hear., 3,* 110–117.

Palva, A., & Jokinen, K. (1975). The role of the binaural test in filtered speech audiometry. *Acta Otolaryngol., 79,* 310–314.

Pinheiro, M. L. (1978). Central auditory evaluation of adults and learning disabled children. Workshop presented at the Annual Convention of the New York State Speech–Language–Hearing Association, Kiamesha Lake, New York.

Porter, R. J., Jr. (1975). Effect of delayed channel on the perception of dichotically presented speech and nonspeech sound. *J. Acoust. Soc. Am., 58,* 884–892.

Riensche, L., Konkle, D., & Beasley, D. (1976). Discrimination of time-compressed CNC monosyllables by normal listeners. *J. Aud. Res., 16,* 98–101.

Rintelmann, W. F. (1985). Monaural speech tests in the detection of central auditory disorders. In M. L. Pinheiro & F. E. Musiek (eds.), *Assessment of central auditory dysfunction: Foundations and clinical correlates,* pp. 173–200. Baltimore: Williams & Wilkins.

Rintelmann, W. F., & Lynn, G. E. (1983). Speech stimuli for assessment of central auditory disorders. In D. F. Konkle & W. F. Rintelmann (eds.), *Principles of speech audiometry,* pp. 231–383. Baltimore: University Park Press.

Roeser, R. J., Johns, D. F., & Price, L. L. (1976). Dichotic listening in adults with sensorinerual hearing loss. *J. Am. Audiol. Soc., 2,* 19–25.

Rossi, G. T., & Britt, R. H. (1980). Neural generators of brainstem auditory evoked responses. II. Electrode recording studies. *Neurosci. Abstr., 6,* 595.

Russolo, M., & Poli, P. (1983). Lateralization, impedance, auditory brainstem response and synthetic sentence audiometry in brainstem disorders. *Audiology, 22,* 50–62.

Roush, J., & Tait, C. A. (1984). Binaural fusion, masking level differences, and auditory brain stem responses in children with language-learning disabilities. *Ear Hear., 5,* 37–41.

Shirinian, M. & Arnst, D. (1982). Patterns in the performance–intensity functions for phonetically balanced word lists and synthetic sentences in aged listeners. *Arch. Otolaryngol., 108,* 15–20.

Smith, B. B., & Resnick, D. M. (1972). An auditory test for assessing brainstem integrity: Preliminary report. *Laryngoscope, 82,* 414–424.

Sparks, R., & Geschwind, N. (1968). Dichotic listening in man after section of neocortical commissures. *Cortex, 4,* 3–16.

Sparks, R., Goodglass, H., & Nickel, B. (1970). Ipsilateral versus contralateral extinction in dichotic listening resulting from hemisphere lesions. *Cortex, 6,* 249–260.

Speaks, C. E. (1975). Dichotic listening: A clinical or research tool? In M. D. Sullivan (ed.), *Proceedings of a symposium on central auditory processing disorders,* pp. 1–25. Omaha: University of Nebraska Medical Center.

Speaks, C. (1980). Evaluation of disorders of the central auditory system. In M. M. Paparella & D. A. Shumrick (eds.), *Otolaryngology,* Vol. 2, 2d ed., pp. 1846–1860. Philadelphia: Saunders.

Speaks, C., & Jerger, J. (1965). Method for measurement of speech identification. *J. Speech Hear. Res., 8,* 185–194.

Speaks, C., Rubens, A. B., Podraza, B., & Kuhl, P. (1973). Dichotic listening and two variaties of conduction aphasia. Paper presented at the Meeting of the Academy of Aphasia, Albuquerque, New Mexico.

Stach, B. A., Jerger, J. F., & Fleming, K. A. (1985). Central presbycusis: A longitudinal case study. *Ear Hear., 6,* 304–306.

Sticht, T. G., & Gray, B. B. (1969). The intelligibility of time-compressed words as a function of age and hearing loss. *J. Speech Hear. Res., 12,* 443–448.

Studdert-Kennedy, M., Shankweiler, D., & Schulman, S. (1970). Opposed effects of a delayed channel on perception of dichotically and monotically presented CV syllables. *J. Acoust. Soc. Am., 48,* 599–602.

Thompson, C. L., Stafford, M., Cullen, J. K., Jr., Hughes, L., Lowe-Bell, S. S., & Berlin, C. I. (1972). Interaural intensity differences in dichotic speech perception. Paper presented at the Eighty-Third Meeting of the Acoustical Society of America, Buffalo, New York.

Thorndike, E. L., & Lorge, I. (1944). *The teacher's word book of 30,000 words.* New York: Teachers College, Columbia University.

Thornton, A. R., & Raffin, M. J. M. (1978). Speech discrimination scores modeled as a binomial variable. *J. Speech Hear. Res., 21,* 507–518.

Tobin, H. (1985). Binaural interaction tasks. In M. L. Pinheiro & F. E. Musiek (eds.), *Assessment of central auditory dysfunction: Foundations and clinical correlates,* pp. 155–172. Baltimore: Williams & Wilkins.

Willeford, J. (1968). Competing sentences for diagnostic purposes. Unpublished manuscript. Fort Collins: Colorado State University.

Willeford, J. A. (1977). Assessing central auditory behavior in children: A test battery approach. In R. W. Keith (ed.), *Central auditory dysfunction,* pp. 43–72. New York: Grune & Stratton.

Willeford, J. A. (1985). Assessment of central auditory disorders in children. In M. L. Pinheiro & F. E. Musiek (eds.), *Assessment of central auditory dysfunction: Foundations and clinical correlates,* pp. 239–256. Baltimore: Williams & Wilkins.

Willeford, J. A., & Billger, J. M. (1978). Auditory perception in children with learning disabilities. In J. Katz (ed.), *Handbook of clinical audiology,* 2d ed., pp. 410–425. Baltimore: Williams & Wilkins.

BRAINSTEM AUDITORY-
EVOKED POTENTIALS

The brainstem auditory-evoked potential (BAEP) or short-latency (early) potential represents a series of neuroelectric potentials recorded from electrodes placed on the scalp (far field) with response latencies within 10 ms. Research on the BAEPs has proliferated following the reports by Sohmer and Feinmesser (1967) who observed 4 peaks following auditory stimulation and by Jewett, Romano, and Williston (1970) and Jewett and Williston (1971) who described a series of 7 peaks following auditory stimulation that are now referred to as the "Jewett bumps." The BAEPs are characterized by small amplitudes, and are elicited by short rise-time and short duration signals with at least some energy spread away from the nominal frequency of the signal. The BAEPs are relatively unaffected by patient state of arousal or sedation.

Since Hecox and Galambos (1974) and Hecox (1975) reported on the effectiveness of the BAEPs in infants, the use of BAEP testing in this population has proliferated. BAEP assessment with clicks enables gross estimation of the magnitude of hearing impairment (although the portion of the frequency range responsible for the BAEP is difficult to establish).

BAEP assessment is useful for early detection of hearing impairment in high-risk infants and multiply or neuro-developmentally handicapped children so habilitation can be initiated by 6 months of age. In children less than 5 months of age and in older multiply or neurodevelop-mentally handicapped children, behavioral observation audiometry (BOA) is often unreliable or yields responses only at moderate to high intensities.

BAEPs have proven to represent a successful electrophy-siologic technique for the assessment of the integrity of the peripheral auditory system and the brainstem auditory pathway from the level of the auditory nerve to the lateral lemniscus in neonates, infants, and children as well as adults. The BAEP test, in comparison with other audiologic tests, has the highest hit rate with respect to auditory ner-vous system pathology to the level of the auditory brainstem (see Chapters 5 and 9). The BAEP hit rate is approximately 95% as opposed to approximately 85% for

the combined acoustic-reflex threshold and decay test; the false-positive rates for these two tests is essentially the same (see Chapter 9). The traditional behavioral site-of-lesion tests and the combined acoustic-reflex threshold and decay test are relatively insensitive to lesions rostral to the superior olivary complex. On the other hand, the BAEP test is able to identify pathologies directly and indirectly im-pinging on the auditory system to the level of the lateral lemniscus. The central auditory speech tests may identify some rostral lesions of the central auditory nervous system; nevertheless, central auditory speech tests cannot be em-ployed in infants or very young children. Furthermore, the sensitivity and specificity rates for the central auditory speech tests are substantially poorer than for the BAEP test (see Chapters 6 and 9).

I. OVERVIEW OF THE AUDITORY-EVOKED POTENTIALS

There are several classes of auditory-evoked potentials, that is, small changing voltages elicited using auditory stimuli. Table I shows the latency, amplitude, and origin of the various classes of auditory evoked potentials. Figure 1 shows a representative waveform for each of the classes of auditory-evoked potentials.

Within the cochlea, there are several types of electrical potentials elicited by auditory stimulation. If an electrode is placed on the round window of the cochlea, an alternating current (AC) potential with a waveform that mirrors that of the acoustic stimulus can be observed. This potential, known as the cochlear microphonic (CM), originates from the cochlea and is dependent on the integrity of the hair cells. The latency (time between stimulus onset and onset of the response) is close to 0 ms, reflecting only the stimulus travel time through the outer and middle ear. The CM is a sustained response since the entire duration of the stimulus contributes to the response. One limitation of the CM is that it is dominated by the haircells closest to the placement of the electrode. Another limitation is that, as the electrode

Table I Latencies, Amplitudes, Peak Components, and Origins of the Various Classes of Auditory-Evoked Potentials

Potential	Peak components	Origin	Latency (ms)	Amplitude (μV)
Very early				
Summating potential (SP)	DC wave	Cochlear haircells	~0.13	0.05–0.5
Cochlear Microphonic (CM)	Waveform mirrors stimulus waveform	Cochlear haircells	~0.13	0.4–350
Compound action potential (AP)	N_1 N_2	Auditory nerve	1.5–4.5	0.1–20
Early/Short				
Brainstem auditory evoked potentials (Jewett waves)	I, II, III, IV, V, VI, VII	Brainstem, auditory nerve	1.3–8.1	0.05–1.0
Frequency following response (FFR)	Waveform mirrors stimulus waveform	Brainstem, auditory nerve, cochlea	7.0–10	0.2–1.0
Slow negative 10 (SN10)	$V(P6)$–N_1	Brainstem	6.0–17	0.05–1.0
Middle				
Middle latency response (MLR)	P_o, N_a, P_a, N_b, P_b, N_c, P_c, N_d	Auditory cortex	8.0–80	0.5–3.0
40-Hz Event-related potential (ERP)	N^a, P_a, N_b, P_b, N_c, P_c, N_d	Classical auditory pathway, reticular formation	12–50	0.1–3.0
Late/Long				
Slow vertex response (SVR)	P_1, N_1, P_2, N_2	Primary and association areas of the cerebral cortex	50–250	3.0–15
Long (P300)	N_1, P_2, P_3	Subcortical brain structures e.g., hippocampal formation and amygdala	250–400	5.0–20
Contingent negative variation (CNV)	DC wave	Association area of the cerebral cortex	>300	10–30

placement becomes more lateral, the amplitude of the response decreases from millivolts to microvolts. To detect a CM having a microvolt amplitude, a relatively high intensity signal must be employed. The use of high-intensity low-frequency signals, however, creates disturbances along the entire basilar membrane so the frequency region responsible for the CM cannot be determined.

The summating potential (SP) is a direct current (DC) sustained potential which usually accompanies the CM. It is elicited with auditory stimulation and originates from the hair cells of the cochlea. The amplitude of the SP is even smaller than that of the CM, ranging from about 0.05 to 0.5 μV. It can be detected, for example, by reversing the stimulus polarity to eliminate the CM from the recording. The limitations associated with the SP are essentially the same as those for the CM.

The compound action potential (AP) can be recorded using an electrode placed near the cochlea. This compound or whole nerve AP represents the aggregate of the spikes from the individual nerve fibers. It is best elicited with stimuli which have a brief rise time, for example, clicks. These stimuli result in more synchronous spike discharge from the individual neurons leading to a larger compound AP. The compound AP is a transient response, that is, only the onset of the stimulus determines the response. Using

electrocochleography, the CM, AP, and SP can be obtained. The best recordings can be obtained with the transtympanic approach, in which a needle electrode is passed through the tympanic membrane using a local or general anesthetic. The major limitation of this approach is that it is invasive. If general anesthesia is employed, the procedure must be performed in the operating room or other facility with life-support equipment and an anesthesiologist, and hospital inpatient time may be necessary during recovery from the anesthesia. Recordings can also be made with an electrode placed in the external auditory meatus near the tympanic membrane or with surface electrodes clipped to the earlobe. Using the more distant (lateral) recording sites, however, the amplitude of the response is decreased.

The BAEP consisting of 5 to 7 peaks occurring within the first 10 ms of stimulus onset depending on intensity has been labeled a far-field recording, since surface electrodes are attached to the scalp distant from the generator source. The response is termed the BAEP to reflect the fact that various sites within the auditory brainstem pathway are generators of the BAEP waves. In fact, the generator of waves I and II is the auditory nerve (Moller, A., & Jannetta, 1982a; Moller, A., Jannetta, Bennett, & Moller, 1981a; Moller, A., Jannetta, & Moller, 1981b,1982; Moller, M., Moller, & Janetta, 1982). The BAEPs, which have been

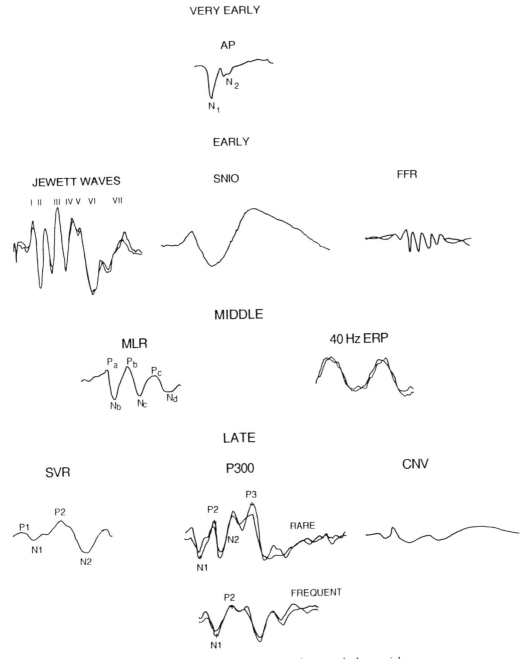

Figure 1 Waveforms of the various auditory-evoked potentials.

studied extensively, are obtained using a noninvasive technique, and are relatively unaffected by sedation, patient alertness, or sleep state. Thus, this chapter will focus on the clinical applicability of the BAEPs in site-of-lesion testing and the prediction of hearing loss.

Another potential generated in the auditory brainstem pathway is classified as the frequency following response (FFR) (Worden & Marsh, 1968). The FFR is a sustained potential which can be elicited using low-frequency tone-bursts or continuous tones. Its waveform mimics that of the

stimulus. The FFR usually cannot be observed using stimulus frequencies above 1500 Hz. One limitation of the FFR is that is usually appears only when the intensity level of the stimulus exceeds 30–40 dB SL. Moreover, both the basal and apical regions of the cochlea contribute to the response, so the FFR does not necessarily reflect low-frequency hearing sensitivity (Marsh, Smith, & Brown, 1976).

The slow negative ten (SN10) potential is a broad negative transient potential. It is a broad response from the peak to the trough of the wave. It has a latency of approximately

10 ms provided the low-frequency cutoff of the bandpass filter is lowered to approximately 30–50 Hz and the high-frequency cutoff is set to 1700–4000 Hz (Davis & Hirsh, 1976; Suzuki & Horiuchi, 1977; Suzuki, Hirai, & Horiuchi, 1977). The SN10 originates within the brainstem (Hashimoto, 1982). Consequently, it is resistant to the effects of sleep state, sedation, and anesthesia. According to several investigators, the tone-elicited SN10 can be used to obtain information concerning a patient's low-frequency as well as high-frequency hearing sensitivity (Davis & Hirsh, 1979; Davis, Hirsh, Turpin, & Peacock, 1985; Davis, Hirsh, Popelka, & Formby, 1984; Suzuki et al., 1977).

Geisler, Frishkopf, and Rosenblith (1958) identified a series of transient small waves with a latency of 12–50 ms which were originally labeled the early response and then relabeled the middle response after the discovery of the Jewett bumps. Bickford, Jacobson, and Cody (1964) and Mast (1965) originally concluded that the middle-latency response (MLR) had a myogenic origin. It is now believed that the MLR is neurogenic in origin, at least for low- to moderate-intensity stimuli (Harker, Hosick, Voots, & Mendel, 1977; Horwitz, Larson, & Sances, 1966; Ruhm, Walker, & Flanigin, 1967). The MLR has been defined and labeled differently by different investigators. Some have labeled the 4 positive peaks as P_0, P_a, P_b, and P_c and the three negative peaks as N_a, N_b, and N_c. Musiek and Geurkink (1981) suggest labeling only the positive waves (P_o–P_c) for convenience. Other investigators include the N_c or P_c waves as part of the late auditory-evoked potentials. The origin of at least some of the MLR waves appears to be the auditory cortex (Celesia, 1968; Graham, Greenwood, & Lecky, 1980; Kaga & Tanaka, 1980; Kraus, Ozdamar, Hier, & Stein, 1982; Ozdamar, Kraus, & Curry, 1982). Although the MLR appears not to be affected by light sleep or light sedation (Mendel, 1980; Mendel, Hosick, Windman, Davis, Hirsh, & Dinges, 1975), it is influenced by deep sedation or sleep (Davis, 1976a). Prosser and Arslan (1985) reported that the MLR was grossly affected by general anesthesia in normal-hearing children. At this time, the MLR has not been studied as extensively as the BAEPs, particularly in the hearing impaired, because of the previously held assumption that the MLR was myogenic in origin.

Galambos, Makeig, and Talmachoff (1981) described a brainstem potential that was labeled the 40-Hz event-related potential. This potential resembles a sine wave with a period of 25 ms and appears when click or tone burst stimuli are presented at a rate approximating 40 Hz. The 40-Hz potential represents the superimposition of the MLR and BAEP components. Galambos (1982) theorized that the origin of the 40-Hz response was the reticular formation in addition to the classical auditory pathway. Advantages of the 40-Hz potential over the MLR include the former's larger amplitude in adults and greater ease of detectability

because of its configuration. Galambos et al. (1981) demonstrated that the 40-Hz potential is abolished by surgical anesthesia. Davis, Hirsh, and Turpin (1983) and Davis et al. (1984) reported that the 40-Hz potential is greatly reduced in amplitude and detectability under sedation and sleep states. Kileny and Shea (1986) reported that the 40-Hz potential enabled accurate prediction of the hearing threshold at 500 Hz in normal-hearing adults. There is some research that indicates that the 40-Hz potential may predict the hearing sensitivity in the low frequencies as indicated by Lynn, Lesner, Sandridge, and Daddario (1984), who reported a confidence interval of −10 to +30 dB at 500 Hz. Nevertheless, further research on the 40-Hz potential using larger sample sizes in the hearing-impaired adult and pediatric populations is needed.

The late wave, also referred to as the slow vertex response (SVR), has a latency of 50–250 ms. It is a transient response, consisting of two positive waves (P_1 and P_2) and two negative waves (N_1 and N_2). The SVR is relatively large in amplitude (3–15 μV) and is best elicited with pure-tone stimuli. The SVR is seriously modified by state of subject awareness, attention, sleep, and sedation. The origins of this potential are thought to be the primary and association areas of the cerebral cortex (Goff, 1978; Goff, Allison, & Vaughan, 1978; Knight, Hillyard, Woods, & Neville, 1980; Vaughan & Ritter, 1970).

The P3 or P300 potential has been termed the long-latency wave or the late positive wave. It is observed under conditions in which the subject must process task-relevant information such as the "oddball" paradigm. In this paradigm, the subject counts the rare occurrences of a target tone embedded in a series of frequently occurring tones. It is believed that the P300 originates at subcortical brain structures such as the hippocampal formation and the amygdala (Halgren, Squires, Wilson, Rohrbaugh, Babb, & Crandall, 1980).

The contingent negative variation (CNV) potential, also termed the "very slow response," is a broad negative DC potential (Walter, 1964). The CNV is elicited by cognitive tasks in which a "conditional" stimulus is associated with another "imperative" stimulus requiring a mental decision or motoric action. It has a latency of more than 300 ms and an amplitude of approximately 20 μV. The origin of the CNV appears to be the association area of the cerebral cortex.

II. INSTRUMENTATION AND SIGNAL PROCESSING

The magnitude of the BAEP is very small, approximately 0.01–1 μV. This small potential is masked by the larger background activity generated by several sources such as the random, ongoing electrical activity (EEG) within the brain, muscular (myogenic) activities in the skull region, electrical radiation from electronic devices in the environment such as the 60-Hz hum, and other artifacts produced while generating the stimuli or recording the potentials. Therefore, in order to identify the BAEP, special equipment is required.

A typical BAEP device is shown in Figure 2. The system usually consists of three major components. The first component, labeled "1," is the signal generating component. This component generates the type of signal desired, for example, click, tone pip, or toneburst. The second components, labeled "2," is the amplifier and filter component. The physiological amplifier is designed to amplify the BAEP from the scalp so the BAEP can be processed easily by the signal averager and filter. The computer averager, labeled "3," is the third component of the BAEP instrument. Its function is to store electrical responses that are time-locked to the stimulus and to cancel out the ongoing EEG activity.

A. AMPLIFIER AND FILTER

The physiological amplifier must be able to eliminate the 60-Hz hum. This could be done using a differential physiological amplifier. The differential amplifier has two stages. The first stage, called the preamplifier stage, receives three inputs. The first input to the preamplifier is from the vertex of the scalp and called the noninverting, or positive, waveform. It is called the noninverted waveform because the signal polarity is unchanged when it reaches the preamplifier stage. (This input has also been referred to as the positive waveform since the first wave has a positive-going direction. It has also been called the active input.) The second input, from the reference site of the scalp to the preamplifier, is the inverted or negative waveform. It is called the inverted input because the signal polarity is reversed when it reaches the preamplifier stage. (This input

has also been referred to as the negative input since the first wave has a negative-going direction. This input has also been called the reference input). The third input to the preamplifier is called the common or neutral input. The inverted and noninverted inputs are compared or referenced against the common input. The common input is also referred to as the neutral or ground input.

The inverted input is then added to the noninverted input, each referenced to the common input. This resulting waveform, the output of the preamplifier stage, is the input to the second amplifier stage. This additive process is shown in Figure 3. If the noninverted and inverted inputs to the first stage of amplification are identical, they will cancel. Since the 60-Hz hum is equal in amplitude but opposite in polarity at the noninverting and inverting electrodes, the 60-Hz hum will be canceled out, so the input to the second stage of amplification will consist of only the resultant BAEP waveform (inverted waveform added to the noninverted waveform). Since the BAEP waveform at the noninverting electrode is larger than that at the inverting electrode, there is only partial cancellation of the BAEP waveform when the inverted and noninverted inputs are added.

The second stage of the amplifier amplifies the input approximately 100,000 times (10^5). The output of the second stage passes through the filter. This filter is designed to increase the signal-to-noise ratio prior to signal averaging. The bandpass of the filter is adjusted to reject background activity unrelated to the potential. For example, the BAEP device can be set to reject frequencies below 100 Hz and above 3000 Hz. Thus, only frequencies between 100 and 3000 Hz will be passed.

B. COMMON MODE REJECTION RATIO

The common mode rejection ratio (CMRR) is used to describe the extent to which the common inputs, such as the 60-Hz hum at the inverting and noninverting electrodes, are canceled out. A CMRR of 100 dB means that the common input is attenuated by a factor of 100,000 (every 20 dB is equivalent to a factor of 10) relative to the differential

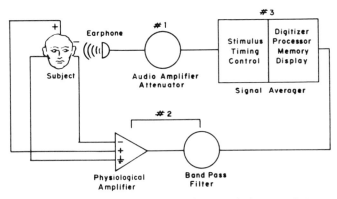

Figure 2 Schematic of a brainstem auditory-evoked potentials instrument. The part labeled "#1" is the signal generating component. The part labeled "#2" is the amplifier and filter components. The part labeled "#3" is the computer averager component. Adapted from Nicolet Instrument Corporation (1979).

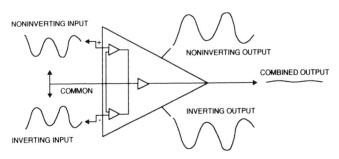

Figure 3 The noninverting and inverting inputs to the differential amplifier and the output of the differential amplifier.

input. A 60-Hz hum of 1.0 V would be amplified by a differential amplifier gain of 10^5 to a value of 100,000 V which is then reduced by a factor of 100,000 (CMRR of 100 dB) to 1.0 V. A differential input of 10 μV is amplified by a differential gain of 10^5 to a value of 1.0 V. Thus, the common input has to be as large as 1 V to have the same effect as a differential input as small as 10 μV. An electrode impedance imbalance will decrease the effect of the CMRR.

C. SIGNAL AVERAGER

The computer or signal averager's function is to store electrical responses that are time-locked to the stimulus and to cancel out the ongoing EEG activity. The principles of the computer averager are based on the concept that a response which is time-locked to the stimulus is consistent in polarity and that electrical activity of the background EEG is randomly changing in polarity. If acoustical stimulation is repeated over and over and a series of time-locked potentials are obtained, the addition of these time-locked potentials and ongoing random electrical activity results in the preservation of the time-locked responses (since they are similar in polarity) and elimination of the ongoing EEG activity (since the activity is random in polarity and addition of random activity leads to cancellation).

Figure 4 shows the major components of the signal averager. The first part of the averager is the analog-to-digital (A–D) converter which converts the responses (potentials) into numbers representing the amplitude of the response, which are then summed and placed in the digital memory of the data processor (computer). In order for the A–D con-

verter to accurately convert the continuous responses into discrete number equivalents and the number equivalents back into analog form (the continuous waveform), the A–D converter must have a sufficient intersample interval (the dwell time or horizontal resolution) and adequate vertical (amplitude) resolution. The continuous response is accurately represented as discrete numbers and vice versa if the intersampling interval is fast. Figure 5A is the initial analog (continuous waveform before it goes to the A–D converter) and Figures 5B and C are the final analogs (after the waveform was analyzed into digital and then back to analog by the A–D converter). In Figure 5B, the intersample interval is short (fast); in Figure 5C, the intersample interval is long. As you can see, a short intersample interval leads to better analog representation of the waveform. In order for the intersample interval to be considered sufficiently short, it must be much smaller than the duration of a wave within the waveform divided by the number of points needed to represent the wave. For example, if the duration of peak I is 1 ms and 100 points are required to faithfully represent this wave, then the required intersample interval should be less than or equal to 1/100 ms or 0.01 ms. Thus, the time between the points at which analysis occurs is 0.01 ms. The second requirement for an A–D converter is adequate vertical resolution (analysis of the waveform amplitude). The number of bits in the computer averager determines how accurately the amplitude of the waveform of interest can be measured and the smallest amplitude of the waveform

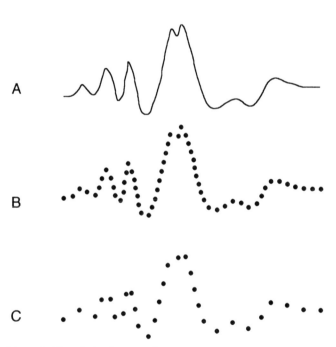

Figure 5 The relation between the analog and digital waveform. (A) The initial analog signal. (B) The digital waveform obtained with a short intersample interval. (C) The digital waveform obtained with a long interwave interval. Adapted from Nicolet Instrument Corporation (1979).

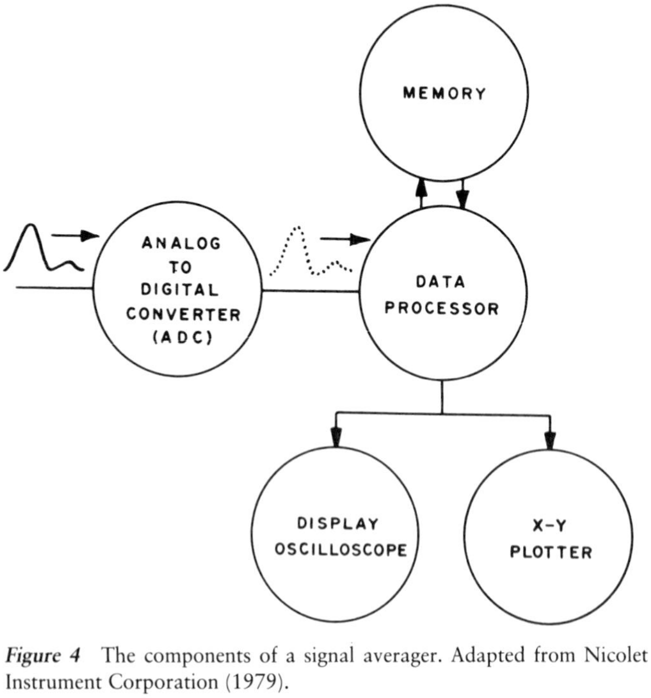

Figure 4 The components of a signal averager. Adapted from Nicolet Instrument Corporation (1979).

Table II The Relation between Analog-to-Digital Converter Vertical Resolution and Digitizer Size[a]

Digitizer resolution	Digitizer size (bits)
1 part in 2	1
1 part in 4	2
1 part in 16	4
1 part in 256	8
1 part in 1024	10
1 part in 4096	12

[a] Modified from Nicolet Instrument Corporation (1979) with permission.

which can be detected. Table II shows the relation between the number of computer bits and the vertical resolution. Let us assume that the A–D converter of a computer averager has 4 bits. This means that the voltage range of the waveform is divided into 16 parts. If the range of the electrode voltage is 1 μV, the smallest potential which can be detected by the computer averager if 1/16 or 0.06 μV. Thus, for a 4-bit computer averager, potentials with values less than 0.06 μV cannot be detected.

III. EFFECTS OF TECHNICAL AND SUBJECT PARAMETERS

A. TECHNICAL PARAMETERS

1. FILTER SETTING

The choice of filter setting is important. The purpose of the filter is to eliminate the contaminating effects of electromyographic noise and to reduce the amplitude of the ongoing electroencephalographic activity without significantly affecting the brainstem auditory-evoked potentials.

As the low-frequency cutoff of the bandpass filter is increased to 300 Hz, the latencies of all the waves decrease and the amplitude of wave V decreases relative to that of wave IV (Laukli & Mair, 1981; Stockard, Stockard, & Sharbrough, 1978b). The effect on the amplitude of wave V is most marked as the low-frequency cutoff is increased from 100 to 300 Hz. Thus, a low-frequency cutoff of 100–150 Hz is preferred (Stockard *et al.*, 1978).

As the high-frequency cutoff of the bandpass filter is increased from 300 to 3000 Hz, the latencies of all the waves decrease and there is improvement in the resolution of waves IV and V. As the high-frequency cutoff increases beyond 3000 Hz, the resolution of waves IV and V is not improved further and high-frequency noise is added to the waveform (Stockard *et al.*, 1978b). The effect of various filter settings on the BAEP waveform is shown in Figure 6.

Most clinicians and researchers use a bandpass filter of 100 to 3000 Hz or 150 to 3000 Hz. A wide bandpass filter is

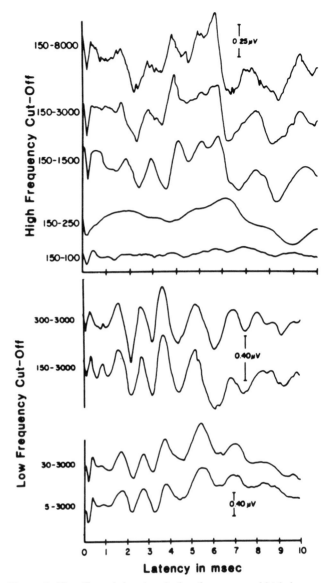

Figure 6 The effect of changing the low-frequency and high-frequency filter cutoff on the BAEP measurement parameters. From Schwartz & Berry (1985) with permission.

recommended to avoid distortion of the BAEP amplitudes and latencies (Laukli & Mair, 1981).

2. SAMPLE SIZE

The electrical activity recorded following auditory stimulation consists of both the time-locked response to the signal and the ongoing electroencephalographic activity (the "noise"). In the averaging process, auditory stimuli are repeatedly presented to an ear and the waveforms elicited by each stimulus are averaged. If one assumes the noise to be random and the time-locked stimulus to be constant, then the averaging process should reduce the noise amplitude and thereby improve the signal-to-noise ratio. The decrease in the noise amplitude related to the number of sweeps is given by the formula $1/(N^{1/2})$. Thus, as the number of sweeps increases from 1 to 2, the noise is reduced in amplitude by a factor of 0.707. As the number of sweeps increases from 2000 to 4000, the noise amplitude is reduced by a factor of 0.0066. The greatest enhancement in the signal-to-noise ratio occurs in the first 500–1000 samples. Stockard *et al.* (1978b) and others recommend the use of at least 2000 samples per average. Figure 7 shows the effect of sample size on the BAEP waveform.

3. Stimulus Rate

As the click rate (number of clicks per second, also referred to as the repetition rate, RR) increases, the absolute latencies of all the BAEP components and the interpeak latencies (IPLs) increase (Don, Allen, & Starr, 1977; Jewett & Williston, 1971; Stockard, Stockard, Westmoreland, & Corfits, 1979). Nevertheless, the absolute latency of wave V is not substantially prolonged until RRs exceeding 30 Hz are obtained.

At high RRs, waves IV and V often merge. Also, as the RR increases, the amplitude of the BAEP components decreases, particularly for the earlier components (Pratt & Sohmer, 1976). At high RRs, the IV–V:I amplitude ratio increases since the amplitude of wave I is more adversely affected than that of the IV–V complex by the rate increase.

The BAEP waveform may be unidentifiable at high RRs. Repetition rates below 33 Hz are recommended for routine clinical use, particularly for the identification of wave I in neurotologic diagnosis. To prevent the appearance of the 60-Hz hum in the BAEP waveform, the stimulus rate should not be a multiple or harmonic of 60 Hz. Thus, RRs of 11.4 or 33.1 are acceptable. RRs of 30 or 10 Hz are unacceptable.

When click rate is increased, the absolute latencies of waves I and V are increased. Wave V is prolonged to a greater extent than wave I so the I–V IPL increases. The increase in IPL with stimulus rate increases is smaller at moderate (50 dB SL) than at high (70 dB SL) intensities, since wave I is more affected than wave V by the rate increase at moderate than at higher intensities.

Chiappa, Gladstone, and Young (1979) reported that the frequency of recognizability of the earlier waves decreases at high RRs. The stimulus rate has little effect on the BAEP threshold. Figure 8 shows the effect of RR on the BAEP waveform.

4. Stimulus Polarity

Rarefaction (R), condensation (C), or alternating (A) polarity (phase) signals are employed in BAEP assessment. Rarefaction clicks tend to be associated with shorter absolute peak latencies than condensation (C) clicks presented at 70 dB SL (Stockard *et al.*, 1979). As shown in Table III, the difference between the peak latencies obtained with C and R clicks is greatest for wave I and smallest for wave V. In 61% of the 64 subjects investigated by Stockard *et al.* (1979), shorter latencies for wave I were obtained with R clicks than with C clicks; in 22%, there were no differences between the peak latencies for wave I with the C and R clicks; in 17%, shorter peak latencies for wave I were ob-

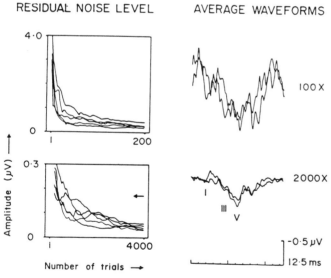

Figure 7 The process of averaging ABRs to 70 dB nHL clicks. Clicks were recorded using electrodes on the vertex and mastoid. Negativity at the vertex is represented by an upward deflection of the recording. *Left,* Graphs showing the decrease in the amplitude of the residual noise level [estimated using the (+) reference] as averaging proceeds over 200 trials (*upper graph*) or 4000 trials (*lower graph*). The results are shown for averaging the ABRs from five different subjects. *Right,* The replicate average responses obtained after 200 trials (100 for each tracing) and after 4000 trials (2000 for each tracing). From Picton *et al.* (1983) with permission.

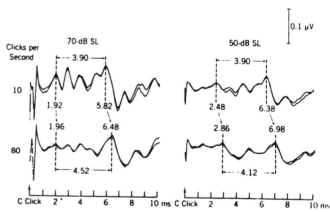

Figure 8 Effect of stimulus intensity on rate-related latency shift of wave I and resultant alteration of rate effect magnitude in I-V interpeak latency in a 25-year-old woman. *Left,* Shift is smaller at 70-dB sensation level (SL) as compared with 50-dB SL (*right*), which is in an intensity range where large jumps in latency occur in latency–intensity function. Stimulation was to right ear. Condensation (C) response shown for better definition of peak V. From Stockard *et al.* (1979) with permission.

Table III The Effect of Acoustic Phase on Peak and Interpeak Latencies of Brainstem Auditory-Evoked Potentials[a]

	I		II		III		IV		V		VI		Vn		I–III		I–V		III–V	
	C	R	C	R	C	R	C	R	C	R	C	R	C	R	C	R	C	R	C	R
Adults																				
Mean	1.69	1.62	2.78	2.80	3.77	3.75	4.92	4.89	5.64	5.62	7.26	7.14	6.35	6.26	2.08	2.13	3.95	4.02	1.92	1.94
SD	0.19	0.12	0.19	0.19	0.20	0.17	0.25	0.23	0.25	0.23	0.36	0.29	0.31	0.25	0.20	0.15	0.26	0.24	0.37	0.38
t	4.13		0.57		0.88		0.57		0.98		2.68		2.83		1.99		2.70		0.62	
df	46		27		46		24		37		30		30		41		35		35	
p	<.001		>.50		>.30		>.50		>.30		<.02		<.01		>.10		<.02		>.50	
Newborns																				
Mean	1.94	1.81	3.15	3.11	4.66	4.62	5.78	5.73	6.71	6.72	8.31	8.20	7.61	7.60	2.72	2.80	4.79	4.92	2.08	2.13
SD	0.25	0.22	0.40	0.28	0.25	0.29	0.41	0.35	0.27	0.32	0.33	0.43	0.34	0.39	0.17	0.21	0.30	0.26	0.24	0.23
t	4.01		0.49		1.11		0.86		0.55		2.40		0.45		2.80		3.46		1.39	
df	54		32		52		18		49		31		52		53		50		48	
p	<0.11		>.60		>.20		>.40		>.50		<.02		>.60		<.01		<.005		>.20	

[a] From Stockard *et al.* (1979) with permission.
[b] C is condensation phase and R is rarefaction phase.

tained with C clicks than with R clicks. Because of the shorter latencies obtained with the R clicks for wave I and the lesser effect of polarity on the peak latency of wave V, the interpeak latencies involving wave I are longer for R clicks than for C clicks.

Stockard *et al.* (1979) also reported that click phase is an important factor contributing to intrasubject variability in amplitude, morphology, and interpeak latencies of the BAEPs. They found that in 70% of their subjects, wave IV was more prominent than wave V with R clicks whereas wave V was more prominent than wave IV with C clicks presented at 70 dB SL. The wave V amplitude was increased with C clicks compared with R clicks presented at 70 dB SL in 80% of their subjects. Some investigators have reported increased amplitude and resolution of wave I with R clicks (Kevanishvili & Aponchenko, 1981; Ruth, Hildenbrand, & Cantrell, 1982). Many of the normal variant morphologic patterns based on the relative amplitudes of waves IV and V (Chiappa *et al.*, 1979) can be attributed to the differential effects of phase (Stockard *et al.*, 1979). At 50 dB SL, a moderate intensity level, waves I and III often appeared as broad and double peaked with R clicks. No morphologic differences with R as opposed to C clicks were apparent at 30 dB SL (Stockard *et. al.*, 1979).

The increase in interpeak latency with increases in stimulus rate is more pronounced for R than for C clicks (Stockard *et al.*, 1979). At high RRs, wave I peak latency remains essentially unchanged or decreased in latency with R clicks whereas it is increased with C clicks. Because of the differential effects of stimulus polarity at high RRs, the use of alternating polarity clicks may result in a spurious wave I, reflecting the summation of the prolonged wave I for C clicks and the early wave II response for R clicks (Stockard *et al.*, 1979). Some clinicians use alternating polarity clicks when the electrical artifact and the cochlear microphonic impinge on wave I; this effect is more apparent at high stimulus presentation levels. The use of separate recordings of both R and C clicks to facilitate resolution of the BAEP

components has been suggested (Stockard *et al.*, 1979).

According to Stockard *et al.* (1979), phase effects are enhanced in the hearing impaired.

Although Stockard *et al.* (1979) and others have observed polarity effects on the latencies and amplitudes of the BAEP components, other investigators (Rosenhamer, Lindstrom, & Lundborg, 1978; Terkildsen, Osterhammel, & Huis in't Veld, 1973) have failed to observe any polarity effects. Stockard *et al.* (1979) suggested that many of the previous studies on the effects of stimulus polarity were done using small sample sizes and that discrepancies may reflect differences in stimulus intensities and ages of the subjects. However, recently Gorga, Kaminski, and Beauchaine (1991) in a convincing article demonstrated that stimulus phase effect on wave V latency is frequency dependent. The effect was shown to be strongest at low frequency (250 Hz) stimulus and diminished as the frequency of the stimulus decreased (2000 Hz). This suggests that the effect of click polarity on ABR latency will depend on the configuration of the hearing. For a further discussion of stimulus polarity effects on the BAEPs, see Gorga and Thornton's (1989) excellent tutorial.

5. ANALYSIS TIME

The analysis time or sweep time is the number of milliseconds after the stimulus onset that the signal averager continues to sample the responses. In adults, the recommended analysis time is 10 ms. In neonates, because of the prolonged peak latencies compared with those of adults, the preferred analysis time is 14–15 ms. Some researchers suggest an analysis time of 20 ms in neonates.

6. ELECTRONIC FILTERING

Electronic filtering causes a shift in the peaks over time. The extent of the shift is related to the spectrum of the peaks and is not the same for all peaks (Doyle & Hyde, 1981a; Dawson & Doddington, 1973). Moreover, the peak spectrum has considerable intersubject variability.

The Bessel filter, an electronic filter with linear phase shift, and the digital filter have been developed to overcome the phase shift limitations of electronic filtering (Doyle & Hyde, 1981a,b; Moller, 1983; Moller, Moller, & Millner, 1981c). Digital filtering is more flexible and economic than the Bessel filter (Moller, M., & Moller, 1985).

7. ELECTRODE IMPEDANCE

Electrode impedance values should not exceed 5000 ohms in adults; below 3000 ohms is preferable. Differences between electrode impedances ideally should not exceed 1000 ohms. In infants, electrode impedance values may reach 10,000 to 15,000 ohms.

8. PLOTTING CONVENTION

When the positive input to the signal averager has a greater magnitude than the negative input, the deflection is directed upward on the oscilloscope. In BAEP assessment, the vertex and ipsilateral earlobe (or mastoid) are common recording sites for the noninverting and inverting electrodes, respectively; thus, if the vertex electrode lead is plugged into the "+" input and the earlobe lead is plugged into the "−" input, the potential which is positive at the vertex relative to the earlobe will be represented as an upward deflection on the oscilloscope; this situation is referred to as "vertex positive and up." If the vertex electrode is plugged into the negative input and the earlobe lead is plugged into the positive input, a potential which is positive at the vertex relative to the earlobe will be represented as a downward deflection; this situation is referred to as "vertex positive and down."

9. RECORDING MONTAGE

Various sites for placement of the noninverting, inverting, and common electrodes have been reported. Although electrode location can affect waveform morphology (Martin & Moore, 1977; Parker, 1981; Picton, Hillyard, Krausz, & Galambos, 1974; Streletz, Katz, Hohenberger & Cracco, 1977; van Olphen, Rodenburg, & Verwey, 1978), investigators disagree on the preferred electrode location.

The vertex site is commonly employed for the noninverting electrode. Several investigators have reported that movement away from the vertex by 6–10 cm in any direction has essentially no effect on the brainstem auditory-evoked potential (Martin & Moore, 1977; Parker, 1981; Terkildsen, Osterhammel, & Huis in't Veld, 1974; van Olphen et al., 1978). Some investigators have recommended the upper forehead site for the noninverting electrode since that site is free of hair and convenient for cleaning and electrode application (Beattie & Boyd, 1984; Coats, 1983; Rosenhamer, 1977; Suzuki, Hirai, & Horiuchi, 1981). The upper forehead site is also more comfortable than the vertex site since it does not cause the electrode to be compressed between the skull and earphones.

The inverting electrode is commonly placed on the mastoid or earlobe ipsilateral to the ear receiving the stimuli (Berlin & Dobie, 1979; Chiappa et al., 1979; Davis, 1976b; Rowe, 1981; Sohmer, 1983; Stockard, J. E., & Stockard, 1983), the ipsilateral neck (Berlin & Dobie, 1979; Davis, 1976b; Glasscock, Jackson, & Josey, 1981; Glattke, 1983; Terkildsen & Osterhammel, 1981; Terkildsen et al., 1974) and on the spinous process of the seventh cervical vertebra (Howe & Decker, 1980; Hughes, Fino, & Gagnon, 1981). According to Berlin and Dobie (1979), wave I is enhanced with the mastoid placement whereas wave V is enhanced with the neck placement. According to Stockard et al. (1978b), wave I is enhanced (i.e., the trough following the peak is increased) with placement on the medial surface of the earlobe compared with other periaural recording sites such as the mastoid. Hecox (1980) and Stockard, Stockard, & Coen (1983a) reported that, with a horizontal recording in which the noninverting electrode is placed on the contralateral mastoid or earlobe and the inverting electrode is placed on the ipsilateral mastoid or earlobe with the common electrode on the forehead, the amplitude of wave I is enhanced. On the other hand, Ruth et al. (1982) found that this montage did not enhance wave I. (The vertex-to-earlobe arrangement is referred to as the vertical montage.) Electrically linked electrodes on the lateral part of the neck rather than electrodes on the mastoid or earlobe were preferred by Terkildsen and Osterhammel (1981) as the inverting electrode site because earphones placed over the ears do not interfere with electrode placement when the electrodes are on the neck. Nevertheless, Glasscock et al. (1981) noted that the neck site was susceptible to neuromuscular potentials. Kevanishvili (1981) reported that when the inverting electrode was placed on the spinous process of the seventh cervical vertebra, larger responses resulted than when the inverting electrode was placed on the mastoid.

Typical electrode locations for the common electrode include the mastoid, earlobe, or neck on the side contralateral to the ear receiving the stimuli or on the forehead (Berlin & Dobie, 1979; Chiappa et al., 1979; Glasscock et al., 1981; Glattke, 1983; Hall, Morgan, Mackey-Hargadine, Aguilar, & Jahrsdoerfer, 1984; Rowe, 1981; Terkildsen & Osterhammel, 1981).

Beattie, Beguwala, Mills, & Boyd (1986) evaluated the effort of electrode placement on the amplitude and latencies of the brainstem auditory-evoked potentials when clicks of alternating polarity were presented at 70 dBnHL to young adults. Ten electrode combinations were evaluated. The noninverting electrode was placed on the vertex for half of the subjects and on the upper forehead for the other half of the subjects. The location for placement of the inverting electrode included the ipsilateral mastoid, the ipsilateral neck, or the seventh cervical vertebra. The various locations for the placement of the common electrode included the contralateral mastoid, the lower forehead, and the contralateral side of the neck. Beattie *et al.* reported that these electrode placements did not significantly affect the latencies of waves I, III, or V. Electrode placement did, however, affect the amplitudes of the brainstem auditory-evoked potentials. The vertex placement for the noninverting electrode resulted in larger amplitudes for wave V ($\overline{X} = 0.527$ μV) than the lower forehead placement ($\overline{X} = 0.385\ \mu V$). Also, for wave V, greater amplitudes were obtained with the following electrode placement locations: (a) inverting on the seventh cervical vertebra and common on the lower forehead ($\overline{X} = 0.525\ \mu V$); (b) inverting on the ipsilateral neck and the common on the lower forehead ($\overline{X} = 0.480\ \mu V$); and (c) inverting electrode on the ipsilateral neck and the common on the contralateral neck ($\overline{X} = 0.483\ \mu V$). Lower amplitudes for wave V were obtained under the following conditions: (a) inverting on the ipsilateral neck and common on the contralateral neck ($\overline{X} = 0.393\ \mu V$), and (b) inverting on the mastoid and common on the lower forehead ($\overline{X} = 0.401\ \mu V$). Electrode placement did not affect the amplitudes of waves I or III.

Since electrode placement did not affect the BAEP latencies for the 10 recording montages evaluated, Beattie *et al.* (1986) concluded that "electrical activity is distributed simultaneously through the head and neck region" (p. 67). In contradiction to Beattie *et al.* (1986), other investigators reported latency differences for various electrode placement sites (Barratt, 1980; Hughes *et al.*, 1981; Kevanishvili, 1980, 1981; Prasher, 1981; Prasher & Gibson, 1980). These studies which found latency effects used electrode placement sites different from those employed by Beattie *et al.* (1986).

Kavanagh and Clark (1989), who compared the mastoid to vertex with the mastoid to high forehead electrode array, obtained findings similar to those of Beattie *et al.* (1986) regarding the lack of latency differences between these arrays. Unlike Beattie *et al.* (1986), however, Kavanagh and Clark (1989) found no significant peak amplitude difference between the vertex and high forehead noninverting electrode sites. Kavanagh and Clark (1989) attributed the discrepancy between their amplitude results and those of Beattie *et al.* (1986) to the former's measurement of peak amplitude from the peak of the IV–V complex in contrast with the latter's measurements from wave V just before the rapid negative deflection.

Beattie *et al.* (1986) stated that the vertex (noninverting)–7th cervical vertebra (noninverting)–forehead (common) placement is preferred for maximizing the amplitude of wave V; since electrode leads do not have to be switched when switching test ears, this montage is employed for investigating binaural interaction; this placement is also preferred since only three electrodes are needed. Previous investigators have also reported increased amplitude for wave V with noncephalic inverting electrode placement

sites than with cephalic inverting electrode placement sites (Berlin & Dobie, 1979; Hall *et al.*, 1984; Kevanishvili, 1981; Streletz *et al.*, 1977). Some investigators have related the noncephalic advantage to the fact that the noncephalic site may be more electrically silent than the cephalic site for the inverting electrode leading to a larger difference between the noninverted waveform and the inverted waveform shifted by 180°. The wave V amplitude difference may be accounted for by the varying impedances of the neural, fluid, bone, fat, and skin tissues of the head and neck regions (Abraham & Ajmone-Marsan, 1958; Beattie *et al.*, 1986; Davis, 1976a,b; Gabor, 1979; Howe & Decker, 1980; Parker, 1981). Because electrode montage varies from clinic to clinic, each clinic must generate its own normative data for the selected electrode montage.

Figure 9 shows the International 10–20 system for electrode placement. Under this system, the vertex electrode site is labeled Cz, the forehead site is labeled Fz, the earlobe site is labeled A (A$_1$ for the left ear and A$_2$ for the right ear), and the mastoid site is labeled M.

10. TWO-CHANNEL RECORDINGS

Simultaneous ipsilateral and contralateral (two-channel) recordings using the vertex as the noninverting site, the ipsilateral and contralateral earlobes (or mastoids) as the inverting site, and the forehead as the common electrode site can facilitate identification of the peaks. With the contralateral recording, peaks I and III are reduced in amplitude (although I′, the negative trough following the positive peak of wave I, amplitude remains essentially the same), the II–III IPL is shortened, and the I–V IPL, the IV–V IPL, and wave V peak latency are increased with the contralateral compared with the ipsilateral recordings (Stockard, J. E., & Stockard, 1983). The increased IV–V IPL in the contralateral recording helps to resolve wave V in the ipsilateral

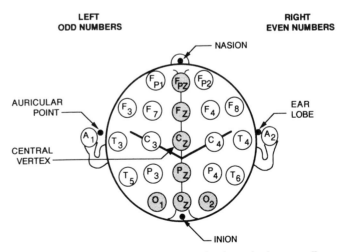

Figure 9 The international 10–20 system for electrode placement. From Nicolet Instrument Corporation (1985) with permission.

recording since waves IV and V may be difficult to identify in the ipsilateral recording derivation. The preservation of wave II with the reduction in the amplitude of waves I and III in the contralateral recording similarly assists in resolving peaks I, II, and III in the ipsilateral recording derivation. Figure 10 shows the ipsilateral and contralateral recording derivations obtained simultaneously.

11. Ipsilateral Masking

Burkard and Hecox (1983a) investigated the effect of ipsilateral broad-band noise (BBN) masking on the latency and amplitude of the click-evoked BAEP. They found that above approximately 10 dB EML effective masking or noise level required to perceptually mask a click of the same nominal intensity level in dBnHL, the ipsilateral noise resulted in increased wave V latencies for click intensities between 20 and 60 nHL (0 dB EML was equivalent to 26 dB SPL). The wave V amplitude decreased as a function of ipsilateral noise level above approximately 20 dB EML for click intensities between 20 and 60 dBnHL. As click RR was increased, the absolute ipsilateral noise-induced wave V latency shift decreased. Burkard and Hecox (1983a) concluded that these effects of ipsilateral noise had implications for BAEP assessment in nonsound attenuated test environments. That is, the wave V latency and amplitude are affected whenever BBN levels (ambient noise levels) measured under the earphones exceed approximately 10 dB EML (36 dB SPL) and 20 dB EML (46 dB SPL), respectively. Since the earphones provide approximately 30 dB attenuation of ambient noise, noise levels in the test suite would have to reach 66 and 76 dB SPL to affect the BAEP latencies and amplitudes, respectively. Another implication of their study concerns the effect of crossover of masking noise from the

nontest ear to the test ear. That is, when crossover yields approximately 40 dB SPL of BBN in the test ear, the amplitude and latency of wave V will be prolonged and so cause a higher false-positive rate to occur.

Burkard and Hecox (1983b) investigated the effects of ipsilateral BBN on the 1000- and 4000-Hz toneburst on the BAEPs. They found that as the ipsilateral noise level increased, the identifiability and response reliability of wave V decreased. Wave V latency was markedly prolonged for ipsilateral noise levels of 20 dB EML and 30 dB EML for the 1000- and 4000-Hz tonebursts, respectively. The amplitude of wave V decreased as a function of noise level above 20 dB EML for both toneburst stimuli. Burkard and Hecox (1983b) also reported that the noise-induced shifts in latency and amplitude were greater for the higher derived bands than for the lower derived bands when clicks were employed as stimuli (i.e., the derived band subtractive masking technique was employed to yield responses for the specific location of the cochlear partition–derived bands).

12. Contralateral Masking

Finitzo-Hieber, Hecox, and Cone (1979) recorded the BAEPs from two adults with unilateral profound hearing impairment. BAEPs were absent even when the hearing-impaired ear was stimulated up to 117 dBpeSPL. They concluded that contralateral masking was unnecessary in BAEP assessment.

Chiappa et al. (1979) obtained findings that contradicted those of Finitzo-Hieber et al. (1979). They recorded the BAEPs from a few patients with unilateral profound hearing impairment. The BAEPs were present when the poorer ear was stimulated but were abolished with BBN masking in the nontest ear at 60 dB SL (the reference level for the SL was unspecified). The contralateral masker did not affect the latencies or amplitudes of the BAEP components in normal listeners, although in several subjects the contralateral masking resulted in a change in waveform morphology. Therefore, they concluded that contralateral masking needed to be employed during BAEP assessment.

Humes and Ochs (1982) recorded the BAEPs for clicks using contralateral masking with BBN in four unilaterally deaf subjects. They reported that the BAEPs recorded from the deaf ear was abolished when sufficient masking was applied to the good ear. The interaural attenuation (IA) values (the difference between the behavioral thresholds for the two ears) ranged from 70–75 dB. They concluded that contralateral masking with BBN does not affect the latency or amplitude of the BAEP. High masking levels are unlikely to ever be employed clinically since—assuming an average IA of 70–75 dB, an average behavioral threshold for clicks of 42 dBpeSPL in normal listeners, and a maximum click intensity of 135 dBpeSPL—more than sufficient masking can be obtained with just 40 dB EML of BBN (one that could mask a 40 dB SL click in normal-hearing listeners.

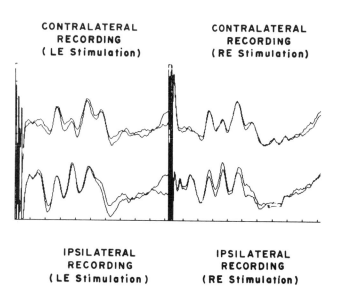

Figure 10 Two-channel, ipsilateral and contralateral recording for left-ear stimulation (left side) and right-ear stimulation (right side).

Moreover, 40 dB EML can never result in interference with the BAEP from the test ear. Humes and Ochs do not recommend assuming that the IA value for all clicks is 70–75 dB since the clicks vary in spectra and the spectra of the maskers differ from instrument to instrument. They attributed the difference in the latency, amplitude, and morphology between the BAEPs obtained at maximum click intensity from the poor ear and the BAEPs obtained from the good ear with click intensities at an SL equivalent to the maximum click intensity minus the IA to the frequency dependency of the IA,

> suggesting that the high-frequency energy of the click stimulus would be attenuated by a greater amount than the low-frequency energy. Thus, the crossed stimulus has much more of its energy in the low frequencies and may be expected to produced ABRs of differing latency, amplitude, and morphology. (p. 535)

If clicks are used as stimuli, broad-band noise can be used to mask the nontest ear. If frequency-specific stimuli are used, narrow-band noise can be used to mask the nontest ear provided the spectral envelope is wide enough to mask the sidebands of the frequency-specific stimuli (Gorga & Thornton, 1989).

Insert earphones, such as the Etymotic ER-3A, used with BAEP testing reduce the electrical stimulus artifact and eliminate the problems with collapsed canals. They are also more comfortable to wear than the supra-aural headphones. With insert earphones, however, the peak latencies are delayed by approximately 0.9–1.0 ms because of the tubing length. Van Campen, Sammeth, and Peek (1990) observed that insert earphones do not provide appreciably increased interaural attenuation for BAEP testing as they do for pure-tone behavioral assessment. Van Campen et al. (1990) hypothesized that the lack of increased interaural attenuation for insert earphones as compared with supra-aural earphones may be related to the dependency of the click-elicited BAEPs to the 2000–4000 Hz region of the cochlea. At this frequency region, insert earphones used for pure-tone behavioral assessment provide little additional interaural attenuation beyond that offered by supra-aural earphones.

13. INTENSITY REFERENCE

Three scales of measurement have been employed to describe the amplitude of the click or other short-duration stimulus: sound-pressure level (SPL) or peak-equivalent SPL (peSPL), sensation level (SL), or normal-hearing level (nHL). Many sound level meters cannot measure impulse sounds such as clicks since they do not have a peak hold capacity. Consequently, it is usually not possible to get true dB SPL measures. Therefore, the stimulus is displayed on an oscilloscope. A pure-tone signal is also fed to the oscilloscope and its amplitude (either peak or peak-to-peak) is adjusted until it matches that of the stimulus. Then a sound level meter is used to measure the SPL of the pure-tone signal that has an amplitude set to match that of the click or other short-duration stimulus. This SPL is therefore referred to as dBpeSPL (dB peak-equivalent SPL).

The dBnHL scale is similar to the dB HL reference intensity employed in conventional audiometry. That is, 0 dBnHL is equivalent to the average of the behavioral perceptual thresholds for the click or other short-duration stimulus in a group of young normal-hearing adults. Thus, 60 dBnHL is 60 dB above the average behavioral perceptual threshold for the BAEP stimulus. The dBnHL value must be determined in each clinic by measuring the behavioral perceptual thresholds for the BAEP stimulus in a group of 10–20 young normal-hearing adults. This value is approximately 35 dB SPL for clicks having a duration of 100 μsec.

With the dB SL scale, the stimulus intensity is referenced to the individual's behavioral perceptual threshold for the stimulus. Although sensation level equates stimulus intensity in persons with conductive hearing impairment, it does not do so in subjects with cochlear hearing impairment.

The dBpeSPL and dB SPL scales are absolute whereas the dB SL and dBnHL scales are relative.

14. BINAURAL STIMULATION

In binaural stimulation, clicks are presented simultaneously to both ears and the responses recorded monaurally. Binaural stimulation results in increased amplitudes of the later waves at all intensities. Since binaural stimulation increases the amplitude of wave V but not wave I, the IV–V:I amplitude ratio is increased with binaural as compared with monaural stimulation (Stockard et al., 1978b). The difference between the summed monaural responses from each ear (the predicted binaural waveform) and the binaural evoked responses should be obtained in order to observe the binaural interaction (Dobie & Berlin, 1979; van Olphen et al., 1978). If each ear and its neural connections functioned independently of the other ear and its neural connections, the summed monaural waveform would be equal to the waveform obtained by binaural stimulation. When the predicted binaural waveform is subtracted from the binaurally evoked waveform, the difference waveform is polyphasic, consisting of two positive peaks (P_1 and P_2), each followed by a negative peak (N_1 and N_2). This polyphasic waveform representing binaural interaction may reflect, in a complex way, neural activity underlying binaural processes such as localization and lateralization of binaural stimuli.

15. RECOMMENDED TECHNICAL PARAMETERS FOR BAEP TESTING

Based on the previous discussion, we recommend the following parameters for BAEP testing.

1. The bandpass filter should be 100–3000 Hz or 150–3000 Hz.
2. The sample size should be 2000 sweeps. When testing infants in the nursery and using low click presentation levels, the sample size may need to be increased to 4000 sweeps in order to compensate for the effect of low intensity and ambient noise on the BAEP.
3. The RR should be below 15 Hz for neurologic purposes (11.4 is commonly employed) in order to maximize the clarity of the waves, particularly wave I. For hearing-loss prediction, the RR can be as high as approximately 40 Hz since this rate is more time-saving and does not substantially affect wave V amplitude. To avoid the 60-Hz hum contamination of the BAEP, the RR should never be a multiple or harmonic of 60 Hz.
4. The rarefaction polarity is preferred for clicks since it is associated with shorter peak latencies and increased amplitude and resolution of wave I than condensation clicks. When normative and clinical data are obtained, the polarity should be kept constant. Clinicians should also obtain normative data for alternating polarity for clicks at high presentation levels (e.g., 90 and 100 dBnHL) so that AP clicks can be employed during clinical testing at high click presentation levels when a stimulus artifact is observed. For short-duration tonal stimuli, alternating polarity should be employed in order to reduce the effect of stimulus artifact.
5. The analysis time (time window) should be 10 ms in adults and 15–20 ms in neonates.
6. Electrode impedance values below 3000 ohms are preferred and should not exceed 5000 ohms in adults. In children, high electrode impedance values are common but should not exceed 15,000 ohms. In any case, differences between electrode impedances should not exceed 1000 ohms.
7. The plotting convention for BAEP testing should be vertex positive and up.
8. Based on Beattie et al.'s (1986) and Kavanagh and Clark's (1989) results, electrode montage does not have a significant effect on BAEP latencies. Therefore, for otoneurologic purposes and single-channel recordings, we recommend the upper forehead (noninverting)–medial earlobe (inverting)–lower forehead (common) electrode array. For the purpose of prediction of hearing impairment, the electrode montage which maximizes the amplitude of wave V should be employed. Based on Beattie et al.'s (1986) results, wave V amplitude is maximal with the vertex–7th cervical vertebra–lower forehead, vertex–ipsilateral neck–lower forehead, or the vertex–ipsilateral neck-contralateral neck electrode arrays.
9. Two-channel recordings (ipsilateral and contralateral) are preferred over one-channel recordings (whenever possible) to aid in the identification of the BAEP peaks.
10. Contralateral masking for BAEP testing should be employed using the initial masking formula for suprathreshold speech-recognition testing (see Chapter 5), conservatively estimating interaural attenuation for clicks to be 50 dB. (Each clinic should obtain its own norms for interaural attenuation of clicks but the 50 dB value can be used in the interim.)

B. SUBJECT PARAMETERS

1. GENDER

Stockard et al. (1979) reported that the interpeak latencies of male adults exceed those of female adults. This effect was attributed to differences in head/brainstem size, length of the external auditory meatus, and auditory nerve diameter. Jerger and Hall (1980) reported that the absolute peak latencies are shorter and the peak amplitudes are larger in females than in males. On average, the wave V peak latency is approximately 0.2 ms shorter and the wave V amplitude is approximately 25% larger in females than in males. Thus, separate norms should be generated for males and females. If gender is not taken into consideration, then the false-negative rate for females and the false-positive rate for males may be increased.

2. DRUGS

It has been reported that sedation does not affect the BAEPs. In fact, sedatives such as chloral hydrate, secobarbitol, and DPT (Demerol, Phenergan, and Thorazine) reduce the muscle artifact, thereby enhancing the BAEP waveform. Starr and Achor (1975) reported that the BAEPs are unaffected even in cases of drug-induced coma. Anticonvulsants such as Dilantin, administered at therapeutic levels, essentially have no effect on the BAEPs (Stockard, Rossiter, Jones, & Sharbrough, 1977a). Anesthetics such as halothane, ethrane, isoflurane, fentanyl, nitrous oxide, meperidine, thiopentene, and diazepam have little effect on the BAEPs (Duncan, Sanders, & McCullogh, 1979; Goff, Allison, Lyons, Fisher, & Conte, 1977; Manninen, Lam, & Nicholas, 1985; Samra, Lilly, Rush, & Kirsh, 1984; Stockard, Stockard, & Sharbrough, 1980). Since anesthesia has a minimal effect on BAEPs, intraoperative monitoring of BAEPs is being increasingly employed. It has also been reported that neuromuscular blocking agents such as pancuronium do not affect the BAEPs (Harker et al., 1977; Kileny, Dobson, & Gelfand, 1983).

Certain drugs do affect the BAEPs. Acute alcohol intoxication is associated with an increased I–V IPL (Chu, Squires, & Starr, 1978; Stockard, Rossiter, & Weiderholt, 1976). Lidocaine, a local anesthetic, has been found to affect the absolute and interpeak latencies and amplitudes of the BAEPs (Shea & Harrell, 1978). Similarly, phenytoin, an anticonvulsant, has been found to cause increased interpeak latencies (Green, Walcoff, & Lucke, 1982). Cholinergic drugs affect the peak amplitudes of the BAEPs (Bhargava, Salamy, & McKean, 1978). In conclusion, BAEP measurement is unaffected by most drugs including anesthetics. Thus, BAEPs can be accurately obtained in sedated children and adults. Acute alcohol intoxication should be ruled out before administering the BAEP test.

3. TEMPERATURE

Hypothermia is associated with increased interpeak latencies (Stockard, Sharbrough, & Tinker, 1978a). Lutschig, Pfenninger, Ludin, and Fassela (1983) suggested subtracting 0.15 msec from the obtained I–V IPL for every °C that the body temperature falls below 36°C. Decreased body temperatures are commonly observed during surgical procedures involving cardiopulmonary bypass or total circulatory arrest, and coma and drug intoxication cases. The BAEPs may be affected when increased body temperature is induced in patients suspected of having multiple sclerosis. Esophageal temperature measured at the level of the left atrium corresponds better with BAEP latency changes than rectal temperature. In summary, body temperature does not affect the BAEP unless it drops below 36°C. The effect of temperature needs to be considered only during special surgical procedures and coma and drug intoxication cases.

4. AGE

The effect of age on amplitude and latencies of the BAEPs is inconclusive. For example, Beagley and Sheldrake (1978) reported a slight, nonsignificant age effect on the peak latency of wave V. Similar findings were obtained by Otto and McCandless (1982), who reported the absence of a significant age effect on the BAEP latencies. Rosenhall, Bjorkman, Pedersen, and Kall (1985) observed the absence of an age effect on the BAEP interwave latencies.

Rowe (1978) reported that the peak latencies and the I–III interpeak latency increased with age as shown by their comparison of 25 young (17–33 years) and 25 older (51–74 years) adults. Thomsen, Terkildsen, and Osterhammel (1978) reported that the peak latency of wave V increases by approximately 0.1 ms per decade. Jerger and Hall (1980) examined the effect of age on the BAEP amplitudes and latencies in 98 normal-hearing adults and 221 sensorineural hearing-impaired adults ranging in age from 20 to 79 years. They reported that the peak latency of wave V increased by 0.20 ms, on average, over the age range from

25 to 55 years. The peak amplitude of wave V decreased, on average, by about 0.05 μV over the same age range. The age effect was present in both males and females. Maurizi, Altissimi, Ottaviani, Paludetti, and Bambini (1982) reported that the average peak latencies were increased by approximately 0.20 ms in their old subjects when compared with their young normal-hearing subjects. Similar age effects on the absolute and interwave BAEP latencies were also reported by other investigators (Allison, Hume, Wood, & Goff, 1984; Chu, 1985; Kelly-Ballweber & Dobie, 1984).

Rosenhamer, Lindstrom, and Lundborg (1980) reported that the gender effect present in young adults was absent in their older (50–65 years) adults. They also found that the peak latencies but not the interpeak latencies were increased in the older female adults compared with the younger female adults; no differences between the peak or interpeak latencies were found between the younger and older male adults. Jerger and Johnson (1988) found an interaction among age, gender, and high-frequency hearing sensitivity. In young adults, females had shorter absolute wave V latencies than males. As the hearing sensitivity at 4000 Hz increased, however, the absolute latency of wave V in females remained constant whereas it increased in males. Similar findings were obtained in the elderly. In contrast with the young adults, however, the gender effect, although present, was reduced in the normal-hearing older adults.

Since some of the studies reported a slight age effect (on the order of 0.2 ms) the age effect must be considered when collecting normative data. As shown by Jerger and Hall (1980) and Maurizi et al. (1982), the age effect becomes apparent after age 50. Therefore, separate norms should be obtained for subjects under 50 years of age and subjects over 50 years of age.

5. SIZE OF NORMATIVE DATA BASE

Most clinical laboratories have based their normative data base on a small sample size of 10–30 subjects. Chiappa (1983) suggested a sample size of 35 whereas Stockard et al. (1978b) recommended an N of 100 to ensure a normal distribution. Sklare (1987) proposed that the standard error of mean be utilized to determine the sample size for a normative data base. He suggested that the N should be sufficiently large to yield a standard error of mean less than the resolution used for measuring BAEPs in the time domain. When latency measurements are determined using cursors on an oscilloscope, the resolution is equal to the sampling interval (dwell time) of the computer averager or the time elapsing between adjacent data samples (points). The standard error of mean of the normative data base should be less than the dwell time. Therefore, as the data base grows, the standard error of mean should be calculated until the N has been reached that yields a standard error of mean (for all BAEP absolute and interpeak latencies evaluated) that is smaller than the time elapsing between adjacent data points.

IV. NORMATIVE DATA

A. BAEP COMPONENTS

Hecox and Galambos (1974) reported that wave V is the most stable of the BAEP components. Starr and Achor (1975) obtained similar findings and found that the IV–V complex was present even at intensity levels as low as 5 dB SL in normal-hearing subjects. Stockard *et al.* (1978b) observed that a bifid wave III and a wave VI with a sharp downward slope are common normal variant morphologic patterns.

Chiappa *et al.* (1979) evaluated the BAEPs in 50 normal adults. They identified 6 morphologic patterns (Types A through F) in which the shape of waves III and the IV–V complex varied. Figure 11 shows these 6 morphologic patterns. Pattern A was characterized by a single peak for the IV–V complex. Pattern B was characterized by separate peaks for waves IV and V with the wave IV peak lower than the wave V peak. Pattern C was similar to pattern B except

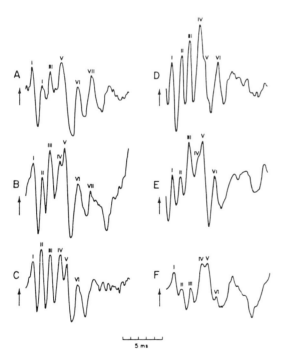

Figure 11 Different wave IV–V complex configurations at ten clicks per second. Each trace is the sum of 2048 to 4096 responses from a single ear of the subject recorded in separate trials of the 1024 clicks each. Separate trials also showed the wave IV–V complex shape shown here. Vertex positivity produces upward deflection. From Chiappa *et al.* (1979) with permission.

that the wave IV peak is higher than the wave V peak. In pattern D, the peaks for IV and V are superimposed, with wave V appearing as a bump on the downward slope following wave IV. In pattern E, the peaks of waves IV and V are also superimposed except that wave IV appears as a bump on the upward slope preceding the peak of wave V. In pattern F, the peaks for waves IV and V are superimposed with bumps of equal heights. The most frequently occurring patterns were B and C (occurring 38 and 33% of the time, respectively) with patterns D and F occurring least frequently (1 and 4% of the time, respectively). Subjects did not always have the same pattern in both ears—only 42% had the same pattern, bilaterally. A bidfid wave III occurred in 5.8% of the subjects and the first peak or the midpoint of the two peaks corresponded to the mean peak latency for wave III seen in other subjects. Chiappa *et al.* (1979) were unable to posit a hypothesis to account for the various common normal variant morphologic patterns. On the other hand, Stockard *et al.* (1979) recorded the BAEPs in 64 normal-hearing adults using rarefaction clicks presented at 70 dB SL. They found that the morphology was dependent upon the click phase. That is, wave IV was more prominent than wave V in 70% of the BAEPs to rarefaction clicks. Stockard *et al.* (1979) contended that Chiappa *et al.* (1979) failed to control for phase of stimulation, which affects the morphologic patterns. According to Stockard *et al.* (1979), the E pattern reported by Chiappa *et al.* (1979) can be obtained with condensation clicks and the D pattern can be obtained with rarefaction clicks.

Hecox and Moushegian (1981) observed that waves IV and V are fused at high intensities with ipsilateral recordings and that wave III has an amplitude exceeding that of wave V at intensities above 70 dBnHL. They also observed that wave I is often notched or bidfid, reflecting the N_1 and N_2 from the eighth-nerve action potential; N_1 is more apparent at intensities above 60 dBnHL whereas N_2 is more apparent at intensities below 60 dBnHL. This factor must be considered when determining the peak latency of wave I.

B. INTENSITY

Chiappa *et al.* (1979) reported that waves I, II, III, and V can be detected more than 90% of the time at 60 dB SL for clicks presented at a repetition rate of 10/s or 30/s. Also, at that sensation level, waves IV and VI can be detected 88 and 84% of the time, respectively, when clicks are presented at a repetition rate of 10/s, but can be detected only 67% of the time when clicks are presented at a repetition rate of 30/s. At the repetition rate of 70/s, only wave V continues to be highly recognizable (99% recognizability). At the repetition rate of 70/s wave III is the next most recognizable of the BAEP components, having an 85% frequency of detectability. The frequency of recognizability of the other waves was below 80%, approaching 34% for wave IV.

Kavanagh and Beardsley (1979) reported that, in their group of 15 normal-hearing subjects, wave V was present at intensity levels as low as 10 dB HL. Other waves could not be elicited at low intensity levels. The presence of other waves was always accompanied by the presence of wave V. Wave II was observed only at high intensity levels. Worthington and Peters (1980a) reported that wave III was present at intensity levels as low as 30 dB SL in approximately 50% of their subjects. Wave I was present at intensity levels as low as 50 dB SL in 75% of their subjects. Therefore, in order to elicit a waveform which contains wave I as well as the other waves, intensity levels of at least 70 dBnHL and low repetition rates should be employed.

C. LATENCY–INTENSITY FUNCTION

Starr and Achor (1975) reported that the mean latency of wave V increases from 5.4 ms at 75 dB SL to 8.1 ms at 5 dB SL. The peak latency of wave III increases from 3.7 ms at 75 dB SL to 5.6 ms at 5 dB SL. From 75 to 25 dB SL, the peak latency for wave I increases from 1.4 to 2.9 ms. Figure 12 shows the change in peak latencies as a function of intensity changes. Changes in intensity have a greater effect on wave I than on the later components. Stockard *et al.* (1979) reported that the peak latency of wave I is most affected by phase and the peak latency of wave V is least affected by phase.

The I–V IPL is also called the brainstem conduction time or the central transmission time. Stockard *et al.* (1979)

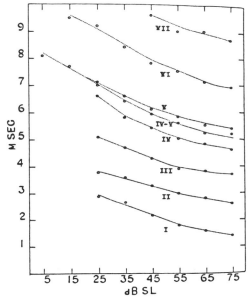

Figure 12 Latency measures of seven components (I to VII) and IV–V complex of auditory brainstem response as a function of signal intensity. Data are means of measures from six subjects with normal hearing in response to monaural click signals. From Starr & Achor (1975) with permission.

reported that the I–III and the I–V IPL decrease with intensity decrease from 70 to 30 dB SL, with latency shifts as large as 0.73 ms occurring for the I–V IPL. The III–V IPL shows a much smaller decrease with intensity. The decrease in the I–III and I–V IPLs with intensity decreases reflects the change in peak latency of wave I. Wave I is particularly affected by intensity because it becomes bifid at higher intensities and because of the large transition between 40 and 60 dB SL. Stockard *et al.* (1979) concluded that the change in IPLs with intensity reflects the behavior of wave I, which is the surface reflection of the eighth-nerve action potential (AP). The two peaks of the action potential represent activity from neurons with high and low thresholds. At 40–60 dB SL (the transition zone), the thresholds for both neuron groups are activated and the AP amplitude dominance shifts from one peak to the other. This shift occurs to a lesser degree for wave III and hardly at all for the peak latency of wave V. Hence, the IPLs, particularly the I–III and the I–IV, increase with intensity.

Stockard *et al.* (1979) also showed that the inversion of phase from rarefaction to condensation clicks results in shifts in the I–III IPL by more than one standard deviation of the mean in the direction of smaller IPLs for the condensation clicks. This trend was reflected to a lesser extent in the I–V IPL and to a still lesser extent in the III–V IPL.

Stockard *et al.* (1979) also reported that the intersubject variability in the IPLs is large, ranging from 0.15 to 0.38 msec for one standard deviation. Eggermont, Don, and Brackmann (1980) reported that the distribution for the I–III and I–V IPLs was Gaussian, with a mean and standard deviation of 2.07 ms and 0.13 ms, respectively, for the former and 4.01 ms and 0.16 ms, respectively, for the latter IPL. Because of the larger intersubject variability and the effects from variation in the technical parameters, clinicians should develop their own IPL norms and not depend on published IPL norms.

The slope of the latency–intensity function is a measure of the steepness of the function. It is calculated by subtracting the latency at the higher intensity from that at the lower intensity and then dividing that remainder by the dB difference in the intensity levels. Slopes of less than or equal to 60 μs/dB are considered to be normal. Values of less than 30 μs/dB, seen in persons with high-frequency hearing loss, are also seen in normal-hearing persons when the slope calculation is made over the shallow portion of the latency–intensity function, that is at high intensities. Since the latency–intensity function is nonlinear, even in normal-hearing subjects, it is an unreliable measure for differential diagnosis.

D. AMPLITUDE

The amplitudes of the brainstem auditory-evoked potentials decrease as signal intensity decreases. There is considerable intersubject variability in amplitude. The amplitude of wave I increases gradually up to 55 dB SL and then increases rapidly at higher intensities. On the other hand, the amplitude of the IV–V complex increases linearly with intensity (Starr and Achor, 1975). In general, the amplitude of the IV–V complex is greater than that of wave I. For example, Chiappa *et al.* (1979) reported that, when clicks were presented at a repetition rate of 10/s at 60 dB SL, the mean amplitude of the IV–V complex was 0.47 μV, the mean amplitude of wave I was 0.28 μV, and the mean amplitude of wave III was 0.23 μV. Chiappa *et al.* (1979) reported, however, that the amplitude of wave I exceeded that of the IV–V complex in approximately 10% of his subjects. As the repetition rate increases, the amplitude of all the waves decreases.

Several researchers (Chiappa *et al.*, 1979; Rowe, 1978; Starr & Achor, 1975) have reported that the absolute amplitude of wave V is too unreliable for assessing the normalcy of wave V. Starr and Achor (1975) suggested using the IV–V:I amplitude ratio (amplitude of the IV–V complex divided by the amplitude of wave I). The IV–V:I amplitude ratio should be measured at moderate intensity levels, not exceeding 70 dBnHL. Starr and Achor (1975) reported that at intensities less than or equal to 65 dB SL, a IV–V:I amplitude ratio less than 0.5 was abnormal.

E. REPLICABILITY

Hecox and Galambos (1974) evaluated the peak latency of wave V in 3 young normal adults over an 8 month period. The combined intrasession, intersession, and intersubject variability ranged from 0.09 to 0.31 ms; the larger end of the range of variability occurred near threshold. Hecox and Moushegian (1981) contend that peak latencies should be replicable within 0.2 ms for clicks presented at low to moderate intensity levels at click rates between 30 and 90 per second. Better replicability can be obtained at lower repetition rates and higher intensity levels. Chiappa *et al.* (1979) reported that, when 8 subjects were retested between 2 and 9 months later, no statistical differences in peak latencies or amplitudes resulted. Thus, the BAEPs are stable over time.

V. GENERATOR SITES

Several investigators have stated that each wave of the BAEP waveform is generated by specific nuclei along the auditory pathway (Lev & Sohmer, 1972; Stockard *et al.*, 1977a). These investigators indicated that wave I is generated from the auditory nerve, wave II is generated by the cochlear nuclei, wave III is generated from the superior olivary complex, and waves IV and V are generated from the lateral lemniscus and the inferior colliculus, respectively.

Moller and Jannetta (1985) contended that hypotheses or theories regarding the origin of the BAEP components in humans based on experiments in animals such as cats, rats, and guinea pigs should be seriously questioned. That is, the BAEP components (except peak I) in animals are generated from sites different from those in humans and the auditory nerve in humans is much longer (2.5 cm long in humans) than in cats, rats, and guinea pigs (0.3 to 0.5 cm long). Since the conduction velocity of the nerve fiber is slow in both humans and animals, the conduction time is much longer in humans than in animals (1 ms as opposed to 0.1–0.3 ms). Bearing this in mind, several investigators (Moller & Jannetta, 1981, 1982a,b, 1983a,b,c; Moller *et al.*, 1981a,b) conducted studies using microelectrodes comparing the BAEPs recorded at far field (vertex and earlobe) and the BAEPs recorded directly along the auditory pathway. From these studies, the following conclusions were drawn.

1. Peaks I and II are generated by the auditory nerve. Peak I is generated at the distal part of the auditory nerve and peak II is generated primarily from the proximal part of the auditory nerve. Recent studies (Wada & Starr, 1983) supported the findings of Moller and his colleagues regarding the generation of waves I and II.
2. Peak III is generated mainly by the ipsilateral cochlear nuclei and may receive a small contribution from the eighth-nerve fibers entering the cochlear nuclei.
3. Peak IV is generated by the third-order neurons, that is, the superior olivary complex. Also contributing to wave IV are the cochlear nuclei and probably the lateral lemniscus nuclei.
4. The origin of the positive component of wave V is the lateral lemniscus. Other nuclei in the vicinity have a minor contribution to the positive component of wave V. The origin of the negative component of wave V is the inferior colliculus.

In terms of clinical applications, since waves III, IV, and V have major and minor generators, if the latency and amplitude of these waves are substantially affected, one can assume that the major generators are impaired. When the latency and amplitude of waves III–V are only slightly affected, a conclusion cannot be drawn regarding the generator site damaged since either the major or minor generator may be responsible for the latency and amplitude effects.

VI. PREDICTION OF HEARING THRESHOLD LEVEL FROM THE BAEP THRESHOLD

Several investigators (Coats & Martin, 1977; Moller, K., & Blegvad, 1976; Stapells, 1989) reported that the BAEP threshold in sensorineural hearing-impaired subjects is correlated with the behavioral hearing threshold levels at frequencies between 2000 and 4000 Hz if the hearing sensitivity is best in that region. Thus, if there are normal-hearing thresholds between 2000 and 4000 Hz with hearing impairment above or below this frequency range, the BAEP threshold will generally reflect the normal-hearing region and hearing impairment will be missed at the other frequencies (Stapells, 1989).

The correlation between the click-elicited BAEP threshold and the hearing thresholds between 2000 and 4000 Hz is low, approximately 0.49 Hz (Jerger & Mauldin, 1978), because the 2000–4000 Hz region may not be the frequency region with the lowest hearing-threshold levels. When the 2000–4000 Hz frequency region is not the region of best hearing sensitivity, the BAEP threshold may be consistent with hearing thresholds in the frequency region of best hearing sensitivity, that is, frequencies not between 2000 and 4000 Hz (Stapells, 1989). For example, Glattke (1983) reported that the BAEP threshold in a patient with a rising configuration that was profound at the low frequencies and became normal-hearing at 8000 Hz was present at 25 dBnHL, reflecting the normal hearing threshold at 8000 Hz. Thus, the BAEP threshold often misses or underestimates hearing sensitivity in the low, mid, or high frequencies. If the BAEP threshold for the click is elevated, it can be concluded that there is hearing impairment at least of the degree indicated by the BAEP threshold in the frequency region with the best hearing sensitivity. Despite the limitations of the click-elicited BAEP threshold, it is a valuable tool for gross prediction of hearing impairment in the difficult-to-test. According to Stapells (1989), the click-elicited BAEP threshold is approximately consistent with the puretone average within one category of normal, mild, moderate, severe, or profound hearing impairment in 90–95% of the cases. Stapells (1989) maintained that most of the time, the BAEP threshold for the click corresponds to the average of the hearing thresholds between 1000 and 4000 Hz or to the best hearing threshold in that range.

VII. ABSENT BAEPS

Schulman-Galambos and Galambos (1979) found that, in one case, no BAEPs could be elicited despite the presence of normal-hearing sensitivity. They attributed their finding to undetected technical error. Worthington and Peters (1980b), however, presented four cases with no neurological evidence of brainstem dysfunction in which hearing-threshold levels were normal or no-worse-than-severe and BAEPs were absent even at maximum intensity levels on two separate occasions in two of the four cases. They suggested that an absent BAEP might indicate that "the ABR is generated only by a portion of the auditory system which is not essential for hearing, i.e., it is an epiphenomena [sic]"

(p. 284). Because absent BAEPs can result despite normal-hearing sensitivity, they advise against employing BAEPs as the sole measure of hearing sensitivity. Davis and Hirsh (1979) reported that BAEPs could not be elicited in some children who responded to sounds at low or moderate intensities.

Davis and Hirsh (1979) proposed that cochlear impairment could result in desynchronization and consequently absent BAEPs. Some other proposed causes for absent BAEPs in cases with normal or near-normal hearing include absence of neural activity, a nerve-conduction block, or desynchronization or discharges in the eighth nerve. The hypothesis concerning desynchronization evolved from findings of abnormal BAEPs in multiple sclerosis (MS) patients with normal hearing sensitivity since MS is associated with demyelination or lack of myelination of the eighth nerve (Naunton & Fernandez, 1978).

Kraus, Ozdamar, Stein, and Reed (1984) reported on seven cases with absent BAEPs or absent wave III or V on repeat testing, absence of clinical signs of brainstem neuropathy, and normal to no-worse-than-moderate hearing-threshold levels. The results of testing with the ITPA (Illinois Test of Psycholinguistic Abilities) and the Wepman Perceptual test battery revealed below age-level scores and poorer performance on the subtests dealing with auditory skills than on those dealing with visual skills. All experienced speech and language delays and formal intelligence testing in five cases revealed four normal scores and one borderline normal score. The investigators suggested that an absent BAEP in the presence of no-worse-than-moderate hearing-threshold levels in cases with absence of clinical signs of brainstem dysfunction may be indicative of communicative and/or learning disorders which may result from subtle brainstem dysfunction. This finding has not yet been verified by other large-scale studies.

VIII. BAEPS ELICITED WITH BONE-CONDUCTED SIGNALS

Yoshie (1973) employed bone-conducted signals in electrocochleography. He observed that the latency–intensity function for bone-conducted signals differed from that for air-conducted signals. Yoshie (1973) attributed this finding to differences between the spectra for air- and bone-conducted clicks. For bone-conducted clicks, the spectrum is low-frequency in comparison with the predominantly high-frequency spectrum for air-conducted clicks.

Mauldin and Jerger (1979) found that the peak latency of wave V was, on average, 0.46 ms longer for bone-conducted signals than for air-conducted signals at equivalent sensation levels. Boezeman, Kapteyn, Visser, and Snel (1983) reported that the latencies for wave V with bone-conducted clicks were, on average, 0.9 ms longer than with air-conducted clicks. Thus, there is considerable variability from clinic to clinic in the latency values of the BAEPs elicited by bone-conducted signals. Therefore, each clinic must obtain its own normative data for BAEPs elicited with bone-conducted signals.

One major limitation of bone-conducted BAEPs is the reduced maximum intensity output compared with air-conducted BAEPs. The intensity output is reduced even further for forehead placement than for mastoid-process placement. At intensities beyond 50 dBnHL, nonlinearities occur that affect the BAEPs (Gorga & Thornton, 1989).

Kavanagh and Beardsley (1979) evaluated the BAEPs to bone-conducted clicks. With bone-conducted clicks, only wave V and occasionally wave III could be identified. Wave I was present in only 5 of the 15 normal-hearing subjects tested. Moreover, the amplitude of wave V for the bone-conducted clicks was smaller than that for the air-conducted clicks. When the click generator was set to 95 dB, the amplitude of the response to the bone-conducted stimulus corresponded to that for an air-conducted stimulus of 35 dB. When intensity of the bone-conducted signal was decreased from 95 to 55 dB (the bone-conducted BAEP threshold), the latency increase was only 0.66 ms, as opposed to 2.14 ms when the intensity of an air-conducted signal was decreased from 50 to 10 dB (air-conducted BAEP threshold).

Mauldin and Jerger (1979) suggested the use of bone-conducted BAEPs in children with congenital atresia who cannot be evaluated using air-conducted signals. They maintained that bone-conducted BAEPs are also valuable to obtain in patients with closed-head injury who have had craniectomies, since the dressing interferes with earphone placement. Mauldin and Jerger (1979) advised clinicians to appropriately employ contralateral masking when obtaining BAEPs with bone-conducted signals.

Gorga and Thornton (1989) reported elevated BAEP thresholds for air-conducted clicks but a BAEP threshold for bone-conducted clicks at 30 dBnHL in a patient with bilateral atresia. In this case, the BAEP threshold for the bone-conducted click enabled assessment of cochlear reserve.

In summary, bone-conducted BAEPs are characterized by higher thresholds, longer latencies, smaller amplitudes, and poorer morphologies than air-conducted BAEPs. The dynamic range of the bond-conducted clicks is reduced to only approximately 30 dB compared with the range of air-conducted clicks. Some clinicians may find it feasible to obtained bone-conducted BAEPs in patients with congenital atresia or stenosis.

IX. FREQUENCY SPECIFICITY

The issue of frequency specificity concerns the ability of the BAEP test to accurately determine the hearing threshold level at a specific frequency independent of the hearing sensitivity at other frequencies. In order to use BAEP testing for frequency-by-frequency prediction of hearing loss, it must satisfy the requirement of frequency specificity.

The BAEP is an onset potential, that is, the response is to the first few milliseconds of the stimulus duration. Also, the BAEP represents the synchronous firing of neurons. Therefore, a stimulus is needed for BAEP testing which is of short duration and rapid onset such as a click, toneburst/tonepip, or logon (Burkard, 1984). A stimulus which is too brief, however, will result in spectral splatter. If spectral splatter occurs, it is difficult to determine which part of the basilar membrane is responsible for the response. In prediction of hearing loss (but not in differential diagnosis), it is important to know which part of the basilar membrane is responsible for the potential.

Most of the BAEP studies have employed clicks. Recall from Section VI that the click-elicited BAEP in normal-hearing subjects generally represents the synchronous firing of neurons in the 2000 to 4000 Hz range so the neurons from the basal end of the basilar membrane are involved in producing the BAEP. Recall also that the click-evoked BAEP threshold fails to yield information about low-frequency hearing sensitivity and may miss or underestimate mid- or high-frequency hearing impairment. A normal BAEP threshold and latency–intensity function can be obtained even when normal hearing is present at only a single frequency in the 2000 to 8000 Hz range (Glattke, 1983). Kiang, Maxon, and Kahn (1976) reported that only 20 neurons are necessary for the synchronous neural discharges that yield a normal BAEP threshold.

Researchers have attempted to improve the frequency specificity of the BAEP test using filtered clicks, tonebursts/tonepips, and logons. The use of filtered clicks has largely been abandoned since, as Burkard (1984) showed, the acoustic spectrum of the filtered click increases as the nominal frequency of the filtered click increases. A limitation of tonebursts/tonepips and logons is that the sidebands are 28–30 dB down in intensity and 35 dB down in intensity, respectively, from the center lobe of the acoustic spectrum. Therefore, in cases of both rising and sloping hearing loss, the BAEP threshold obtained using tonebursts/tonepips or logons does not reflect the response of neurons at the center lobe frequency; rather, it reflects the response of neurons at the sidelobe frequencies. Therefore, the BAEP threshold underestimates the hearing loss at the nominal frequency of the toneburst/tonepip or logon. In normal-hearing subjects, this limitation of tonebursts/tonepips and logons is not encountered since the signal intensity is generally not increased to a level at which sidelobes are produced. Another limitation in using tonebursts/tonepips and logons is that, when the signal intensity reaches a high level, the BAEP response represents the firing of high-frequency neurons from the basal end of the basilar membrane.

Jacobson (1983) recorded BAEPs using 500-Hz tone-bursts/tonepips at moderate-to-high intensities. He found that, when high-pass ipsilateral maskers with a cutoff frequency at 1000 Hz were employed simultaneously with the toneburst/tonepip, the peak latencies increased compared with the peak latencies obtained without the high-pass ipsilateral masker. The increased peak latencies when the 500-Hz toneburst/tonepip is presented with masking suggests:

1. The BAEP for the 500-Hz toneburst/tonepip that is obtained without masking is derived primarily from the basal end of the cochlear partition.
2. The BAEP for the 500-Hz toneburst/tonepip that is obtained with masking is derived primarily from the apical end.

Stapells, Picton, Perez-Abalo, Read, and Smith (1985), using tonebursts/tonepips presented simultaneously with notched noise as an ipsilateral masker in which the broadband noise is filtered only around the toneburst/tonepip frequency, obtained findings similar to those reported by Jacobson (1983) (see Figure 13). The purpose of the high-pass ipsilateral masker in the case of Jacobson (1983) and the ipsilateral notched noise in the case of Stapells *et al.* (1985) was to prevent the response of the neurons at frequencies that comprise the masker so that only the neurons at the toneburst/tonepip or logon nominal frequency can respond.

Although the frequency-selectivity experiments were successful in normal-hearing subjects using low-to-moderate intensity stimuli, few studies have been done in the hearing-impaired population. The applicability to hearing-impaired subjects of the findings of the frequency-selectivity studies employing ipsilateral masking in the normal-hearing subjects has been questioned on theoretical grounds by Gorga and Worthington (1983). According to Gorga and Worthington (1983), frequency selectivity as achieved using tonebursts/tonepips in the presence of ipsilateral maskers is confounded by an important neural phenomenon: the tuning curve of the high-frequency neurons (see Figure 14). In Figure 14, a set of tuning curves for various single neural fibers are shown. As illustrated in this figure, there is a particular characteristic frequency at which the neuron fires best. At frequencies below the best frequency, the neuron still fires but the threshold of activation at these frequencies is substantially higher. It is possible to mask the characteristic frequency of the neuron using high-frequency noise as suggested by Jacobson (1983) and Folsom (1984) or notched noise as suggested by Stapells *et al.* (1985). The masking of the best frequency of the neuron using such maskers can be implemented in normal-hearing but not in hearing-impaired subjects because:

1. The threshold of the best frequency is elevated in hearing-impaired subjects.
2. The slope of the tuning curve of both the low-frequency and high-frequency sides of the best frequency is shallower in hearing-impaired persons than in normal-hearing persons.
3. The ratio of the thresholds for the frequencies below the best or characteristic frequency (CF) of the neuron to the threshold of characteristic frequency (called the tail to tip ratio) is decreased in cochlear hearing-impaired subjects compared with normal-hearing subjects.

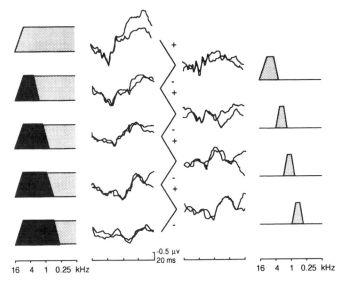

Figure 13 Derived brainstem responses obtained using high-pass masking. *Left,* The brainstem responses to 70-dB nHL clicks presented at a rate of 39/s either alone or in the presence of high-pass masking with the cutoff settings at 4000, 2000, 1000, and 500 Hz. Each tracing represents the average of 2000 responses recorded from vertex to mastoid, with negativity at the vertex represented by an upward deflection. The diagrams to the left of the tracings represent the spectra of the click (gray) and the masking noise (black). *Right,* The derived responses obtained by sequential subtraction of the responses obtained using decreasing filter settings for the high-pass noise. On the far right of the figure are shown diagrammatically the narrow-band frequency areas that theoretically activate the derived responses. From Stapells *et al.* (1985) with permission.

Such alterations in the tuning curves of the cochlear hearing-impaired subjects will reduce the efficiency of masking (Gorga & Worthington, 1983). That is, the threshold of activation of neurons with high characteristic frequencies when a low-frequency stimulus is employed is shifted only minimally by a high-frequency ipsilateral masker in the hearing impaired. The threshold of activation of high characteristic frequency neurons when a low-frequency stimulus is employed is shifted to a greater extent by a high-frequency masker in the normal-hearing persons. Therefore, in cochlear hearing-impaired persons, the use of a masker to eliminate the participation of high-frequency

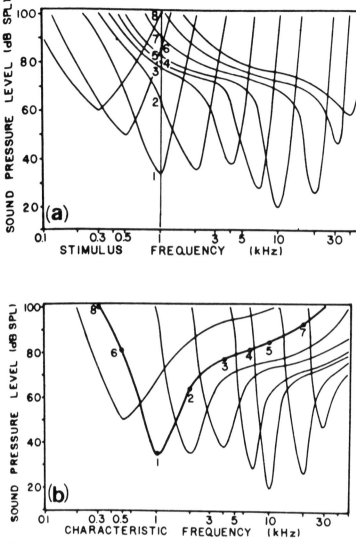

Figure 14 Threshold as a function of frequency for a group of auditory neurons; each neuron innervates a different point along the basilar membrane. Notice that the fibers that innervate the basal end of the cochlea (i.e., high CF fibers) will respond to moderately intense low-frequency stimuli as well. From Gorga & Worthington (1983) with permission.

neurons to the BAEP elicited with low-frequency stimuli is very limited, at least in theory.

Extensive clinical studies on the effect of ipsilateral masking on the BAEPs for low-frequency stimuli in cochlear hearing-impaired subjects are needed to determine if this theoretical argument against the effectiveness of such maskers for frequency selectivity in the hearing impaired is valid. Preliminary data by Stapells (1989) are encouraging. He reported on the results of BAEP testing using frequency-specific stimuli (with ipsilateral notched-noise masking) in a group of normal-hearing children and adults and a group of 20 hearing-impaired children and adults. Stapells (1989) used the following stimulus/instrumentation parameters: (a) 2-1-2 (cycles rise time, cycles plateau, cycles fall time)

linearly gated tones, (b) alternating polarity, (c) repetition rate of 39.1/sec, (d) band-reject (notched) noise with a 1-octave notch centered at the tone frequency (high-pass and low-pass filters, 48 dB/octave slope each, with the intensity of the unfiltered noise set at 20 dB below the peak equivalent intensity of the tone), (e) EEG filter of 30–3000 Hz, (f) analysis time of 25 ms, and (g) 2000 trials per average. A broad vertex positive (wave V) to vertex negative (V′) auditory brainstem response corresponded "reasonably" (p. 240) well with the behavioral thresholds between 500 and 4000 Hz, with better correspondence for the high-frequency than low-frequency stimuli. The tones in notched-noise technique produced BAEP thresholds within 20 dB of the behavioral thresholds in 91% of the cases.

CONCLUSIONS

1. If the click-evoked BAEP threshold is normal, it can be assumed that normal hearing is present for at least one frequency between 250 and 8000 Hz.

2. If the click-evoked BAEP threshold is normal and the latency–intensity function for wave V is normal, it can be assumed that normal hearing is present in at least one frequency between 2000 and 8000 Hz.

3. If the click-evoked BAEP threshold is normal and the latency–intensity function for wave V is abnormal it can be assumed that a significant hearing loss is present throughout the 2000 to 8000 Hz region (with normal hearing present for at least one frequency below 2000 Hz) or normal hearing with retrocochlear impairment is present.

4. If the BAEP threshold elicited with low-frequency tonebursts/tonepips or logons is normal or better than that for high-frequency signals, it can be assumed that the BAEP threshold for the low-frequency stimuli reflects the hearing threshold level at the nominal frequency of the stimulus. The BAEP threshold for the high-frequency stimuli may underestimate the hearing threshold level at the high-frequencies if normal low-frequency hearing sensitivity is present.

5. If the BAEP threshold elicited with low-frequency tonebursts/tonepips or logons is elevated and the BAEP threshold elicited with high-frequency stimuli is normal, it cannot be assumed that the BAEP threshold for low-frequency stimuli represents the hearing threshold at the nominal frequency of the stimulus. That is, the BAEP threshold for the low-frequency stimulus may underestimate the hearing-threshold level at the nominal frequency of the stimulus if normal hearing-threshold levels at the high frequencies are present.

6. It is recommended that, for prediction of hearing loss, the clinician obtain the BAEP threshold and latency–intensity function for wave V using the click and the 500-Hz toneburst/tonepip or logon.

X. EFFECT OF AUDITORY PATHOLOGY ON THE BAEP

A. CONDUCTIVE HEARING IMPAIRMENT

Kavanagh and Beardsley (1979) evaluated the BAEPs elicited with clicks in conductive hearing-impaired subjects. The latency–intensity functions for the seven subjects with conductive hearing impairment is shown in Figure 15. This figure shows that the wave V latency–intensity function for conductive hearing-impaired persons is shifted to the right of that for normal-hearing subjects. The slope of the function is the same as for normal-hearing subjects. The amount of shift in the latency–intensity function (and hence, the

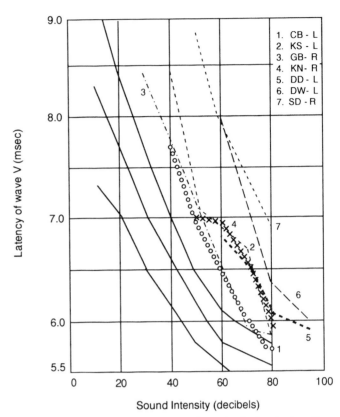

Figure 15 Various BAEPs in patients with conductive hearing loss. Normal mean latency of 15 control subjects is represented by the center solid line; ± 2 SD are shown by the two outer solid lines. From Kavanagh & Beardsley (1979) with permission.

BAEP threshold) generally corresponds to the degree of hearing impairment in the high frequencies (Borg, Lofqvist, & Rosen, 1981; Hecox & Galambos, 1974). Because of the shift of the latency–intensity function to the right in conductive-impaired persons, the peak latencies of the BAEP components are prolonged at a given intensity level relative to those in normal-hearing subjects. This prolonging of peak latencies and elevation of the BAEP threshold occurs because a conductive hearing impairment reduces the effective intensity of a sound. Several investigators (Galambos & Hecox, 1978; Yamada, Yagi, Yamane, & Suzuki, 1975) reported that the prolonged latency values in conductive hearing-impaired listeners are similar to those seen in retrocochlear-impaired listeners.

Although several researchers have suggested that the amount of peak latency delay can be predicted by the magnitude of the conductive component, other researchers (Clemis & Mitchell, 1977; Mendelson, Salamy, Lenoir, & McKean, 1979; Yamada *et al.*, 1975), on the other hand, have reported that the latency delay cannot be predicted from the size of the conductive component. The results of these studies, however, were confounded by technical and procedural factors.

McGee and Clemis (1982) obtained BAEPs elicited with 1000, 2000, and 4000 Hz tonebursts (1 ms rise–decay time, no plateau) in 23 subjects with various kinds of conductive pathologies. For each subject, the air–bone gap was calculated from the audiogram. The degree of conductive hearing loss was estimated from the latency–intensity function (see Figure 16). The latency–intensity function for a toneburst at a given nominal frequency from a particular subject and the mean latency–intensity function for normal-hearing subjects were plotted on the same graph. The dB difference between a given latency on the conductive function and the same latency on the normal function was then measured. This was done for all the points on the conductive latency–intensity function. Then the dB difference values were averaged to obtain a mean latency–intensity function (LIF) shift value in dB. Figures 17 and 18 show the LIF shift as a function of the air–bone gap for the various types of conductive pathologies. As illustrated in these figures, most of the data points fall within 10 dB of the predicted line (slope of +1) although the LIF shift overestimates the air–bone gap by more than 10 dB in cases of ossicular chain disorders (otosclerosis and ossicular discontinuity). Thus, the results only grossly support the conclusion that the prolonged latencies reflect the size of the air–bone gap in conductive disorders resulting from middle-ear effusion and earplugs. There is a substantial lack of agreement between the LIF shift and the size of the air–bone gap in cases of conductive impairment resulting from ossicular chain disorders; the air–bone gap seen in the audiogram does not accurately reflect the attenuation in sound caused by the conductive hearing impairment because of the elevated bone-conduction thresholds resulting from purely mechanical factors. Hence, the air–bone gap will underestimate the true sound attenuation resulting from the conduc-

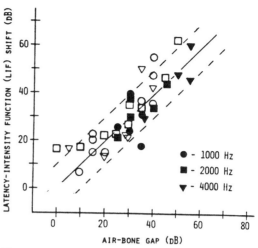

Figure 17 Latency–intensity function shift vs. air–bone gap; losses induced with earplugs (closed symbols) and middle-ear effusion (open symbols). From McGee & Clemis (1982) with permission.

tive component and the LIF shift will reflect the actual sound attenuation.

McGee and Clemis (1982) claim that the accuracy in determining the LIF shift resulting from the presence of air–bone gaps is sufficient to enable the clinician to determine which part of the prolonged wave V peak latency, in cases of combined conductive pathology not due to ossicular chain disorder and retrocochlear pathology, results from just the conductive component. Eggermont (1982) contends that the error in prediction of conductive hearing loss from the LIF can be as large as 20 dB since a given latency

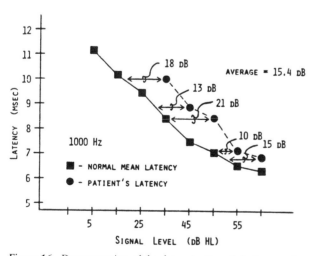

Figure 16 Demonstration of the determination of the latency–intensity function shift in order to estimate the degree of conductive loss. From McGee & Clemis (1982) with permission.

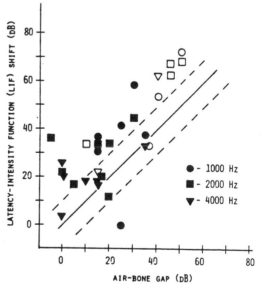

Figure 18 Latency–intensity function shift vs. air–bone gap; ossicular-chain disorders. Otosclerosis (closed symbols) and ossicular discontinuity (open symbols). From McGee & Clemis (1982) with permission.

value may be associated with a range of intensity values as large as 20 dB. Hence, one may not be able to detect the presence of a mild conductive impairment on the basis of the LIF.

McGee and Clemis (1982) suggest that, in cases in which the latency prolongation resulting from the retrocochlear pathology is slight, it is difficult to sort out the portion of the latency delay attributable to just the conductive pathology in cases of combined conductive and retrocochlear disorders. If the clinician attempts to predict the air–bone gap from the LIF in such cases, the retrocochlear disorder may not be detected. Thus, wave I needs to be recorded so the I–V IPL can be determined for differential diagnosis. McGee and Clemis (1982) reported that wave I could be recorded in only 15 of their 32 ears with conductive pathology. In all of these 15 ears, the I–V IPL was essentially normal, as is also the case in cochlear-impaired ears, in contrast with retrocochlear-impaired ears, which are characterized by a prolonged I–V IPL.

In summary, the following conclusions can be drawn with respect to conductive-impaired ears:

1. The latency–intensity function is shifted to the right of the LIF for normal-hearing subjects; the slope of the function is essentially similar to that for normal-hearing subjects.
2. The LIF shift in dB (and hence, the BAEP threshold elevation) only roughly corresponds to the air–bone gap (within 20 dB), except in cases of ossicular chain disorders, in which case the LIF shift overestimates the apparent air–bone gap as observed on the audiogram.
3. The I–V IPL is essentially normal, similar to that in cochlear-impaired ears. It is not always possible to obtain the I–V IPL since wave I often cannot be recorded in conductive-impaired ears.
4. The latency–intensity function for wave V resembles that LIF in retrocochlear-impaired ears.

B. COCHLEAR HEARING IMPAIRMENT

Galambos and Hecox (1978) reported that the BAEP threshold in patients with cochlear hearing impairment is elevated, as is the case for patients with conductive hearing impairment. In general, the latency–intensity function for wave V has a steep slope, that is, the latency values are prolonged at low intensities and become or approach normal values at high intensities. This latency–intensity function is illustrated in Figure 19. This latency–intensity function is most characteristic of flat or mild-to-moderate sloping cochlear hearing impairment. Subjects with significant sloping hearing impairment often demonstrate a latency–intensity function which is two-legged (Galambos & Hecox, 1978). The average value of the L–I slope in

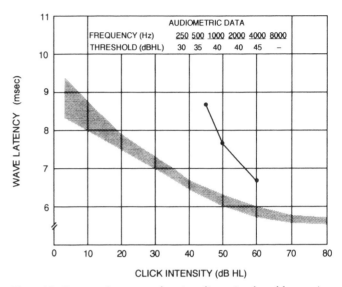

Figure 19 Response latency as a function of intensity plotted for a patient with sensorineural recruiting hearing loss due to Meniere's disease. Note the rapid change in the slope of the latency–intensity function at intensities near threshold; this finding is characteristic of patients with recruiting hearing losses, regardless of etiology. From Galambos & Hecox (1978) with permission.

persons with significant sloping cochlear impairment may be similar to that for normal-hearing persons, since the function is two-legged—one leg with a steep slope followed by a leg with a shallow slope—and the slope is determined on the basis of latencies at a high intensity (where the slope is steep) and at a low intensity (where the slope is shallow). A two-legged latency–intensity function for a person with a high-frequency sensorineural hearing impairment is shown in Figure 20. Subjects with hearing impairment which is precipitously sloping above 1000 Hz may demonstrate a latency–intensity function that is shifted upward of that in normal-hearing persons (Stapells et al., 1985). Figure 21 illustrates a latency–intensity function obtained from a person with a cochlear hearing loss precipitously sloping above 1000 Hz. In such cases, the BAEP threshold may be obtained at normal threshold levels (although the latency will be prolonged), reflecting the contribution of intact nerve fibers from the apical end of the basilar membrane. The peak latency of wave V never approaches values seen in normal-hearing persons since the response is always dominated by apical fibers. As the intensity increases, there is a basalward shift in the fibers dominating in the response, but the intensity never reaches a level sufficient to stimulate the basal fibers.

If the slope of the latency-intensity function exceeds 60 μs/dB (the slope is obtained by subtracting the latency value obtained at the higher intensity from that obtained at a lower intensity and then dividing the difference by the

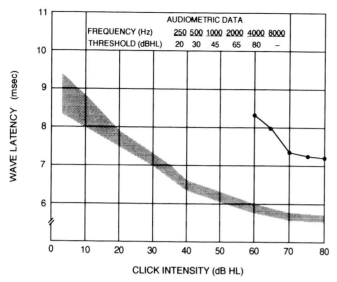

Figure 20 Response latency as a function of intensity plotted for a patient with a sensorineural recruiting loss involving predominantly high-frequency fibers, as shown in the audiogram. The latency–intensity curve shows the steep slope seen in Figure 19 followed by a flat region elevated above the normal. From Galambos & Hecox (1978) with permission.

decibel difference in the intensity levels), cochlear hearing impairment is likely to be present. If the slope is less than 30 μs/dB, one can conclude that the patient either has normal hearing-threshold levels or a significant sloping high-frequency hearing impairment. If the slope is normal, that is, between 30 and 60 μs/dB, then one can conclude that either the patient has a significant high-frequency cochlear hearing impairment and the slope was determined over the steep and shallow legs of the function or that the patient

has normal hearing and the slope was determined based on the latency values at the higher intensities. The slope values for a person with a precipitously sloping cochlear hearing impairment are similar to those for normal-hearing persons. Thus, cochlear hearing impairment cannot be ruled out on the basis of a normal slope value. Also, slope values which are normal or less than 30 μs/dB may also be encountered in cases of retrocochlear pathology. Thus, only slope values exceeding 60 μs/dB can be considered diagnostically significant. The clinicians should carefully delineate the latency–intensity function over several intensity levels and a wide range in intensity. If too few data points are obtained, the shape of the latency function obtained may be inaccurate and the slope may be calculated over inappropriate intensity levels, leading to a nondiagnostically significant slope value.

Coats (1978) evaluated the latency–intensity function in subjects with cochlear pathology. He subdivided his 37 cochlear-impaired ears according to the average of the hearing threshold levels in the 4000 to 8000 Hz range. The latency–intensity functions for wave V, the I–V IPL, and wave I for these cochlear-impaired ears were then superimposed on the plot showing the limits of the latency–intensity function in normal-hearing ears. Figure 22 shows these latency–intensity functions for the cochlear-impaired ears subdivided into four hearing-loss groups on the basis of the average hearing threshold levels in the 4000 to 8000 Hz range. This figure illustrates the shift upward in the latency–intensity function as the magnitude of the hearing loss increases. The latency–intensity function for the I–V IPL, on the other hand, approaches the lower limit of the normal-hearing limits as the magnitude of the hearing loss increases. It can be seen that the effect of hearing impairment is most striking on the latency–intensity function for wave I, which clearly shifts substantially above the upper limit of normalcy as the hearing loss increases. The latency prolongation seen in the latency–intensity functions for waves I and V is most noticeable at the lower stimulus intensities and approaches more normal values at the higher intensities. The steepness of the latency–intensity function increases as the magnitude of the hearing loss increases and is greater for wave I than for wave V. As a result of the high-frequency cochlear hearing loss effects on the peak latencies of waves I and V, the tendency seen in normal-hearing persons for the I–V IPL to increase slightly as stimulus intensity increases is exaggerated in the cochlear-impaired group. Thus, the slight upward slope of the I–V latency-intensity function in normal-hearing ears increases (steepens) as the hearing loss in the 4000 to 8000 Hz range increases.

Gorga, Reiland, and Beauchaine (1985a) tested the hypothesis raised by Gorga, Worthington, Reiland, Beauchaine, and Goldgar (1985b) that the latency–intensity function for wave V is determined by the audiometric con-

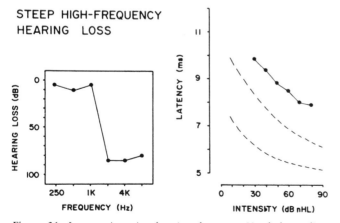

Figure 21 Latency–intensity function for wave V of the auditory brainstem response. On the latency–intensity graph the dashed lines represent the normal values obtained in our laboratory plotted at ± 2 SD. Shown are the results obtained in a patient with a steep high-frequency hearing loss. From Stapells *et al.* (1985) with permission.

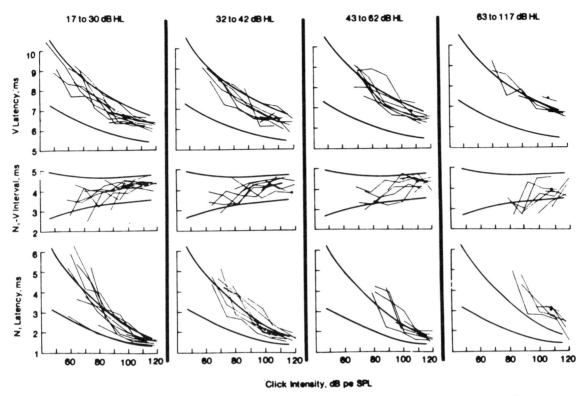

Figure 22 Latency–intensity curves from 37 cochlear-loss ears (fine lines) superimposed on estimated normal ranges (heavy lines). Cochlear-loss L–I curves are divided into four groups based on average 4 to 8 kHz hearing level (HL), shown at tops of columns. From Coats (1978) with permission.

figuration. The hypothesis rests on the assumption that the peak latency of wave V is related to the region of the cochlea which predominates in the response. In normal-hearing persons and persons with mild-to-moderate flat or high-frequency hearing impairment, the latency of wave V at high intensities is determined by the basal region of the cochlea. At lower stimulus intensities in normal-hearing persons and persons with flat hearing impairment, the latency of wave V is dominated by slightly more apical regions of the cochlea. At lower stimulus intensities in persons with significant high-frequency hearing loss, the cochlear region which predominates in the response is shifted significantly in the apical diretion so substantially prolonged latencies are obtained, reflecting longer travel times to the apical site where maximal disturbance of the basilar membrane occurs.

Gorga *et al.* (1985a,b) obtained the latency–intensity function for wave V in a patient with a high-frequency conductive hearing loss. The steep latency–intensity function obtained supported the hypothesis that the wave V latency is determined by the audometric configuration and challenges the contention made by Galambos and Hecox (1977, 1978) that a steep latency–intensity function for wave V is associated with the presence of behavioral recruitment.

Keith and Greville (1987) obtained BAEPs at several intensity levels from 47 high-frequency cochlear hearing-impaired ears, 8 low-frequency cochlear hearing-impaired ears, 44 flat cochlear hearing-impaired ears, 27 notched high-frequency hearing-impaired ears, and 28 normal-hearing ears. The absolute latencies of waves I and V and the I–V interpeak latencies were measured. The results revealed that, in the high-frequency group, wave I latency tended to be dalayed at all intensity levels (70, 80, and 90 dBnHL), wave V tended to be delayed at low intensity levels but normal or near normal at high intensity levels, and the I–V interpeak latency tended to be approximately normal or reduced. In the low-frequency group (with a greater magnitude of hearing impairment in the low than high frequencies), wave I latency tended to be normal, wave V latency tended to be normal or earlier than normal (at the low intensities), and the I–V interpeak tended to be normal or reduced (especially at lower intensities). In the flat group, wave I latency, wave V latency, and the I–V interpeak latency tended to be normal. In the notched group, wave I latency tended to be normal or early, wave V latency tended to be delayed, and the I–V interpeak latency tended to be prolonged (particularly at low intensities). Keith and Greville (1987) concluded that the I–V interpeak latency was more prolonged in cases of notched hearing impairment than in cases of high-frequency cochlear hearing impairment. In the former but not in the latter case, wave I latency is earlier than normal because of the absence of the longer latency contributions from the 3000–4000 Hz region of the cochlea together with the presence of the shorter latency contributions form the 4000–8000 Hz region of the cochlea.

The results of Keith and Greville (1987) also revealed that, at intensities between 70 and 90 dBnHL, the limit that was 2 standard deviations below the mean for wave I latency in the normal hearing group was 1.34 ms. The limit that was 2 standard deviations above the mean for wave I latency in the high-frequency hearing-impaired group (the cochlear group with the longest wave I latency) was 2.35 ms.

In summary, the following conclusions can be drawn about subjects with cochlear hearing impairment:

1. The BAEP threshold is elevated as it is for conductive hearing-impaired persons.
2. The latency–intensity function for wave V has a steep slope. That is, the latencies are prolonged at lower intensities and become or approach normal values at high intensities. This type of latency–intensity function is most commonly observed in persons with flat or mild-to-moderate sloping cochlear hearing impairment. Persons with more severe high-frequency hearing loss may demonstrate a two-legged latency–intensity function in which the first leg, over the lower intensities, is steep and the second leg, over the higher intensities, is shallow. The latency–intensity function in persons with hearing loss precipitously sloping above 1000 Hz (but sloping below 4000 Hz) often demonstrates a latency–intensity function which is shifted upward with respect to that seen in normal-hearing persons. The clinician is reminded that the likelihood of obtaining a latency–intensity function decreases as the hearing loss increases beyond approximately 80 dB HL and the BAEP may be absent even at the maximum output levels.
3. If the slope of the latency–intensity function for wave V exceeds 60 μs/dB, it is diagnostic of cochlear pathology. Smaller slope values are nondiagnostic.
4. If the latency–intensity function is obtained, it should be based on several intensity levels over a wide intensity range so that the shape can be accurately defined and appropriate intensity levels can be selected for determination of the slope value.
5. The hearing impairment has a greater effect on the latency of wave I than on that of wave V, that is, the latency of wave I is prolonged more than that of wave V as a result of the hearing loss. In cases of flat cochlear hearing impairment, the latencies of I and V are normal once threshold is exceeded. In cases of

notched high-frequency cochlear hearing impairment, wave V is prolonged but wave I latency tends to be earlier than normal.
6. The I–V IPL is reduced (as it is in conductive hearing-impaired persons) or normal compared with that in normal-hearing persons. Nonetheless, the I–V interpeak interval may be prolonged in cases of notched high-frequency hearing impairment or normal in cases of flat cochlear hearing impairment.

C. RETROCOCHLEAR IMPAIRMENT

The use of BAEP testing for the identification of retrocochlear site of pathology is becoming an increasingly popular challenge for the audiologist. Various BAEP measures, either singly or in combination, have been employed for the detection of the presence of retrocochlear pathology: (a) prolonged wave V, (b) long interaural wave V difference, (c) prolonged I–V interpeak latency (IPL), (d) absence of the later waves, (e) absence of the BAEP waveform, (f) absence of waveform reproducibility, (g) abnormal IV–V:I amplitude ratio, (h) prolonged interaural I–V IPL, (i) abnormalities at high repetition rates, (j) contralateral ear effects, and (k) abnormal waveform morphology.

1. PROLONGED WAVE V LATENCY

Coats (1978) investigated the latency–intensity functions for wave V in 14 retrocochlear-impaired ears with varying degrees of hearing loss. Figure 23 shows the latency–intensity functions for the retrocochlear-impaired ears superimposed against the two standard deviation limits for the cochlear hearing-impaired and normal-hearing ears. These results confirm the findings of previous investigators (Coats & Martin, 1977; Selters & Brackmann, 1977; Stockard & Rossiter, 1977) that the effect of retrocochlear pathology is to prolong the peak latency for wave V. Also, the peak latency of wave V is prolonged in a retrocochlear ear with hearing impairment beyond that seen in a cochlear hearing-impaired ear with an equivalent degree of hearing impairment. Table IV shows the clinical utility of each of the various BAEP measures in differential diagnosis. For a particular measure, the percentage of the retrocochlear population identified by that measure and the percentage of the total cochlear population which is wrongly identified as retrocochlear impaired based on that measure are shown. The percentage of retrocochlear-impaired ears identified by the measure is not the hit rate since it was calculated on the basis of the total retrocochlear population investigated and not on the total number of retrocochlear-impaired ears in which the measure could be obtained. For the same reason, the percentage of the total cochlear population wrongly demonstrating the presence of a particular BAEP measure cannot be considered the false-alarm rate.

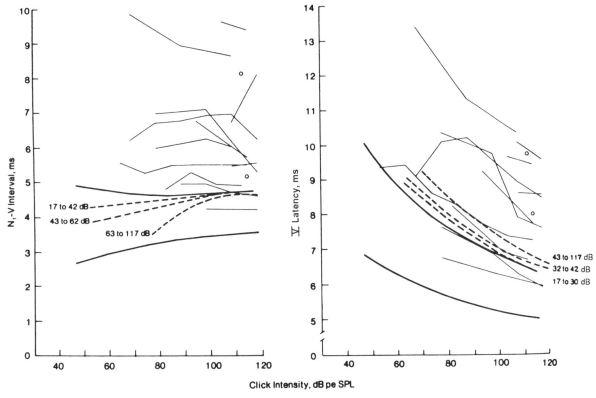

Figure 23 Retrocochlear N_1–V interval and V latency L–I functions (fine lines and, for ears giving only one data point, small circles) superimposed on normal (heavy solid lines) and upper cochlear-loss (heavy dashed lines) limits. From Coats (1978) with permission.

As can be seen from Table IV, Bauch, Rose, and Harner (1982) found that the presence of a bilaterally delayed wave V was the least clinically useful measure compared with the absence of the BAEP or the prolonged interaural wave V measure. Their findings showed that bilateral prolongation of wave V occurred in only 3% of their retrocochlear ears; an absent BAEP was present in 50% and the prolonged interaural wave V was present in 43% of their retrocochlear-impaired ears. The primary factor accounting for their low rate was that the peak latency of wave V was not considered prolonged unless it was prolonged bilaterally. It is probable that they employed this measure to detect the presence of bilateral tumors which would otherwise be missed with the interaural wave V latency difference.

The results of the study by Clemis and McGee (1979) indicated that the unilaterally or bilaterally prolonged wave V latency measure was clinically useful; this measure detected 70% of retrocochlear-impaired ears, compared with the absence of the BAEP waveform measure, which detected only 15% of the retrocochlear-impaired ears. Clemis and McGee's identification rate for the prolonged wave V measure was similar to that for the prolonged interaural wave V measure (74%). Coats (1978) found that wave V latency was prolonged in 79 to 86% of his retrocochlear-

impaired ears (depending upon whether the degree of hearing loss in the high frequencies was considered). This high identification rate at least partially reflects the fact that ears were excluded from the study if the BAEP waveform was absent.

Coats (1978) showed that the percentage of cochlear-impaired ears having a significantly prolonged peak latency of wave V could be decreased if the hearing loss in the 4000 to 8000 Hz region was considered. When the individual latency–intensity functions for retrocochlear-impaired ears with hearing loss were superimposed against the two-standard-deviation limits for cochlear-impaired ears with an equivalent magnitude of hearing loss in the 4000 to 8000 Hz region, fewer retrocochlear ears had data points falling out of the two-standard-deviation limits for cochlear-impaired ears. As Table IV shows, the percentage of cochlear ears with significantly prolonged wave V peak latency decreased from 14 to 0% when the peak latency was compared with the two-standard-deviation limits for cochlear-impaired rather than normal-hearing ears. The percentage of retrocochlear-impaired ears demonstrating a prolonged wave V peak latency was decreased, but only slightly (7%), as a result of comparing the wave V peak latency against the two-standard-deviation limits for cochlear-impaired rather than normal-hearing ears.

Table IV Percentage of Retrocochlear-Impaired Ears and Cochlear-Impaired Ears Showing a Positive Result for Each of the BAEP Measures, as Reported by Various Investigators

Investigator	Criteria	Positive result	
		Retrocochlear-impaired ears (%)	Cochlear-impaired ears (%)
1. Prolonged peak latency of wave V			
Selters & Brackmann (1977)	Positive if wave V is absent	46	0
Coats (1978)[a]	Positive if at least 50% of the data points on the wave V L-I function exceed the normal limits	86	14
Coats (1978)[a]	Positive if at least 50% of the data points on the wave V L-I function exceed the cochlear limits	79	0
Clemis & McGee (1979)	Positive if significantly different from the normal mean	70	38
House & Brackmann (1979)	Positive if >6.0 ms or absent	98[b] 75[c]	10 CND[d]
Bauch, Rose, & Harner (1983)	Positive if >6.1 ms bilaterally, after adjusting for hearing loss	3	3
2. ILD for wave V			
Selters & Brackmann (1977)	Positive if >0.2 ms up to 50 dB HL, >0.3 ms 55–65 dB HL, >0.4 ms for 70+ dB HL	46	12
Clemis & McGee (1979)	Positive if >0.3 ms (>0.4 ms when the HL is 65+ dB HL)	74	CND
Bauch, Rose, & Harner (1983)[e]	Positive if >0.2 ms after adjusting for 4000-Hz HL following Selters & Brackmann (1979)	43	10
Moller & Moller (1983)[f]	Positive if >0.3 ms	91	CND
Musiek, Josey, & Glasscock (1986a)[g]	Positive if >0.3 ms	100	6
3. Prolonged I–V IPL			
Coats (1978)[a]	Positive if exceeds 2 SD on normals	86	0
Coats (1978)[a]	Positive if exceeds 2 SD on cochlear ears	93	0
Eggermont, Don, & Brackmann (1980)[e]	Positive if exceeds 2 SD	60	5
Musiek, Josey, & Glasscock (1986)[g]	Positive if exceeds 2 SD	75	0
4. Absence of the BAEP			
Clemis & McGee (1979)	Absent even at high intensities	15	CND
Bauch, Olsen, & Harner (1983)	Absent even at high intensities	50	10
Eggermont, Don, & Brackmann (1980)[e]	Absent even at high intensities	16	CND
5. Reduced IV/V:I AR			
Musiek, Kibbe, Rackliffe, & Weider (1984)[h]	Positive if AR <1.00	44	4
6. Lack of replicability			
Musiek, Josey, & Glasscock (1986a)[g]		74	Cochlear ears excluded if the BAEPs were nonreplicable

[a] Ears excluded from study if the BAEP could not be obtained. EcOG was employed to record wave I.
[b] Based on ears with acoustic neuroma.
[c] Based on ears with cerebellopontine angle tumors not originating in the internal auditory meatus.
[d] Could not determine.
[e] EcOG employed to record wave I.
[f] Statistic based on population on whom the ILD could be obtained.
[g] Criterion for selection was replicable waves I, III, and V. Control subjects were normal hearing or cochlear hearing-impaired.
[h] Criterion for selection was readable waves I and V. Control subjects were normal hearing or cochlear hearing-impaired.

Clemis and McGee (1979) reported that a very large percentage of cochlear hearing-impaired ears—38%—demonstrated a prolonged wave V peak latency. As Table IV shows, the peak latency of wave V was considered significantly delayed by Clemis and McGee if it exceeded the two-standard-deviations-from-the-mean limit for normal-hearing persons. This high rate is probably related to the fact that Clemis and McGee did not consider the effect of hearing impairment on the peak latency of wave V. This rate would probably have been decreased had they compared the peak latency of wave V against the two-standard-deviations-from-the-mean limit for cochlear hearing-impaired ears, following Coats (1978).

The wide disparity in the percentage of cochlear hearing-impaired persons demonstrating a prolonged wave V latency may be due in part to the differences in hearing threshold levels between samples; a cochlear group with a high average degree of hearing impairment in the high frequencies would be more likely to demonstrate a significantly prolonged wave V peak latency than a cochlear group with a low average degree of hearing impairment in the high frequencies. To offset the effect of hearing impairment, Jerger and Mauldin (1978) suggested that 0.2 ms be added to the tolerance limit for the peak latency for wave V for each 30 dB difference between the hearing thresholds at 1000 and 4000 Hz. Selters and Brackmann (1977) suggested that 0.1 msec be added to the tolerance limit for the peak latency for wave V for each 10 dB the hearing-threshold level at 4000 Hz exceeds 50 dB HL. Josey (1985) and D. M. Schwartz (personal communication) suggest not employing any corrections for hearing impairment. D. M. Schwartz (personal communication) cautions that the use of such formulas may lead the clinician to label a combined retrocochlear–cochlear hearing impaired ear as negative with respect to retrocochlear pathology since the presence of high-frequency hearing impairment does not always prolong the peak latency of wave V. Because of this, Schwartz prefers other BAEP measures which are less susceptible to the effect of hearing impairment for differential diagnosis.

2. Prolonged Interaural Latency Difference for Wave V

The presence of an interaural difference in the peak latency of wave V has been used as an indicator of retrocochlear pathology. With this measure, the ear not at risk for retrocochlear pathology serves as the control ear. Thus, the subject serves as his or her own control. Selters and Brackmann (1977) described the distribution of interaural latency differences (ILDs) for ears with retrocochlear pathology (tumors) and ears with cochlear hearing impairment. This distribution is shown in Figure 24. Figure 24 shows that the most common ILD in the nontumor group

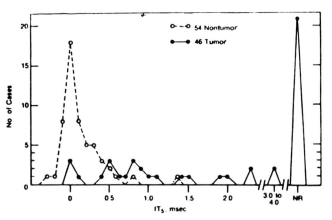

Figure 24 Distribution of IT5 for tumor group (closed circles) and nontumor group (open circles). From Selters & Brackmann (1977) with permission.

was 0 ms, that is, many of the cochlear-impaired ears had equal latencies in both ears despite the presence of a unilateral cochlear hearing impairment. In contrast, in the retrocochlear-impaired group, there was a wide distribution of ILDs; 21 of the 46 retrocochlear-impaired ears had ILDs of at least 0.4 msec.

As can be seen in Table IV, Selters and Brackmann (1977) reported that the ILD measure was as good as the absence of response measure in detecting the presence of retrocochlear pathology; they reported that 46% of their retrocochlear-impaired ears had significantly prolonged ILDs. Bauch, Rose, and Harner (1982) obtained similar findings; the ILD measure was prolonged in 43% of their retrocochlear impaired ears. Musiek, Josey, and Glasscock (1986a) reported that more of their retrocochlear-impaired ears had a prolonged ILD than had a prolonged I–V IPL: the former measure identified 25% more ears than the latter measure. Clemis and McGee (1979) reported that a prolonged ILD was present in essentially the same proportion of retrocochlear-impaired ears as the prolonged absolute wave V peak latency measure.

Once wave V can be measured bilaterally, the percentage of retrocochlear-impaired ears with significantly prolonged ILDs has been reported to be very high—as high as 100% as reported by Musiek et L. (1986b) and as high as 90% as reported by Eggermont et al. (1980).

Selters and Brackmann (1977) investigated the effect of high-frequency hearing impairment on the ILD. Figure 25 shows the ILD as a function of hearing-threshold level at 4000 Hz for the cochlear hearing-impaired ears and retrocochlear hearing-impaired ears. They drew the dashed line, the tolerance limit, such that the maximum number of cochlear-impaired ears would fall below the line and all of the retrocochlear-impaired ears would fall above the line.

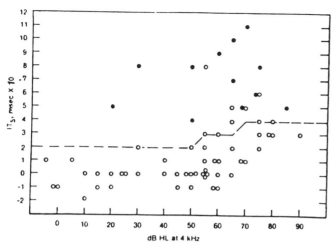

Figure 25 IT5 vs. pure-tone threshold at 4 kHz. Nontumor group (open circles) and acoustic tumor group (filled circles). From Selters & Brackmann (1977) with permission.

This figure clearly shows that the ILD increases as the hearing-threshold level at 4000 Hz increases.

The ILD measure has a drawback in cases of bilateral retrocochlear impairment, which would have an effect on the peak latency of wave V in both ears, so the interaural difference would not be significant. Another disadvantage of the ILD measure is that it may be influenced by asymmetrical hearing impairment.

Bauch, Rose, and Harner (1982) reported that 10% of their cochlear hearing-impaired ears demonstrated significant ILDs; the same percentage had absent BAEPs. Musiek *et al.* (1986b) reported that only 6% of their cochlear-impaired ears had prolonged ILDs, compared with 0% who had a prolonged I–V IPL. Selters and Brackmann (1977) reported that more of their cochlear-impaired ears had a prolonged ILD (12%) than had an absent BAEP (0%).

Moller and Moller (1983) obtained the ILD for wave III as well as for wave V in their group of 23 patients with cerebellopontine angle tumors. In 11, the ILD for wave III was the same as for wave V. In 4 ears, the ILD for wave III was larger than for wave V and in another 4 ears, the reverse finding was obtained. Thus, Moller and Moller suggested that the ILD for wave III may be a useful indicator of retrocochlear pathology.

Musiek, Johnson, Gollegly, Josey, and Glasscock (1989) observed that in persons with bilaterally symmetrical hearing thresholds, an ILD for wave V exceeding 0.3 ms occurred in none of their normal-hearing ears, 21% of their cochlear-impaired ears, 100% of their 15 cases with eighth-nerve or cerebellopontine-angle tumors, and 47% of their 15 cases with brainstem lesions. If the ILD of 0.4 ms was considered significantly prolonged, a significantly pro-

longed ILD occurred in none of their normal group, 6% of their cochlear-impaired group, 100% of their eighth-nerve/ cerebellopontine-angle group, and 40% of their brainstem group. Thus, the ILD for wave V appears to be less sensitive to brainstem than to eighth-nerve or cerebellopontine-angle lesions.

3. I–V Interpeak Latency

The presence of a prolonged I–V interpeak latency (IPL) or interwave interval (IWI) has been commonly employed as an indicator of retrocochlear pathology. Coats (1978) investigated the I–V latency–intensity functions in 14 retrocochlear impaired ears with varying degrees of hearing impairment. Figure 23 shows the individual functions superimposed against the upper normal and cochlear limits. This figure shows that the I–V latency functions are markedly shifted upward in comparison with the normal-hearing and cochlear hearing-impaired limits. Thus, at a given click intensity level, the I–V IPL is markedly prolonged in a retrocochlear-impaired ear in comparison with a normal-hearing ear. Moreover, the figure shows the opposing effects of retrocochlear and cochlear hearing impairment on the I–V IPL. In retrocochlear-impaired ears, the I–V IPL is prolonged whereas in cochlear-impaired ears, the I–V IPL is reduced. The differing effects of retrocochlear and cochlear pathology become more apparent as the degree of cochlear hearing impairment is increased. Coats (1978) employed electrocochleography in order to record wave I so the I–V IPL could be determined.

The drawback of the I–V IPL is that it is often difficult to record wave I during BAEP testing, particularly when hearing impairment is present. Eggermont *et al.* (1980) reported that 30% of their 45 patients with cerebellopontine angle tumors did not show a wave I. Cashman and Rossman (1983) reported that interwave measurements were unobtainable in 86% of their group of 35 patients with acoustic tumors. Hyde and Blair (1981) reported that wave I was present in only 42% of their patients with sensorineural hearing impairment. Bauch *et al.* (1982) did not employ the I–V IPL measure because many of the early waves could not be detected, even in normal-hearing listeners (Bauch, Rose, & Harner, 1980), and, in cochlear hearing-impaired ears, these components were even more difficult to identify.

Moller and Moller (1983) demonstrated that the peak latency of wave I is normal although the peak latencies of waves II and III are prolonged in cases of acoustic neuroma. The presence of a prolonged peak latency for wave II or III is then reflected as a prolonged peak latency for wave V. Therefore, the I–V IPL is prolonged. The peak latency of wave I is normal since it comes from the part of the auditory nerve which is distal to the brainstem and acoustic neuromas are usually proximal to the brainstem. Since wave II is generated from the proximal portion of the eighth nerve, the peak latency of wave II is prolonged in cases of tumors affecting the auditory nerve.

As can be seen in Table IV, 60% of Eggermont et al.'s (1980) retrocochlear-impaired ears had a prolonged I–V IPL.

When waves I and V can be recorded, the percentage of retrocochlear-impaired ears demonstrating a prolonged I–V IPL is relatively high. For example, Eggermont et al. (1980) reported that 93% of the retrocochlear-impaired ears for which waves I (via electrocochleography) and V could be recorded had prolonged I–V IPLs. Rosenhall, Hedner, and Bjorkman (1981) reported that 80% of their patients with brainstem lesions had increased I–V IPLs. Coats (1978) reported that 93% had prolonged I–V IPLs (when the IPL was compared against the tolerance limits for cochlear-impaired ears).

Eggermont et al. (1980) found that the I–V IPL measure identified substantially more retrocochlear-impaired ears than the absent BAEP measure. Coats (1978) found that the I–V IPL was a slightly more sensitive indicator of retrocochlear pathology than the prolonged wave V peak latency measure. Musiek et al. (1986b) found that more retrocochlear-impaired ears had prolonged ILDs (100%) than had prolonged I–V IPLs (75%). Musiek et al. (1986b) found that 100% of their retrocochlear-impaired ears had a prolonged I–III or III–V IPL. In some cases, one of the intervals would be long and one would be sufficiently short to produce a I–V IPL that was not prolonged beyond the normal limits. Moller and Moller (1983) reported that the I–III IPL was prolonged in 85% of their retrocochlear-impaired patients in whom the interwave interval could be recorded. In only 2 cases was the III–V IPL prolonged and the I–III IPL normal.

Table IV also shows that most investigators found that none of their cochlear-impaired ears had prolonged I–V IPLs. This was in striking contrast to other BAEP measures. For example, a prolonged wave V peak latency was reported to be present in up to 38% of the cochlear-impaired sample (Clemis & McGee, 1979).

As shown in Table IV, most investigators who evaluated the clinical utility of several BAEP measures within the same study found that the I–V IPL measure is one of the more powerful for differential diagnosis since more retrocochlear ears and fewer cochlear hearing-impaired and normal-hearing ears are labeled positive by this measure than by the other BAEP measures. Although the ILD measure identified more retrocochlear-impaired ears than the I–V IPL measure, the ILD test is positive in substantially more cochlear-impaired and normal-hearing ears than the I–V IPL measure.

To improve the clinical utility of the I–V IPL measure, clinical techniques must be employed to enhance wave I. Some of the existing techniques to enhance wave I are

unsatisfactory. For example, electrocochleography is invasive and controversy exists regarding the enhancement of wave I with the horizontal montage. A promising technique for the identification of wave I is the ear-canal electrode, for example, the Nicolet Tiptrode. Another promising technique for the enhancement of wave I involves the use of digital filtering rather than the currently employed electronic filtering (Moller, 1983). Figure 26 shows the enhancement of wave I in a retrocochlear-impaired ear as a result of the use of digital filtering. The use of two-channel recordings (ipsilateral and contralateral) also aids in the identification of wave I.

In patients with high brainstem lesions, the III–V rather than the I–III IPL is commonly prolonged (Lynn & Verma, 1985).

Sturzebecher, Kevanishvili, Werbs, Meyer, & Schmidt (1985) suggested that the interaural I–V IPL measure was useful for the detection of retrocochlear pathology since no correction factor is required for interaural differences in hearing threshold level. Weber (1983) and Stockard and

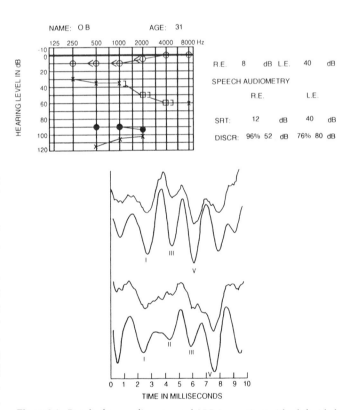

Figure 26 Results from audiometry and ABR in a patient with a left-sided acoustic nerve tumor. Upper tracings show unfiltered and digitally filtered recordings from the unaffected side; lower tracings show unfiltered and filtered recordings from the tumor side. Wave II shows both prolonged latency and decreased amplitude, while the IPL for waves III–V is normal. From Moller & Moller (1983) with permission.

Stockard (1983), on the other hand, maintain that inter-aural threshold differences contaminate the interaural I–V interpeak latency difference. They reported that the 95th percentiles for interaural I–V IPL do not exceed 0.2 ms in normal-hearing persons or persons with unilateral or symmetrical hearing loss and do not exceed 0.3 msec in patients with asymmetrical or noise-induced hearing loss. Eggermont *et al.* (1980) considered interaural I–V IPLs exceeding 0.4 ms to be positive. Further study on the interaural I–V IPL is needed before judgment can be made regarding the clinical utility of this measure.

4. Absent BAEP

Absence of the BAEP waveform even at the maximum-output levels of the instrument has been interpreted as consistent with the presence of retrocochlear pathology. As can be seen in Table IV, Clemis and McGee (1979) and Eggermont *et al.* (1980) reported that the BAEP waveform could not be obtained, that is, all waves were absent, in approximately 15% of their retrocochlear-impaired ears. Of the retrocochlear-impaired ears investigated by Bauch *et al.* (1982), approximately half had absent BAEP whereas 43% had a prolonged wave V interaural latency difference. The BAEPs were also absent in 10% of Bauch *et al.*'s (1983) cochlear hearing-impaired ears.

5. IV/V:I Amplitude Ratio

The presence of abnormal amplitude ratio (AR) as an indicator of retrocochlear pathology has been employed by some investigators (Musiek, Kibbe, Rackliffe, & Weider, 1984; Stockard & Rossiter, 1977). Hecox (1980) reported that a IV–V:I AR was suggestive of retrocochlear pathology if it was between 0.5 and 1.0 and was diagnostic of retrocochlear pathology if it was less than 0.5. He recommended that the AR be calculated at intensity levels not exceeding 80 dBnHL, for example, 60–70 dBnHL, since the AR decreases at the higher intensity levels. Musiek *et al.* (1984) found that the IV–V:I AR was less than 1.00 in 44% of their retrocochlear-impaired ears. In only 4% of their cochlear hearing-impaired and normal-hearing ears was the AR less than 1.00. Hecox (1983) suggested that, if there is doubt concerning which of the early peaks is wave I, the AR can be considered normal as long as none of the early peaks has an amplitude which exceeds that of wave V. The AR is not a commonly employed criterion for differential diagnosis since it is very sensitive to recording and stimulation variables.

6. Lack of Test–Retest Replicability

Some investigators have suggested that lack of test–retest reproducibility of the BAEPs is predictive of retrocochlear pathology. Musiek, Josey, & Glasscock (1986a) reported that waves I, III, and V were not replicable at the same repetition rate, intensity, and polarity in 74% of their 61

retrocochlear-impaired ears. In many patients with multiple sclerosis, there is lack of replicability. Elidan, Sohmer, Gafni, and Kahana (1982) found that in several of their patients with multiple sclerosis, waveform morphology changed from minute to minute, possibly reflecting the presence of intermittent conduction in a demyelinated fiber. Hecox (1980) contended that lack of replicability should not be considered a powerful predictor of neurologic disease since application of this criterion makes it hard to maintain quality control. Lack of replicability should be considered an indicator of retrocochlear pathology only if all technical and subject factors can be ruled out.

7. Absence of the Later Waves

The presence of wave I only or the presence of the early waves with the absence of the later waves has been employed as an indicator of retrocochlear pathology (House & Brackmann, 1979; Rosenhall *et al.*, 1981; Selters & Brackmann, 1977). Rosenhall *er al.* (1981) reported that wave V was absent in 57% of their retrocochlear-impaired subjects. Selters & Brackmann (1977) reported that in 46% of their retrocochlear-impaired ears and 0% of their cochlear-impaired ears, wave V was absent.

8. Repetition Rate Effects

Some investigators have suggested that the use of high repetition rates of stimulation to stress the auditory system may reveal subtle abnormalities. Since an increased repetition rate may result in increased peak latencies and decreased peak amplitudes in normal-hearing persons, a shift in latency or decrease in amplitude as a result of an increase in repetition rate can be considered significant only if the change is greater than what would be seen in normal-hearing persons.

Musiek and Gollegly (1985) use the following formula to determine whether a shift in the peak latency of wave V as a result of the increased repetition rate is significant: for every 10 Hz increase in the repetition rate, 0.1 ms is added to the tolerance limit and a variability of 0.2 ms around the final result is acceptable. Hecox (1980) uses the formula

$$0.006 \times \text{high click rate} - \text{low click rate} + 0.4 \text{ ms} = \\ \text{maximum acceptable latency shift}$$

for a result that is within normal limits.

There is disagreement in the literature concerning the clinical utility of varying repetition rate to elicit an abnormality. Hecox (1980) reported that only 4% of the neurologically impaired have BAEP abnormalities at high but not at low repetition rates. Elidan *et al.* (1982) reported that, in their group of patients with multiple sclerosis, there was no case in which a normal BAEP was obtained for standard click stimuli (75 dBnHL presentation level, 10–20 clicks/s) and an abnormal response was obtained when the repetition rate was increased to 50 clicks/s or 80 clicks/s and/or the presentation level was lowered. Nevertheless, the intensity and repetition rate manipulations did make any abnormality seen at standard click intensity and repetition rate more pronounced. Chiappa, Harrison, Brooks, and Young (1980) also found that the incidence of BAEP normality did not increase in their sample of 200 multiple sclerosis patients when the repetition rate was increased.

Discrepant findings were obtained by Stockard, Stockard, and Sharbrough (1977b) who evaluated the BAEPs in 100 multiple sclerosis patients. They reported that, as the repetition rate increased, the number of patients showing BAEP abnormalities was increased. Robinson and Rudge (1977) obtained findings similar to those reported by Stockard *et al.* (1977b).

9. Abnormal Waveform Morphology

Starr and Achor (1975) reported that distorted BAEP waveforms may be consistent with the presence of retrocochlear pathology. Eggermont *et al.* (1980) observed that normal BAEP waveform morphology was rarely present in ears with acoustic tumors. Figure 27 shows the BAEP waveform in a normal ear and in five ears with acoustic tumors. As can be seen in this figure, peak identification is a major problem in ears with retrocochlear pathology. Significant

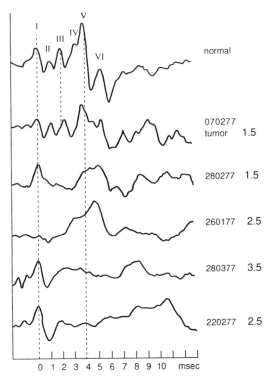

Figure 27 Waveforms of brainstem electric responses in acoustic neuroma cases. The numbers in the far right column represent the tumor size (cm). The normal morphology indicated in the upper trace is only rarely observed in tumor cases. However, the second trace is an example of prolonged I–III and I–V delays. In most cases, identification of the waves, except I, becomes difficult. From Eggermont *et al.* (1980) with permission.

cochlear hearing impairment may also adversely affect waveform morphology.

10. Contralateral Ear Effects

Selters and Brackmann (1977) observed that, when large tumors were present, the peak latency of wave V was prolonged and the wave V peak amplitude was reduced for the ear contralateral to the side of the lesion. The delay in wave V was reflected by the prolonged III–V IPL in the ear contralateral to the side of the tumor. The mean III–V IPL in the nontumor ear in cases in which the tumor size was < 3.0 cm was 1.87 ms as opposed to 2.14 ms in the nontumor ear in cases in which the tumor size was at least 3.0 cm. This difference was statistically significant. Selters and Brackmann (1977) hypothesized that a prolonged III–V IPL in the ear contralateral to the side of the tumor can result when the tumor is large enough to displace the brainstem and compress the contralateral auditory neurons. This hypothesis was confirmed by the results of computerized cranial tomograms.

Musiek, Sachs, Geurkink, and Weider (1980) reported on the BAEP findings in a patient with retrocochlear pathology in which the III–V IPL was prolonged in the ear contralateral to the side with the tumor. The hypothesis of a large tumor pressing against the brainstem was confirmed by radiology and at surgery. The presence of a profound hearing loss in the retrocochlear-impaired ear precluded BAEP testing in that ear; the tumor was detected by doing BAEP testing in the non-retrocochlear-impaired ear. Schwartz (1985) found that the I–V IPL was prolonged in the ear contralateral to the side with a large cerebellopontine angle tumor.

11. Combined BAEP Measures

Several investigators judge the BAEP waveform as normal or abnormal on the basis of several rather than just one BAEP measure. The ear is considered abnormal if abnormal findings are obtained on at least one of the BAEP measures. The hit and false alarm rate for BAEP testing based on the use of combined BAEP measures, as reported by various investigators is shown in Table V. As can be seen in Table V, most investigators have reported hit rates exceeding 90% when the evaluation of the BAEP waveform is based on several BAEP measures. These high hit rates indicate that the BAEP test is highly sensitive to the presence of retrocochlear pathology. This table also shows that BAEP testing is less sensitive to cerebellopontine-angle tumors not originating in the internal auditory meatus than to tumors originating in the internal auditory meatus as evidenced by House and Brackmann's findings.

The false-positive rate ranges from 4 to 30%. Such differences may reflect differences in the hearing sensitivity of the control group, the use of different criteria BAEP measures, and the use of different recording parameters.

Table V Hit and False-Alarm Rates for the BAEP Test Based on Multiple Criteria as Reported by Various Investigators

Investigator	Criteria	Hit rate (%)	False-alarm rate (%)
Selters & Brackmann (1977)[a]	1. ILD >0.2 ms for HL up to 50 dB, >0.3 ms for HL of 55-65 dB, >0.4 ms for HL of 70+ dB 2. Wave V absent	91	11
Clemis & McGee (1979)[b]	1. Wave V latency significantly different from the normal mean latency 2. ILD >0.3 ms (>0.4 ms for HL of 65+dB) 3. Absent BAEP	93	30
Glasscock, Jackson, Josey, Dickens, & Wiet (1979)[c]	1. Wave V latency greater than 2SD 2. I-V IPL greater than 2 SD 3. ILD prolonged following Selters & Brackmann (1977)	98	4
House & Brackmann (1979)	1. Wave V latency greater than 2 SD 2. Wave V absent	98[d](75[e])	10 CND[f]
Eggermont, Don, & Brackmann (1980)[g]	1. Absent wave V 2. Absent BAEP 3. Prolonged ILD 4. I-V IPL greater than 2 SD	95	CND
Bauch, Olsen, & Harner (1983)[h]	1. ILD >0.2 ms for HL up to 50 dB, >0.3 ms for 55-65 dB HL, >0.4 ms for HL of 70+ dB 2. Wave V peak latency >6.1 ms bilaterally 3. Absence of the BAEP	97	23
Musiek, Josey, & Glasscock (1986a)[i]	1. I-III IPL greater than 2 SD 2. III-V IPL greater than 2 SD 3. I-V IPL greater than 2 SD 4. IPL >0.3 ms	100	6

[a] Retrocochlear group consisted of ears with acoustic neuroma, meningioma, facial nerve neuroma, cholesteatoma, hemangioma, arachnoid cyst.
[b] Retrocochlear group consisted of ears with vestibular schwannoma; the control group consisted of ears with asymmetric sensorineural hearing loss or conductive hearing loss.
[c] Retrocochlear group consisted of ears with tumors in the internal auditory canal or cerebellopontine angle; statistic reported for the control group was based on ears with Meniere's disease.
[d] Retrocochlear group consisted of ears with acoustic neuroma.
[e] Retrocochlear group consisted of ears with tumors in the cerebellopontine angle other than acoustic neuromas.
[f] Could not determine.
[g] Electrocochleography was used to record wave I; retrocochlear group consisted of ears with pontine angle tumors.
[h] Retrocochlear group consisted of ears with cerebellopontine angle tumors; subjects in the cochlear and retrocochlear groups were matched for hearing loss.
[i] Subjects had to have replicable waves I, III, and V; retrocochlear group consisted of ears with eighth nerve or cerebellopontine angle tumors.

Another factor which may contribute to the high false-positive rates reported by some investigators is the possibility of undetected retrocochlear pathology, such as head trauma, which may affect various levels of the auditory brainstem pathway in the cochlear-impaired and normal-hearing ears. Moller and Moller (1985) reported that vascular compression at the brainstem in older adults may result from looping of the anterior inferior cerebellar artery in the cerebellopontine angle and the audiovestibular and facial nerve bundles. If these loops become elongated because of arteriosclerosis or deterioration of vascular collagen, BAEP abnormalities may result. Symptoms of this disorder include vertigo, unilateral sensorineural hearing impairment, and reduced speech-recognition ability. This disorder cannot be detected by any existing radiographic technique—only by vascular compression studies.

Because of the effect of hearing impairment on the BAEP waveform, the risk of a false-positive result increases as the magnitude of high-frequency hearing impairment increases beyond 50 dB HL. Another factor which may contribute to the false-positive rate is the inability to record wave I in many cases. Without wave I, the I–V IPL, the most powerful measure, cannot be obtained, leading the investigator to rely on less powerful BAEP measures that are more susceptible to the effects of peripheral hearing impairment.

12. The Effect of Tumor Size and Location on the BAEP

Selters and Brackmann (1977) found that tumor size was highly correlated with the ILD. The BAEPs were absent in 30% of the ears with acoustic tumors less than 2.5 cm in size and were absent in 80% of ears with acoustic tumors greater than 2.5 cm in size.

Clemis and McGee (1979) also reported the presence of a significant correlation between tumor size and the ILD for wave V. Nevertheless, one patient with a small tumor had a substantially prolonged ILD. In cases when no response was present, there was a wide range in tumor size. Thus, it is not only the size of the tumor but also the site of the tumor that determines the strength of the effect on the BAEP. Even a small tumor can have a marked effect on the wave V peak latency if it is strategically placed. In general, however, the larger the tumor, the greater its effect on the BAEP latency.

Musiek, Kibbe-Michal, Geurkink, Josey, & Glasscock (1986b) found no correlation between any of the BAEP indices and tumor size in their group of 16 young adult normal-hearing patients with posterior fossa tumors. They suggested that other factors such as tumor consistency, rate of tumor growth, exact site of the tumor, and neural plasticity influence the BAEP in ears with posterior fossa tumors.

In cases of low brainstem lesions, BAEP abnormalities are usually observed in the ear ipsilateral to the side of the pathology unless the lesion is large enough to compress the brainstem, in which case BAEP abnormalities may be observed bilaterally. In cases of high brainstem lesions, BAEP abormalities may be observed ipsilateral or contralateral to the site of the lesion or bilaterally.

13. Summary

From the previous discussion on the use of BAEP testing in differential diagnosis, the following conclusions can be drawn:

1. The most important BAEP indices are the I–V interpeak latency, the absolute peak latency of wave V, the interaural latency difference for wave V, the absence of later waves, or the absence of a BAEP waveform. If the I–V interpeak latency can be obtained, it is usually very sensitive to the presence of retrocochlear pathology and has a low false-alarm rate. The power of BAEP testing is enhanced when

these measures are employed in combination. Moreover, these multiple measures can be obtained without substantially increasing the test time.

2. The effect of high-frequency hearing impairment on the absolute peak latency of wave V becomes more apparent as the magnitude of the hearing impairment exceeds 50 dB HL. Therefore, the false-positive rate is likely to be increased when the hearing impairment exceeds 50 dB HL if the BAEP indices include the absolute peak latency of wave V and the interaural latency difference for wave V. This is true to a lesser extent when BAEP indices include absence of the BAEP. We recommend that, instead of employing a constant correction factor, tolerance limits (two standard deviations above the mean) be developed based on normative data from ears with varying degrees of hearing impairment (particularly exceeding 50 dB HL at 4000 Hz). The tolerance limits should be developed from normative data obtained from one's own clinic. For high-frequency hearing impairment less than 50 dB HL, the interaural latency difference for wave V and absolute peak latency of wave V measures (as well as the I–V interpeak latency) are sensitive to the presence of retrocochlear pathology. If the peak latencies are prolonged at one intensity, BAEP testing should be repeated at a higher intensity (up to a maximum intensity of 95 dBnHL) to see if the latencies normalize.

3. The strength of the I–V interpeak latency becomes particularly apparent as the hearing impairment increases (provided wave I can be recorded). The greater the magnitude of hearing impairment, the greater the difference in the I–V interpeak latency between the cochlear and retrocochlear groups. Since the use of the I–V interpeak latency requires that wave I be recorded, we recommend that techniques be employed which enhance wave I as mentioned in Section X,C,3. If the I–V interpeak latency can be obtained, it is preferred to the ILD and peak latency for wave V measures when the hearing impairment in the high frequencies exceeds 50 dB HL.

4. Bilateral lesions can be detected by the presence of bilaterally abnormal BAEP results; the ILD measure is insensitive to the presence of bilateral lesions.

5. Large tumors pressing on the brainstem can sometimes be detected on the basis of the BAEP from the ear contralateral to the lesion when auditory stimulation is presented to the ear contralateral to the side of the lesion. This effect is particularly important in cases when the BAEP cannot be elicited from the ear ipsilateral to the lesion.

6. There are some drawbacks to the use of the following measures for differential diagnosis: IV–V:I AR, nonreplicability, waveform distortion, and high repetition rates. The AR is also susceptible to

recording and stimulation variables. The nonreplicability measure makes it difficult to maintain quality control. Waveform distortion is difficult to quantify. There is disagreement in the literature regarding the utility of repetition rates. At this time, we recommend that abnormalities seen at high repetition rates not be considered pathological unless they enhance abnormalities seen at low repetition rates. Clinicians who choose to use these BAEP measures for differential diagnosis should exercise caution.

7. Before considering a BAEP abnormality in a presumably cochlear ear as indicative of a false-positive result when tumors have been ruled out on the basis of definitive medical tests, other factors should be considered, such as the possibility of vascular disorder in the brainstem, head trauma, or neurologic disease affecting the brainstem.

XI. PITFALLS IN BAEP TESTING AND INTERPRETATION

Although BAEP testing involves measurement of an objective response, it involves subjective interpretation since the clinician must make a decision regarding the presence/absence of the response and the components of the response. Weber (1983) noted that one of the problems with BAEP assessment was that repeating stimulus conditions prolongs the test time, an important consideration since a time-consuming procedure may result in the patient's awakening or becoming restless. Obtaining only fair agreement between replications makes it difficult for the examiner to determine the next step: to obtain another replication or to proceed without another replication. Weber (1983) contended that the absence of a BAEP at a given intensity did not necessarily mean that the response was absent. Factors to be ruled out include restlessness of the patient and extrapatient contamination, for example, 60-Hz interference. Even when a BAEP is present, it may not be possible to determine a latency value precisely because of poor waveform morphology, for example, a mound-shaped peak reflecting fusing of waves IV and V (particularly at high intensity levels), multiple bumps in the region of wave V, poor test–retest reliability, and cyclic appearing waves in infants.

Extrapolation of the BAEP threshold from the response latencies is complicated when adequate normative data are unavailable. Moreover, latency does not change with intensity in many sensorineural hearing-impaired subjects in the same manner that it does in normal-hearing subjects. Hence, it is difficult to extrapolate the BAEP threshold from the latency values in such cases. Furthermore, since only the high-intensity fibers (and not also the low-intensity fibers)

are activated at high intensities in persons with sensorineural hearing impairment, the latency calculated at such high intensities may result in miscalculation of the BAEP threshold.

Control runs (recordings obtained at the lowest intensity limits of the instrument) are usually obtained in order to rule out extrapatient sources of the BAEP waveform. Hence, a component appearing during stimulation but not during the control run is assumed to originate from intrapatient sources. Weber cautions that a stimulus run may differ from a control run because of the presence of a stimulus artifact with a shape similar to wave I in a stimulus run conducted at high intensities. Another problem with respect to control runs, which Weber noted, is that many clinicians terminate a control run when movement artifacts are seen. When a stimulus run is done at high-intensity levels, the clinician is less likely to terminate the run since the artifacts are highly likely to be mistaken for responses.

> As a result, a stimulus run containing artifact contamination (but no response) could be erroneously scored as a response because it differs markedly from the much less contaminated control runs. If a more stringent criterion for acceptance is applied to the control runs than to the stimulus runs, serious interpretation errors can result. (Weber, 1983, p. 181)

The artifact-reject function discards any sweep containing an amplitude exceeding some preset voltage. According to Weber (1983), some clinicians have assumed that the BAEP record quality is inversely related to the number of rejected sweeps during a stimulus run. If the electrophysiologic voltage is markedly smaller than the preset voltage amplitude required to trigger the artifact-reject function, then movement artifacts in addition to the response may not trigger the artifact-reject function. Consequently, the stimulus run will be characterized by few rejected sweeps but many artifacts. On the other hand, if the electrophysiologic voltage is close to that of the preset voltage of the artifact-reject function, then a movement artifact will usually trigger the artifact-reject function. Hence, the stimulus run will be characterized by many rejected sweeps but few artifacts. Thus, lowering the amplifier gain to reduce the number of rejected sweeps will create the spurious impression of a better quality BAEP recording. Lowering the amplifier gain will cause the amplitude of the response and the artifact to be reduced so that the artifact-reject function will not be triggered. Consequently, the stimulus run will be more contaminated by artifacts. Weber reminds the clinician that the artifact-reject function reduces but does not eliminate artifacts, as evidenced by contamination of tracings resulting from swallowing, chewing, and eyeblinks.

Concerning the use of BAEPs for differential diagnosis, Weber provides the following remarks. First, the use of clicks presented at equal sensation levels (SLs) relative to the behavioral threshold for the click stimulus to the two ears does not rule out the effects of asymmetrical hearing levels and is not always feasible. That is, such SLs may result in presentation levels beyond the equipment limits and the use of a lower SL to accommodate equipment limits may result in a less effective stimulus. Second, since a patient with a sharply sloping loss may have a low behavioral threshold for clicks because of good low-frequency hearing, the use of a stimulus intensity based on SL in this patient may not effectively elicit a BAEP which contains its primary energy in the 2000- to 4000-Hz region. Moreover, the use of equivalent SLs may result in near-normal latency values, evidence of recruitment-like behavior, in a person with sensorineural hearing impairment; consequently, less asymmetry in the peak latencies would exist at high than at low intensity levels. Therefore, presentation at equal SLs does not necessarily result in equal loudness. The use of equal hearing levels results in equivalent physical stimulation of the two ears.

Weber (1983) addressed the problem of identifying the BAEP components, particularly in subjects with high-frequency hearing impairment. In such patients, wave I is difficult to detect and the peaks are often rounded rather than sharply defined. Weber advises against reporting peak latency values to the nearest 0.01 ms when ambiguity regarding peak location exists. The problem is compounded when waveform morphology differs in the two ears, complicating the comparison of the peak latencies from the two ears. The I–V IPL is not free of peripheral influences, as evidenced by the presence of reduced I–III and I–V IPLs in cochlear hearing-impaired ears. In some cases, combined cochlear and retrocochlear pathologies in the same ear may result in a normal I–V IPL, since the effect of cochlear pathology may offset, at least to some extent, the effect of retrocochlear pathology on the IPL. Thus, this finding may occur in cases of retrocochlear lesions that disrupt the blood supply to the cochlea, resulting in a combined cochlear and retrocochlear disorder. Stockard and Stockard (1983) suggested that the clinician should not attempt to compare the interpeak latencies from the two ears unless the interaural wave I peak latency difference does not exceed 0.1 ms. Weber (1983) feels this criterion is difficult to uphold since most patients referred for BAEP testing have asymmetrical audiometric configurations.

Weber (1983) observed that wave I cannot always be obtained, so heavy reliance must be placed on the absolute peak latency of wave V in such cases. When the absolute latency of wave V is employed, corrections for high-frequency hearing impairment are made. Weber (1983) proposed that such corrections are not always adequate. The use of such formulas may result in overcorrected or undercorrected results. Moreover, the presence of even a minor conductive component can prolong wave V latency so that it becomes difficult to determine whether any part of

the delay is attributable to the presence of retrocochlear pathology. Weber (1983) noted that the delay can be estimated from the air–bone gap in cases of middle-ear effusion but not in cases of ossicular-chain disorders.

Criteria for detection of retrocochlear pathology have included reproducibility, amplitude, morphology, and absence of waves. Nevertheless, as Stockard et al. (1978b) have shown, alterations in these aspects of the BAEPs can also result from peripheral hearing impairment and technical or stimulus factors. Since waveform morphology and reproducibility cannot be determined completely objectively, Weber (1983) suggested that waveform morphology and reproducibility not be considered pathognomic of retrocochlear lesions. Tinnitus, for example, can affect the BAEP as a result of its masking effects (Seitz, Mundy, & Pappas, 1981).

XII. BAEPs IN INFANTS

A. THRESHOLD

Wave I first appears at 27–30 weeks conceptional age (Stockard et al., 1983a). By the conceptional age of 32 weeks, the average threshold for wave I is 85 dBpeSPL. At the conceptional age of more than 32 weeks, the wave I threshold is less than or equal to 75 dBpeSPL at low repetition rates and with large sampling sizes. (Conceptional age is the gestational age as estimated from the first day of the mother's last menses added to the postnatal age.) Stockard et al. (1983a) also reported that a single long duration of the late component with a late (greater than 9 ms) vertex peak, termed wave Vn, appears at 27–30 weeks. Wave V lags behind waves I and Vn in peak definition. Wave V is easily discernible after 32 weeks. Some typical infant BAEPs are shown in Figure 28. The neonate BAEP differs from the adult BAEP in that it consists primarily of waves I, III, and V, and the amplitude of wave V is reduced whereas the amplitude of wave I is increased in comparison with the adult peak amplitudes. When wave II is present in infant BAEP waveforms, it is usually superimposed on the negative slope following wave I (Stapells, 1989).

B. PEAK LATENCY

The results of studies on the peak latencies of the BAEPs indicated that auditory maturation is incomplete at birth (Salamy & McKean, 1976; Starr, Amlie, Martin & Sanders, 1977). Fria and Doyle (1984) reported that the peak latencies for waves I, III, and V decreased with age in infants between 32 weeks conceptional age and 36 months as seen for click stimulation at 60 dBnHL. The maturational process was completed by 2 years of age. The most rapid changes were seen at conceptional ages between 23 and 44 weeks. The peak latency for wave I, however decreased

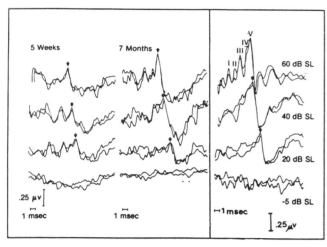

Figure 28 Brain stem evoked responses at three age levels. Each tracing represents the sum of 1000 to 2000 responses to 0.1-ms monaural click, delivered 30 times per second at the intensity level (with respect to adult threshold) shown on right; superimposed tracings are replications. Vertex positive is plotted upward. Successive waves are designated I–V on 60 dB SL adult record according to the convention of Jewett and Williston (1971). Note stability of wave V (arrows) and increase in latency with decreased stimulus intensity in all subjects. From Hecox & Galambos (1974) with permission.

from birth to 8–10 weeks with no further changes thereafter. Thus, there are two stages of maturation of peak latencies: (a) a very rapid stage up to 8–10 weeks postnatally, which reflects both peripheral and central changes; and (b) a less rapid stage plateauing at about 110 weeks postpartum (2.1 years) which reflects the maturation of the central components. Gorga, Kaminski, Beauchaine, Jesteadt, and Neely (1989) reported the absence of maturational effects on the interaural latency difference for wave V.

Fria and Doyle (1984) concluded that two exponential models were required to account for the maturational effects on the wave V latencies. Gorga et al. (1989), on the other hand, concluded that a single exponential model could describe the maturational effects of wave V latency.

C. INTERPEAK LATENCY

Stockard et al. (1983a) reported that the I–V IPL in infants was characterized by great intersubject variability. The mean I–V IPL at 110 dBpeSPL for rarefaction clicks presented at a rate of 10/s was 7.3 ms. Hence, the infant IPL is increased, compared with that in adults. Before term, the major decrease in the I–V IPL with age occurs prior to 33 weeks. Fria and Doyle (1984) also reported that the I–V IPL decreases with age and does so in a manner similar to the decrease in the peak latencies of waves III and V. Stockard et al. (1983a) reported that the I–V IPL values are distributed normally in full term but not in high-risk premature infants.

D. LATENCY–INTENSITY FUNCTION

At gestational ages of less than 32 weeks, the slopes of the latency–intensity functions for waves I and V are steeper than in full-term infants; by 36 weeks gestational age, the slope of the latency–intensity function is approximately equivalent to that of full-term infants (Stockard, Stockard, Kleinberg, and Westmoreland, 1983b). The intersubject variability in slope decreases with gestational age. By 1–2 months postnatal age, the slope of the latency–intensity function is similar to that in adults.

E. RECORDING TECHNIQUES

Because peak latencies are prolonged in newborns and infants, the sweep duration is increased to 10–32 ms (Hecox & Galambos, 1974; Mokotoff, Schulman-Galambos, & Galambos, 1977; Starr et al., 1977) with the sweep time of approximately 20 ms most commonly employed. Stapells (1989) recommends an analysis time of 15 ms for click-elicited BAEPs and 25 ms for tone-elicited BAEPs. Routine repetition rates generally range from 5 to 40 per second (Frye-Osier, Goldstein, Hirsch, & Weber, 1982; Starr et al., 1977; stockard et al., 1983a).

The bandpass filter commonly employed in the pediatric population is 100–3000 Hz although lower low-frequency cutoffs have been employed (Hecox, Cone, & Blaw, 1981; Hecox & Galambos, 1974; Stockard et al., 1979). Low-frequency cutoffs are sometimes used when tone pips are employed. Nevertheless, such low-frequency cutoffs below 100 Hz are infeasible when testing in a noisy environment such as a nursery (Stockard et al., 1983b).

Sample sizes of at least 2000 and up to 8000 have been employed (Starr et al., 1977; Stockard et al., 1979; Stockard et al., 1983b) because response amplitudes are smaller in infants and because noise levels are higher in the nursery test environment than in a sound-treated audiometric booth.

Rarefaction phase is most commonly employed for click-elicited BAEPs in infants because of greater response stability and better resolution of wave I, although alternating phase is more commonly employed for tone-elicited BAEPs.

Electrode impedance values are often higher in infants than in adults. It is desirable to have electrode impedance values below 5000 ohms. Electrode impedance values should not exceed 10,000 ohms. Interelectrode impedances should be kept below 1000 ohms, whenever possible.

Mild sedation is generally employed in uncooperative children and infants more than 6–12 months of age in BAEP testing to reduce the effect of muscle activity on the recording. The most commonly employed sedatives include chloral hydrate (taken orally), secobarbitol (administered intramuscularly), DPT (combination of Demerol, Phenergan, and Thorazine), and nembutal. The use of a sedative combined with sleep deprivation the night before the test often ensures that the sleep induced by the drug is of sufficient length to enable completion of the BAEP test.

The Committee on Hearing, Bioacoustics, and Biomechanics (CHABA) (1987) recommended the following recording techniques for BAEP testing of infants: (a) the use of an earphone with a known high-frequency acoustical response as a transducer: (b) controlling for ear-canal collapse resulting from placement of the headphones; (c) testing when subjects are asleep, resting comfortably, or under sedation if artifact potentials from eyes, jaw, head, or body movement cannot otherwise be reduced; (d) controlling for acoustical leaks of low-frequency energy from the headphones; (e) using a filter frequency range of 100–3000 Hz; (f) employing an instrument with a resolution for each digitized point not greater than 50 ms; (g) employing an instrument with at least a 10-bit A–D converter and preferably a 12-bit A–D converter that can resolve 1 part in 4096 in amplitude; (h) using a sound-treated room meeting ISO (ANSI) standards for hearing testing; (i) using the Cz, Fp, M_1 and M_2 (or A_1 and A_2) sites for electrode placement; and (j) establishing norms with identical equipment and parameters as those used for testing.

F. BAEP SCREENING OF INFANTS

Several centers conduct BAEP screenings of newborns for the purpose of identification of hearing impairment and/or neurologic disorders. Table VI shows the pass/fail criteria employed by seven centers which have newborn BAEP screening programs. As can be seen in this table, some programs have both audiologic and neurologic criteria.

CHABA (1987) made the following recommendations for BAEP newborn screening: (a) intensities less than or equal to 30 dBnHL for full-term infants and 40 dBnHL for less than full-term infants (<35 weeks conceptional age); (b) repetition rate of 10–20/s for full-term infants and less than or equal to 10/s for less than full-term infants; (c) BBN click with a known spectrum and controlled polarity and rate; (d) screening at or near the time of discharge when the infant is healthy, breathes room air, and is free of respiratory distress, systemic illness, apnea, or bradycardia; and (e) screening of all infants failing the High Risk Register developed by the Joint Committee on Newborn Screening and all infants in the intensive care nursery.

CHABA (1987) concluded that the uncertainties in interpretation of BAEPs for infants are greater than those for adults because of the influence of developmental changes: neurologic changes, such as myelination of the central nervous system pathways and growth of neurons and synapses of the central nervous system, and peripheral changes, such as changes in the volume and impedance of the outer and middle ears and structural changes in the cochlea. These physiologic and anatomic developmental changes are asso-

Table VI Loss Criteria of Seven Testing Programs[a]

Program[b]	Peripheral	Central
1	Wave I delayed latency with shift in threshold	(wave V–wave I) Interpeak latency Absence of I, III, and/or V, either ear
2	ABR threshold greater than 30 dB HLn Latency I and V greater than normal but (V–I) normal Get intensity function (3 levels); if intensity function is parallel to normal, then conductive	(V–I) Interpeak latency greater than 2 SD
3	No repeatable response at 20–25 dB HLn	(PASS) Waves I through V present at 60 dB HLn; (V-I) Interpeak latency greater than or equal to 4.8-5.4 ms (term newborns); V/I amplitude ratio equal to or greater than 1/2
4[b]	—	No response at 30 dB HLN, either ear is failure, that ear
5[b]	—	No wave V at 40–60 dB HLn
6[b]	—	No repeatable wave V at 35 dB HLn No wave III with normal interpeak latency
7[b]	—	Two-trial fail, wave V, right or left ear

[a] From CHABA (1987).
[b] Loss criteria for programs 4–7 might occasionally be peripheral in origin.

ciated with developmental changes in the peak latencies and amplitudes.

The issue of the validity of the ABR for infants is more complex than that for adults, since long-term prediction is involved, in addition to measurement of current auditory function. It is now clear that profoundly hearing-impaired infants will not develop adequate social communication without some major form of intervention. Among infants tested in intensive care unit (ICU) populations, a recent review of published reports concludes that 12–17% have abnormal ABR responses on initial tests, and of those, approximately one-third were confirmed later as hearing impaired (Murry, Javel, & Watson, 1985). The working group recognizes, of course, that detection of those infants with auditory dysfunction may justify some significant rate of false-positive testing programs. Current data are inadequate, however, to allow precise estimates of the actual rate of correct detection and false-positives in ABR testing of neonates, primarily because of the lack of adequate follow-up data in the ICU population (Murray et al., 1985).

The submicrovolt magnitudes of the ABR waves, the requirement for sophisticated instrumentation and skill in its proper use, the limited range of acoustical stimuli that evoke clear, unambiguous ABRs, and the inherent difficulties of interpreting physiological responses produced by the summation of electrical activity from large groups of neural elements suggest that great caution should be used in deriving detailed inferences about underlying pathology from the ABR. Despite limitations on the applicability of ABRs and their highly empirical scientific status, in certain circumstances they provide a useful tool for drawing inferences about the state of the auditory nervous system (CHABA, 1987, pp. 48–49).

Stapells (1989) recommends that BAEP testing for hearing-screening purposes be deferred until the neonate is at least 2 months old (corrected age) to avoid failure because of immaturity and transient conductive hearing impairment. Stapells (1989) reported that BAEP testing of infants before this age is generally done to obtain neurologic information. Nevertheless, even BAEPs done for neurologic purposes are not done before the infant attains term age; if any BAEP abnormality is present at this time, the BAEP is repeated after the infant attains 2 months corrected age.

The ASHA (1989) guidelines for audiologic screenings of newborn infants at risk for hearing impairment recommends BAEP screening of infants at risk as defined by the following criteria: (a) familial history of childhood hearing impairment; (b) congenital perinatal infections (e.g., cytomegalovirus, rubella, herpes, toxoplasmosis, syphilis); (c) anatomic malformation involving the head or neck; (d) birthweight <1500 gm; (e) hyperbilirubinemia at levels exceeding indications for exchange transfusion; (f) bacterial meningitis; and (g) severe asphyxia which may include infants with Apgar scores of 0–3 who fail to institute spontaneous respiration by 10 min and those with hypotonia persisting to 2 hr of age. ASHA (1989) recommends BAEP screening of high-risk infants prior to hospital discharge. The ASHA (1989) pass criterion is a response to a ≤ 40 dBnHL click (or tonebursts/tone pips) having energy in the frequency region important for speech recognition, bilaterally. Infants who fail should receive comprehensive and medical intervention. Habilitation of hearing-impaired infants should be instituted by 6 months of age. If an infant fails BAEP screening in only one ear, audiologic monitoring should continue until both ears meet pass criteria or stable unilateral hearing impairment is confirmed. The ASHA (1989) guidelines also recommend professional interpretation of results, parent/caregiver counseling, and screening of infants not at risk for hearing impairment if the parent/caregiver or primary health-care provider has concern about the infant's communicative development.

XIII. SPECIAL APPLICATIONS OF BAEP TESTING

A. COMATOSE POPULATION

One recent application of brainstem auditory-evoked potentials testing is with patients who are comatose. The purpose of BAEP testing in this population is twofold: to determine whether brain death is present and to predict the neurologic prognosis (Keith, Jabre, & Heerse, 1983). Starr (1976) evaluated the BAEPs in 27 patients who met the criteria for brain death. The BAEP was absent in 16 cases and only wave I was present with a prolonged latency in 1 case. He found that serial BAEP recordings in 4 patients with acute anoxia revealed deteriorating BAEPs over time, consistent with brainstem deterioration. He also found that in patients close to anoxia, serial BAEPs revealed that the peak latencies increased and the peak amplitudes decreased over time until the waves disappeared, one at a time, starting with wave V, until only wave I was present, consistent with brain death. Several investigators (Brewer & Resnick, 1981; Hall, Huang-Fu, & Gennarelli, 1982; Keith et al., 1983) reported that absent or markedly abnormal BAEPs were highly correlated with eventual death. Keith et al. (1983) concluded that BAEPs can be used to confirm brain death in cases in which all bioelectric activity is absent. They also concluded that when a series of BAEPs show increasing abnormalities over time, the findings are consistent with deteriorating brainstem function. A normal BAEP, on the other hand, is not as highly predictive of a good neurologic outcome as a markedly abnormal BAEP is of a poor neurologic outcome; almost half of the patients with a normal BAEP eventually died or had a poor neurologic outcome (Brewer & Resnick, 1981; Hall et al., 1982; Keith et al., 1983).

Hall et al. (1982) reported that 60% of their comatose patients had abnormal tympanometric results and 84% had abnormal acoustic-reflex results. Thus, middle-ear abnormalities must be taken into consideration when evaluating BAEPs in patients who are comatose, particularly in those with a recent history of severe head injury. The possibility of the presence of sensorineural hearing impairment must also be taken into consideration when evaluating the BAEPs from comatose patients, particularly when there is a recent history of transverse or longitudinal head injury (Keith et al., 1983). Another factor to consider when evaluating the BAEPs from a comatose patient is the possibility of a previous central nervous system disorder such as multiple sclerosis; a careful history to detect previous central nervous system disorder is important in such cases (Keith et al., 1983). Keith et al. (1983) found that barbiturate coma, intracranial pressures as high as 50 cm H₂0, and hypotension do not significantly affect the BAEPs. Hypothermia, a condition common in comatose patients and those under-going open-heart surgery with cardiopulmonary bypass, results in prolongation of the I–V IPLs by 1.6 msec for every 10°C decrease in esophageal temperature (Stockard *et al.*, (1978a)).

According to Keith *et al.* (1983), variables in the surgical intensive care unit (SICU) which can adversely affect the BAEPs obtained include (a) high ambient noise levels; (b) fluorescent light bulbs and other electrical monitoring equipment resulting in electromagnetic radiation and the 60-Hz hum. To reduce the deleterious effects of the 60-Hz hum, the BAEP device should be well grounded and the electrode leads should be as short as possible.

For BAEP testing in the SICU, one should have a portable BAEP device which is free of shock hazard and has an isolation transformer. The presence of turban bandages, neck collars, electronic monitors, feeding tubes, intravenous lines, or intracranial pressure monitors may interfere with electrode and earphone placement. Keith *et al.* (1983) suggest the use of a hand-held headphone or a high-frequency hearing-aid receiver with a standard earmold, provided the electroacoustic characteristics are known and normative data are available. They also suggest the use of the forehead placement or the site several centimeters posterior to the Cz location when the vertex position is unattainable. Ear clip electrodes are recommended when the mastoid position is unfeasible. An alternative to the forehead site for the ground electrode placement is the shoulder. Keith *et al.* (1983) suggest considering the use of needle electrodes in patients with severe burns.

B. INTRAOPERATIVE MONITORING

Another application of the BAEPs is in intraoperative monitoring of the functional status of the auditory pathway during posterior fossa neurosurgery (Grundy, Lina, Procopio, & Jannetta, 1981; Grundy, Jannetta, Procopio, Lina, Boston, & Doyle, 1982; Levine, 1979). During surgery, serial recordings of the BAEPs are obtained and compared with the preoperative baseline BAEP. A difference between the intraoperative BAEP recordings and preoperative recordings is indicative of disruption of auditory brainstem function and possible injury to the auditory brainstem.

A difference between the intraoperative and preoperative BAEPs can be considered significant only if technical, pharmacologic, and physiologic factors can be ruled out. Schwartz, Bloom, and Dennis (1985) discussed the technical factors to be considered when doing intraoperative monitoring of the BAEPs. One factor is poor or unmatched electrode impedance. To reduce the influence of this factor, Schwartz *et al.* (1985) suggest using collodion to affix electrodes to the scalp and two electrodes at each recording site

in case an electrode becomes dislodged or develops high impedance. Another technical factor to be considered is the 60-Hz hum which can be controlled by shielding electrode cables, braiding, and isolating the electrode cables from other power sources such as power cords. Schwartz *et al.* (1985) also suggest checking to be sure that the transducer is properly positioned, that the electrode leads are intact, and that the stimulus generator is on. They reported that a BAEP device with an internal artifact-reject feature and a pause mode is desirable for preventing BAEPs that are contaminated by high-frequency noise from surgical instruments—such as the bovie, bipolar forceps, drills, or cavitrons—from being averaged. They also recommend obtaining a control run during intraoperative monitoring so the BAEPs elicited with acoustic stimuli can be compared against the averaged electroencephalographic activity without stimulation. Regarding the pharmacologic factors, some pharmacologic agents have a slight effect on the BAEPs (Stockard & Sharbrough, 1980).

The intraoperative BAEP protocol recommended by Schwartz *et al.* (1985) follows. Pairs of electrodes are attached with collodion at the Cz, A_1, and A_2 sites with FPz as the ground. An ear-canal electrode is inserted to enhance wave I. Clicks of alternating polarity are employed. The stimulus is transduced through an Etymotic Research (ER-3) insert transducer fitted into the ear canal with a foam plug. To keep the insert transducer in place, the ear canal is taped or sealed with bone wax. The transducer assembly is taped to the patient's chest and isolated from the electrode and other monitoring leads. Schwartz *et al.* (1985) recommend that the preoperative BAEP be obtained the day before surgery and immediately after anesthesia is administered. The BAEPs are then monitored continuously during surgery. The neurosurgeon is notified of changes in the BAEPs only after technical factors have been ruled out; the contralateral ear is used as a control for detecting technical errors or global ischemia. Changes in the BAEPs are considered significant only if the peak latency is prolonged by at least 2.0 ms and the amplitude is decreased by more than 50%. If these changes occur or the BAEP becomes obliterated without returning before the end of surgery, the patient is at risk for permanent neurologic insult. If these changes or the BAEP absence are transient, there is a lesser risk of permanent neurologic insult.

According to Schwartz *et al.* (1985), BAEP changes can result from surgical manipulations or patient physiologic states such as excessive retractor tension, poorly positioned retractors, stretching of a cranial nerve, placement of cool saline directly on the cranial nerve, hypotension, hypocarbia, trauma to the nervous system during tumor dissection, and so forth.

Several investigators (Grantz, Holliday, Gmuer, & Fisch, 1984; Moller & Jannetta, 1984; Schwartz *et al.*, 1985) suggested recording the motor action potentials of the facial nerve (which can be obtained along with the BAEPs) during surgery that may place the facial nerve at risk for insult or damage, such as acoustic tumor dissection, parotidectomy, facial nerve decompression, and difficult mastoid procedures.

REFERENCES

Abraham, K., & Ajmone-Marsan, C. (1958). Patterns of cortical discharges and their relation to routine scalp electroencephalography. *Electroencephalogr. Clin. Neurophysiol., 10,* 447–461.

Allison, T., Hume, A. L., Wood, C. C., & Goff, W. (1984). Developmental and aging changes in somatosensory, auditory, and visual evoked potentials. *Electroencephalogr. Clin. Neurophysiol., 58,* 14–24.

American Speech–Language–Hearing Association (1989). Audiologic screening of newborn infants who are at risk for hearing impairment. *Asha, 31,* 89–92.

Barratt, H. (1980). Investigation of the mastoid electrode contribution to the brain stem auditory evoked response. *Scand. Audiol., 9,* 203–211.

Bauch, C. D., Olsen, W. O., & Harner, S. G. (1983). Auditory brainstem responses and acoustic reflex test: Results from patients with and without tumor matched for hearing loss. *Arch. Otolaryngol., 109,* 522–525.

Bauch, C. D., Rose, D. E., & Harner, S. G. (1980). Brainstem responses to tone pip and click stimuli. *Ear Hear., 1,* 181–184.

Bauch, C., Rose, D., & Harner, S. (1982). Auditory brainstem response results from 255 patients with suspected retrocochlear involvement. *Ear Hear., 3,* 83–86.

Beagley, H. A., & Sheldrake, J. B. (1978). Differences in brainstem response latency with age and sex. *Br. J. Audiol., 12,* 69–77.

Beattie, R. C., & Boyd, R. (1984). Effects of click duration on the latency of the early evoked response. *J. Speech Hear. Res., 27,* 70-76.

Beattie, R. C., Beguwala, F. E., Mills, D. M., & Boyd, R. L. (1986) Latency and amplitude effects of electrode placement on the early auditory evoked response. *J. Speech Hear. Dis., 51,* 63–70.

Berlin, C. I., & Dobie, R. A. (1979). Electrophysiologic measures of auditory function via electrocochleography and brainstem-evoked responses. In W. F. Rintelmann (ed.), *Hearing assessment,* pp. 425–458. Baltimore: University Park Press.

Bhargava, V. K., Salamy, A., & McKean, C. W. (1978). Effect of cholinergic drugs on the brainstem auditory evoked response (far-field) in rats. *Neuroscience, 13,* 821–826.

Bickford, R. G., Jacobson, J. L., & Cody, T. R. (1964). Nature of averaged evoked potentials to sound and other stimuli in man. *Ann. N.Y. Acad. Sci., 112,* 204–223.

Boezeman, E., Kapteyn, T., Visser, S., & Snel, A. (1983) Comparison of the latencies between bone and air conduction in the auditory brainstem evoked potential. *Electroencephalogr. Clin. Neurophysiol., 56,* 244–247.

Borg, E., Lofqvist, L., & Rosen, S. (1981). Brainstem response (ABR) in conductive hearing loss. *Scand. Audiol. Suppl., 13,* 95–97.

Brewer, C. C., & Resnick, D. M. (1981). Predictive accuracy of ABR in comatose patients. Paper presented at the Annual Convention of the American Speech–Language–Hearing Association, Los Angeles, California.

Burkard, R. (1984). Sound pressure level measurement and spectral analysis of brief acoustic transients. *Electroencephalogr. Clin. Neurophysiol., 57,* 83–91.

Burkard, R., & Hecox, K. (1983a). The effect of broadband noise on the

human brainstem auditory evoked response. I. Rate and intensity effects. *J. Acoust. Soc. Am., 74,* 1204–1213.

Burkard, R., & Hecox, K. (1983b). The effect of broadband noise on the human brainstem auditory evoked response. II. Frequency specificity. *J. Acoust. Soc. Am., 74,* 1214–1223.

Cashman, M., & Rossman, R. (1983). Diagnostic features of the auditory brainstem response in identifying cerebellopontine angle tumors. *Scand. Audiol., 12,* 35–41.

Celesia, G. G. (1968). Auditory evoked responses: Intracranial and extracranial average evoked responses. *Arch. Neurol., 19,* 430–437.

Chiappa, K. (1983). *Evoked potentials in clinical medicine.* New York: Raven Press.

Chiappa, K. H., Gladstone, K. J., & Young, R. R. (1979). Brain stem auditory evoked responses: Studies of waveform variation in 50 normal human subjects. *Arch. Neurol., 36,* 81–87.

Chiappa, K. H., Harrison, J. L., Brooks, E. B., & Young, R. R. (1980). Brainstem auditory evoked potentials in multiple sclerosis. *Neurol., 30,* 110–123.

Chu, N. (1985). Age-related latency changes in the brain-stem auditory evoked potentials. *Electroencephalogr. Clin. Neurophysiol., 62,* 431–436.

Chu, N. S., Squires, K. C., & Starr, A. (1978). Auditory brain stem potentials in chronic alcohol intoxication and alcohol withdrawal. *Arch. Neurol., 35,* 596–602.

Clemis, J. D., & McGee, T. (1979). Brain stem electric response audiometry in the differential diagnosis of acoustic tumors. *Laryngoscope, 1,* 31–42.

Clemis, J. D., & Mitchell, C. (1977). Electrocochleography and brainstem responses used in the diagnosis of acoustic tumors. *J. Otolaryngol., 6,* 447–458.

Coats, A. C. (1978). Human auditory nerve action potentials in brainstem evoked responses: Latency–intensity functions in detection of cochlear and retrocochlear abnormality. *Arch. Otolaryngol., 104,* 709–717.

Coats, A. C. (1983). Instrumentation. In E. J. Moore (ed.) *Bases of auditory brain-stem evoked responses,* pp. 197–220. New York: Grune & Stratton.

Coats, A. C., & Martin, J. L. (1977). Human auditory nerve action potentials and brainstem evoked responses: Effects of audiogram shape and lesion location. *Arch. Otolaryngol., 103,* 605–622.

Committee on Hearing, Bioacoustics, and Biomechanics (1987). Brainstem audiometry of infants. *Asha, 29,* 47–55.

Conraux, C., Dauman, R., & Fablot, Pl. (1981). Potentials evoques auditifs rapides "derives." *Audiology, 20,* 382–393.

Davis, H. (1976a). Brain stem and other responses in electric response audiometry. *Ann. Otol. Rhinol. Laryngol., 85,* 1–12.

Davis, H. (1976b). Principles of electric response audiometry. *Ann. Otol. Rhinol. Laryngol. Suppl., 28,* 1–96.

Davis, H., & Hirsh, S. K. (1976). The audiometric utility of brainstem responses to low-frequency sounds. *Audiology, 15,* 181–195.

Davis, H., & Hirsh, S. K. (1979). A slow brainstem response for low-frequency audiometry. *Audiology, 18,* 445–461.

Davis, H., Hirsh, S. K., & Turpin, L. L. (1983). Possible utility of middle-latency responses in electric response audiometry. *Adv. Oto-Rhino-Laryngol., 31,* 208–216.

Davis, H., Hirsh, S. K., Popelka, G. R., & Formby, C. (1984). Frequency selectivity and thresholds of brief stimuli suitable for electric response audiometry. *Audiology, 23,* 59–74.

Davis, H., Hirsh, S. K., Turpin, L. L., & Peacock, M. E. (1985). Threshold sensitivity and frequency specificity in auditory brainstem audiometry. *Audiology, 24,* 54–70.

Dawson, W. W., & Doddington, A. W. (1973). Phase distortion of biological signals: Extraction of signal from noise without phase error. *Electroencephalogr. Clin. Neurophysiol., 34,* 207–211.

Dobie, R. A., & Berlin, C. I. (1979). Binaural interaction in brainstem evoked responses. *Arch. Otolaryngol., 105,* 391–398.

Don, M., Allen, A. R., & Starr, A. (1977). Effect of click rate on the latency of auditory brainstem responses in humans. *Ann. Otol. Rhinol. Laryngol., 86,* 186–195.

Doyle, D. J., & Hyde, M. L. (1981a). Bessel filtering of brain stem auditory evoked potentials. *Electroencephalogr. Clin. Neurophysiol., 51,* 446–448.

Doyle, D. J., & Hyde, M. L. (1981b). Analogue and digital filtering of auditory brainstem response. *Scand. Audiol., 10,* 31–39.

Duncan, P. G., Sanders, R. A., & McCullough, D. W. (1979). Preservation of auditory-evoked brainstem responses in anesthetized children. *Can. Anesthesiol. Soc. J., 26,* 492–495.

Eggermont, J. (1982). The inadequacy of click-evoked auditory brainstem responses in audiological applications. *Ann. N.Y. Acad. Sci., 388,* 707–709.

Eggermont, J. J., Don, M., & Brackmann, D. E. (1980). Electrocochleography and auditory brainstem electric responses in patients with pontine angle tumors. *Ann. Otol. Rhinol. Laryngol. Suppl., 75,* 1–19.

Elberling, C., & Parbo, J. (1987). Reference data for ABRs in retrocochlear diagnosis. *Scand. Audiol., 16,* 49–55.

Elidan, J., Sohmer, H., Gafni, M., & Kahana, E. (1982). Contribution of changes in click rate and intensity on diagnosis of multiple sclerosis by brainstem auditory evoked potentials. *Acta Neurol. Scand., 65,* 570–585.

Finitzo-Hieber, T., Hecox, K., & Cone, B. (1979). Brain stem auditory evoked potentials in patients with congenital atresia. *Laryngoscope, 89,* 1151–1158.

Folsom, R. C. (1984). Frequency specificity of human auditory brainstem responses as revealed by pure-tone masking profiles. *J. Acoust. Soc. Am., 75,* 919–924.

Fria, T. J., & Doyle, W. J. (1984). Maturation of the auditory brain stem response (ABR): Additional perspectives. *Ear Hear., 5,* 361–365.

Frye-Osier, H. A., Goldstein, R., Hirsch, J. E., & Weber, K. (1982). Early and middle-ABR components to click as response indices for neonatal hearing screening. *Ann. Otol. Rhinol. Laryngol., 91,* 272–276.

Gabor, A. J. (1979). *Physiological basis of electrical activity of cerebral origin.* Quincy, Massachusetts: Grass Instrument Co.

Galambos, R. (1982). Tactile and auditory stimuli repeated at high rates (30–50 per sec) produce similar event-related potentials. *Ann. N.Y. Acad. Sci., 388,* 722–728.

Galambos, R., & Hecox, K. (1977). Clinical applications of the brain stem auditory evoked potentials. In J. E. Desmedt (eds.), *Auditory evoked potentials in man. Psychopharmacology correlates of EPs. Progress in clinical neurophysiology,* Vol. 2, pp. 1–19. Basel, Switzerland: Karger.

Galambos, R., & Hecox, E. (1978). Clinical applications of the auditory brainstem response. *Otolaryngol. Clin. N. Am. 11,* 709–722.

Galambos, R., Makeig, S., & Talmachoff, P. J. (1981). A 40-Hz auditory potential recorded from the human scalp. *Proc. Natl. Acad. Sci. U.S.A., 78,* 2643–2647.

Geisler, C. D., Frishkopf, L. S., & Rosenblith, W. A. (1958). Extracranial responses to acoustic clicks in man. *Science, 128,* 1210–1211.

Glasscock, M. E., Jackson, C. G., Josey, A. F., Dickens, J. R. E., & Wiet, R. J. (1979). Brainstem evoked response audiometry in a clinical practice. *Laryngoscope, 89,* 1021–1035.

Glattke, T. J. (1983). *Short-latency auditory evoked potentials—Fundamental bases and clinical applications.* Baltimore: University Park Press.

Glasscock, M. E., Jackson, C. G., & Josey, A. F. (1981). *Brain stem electric response audiometry.* New York: Brain C. Decker.

Goff, W. (1978). The scalp distribution of auditory evoked potentials. In R. F. Naunton & C. Fernandez (eds.), *Evoked electrical activity in the auditory nervous system,* pp. 505–524. New York: Academic Press.

Goff, W. R., Allison, T., Lyons, W., Fisher, T. C., & Conte, R. (1977). Origins of short latency auditory evoked potentials in man. *Prog. Clin. Neurophysiol., 2,* 30–44.

Goff, W. R., Allison, T., & Vaughan, H. G. (1978). The functional neuroanatomy of event-related potentials. In E. Calloway, P. Tueting, & S. H. Koslow (eds.), *Event-related potentials in man,* pp. 124–138. New York: Academic Press.

Gorga, M. P., & Thornton, A. R. (1989). The choice of stimuli for ABR measurements. *Ear Hear., 10,* 217–230.

Gorga, M. P., & Worthington, D. W. (1983). Some issues relevant to the measurement frequency-specific auditory brainstem responses. *Sem. Hear., 4,* 353–362.

Gorga, M. P., Reiland, J. K., & Beauchaine, K. A. (1985a). Auditory brainstem responses in a case of a high-frequency conductive hearing loss. *J. Speech Hear. Dis., 50,* 346–350.

Gorga, M. P., Worthington, D. W., Reiland, J. K., Beauchaine, K. A., & Goldgar, D. E. (1985b). Some comparisons between auditory brainstem response thresholds, latencies, and the pure-tone audiogram. *Ear Hear., 6,* 105–112.

Gorga, M. P., Kaminski, J. R., Beauchaine, K. L., Jesteadt, W., & Neely, S. T. (1989). Auditory brainstem responses from children three months to three years of age: Normal patterns of response II. *J. Speech Hear. Res., 32,* 281–288.

Gorga, M. P. Kaminski, J. R., and Beauchaine, K. L. (1991). Effects of the stimulus phase on the latency of the auditory brainstem response. *J. Am. Acad. Aud.* **2**(1), 1–6.

Graham, J., Greenwood, R., & Lecky, B. (1980). Cortical deafness: A case report and review of the literature. *J. Neurol. Sci., 48,* 35–49.

Grantz, B. J., Holliday, M., Gmuer, A. A., & Fisch, U. (1984). Electroneurographic evaluation of the facial nerve. *Ann. Otol. Rhinol. Laryngol., 93,* 394–398.

Green, J. B., Walcoff, M., & Lucke, J. F. (1982). Phenytoin prolongs far-field somatosensory and auditory evoked potential interpeak latencies. *Neurol., 32,* 85–88.

Grundy, B. L, Lina, A., Procopio, P. T., & Jannetta, P. J. (1981). Reversible evoked potential changes with retraction of the eighth cranial nerve. *Anesth. Analg., 60,* 835–838.

Grundy, B. L., Jannetta, P. J., Procopio, P. T., Lina, A., Boston, R., & Doyle, E. (1982). Intraoperative monitoring of brain-stem auditory evoked potentials. *J. Neurosurg., 57,* 674–681.

Halgren, E., Squires, N. K., Wilson, C. L., Rohrbaugh, J. W., Babb, T. L., & Crandall, P. H. (1980). Endogenous potentials generated in the human hippocampal formation and amygdala by infrequent effects. *Science, 210,* 803–805.

Hall, J. W., Huang-Fu, M., & Gennarelli, T. A. (1982). Auditory function in acute severe head injury. *Laryngoscope, 92,* 883–890.

Hall, J. W., III, Morgan, S. H., Mackey-Hargadine, J., Aguilar, E. A., & Jahrsdoerfer, R. A. (1984). Neuro-otologic applications of simultaneous multi-channel auditory evoked response recordings. *Laryngoscope, 94,* 883–889.

Harker, L. A., Hosick, E., Voots, R. J., & Mendel, M. I. (1977). Influence of succinylcholine on middle-component auditory evoked potentials. *Arch. Otolaryngol., 103,* 133–137.

Hashimoto, I. (1982). Auditory evoked potentials from the human midbrain: Slow brain stem responses. *Electroencephalogr. Clin. Neurophysiol., 53* 652–657.

Hecox, K. (1975) Electrophysiological correlates of human auditory development. In L. Cohen & P. Salapatek (eds.), *Infant perception: From sensation to cognition,* Vol. 2, pp. 151–191. New York: Academic Press.

Hecox, K. (1980). Brainstem evoked potentials: Neurological applications. Paper presented at the Conference on Auditory Evoked Response in Otology and Audiology, Cambridge, Massachusetts.

Hecox, K., & Galambos, R. (1974). Brain stem auditory evoked responses in human infants and adults. *Arch. Otolaryngol., 99*, 30–33.

Hecox, K., & Moushegian, G. (1981). Brainstem auditory evoked potentials: I. Methods and norms. Paper presented at the auditory brainstem response workshop, Kresge Laboratory, Louisiana State University, Medical Center, New Orleans, Louisiana.

Hecox, K., Cone, B., & Blaw, M. E. (1981). Brainstem auditory evoked response in the diagnosis of pediatric neurologic disease. *Neurol., 31*, 832–840.

Horwitz, S., Larson, S., & Sances, A. (1966). Evoked potentials as an adjunct to the auditory evaluation of patients. *Proc. Symp. Biomed. Eng., 1*, 49–52.

House, J. W., & Brackmann, D. E. (1979). Brainstem audiometry in neurotologic diagnosis. *Arch. Otolaryngol., 105*, 305–309.

Howe, S. W., & Decker, T. N. (1980). Auditory evoked potential: Effects of recording site. *Hear. Instr., 31*, 22–50.

Hughes, J. R., Fino, J., & Gagnon, L. (1981). The importance of phase of stimulus and the reference recording electrode in brain stem auditory evoked potentials. *Electroencephalogr. Clin. Neurophysiol., 51*, 611–623.

Humes, L. E., & Ochs, M. G., (1982). The use of contralateral masking in the measurement of the auditory brainstem response. *J. Speech Hear. Res., 25*, 528–535.

Hyde, M. L., & Blair, R. L. (1981). The auditory brainstem responses in neurotology: Perspectives and problems. *J. Otolaryngol., 10*, 117–125.

Jacobson, J. T. (ed.) (1985) *The auditory brainstem response.* Austin: Pro-Ed.

Jacobson, J. T. (ed.) (1985). *The auditory brainstem response.* San Diego: College-Hill Press.

Jerger, J., & Hall, J. (1980). Effects of age and sex on auditory brainstem response. *Arch Otolaryngol., 106*, 387–391.

Jerger, J., & Johnson, K. (1988). Interactions of age, gender, and sensorineural hearing loss on ABR latency. *Ear Hear., 9*, 168–176.

Jerger, J., & Mauldin, L. (1978). Prediction of sensorineural hearing level from the brainstem evoked response. *Arch. Otolaryngol., 104*, 456–461.

Jewett, D. L., & Williston, J. S. (1971). Auditory-evoked far fields averaged from the scalp of humans. *Brain, 94*, 681–696.

Jewett, D. L., Romano, M. N., & Williston, J. S. (1970). Human auditory evoked potentials: Possible brain stem components detected on the scalp. *Science, 167*, 1517–1518.

Josey, A. F. (1985). Auditory brainstem response in site of lesion testing. In J. Katz (ed.), *Handbook of clinical audiology*, 3d ed., pp. 534–548. Baltimore: Williams & Wilkins.

Kaga, K., & Tanaka, Y. (1980). Auditory brainstem response and behavioral audiometry: Developmental correlates. *Arch. Otolaryngol., 106*, 564–566.

Kavanagh, K. T., & Beardsley, J. V. (1979). Brainstem auditory evoked response. *Ann. Otol. Rhinol. Laryngol., 88*, 1–28.

Kavanagh, K. T., & Clark, S. T. (1989). Comparison of the mastoid to vertex and mastoid to high forehead electrode arrays in recording auditory evoked potentials. *Ear Hear., 10*, 259–261.

Keith, W. J., & Greville, K. A. (1987). Effects of audiometric configuration on the auditory brainstem response. *Ear Hear., 8*, 49–55.

Keith, R. W., Jabre, A. F., & Heerse, M. A. (1983). Auditory brainstem response testing in the surgical intensive care unit. *Sem. Hear., 4*, 385–390.

Kelly-Ballweber, D., & Dobie, R. A. (1984). Binaural interaction measured behaviorally and electrophysiologically in young and old adults. *Audiology, 23*, 181–194.

Kevanishvili, Z. (1980). Sources of the human brainstem auditory evoked potential. *Scand. Audiol., 9*, 75–82.

Kevanishvili, Z. (1981). Considerations of the sources of the human

brainstem auditory evoked potential on the basis of the bilateral asymmetry of its parameters. *Scand. Audiol., 10*, 197–202.

Kevanishvili, Z., & Aponchenko, K. (1981). Click polarity inversion effects upon the human brainstem auditory evoked potential. *Scand. Audiol., 10*, 141–147.

Kiang, N. Y. S., Moxon, E. C., & Kahn, A. R. (1976). The relationship of gross potentials recorded from the cochlea to single unit activity in the auditory nerve. In R. J. Ruben, C. Elberling, & G. Salomon (eds.), *Electrocochleography*, pp. 95–115. Baltimore: University Park Press.

Kileny, P., & Shea, S. L. (1986). Middle-latency and 40-Hz auditory evoked responses in normal-hearing subjects: Click and 500-Hz thresholds. *J. Speech Hear. Res., 29*, 20–28.

Kileny, P., Dobson, D., & Gelfand, E. T. (1983). Middle-latency auditory evoked responses during open-heart surgery with hypothermia. *Electroencephalogr. Clin. Neurophysiol., 55*, 268–276.

Klein, A. J., & Mills, J. G. (1981). Physiological (waves I and V) and psychophysical tuning curves in humans. *J. Acoust. Soc. Am., 69*, 760–768.

Knight, R. T., Hillyard, S. A., Woods, D. L., & Neville, H. J. (1980). The effects of frontal and temporal–parietal lesions on the auditory evoked potentials in man. *Electroencephalogr. Clin. Neurophysiol., 50*, 112–124.

Kramer, S. J., & Teas, D. C. (1979). BSR (wave V) and N1 latencies in response to acoustic stimuli with different bandwidths. *J. Acoust. Soc. Am., 66*, 446–455.

Kraus, N., Ozdamar, O., Hier, D., & Stein, L. (1982). Auditory middle latency response (MLRs) in patients with cortical lesions. *Electroencephalogr. Clin. Neurophysiol., 54*, 275–287.

Kraus, N., Ozdamar, O., Stein L., & Reed, N. (1984). Absent auditory brain stem response: Peripheral hearing loss or brain stem dysfunction? *Laryngoscope, 94*, 400–406.

Laukli, E., & Mair, I. W. S. (1981). Early auditory evoked responses: Filter effects. *Audiology, 20*, 300–312.

Lev, A., & Sohmer, H. (1972). Sources of averaged neural responses recorded in animal and human subjects during cochlear audiometry. *Arch. Klin. Exp. Ohren Nasen Kehlkopfheilkd., 201*, 79–90.

Levine, R. A. (1979). Monitoring auditory potentials during acoustic neuroma surgery. In H. Silverstein & H. Novell (eds.), *Neurosurgery of the ear*, Vol. 2, pp. 287–293. Birmingham, Alabama: Aesculapius.

Lutschig, J., Pfenninger, J., Ludin, H. P., & Fassela, F. (1983). Brain-stem auditory evoked potentials and early somatosensory evoked potentials in neurointensively treated comatose children. *Am. J. Diseases Children, 137*, 421–426.

Lynn, G. E., & Verma, N. P. (1985). ABR in upper brainstem lesions. In J. T. Jacobson (ed.), *The auditory brainstem response*, pp. 203–217. Austin: Pro Ed.

Lynn, J. M., Lesner, S. A., Sandridge, S. A., & Daddario, C. (1984). Electrophysiologic tecniques in audiology: Threshold prediction from the auditory 40-Hz evoked potential. *Ear Hear., 5*, 366–370.

McGee, T. J., & Clemis, J. D. (1982). Effects of conductive hearing loss on auditory brainstem response. *Ann. Otol. Rhinol. Laryngol., 91*, 304–309.

Manninen, H., Lam, A. M., & Nicholas, J. F. (1985). The effects of isoflurane and isoflurane-nitrous oxide anesthesia on brainstem auditory evoked potentials in man. *Anesth. Anal., 64*, 43–47.

Marsh, J. T., Smith, J. C., & Brown, W. S. (1976). Frequency following response to the missing fundamental. *J. Acoust. Soc. Am., 60*, S16.

Martin, M. E., & Moore, E. J. (1977). Scalp distribution of early (0 to 10 ms) auditory evoked responses. *Arch Otolaryngol., 103*, 326–328.

Mast, T. E. (1965). Short latency human evoked response to clicks. *J. Applied. Physiol., 20*, 725–730.

Mauldin, L., & Jerger, J. (1979). Auditory brainstem evoked responses to bone-conducted signals. *Arch. Otolaryngol., 105*, 656–661.

Maurizi, M., Altissimi, G., Ottaviani, F., Paludetti, G., & Bambini, M. (1982). Auditory brainstem responses (ABR) in the aged. *Scand. Audiol., 11,* 213–221.

Mendel, M. I. (1980). Clinical use of primary cortical responses. *Audiology, 19,* 1–15.

Mendel, M. I., Hosick, E. C., Windman, T. R., Davis, H., Hirsh, S. K., & Dinges, D. F. (1975). Audiometric comparison of the middle and late components of the adult auditory evoked potentials awake and asleep. *Electroencephalogr. Clin. Neurophysiol., 38,* 27–33.

Mendelson, T., Salamy, A., Lenoir, M., & McKean, C. (1979). Brainstem evoked potential findings in children with otitis media. *Arch. Otolaryngol., 105,* 17–20.

Mokotoff, B., Schulman-Galambos, C., & Galambos, R. (1977). Brainstem auditory evoked responses in children. *Arch. Otolaryngol., 103,* 38–43.

Moller, A. R., (1983). Improving brain stem auditory evoked potential recordings by digital filtering. *Ear Hear., 4,* 108–113.

Moller, A. R., & Jannetta, P. J. (1981). Compound action potentials recorded intracranially from the auditory nerve in man. *Exp. Neurol., 74,* 862–874.

Moller, A. R., & Jannetta, P. J. (1982a). Auditory evoked potentials recorded intracranially from the brainstem in man. *Exp. Neurol., 78,* 144–157.

Moller, A. R., & Jannetta, P. J. (1982b). Evoked potentials from the inferior colliculus in man. *Electroencephalogr. Clin. Neurophysiol., 53,* 612–620.

Moller, A. R., & Jannetta, P. J., (1983a). Mointoring auditory functions during the cranial nerve microvascular decompression operations by direct recording from the eighth nerve. *J. Neurosurg., 59,* 493–499.

Moller, A. R., & Jannetta, P. J. (1983b). Auditory evoked potentials recorded from the cochlear nucleus and its vicinity in man. *J. Neurosurg., 59,* 1013–1018.

Moller, A. R., & Jannetta, P. J. (1983c). Interpretation of brainstem auditory evoked potentials: Results from intracranial recordings in humans. *Scand. Audiol., 12,* 135–143.

Moller, A. R., & Jannetta, P. J. (1984). Preservation of facial function during removal of acoustic neuromas. *J. Neurosurg., 61,* 757–760.

Moller, A. R., & Jannetta, P. J. (1985). Neural generators of the auditory brainstem response. In J. T. Jacobson (ed.), *The auditory brainstem response,* pp. 13–31. Austin: Pro-Ed.

Moller, A. R., Jannetta, P. J., Bennett, M., & Moller, M. G. (1981a). Intracranially recorded responses from the human auditory nerve: New insights into the origin of brainstem auditory evoked potentials (BSEPs). *Electroencephalogr. Clin. Neurophysiol., 52,* 18–27.

Moller, A. R., Jannetta, P. J., & Moller, M. B (1981b). Neural generators of brainstem evoked potentials. Results from human intracranial recordings. *Ann. Otol. Rhinol. Laryngol., 90,* 591–596.

Moller, A. R., Moller, M. B., & Millner, D. (1981c). A computer system for auditory evoked responses. In B. D. Shriver, T. H. Walker, R. R. Grams, & R. H. Sprague (eds.), *Proceedings of the fourteenth Hawaii international conference on system sciences, Honolulu, Jan. 1981,* pp. 49–53. North Hollywood, California: Western Periodicals.

Moller, A. R., Jannetta, P. J., & Moller, M. B. (1982). Intracranially recorded auditory nerve responses in man: New interpretations of BSER. *Arch. Otolaryngol., 108,* 77–82.

Moller, M., & Moller, A. (1983). Brainstem auditory evoked potentials in patients with cerebellopontine angle tumors. *Ann. Otol. Rhinol. Laryngol., 92,* 645–650.

Moller, M. B., & Moller, A. R. (1985). Auditory brainstem-evoked responses (ABR) in diagnosis of eighth nerve and brainstem lesions. In M. L. Pinheiro & F. E. Musiek (eds.), *Assessment of central auditory dysfunction: Foundations and clinical correlates,* pp. 43–65. Baltimore: Williams & Wilkins.

Moller, M. B., Moller, A. R., & Jannetta, P. J. (1982). Brainstem auditory evoked potentials in patients with hemifacial spasm. *Laryngoscope, 92,* 848–852.

Moller, K., & Blegvad, B. (1976). Brainstem responses in patients with sensorineural hearing loss. *Scand. Audiol., 5,* 15–127.

Murray, A. D., Javel, E., & Watson, C. S. (1985). Prognostic validity of auditory brainstem evoked response screening in newborn infants. *Am. J. Otolaryngol., 6,* 120–131.

Musiek, F. E., & Gollegly, K. M. (1985). ABR in eighth nerve and low brainstem lesions. In J. T. Jacobson (ed.), *The auditory brainstem response,* pp. 181–202. Austin: Pro-Ed.

Musiek, F. E., Kibbe, K., Rackliffe, L., & Weider, D. J. (1984). The auditory brain stem response I-V amplitude ratio in normal, cochlear, and retrocochlear ears. *Ear Hear., 5,* 52–55.

Musiek, F. E., Josey, A. F., & Glasscock, M. E. (1986a). Auditory brain stem responses—Interwave measurements in acoustic neuromas. *Ear Hear., 7,* 100–105.

Musiek, F. E., Kibbe-Michal, K., Geurkink, N. A., & Josey, A. F. (1986b). ABR results in patients with posterior fossa tumors and normal pure-tone hearing. *Otolaryngol. Head Neck Surg., 94,* 568–573.

Musiek, R. E., Sachs, E., Jr., Geurkink, N. A., & Weider, D. J. (1980). Auditory brainstem response and eighth nerve lesions: A review and presentation of cases. *Ear Hear., 1,* 297–301.

Musiek, R. E., Johnson, G. D., Gollegly, K. M., Josey, A. F., & Glasscock, M. E. (1989). The auditory brain stem response interaural latency difference (ILD) in patients with brain stem lesions. *Ear Hear., 10,* 131–134.

Musiek, R., & Geurkink, N. (1981). Auditory brainstem and middle latency evoked response sensitivity near threshold. *Ann. Otol. Rhinol. Laryngol., 90,* 236–240.

Naunton, R. F., & Fernandez, C. (eds.) (1978). *Evoked electrical activity in the auditory nervous system.* New York: Academic Press.

Nicolet Instrument Corporation (1979). *Introduction to evoked potential instrumentation.* Madison, Wisconsin: Nicolet Instrument Corporation.

Nicolet Instrumentation Corporation (1985). *Nicolet Compact Four electrodiagnostic systems reference manual.* (Revised) Madison, Wisconsin: Nicolet Instrument Corporation.

Otto, W. C., & McCandless, G. A. (1982). Aging and the auditory brain stem response. *Audiology, 21,* 466–473.

Ozdamar, O., Kraus, N., & Curry, F. (1982). Auditory brainstem and middle latency responses in patients with cortical deafness. *Electroencephalogr. Clin. Neurophysiol., 53,* 224–230.

Parker, D. J. (1981). Dependence of the auditory brainstem response on electrode location. *Arch. Otolaryngol., 107,* 367–371.

Picton, T. W., Hillyard, S. A., Krausz, H. I., & Galambos, R. (1974). Human auditory evoked potentials. I. Evaluation of components. *Electroencephalogr. Clin. Neurophysiol., 36,* 179–190.

Picton, T. W., Linden, R. D., Hamel, G., & Maru, J. T. (1983). Aspects of averaging. *Sem. Hear., 4,* 327–341.

Prasher, D. K. (1981). Alternative hypotheses concerning the sources of the human brain stem auditory evoked potentials. *Scand. Audiol., 10,* 63–64.

Prasher, D. K., & Gibson, W. P. (1980). Brain stem auditory evoked potentials. Significant latency differences between ipsilateral and contralateral stimulation. *Electroencephalogr. Clin. Neurophysiol., 50.* 240–246.

Pratt, H., & Sohmer, H. (1976). Intensity and rate functions of cochlear and brainstem evoked responses to click stimuli in man. *Arch. Otolaryngol., 212,* 85–92.

Prosser, S., & Arslan, E. (1985). Does general anesthesia affect the child's auditory middle latency response (MLR)? *Scand. Audiol., 14,* 105–108.

Robinson, K., & Rudge, P. (1977). Abnormalities of the auditory evoked potentials in patients with multiple sclerosis. *Brain, 93,* 583–598.

Rosenhall, U., Hedner, M., & Bjorkman, G. (1981). ABR and brainstem lesions. *Scand. Audiol. Suppl., 13,* 117–123.

Rosenhall, U., Bjorkman, G., Pedersen, K., & Kall, A. (1985). Brain-stem auditory evoked potentials in different age groups. *Electroencephalogr. Clin. Neurophysiol., 62,* 426–430.

Rosenhamer, H. J. (1977). Observations on electric brain-stem responses in retrocochlear hearing loss: A preliminary report. *Scand. Audiol., 6,* 179–196.

Rosenhamer, H. J., Lindstrom, B., & Lundborg, J. (1978). On the use of click evoked electrical brainstem responses in audiologic diagnosis. I. The variability of the normal response. *Scand. Audiol., 7.* 193–206.

Rosenhamer, H. J., Lindstrom, B., & Lundborg, T. (1980). On the use of click-evoked electric brainstem responses in audiological diagnosis. II. The influence of sex and age upon the normal response. *Scand. Audiol., 9,* 93–100.

Rowe, M. J., III (1978). Normal variability of the brain-stem auditory evoked response in young and old adult subjects. *Electroencephalogr. Clin. Neurophysiol., 44,* 459–470.

Rowe, M. J. (1981). The brainstem auditory evoked response in neurological disease: A review. *Ear Hear., 2,* 41–51.

Ruhm, H., Walker, E., & Flanigin, H. (1967). Acoustically evoked potentials in man: Mediation of early components. *Laryngoscope, 77,* 806–822.

Ruth, R. A., Hildenbrand, D. L., & Cantrell, R. W. (1982). A study of methods used to enhance wave I in the auditory brain stem response. *Otolaryngol. Head Neck Surg., 90,* 635–640.

Salamy, A., & McKean, C. M. (1976). Postnatal development of human brainstem potentials during the first year of life. *Electroencephalogr. Clin. Neurophysiol., 40,* 418–426.

Samra, S. K., Lilly, D. J., Rush, N. L., & Kirsh, M. N. (1984). Fentanyl anesthesia and human brain-stem auditory evoked potentials. *Anesthesiology, 61,* 261–265.

Schulman-Galambos, C., & Galambos, R. (1979). Brainstem evoked response audiometry in newborn hearing screening. *Arch. Otolaryngol., 105,* 86–90.

Schwartz, D. M. (1985). The contralateral effect of a large CPA tumor. In J. T. Jacobson (ed.), *The auditory brainstem response,* pp. 414–415. Austin: Pro-Ed.

Schwartz, D. M., & Berry, G. A. (1985). Normative aspects of the ABR. In J. T. Jacobson (ed.), *The auditory brainstem response,* pp. 65–97. Austin: Pro-Ed.

Schwartz, D. M., Bloom, M. J., & Dennis, M. J. (1985). Perioperative monitoring of auditory brainstem responses. *Hear. J., 38,* 9–14.

Seitz, M. R., Mundy, M. R., & Pappas, D. G. (1981). The effects of tinnitus on ABR waveforms. Paper presented at the Convention of the American Auditory Society, New Orleans.

Selters, W., & Brackmann, D. (1977). Acoustic tumor detection with brainstem electric response audiometry. *Arch. Otolaryngol., 103,* 181–187.

Shea, J. J., & Harrell, M. (1978). Management of tinnitus aurium with lidocaine and carbamazepine. *Laryngoscope, 8,* 1477–1484.

Sklare, D. A. (1987). Auditory brain stem response laboratory norms: When is the data base sufficient? *Ear Hear., 8,* 56–67.

Sohmer, H. (1983). Neurologic disorders. In E. J. Moore (ed.), *Bases of auditory brain-stem evoked responses,* pp. 317–341. New York: Grune & Stratton.

Sohmer, H., & Feinmesser, M. (1967). Cochlear action potentials recorded from the external ear in man. *Ann. Otol. Rhinol. Laryngol., 76,* 427–438.

Stapells, D. R. (1989). Auditory brainstem response assessment of infants and children. *Sem. Hear., 10,* 229–251.

Stapells, D. R., Picton, T. W., Perez-Abalo, M., Read, D., & Smith, A.

(1985). Frequency specificity in evoked potential audiometry. In J. T. Jacobson (ed.), *The auditory brainstem response,* pp. 147–177. Austin: Pro-Ed.

Starr, A. (1976). Auditory brainstem responses in brain death. *Brain, 99,* 543–554.

Starr, A., & Achor, J. (1975). Auditory brain stem responses in neurological disease. *Arch. Neurol., 32,* 761–768.

Starr, A., Amlie, R. N., Martin, W. H., & Sandars, S. (1977). Development of auditory function in newborn infants revealed by auditory brainstem potentials. *Pediatrics, 60,* 831–839.

Stockard, J. E., & Stockard, J. J. (1983). Recording and analyzing. In. E. J. Moore (ed.), *Bases of auditory brain-stem evoked responses,* pp. 255–286. New York: Grune & Stratton.

Stockard, J. E., Stockard, J. J., Westmoreland, B. F., & Corfits, J. L. (1979). Brainstem auditory evoked responses. Normal variation as a function of stimulus and subject characteristics. *Arch. Neurol., 36,* 823–831.

Stockard, J. E., Stockard, J. J., & Coen, R. W. (1983a). Auditory brain stem response variability in infants. *Ear Hear., 4,* 11–23.

Stockard, J. E., Stockard, J. J., Kleinberg, K. L., & Westmoreland, B. F. (1983b). Prognostic value of brainstem auditory evoked potentials in neonates. *Arch. Neurol., 40,* 360–365.

Stockard, J. J., & Rossiter, V. S. (1977). Clinical and pathologic correlates of brainstem auditory response abnormalities. *Neurol., 27,* 316–325.

Stockard, J. J., & Sharbrough, F. W. (1980). Unique contributions of short-latency auditory and somatosensory evoked potentials to neurologic diagnosis. *Prog. Clin. Neurophysiol., 7,* 231–263.

Stockard, J. J., Rossiter, V. S., & Weiderholt, W. C. (1976). Brainstem auditory evoked responses in suspected central pontine myelinosis. *Arch. Neurol., 33,* 726–728.

Stockard, J. J., Rossiter, V. S., Jones, T. A., & Sharbrough, F. W. (1977a). Effects of centrally acting drugs on brainstem auditory responses. *Electroencephalogr. Clin. Neurophysiol., 43,* 550–551.

Stockard, J. J., Stockard, J. E., & Sharbrough, F. W. (1977b). Detection and localization of occult lesions with brainstem auditory responses. *Mayo Clinic Proc., 52,* 761–769.

Stockard, J. J., Sharbrough, F. W., & Tinker, J. A. (1978a). Effects of hypothermia on the human brainstem auditory response. *Ann. Neurol., 3,* 368–370.

Stockard, J. J., Stockard, J. E., & Sharbrough, F. W. (1978b). Nonpathologic factors influencing brainstem auditory evoked potentials. *Am. J. EEG Technol., 18,* 177–209.

Stockard, J. J., Stockard, J. E., & Sharbrough, F. W. (1980). Brainstem evoked potentials in neurology: Methodology, interpretation, clinical application. In M. J. Aminoff (ed.), *Electrodiagnosis in clinical neurology,* pp. 370–413. New York: Churchill Livingstone.

Streletz, L. J., Katz, L., Hohenberger, M., & Cracco, R. Q. (1977). Scalp recorded auditory evoked potentials and sonomotor responses. An evaluation of components and recording techniques. *Electroencephalogr. Clin. Neurophysiol., 43,* 192–206.

Sturzebecher, E., Kevanishvili, Z., Werbs, M., Meyer, E., & Schmidt, D. (1985). Interpeak intervals of auditory brainstem response, interaural differences in normal-hearing subjects and patients with sensorineural hearing loss. *Scand. Audiol., 14,* 83–87.

Suzuki, T., & Horiuchi, K. (1977). Effect on high-pass filter on auditory brainstem responses to tone pips. *Scand. Audiol., 6,* 123–126.

Suzuki, T., Hirai, Y., & Horiuchi, K. (1977). Auditory brain stem responses to pure tone stimuli. *Scand. Audiol., 6,* 51–56.

Suzuki, T., Hirai, Y., & Horiuchi, K. (1981). Simultaneous recording of early and middle components of auditory electric response. *Ear Hear., 2,* 276–282.

Terkildsen, K., & Osterhammel, P. (1981). The influence of reference electrode position on recordings of the auditory brainstem responses.

Ear Hear., 2, 9–14.

Terkildsen, K., Osterhammel, P., & Huis in't Veld, F. (1973). Electrocochleography with a far field technique. *Scand. Audiol., 2,* 141–148.

Terkildsen, K., Osterhammel, P., & Huis in't Veld, F. (1974). Far field electrocochleography, electrode positions. *Scand. Audiol., 3,* 123–129.

Thomsen, J., Terkildsen, K., & Osterhammel, P. (1978). Auditory brainstem responses in patients with acoustic neuroma. *Scand. Audiol., 7,* 179–183.

Van Campen, L. E., Sammeth, C. A., & Peek, B. F. (1990) Interaural attenuation using Etymotic ER-3A insert earphones in auditory brain stem response testing. *Ear Hear., 11,* 66–69.

van Olphen, A. F., Rodenburg, M., & Verwey, C. (1978). Distribution of brain stem responses to acoustic stimuli over the human scalp. *Audiology, 17,* 511–518.

van Olphen, A. F., Rodenburg, M., & Verwey, C. (1979). Infuence of stimulus repetition rate on brainstem evoked responses in man. *Audiology, 18,* 388–394.

Vaughan, H. G., & Ritter, W. (1970). The sources of auditory evoked responses recorded from the human scalp. *Electroencephalogr. Clin. Neurophysiol., 28,* 360–367.

Wada, S., & Starr, A. (1983). Generation of auditory brainstem responses (ABRs). III. Effects of lesions of the superior olive, lateral lemniscus and inferior colliculus on the ABR in guinea pig. *Electroencephalogr. Clin. Neurophysiol., 56,* 352–366.

Walter, H. (1964). The convergence and interaction of visual, auditory, and tactile responses in human nonspecific cortex. *Ann. N. Y. Acad. Sci., 112,* 320–361.

Weber, B. A. (1983). Pitfalls in auditory brain stem response audiometry. *Ear Hear., 4,* 179–184.

Worden, F. G., & Marsh, J. T. (1968). Frequency following (microphic-like) neural responses evoked by sound. *Electroencephalogr. Clin. Neurophysiol., 25,* 42–52.

Worthington, D. W., & Peters, J. F. (1980a). Electrophysiologic audiometry. *Ann. Otol. Suppl., 74,* 59–62.

Worthington, D. W., & Peters, J. F. (1980b). Quantifiable hearing and no ABR: Paradox or error? *Ear Hear., 1,* 281–285.

Yamada, O., Yagi, R., Yamane, H., & Suzuki, J. I. (1975). Clinical evaluation of the auditory evoked brainstem response. *Auris Nasus Larynx, 2,* 97–105.

Yoshie, N. (1973). Diagnostic significance of the electrocochleogram in clinical audiometry. *Audiology, 12,* 504–539.

CHAPTER 8

ELECTRONYSTAGMOGRAPHY

The auditory and vestibular end-organs occupy the same area within the temporal bone of the skull and are innervated by branches of the eighth cranial nerve, the vestibulocochlear nerve. Because of the geographic proximity of the vestibular system to the auditory system, hearing and balance disorders often coexist. Therefore, the audiologist is often called upon in the evaluation of both the vestibular and auditory systems.

The vestibular system, in conjunction with the ocular and proprioceptive systems, functions to maintain equilibrium. Disturbances in any of these systems result in the perception of dysequilibrium. In cases of vestibular disorders, the dysequilibrium is usually associated with vertigo (hallucination of motion such as the sensation that one's body is moving in space, or the room/space is moving around one's body). Patients often refer to vertigo as dizziness.

Dizziness is a broad term which includes lightheadedness, unsteadiness, ataxia, syncope, giddiness, wooziness, and vertigo. Table I lists the most common causes of dizziness. Patients with vertigo, ataxia, and lightheadedness may describe the sensation of dizziness similarly. Thus, an accurate description of the dizziness is often absent, particularly in children.

Although vertigo is symptomatic of vestibular disorders and may occur in some temporal-lobe disorders, not everyone with a vestibular disorder complains of vertigo. Keim (1985) reported that 66% of his group of 229 dizzy patients with unilateral vestibular abnormalities did not complain of vertigo. Therefore, a technique is needed to differentiate between patients with dizziness related to vestibular disorders and patients with dizziness related to nonvestibular disorders so appropriate medical management can be implemented. Such differentiation serves a medical rather than audiologic function. Audiologists, however, are often involved in this differentiation because of their historical use of electronystagmography (ENG) testing to distinguish between cochlear and retrocochlear sites of lesion. As will be shown in Chapter 8, ENG is not a useful tool for detection of retrocochlear disorders. It also does not enable differentiation between cochlear and retrocochlear disorders. Audio-

logists who do ENG testing do so to assist the physician in (a) differentiation between vestibular and nonvestibular causes of dizziness for the purpose of medical management; (b) differentiation between central and peripheral sites of vestibular disorder for the purpose of medical management; (c) establishment of the etiology of some auditory disorders such as Meniere's disease; and (d) quantification and monitoring of the dizziness for medico-legal purposes and for long-term follow-up in medical management.

Central vestibular, peripheral vestibular, and temporal-lobe causes of vertigo are shown in Tables II, III, and IV, respectively.

Dizziness associated with vestibular disorders, usually manifested as vertigo, may be accompanied by jerk or rhythmic nystagmus. This nystagmus represents a pattern of eye movement which has a fast or quick component and a slow phase. The nystagmus occurs because of the anatomical connection between the vestibular and ocular systems. Rhythmic nystagmus can also occur in some cases of ocular disorders, in some healthy persons, and can be induced in normal persons under certain stimulation conditions. Since eye movements result in changes in the electrical field around the eyes, nystagmus and other related eye movements can be recorded using electronystagmography. Electronystagmography is the primary clinical tool employed by audiologists for the identification of vestibular disorders.

I. ANATOMY AND PHYSIOLOGY OF THE VESTIBULAR SYSTEM

The membranous labyrinth of the inner ear in Figure 1 contains the cochlea, the organ of hearing, in its anterior part and the organ of balance in its posterior part. The vestibular labyrinth, that is, the organ of balance, helps to maintain a balanced position in space. Each vestibular labyrinth (one in each ear) contains three semicircular canals, a utricle, and a saccule, The superior (anterior), posterior, and horizontal (lateral) semicircular canals are located at

Table I Causes of Dizziness

OCULAR	**METABOLIC**
glaucoma	diabetes
refractive errors	thyroid disorders
cataracts	hyperlipidemia
gross ocular muscle imbalance	hypoglycemia
	hypoadrenalism
CENTRAL NERVOUS SYSTEM	
multiple sclerosis	**HEMATOLOGIC**
skull trauma	pernicious anemia
migraine and migraine	polycythemia
equivalents	leukemia
seizure disorders	
ataxic diseases	**DRUGS**
meningitis	streptomycin
encephalitis	kanamycin
tertiary syphilis	diazepam
increased intracranial pressure	sedatives
due to embolism, aneurysm,	opiates
or tumor	alcohol
vertebral-basilar artery	neuroleptics
insufficiency	aspirin
	caffeine
	prochlorperazine
OTOLOGIC	"recreational" drugs
otitis media	
labyrinthitis	**INFECTIONS**
vestibular neuronitis	influenza
cholesteatoma	measles
petrositis	mumps
poststapedectomy syndrome	
perilymph fistula	**CARDIOVASCULAR**
Meniere's disease	cerebral hypoxia
benign paroxysmal positional	arteriosclerosis
vertigo	hypertension
acoustic neuroma (intracanal)	postural hypotension
cerebellopontine angle tumors	arrythmia
impacted wax	aortic stenosis
foreign body in external	atherosclerotic heart disease
auditory meatus	bradycardia
herpes zoster oticus	poor pumping efficiency
	myxoma embolization
PROPRIOCEPTIVE OR	
NEUROMUSCULAR	**OTHER**
Paget's disease	toxic reactions to ingested
spinal degeneration with	foods, environmental fumes
cervical arthritis	heavy metals
tabes dorsalis	autoimmune diseases
	temporomandibular-joint
NECK	syndrome
trauma	heat stroke
osteoarthritis	functional, nonorganic causes
subclavian-steal syndrome	
vertebral-artery insufficiency	
carotid-artery disease	
thyromegaly	

right angles to each other. The enlarged portion of each semicircular canal, the ampulla, is connected to the utricle. The membranous labyrinth is filled with endolymph.

There are two sense organs in the vestibular labyrinth: the crista ampullaris in the semicircular canals, which re-spond to angular acceleration (head turning), and the mac-ulae of the utricle and saccule, which respond to linear acceleration (up and down, forward and backward, and sideways movement). The crista ampullaris in the right and left semicircular canals oriented in the same plane (e.g., the right superior and the left posterior canals, the left posterior and the right superior canals, or the left and right horizontal canals) respond to angular acceleration in that plane.

As illustrated in Figures 1 and 2, the crista ampullaris is shaped like a small hill and contains hair cells from which protrude many stereocilia and a single kinocilium em-bedded in a gelatinous substance called the cupula. As can be seen in Figure 2, the kinocilium is located proximal and the stereocilia are located distal to the utricle of the horizon-tal semicircular canals. In the posterior and superior semi-circular canals, however, the kinocilium is located distal and the stereocilia are located proximal to the utricle. De-flection of the kinocilium toward the utricle in the horizon-tal, superior, and posterior canals results in utriculopetal (ampullopetal) deviation. Utriculopetal deviation is associ-ated with increased electrical activity in the horizontal semi-circular canal and decreased electrical activity in the superior and posterior semicircular canals. Deflection of the kinocilium away from the utricle in the horizontal, superior, or posterior canals results in utriculofugal (ampu-llofugal) deviation. Utriculofugal deviation is associated with decreased electrical output in the horizontal semicir-cular canal and increased electrical output in the superior and posterior semicircular canals.

The maculae shown in Figure 1 contain hair cells and supporting cells. The stereocilia of the hair cells are em-bedded in a gelatinous material. On the surface of the gela-tinous layer are otoconia, composed of calcium carbonate, which transmit the effects of gravity to the underlying hair cells, thereby making the hair cells more sensitive to linear acceleration.

The vestibular branch of the vestibulocochlear nerve in-nervates the five vestibular sense organs: the cristae ampul-laris of the superior, posterior, and horizontal canals and the maculae of the utricle and saccule. The first-order ves-tibular neurons terminate in the vestibular nuclei in the lower brainstem. The vestibular system contains six neuro-nal pathways from the vestibular nuclei to the central ner-vous system: (a) to the cerebellum, which coordinates reflex and other muscular and neural activity required for orienta-tion; (b) to the vestibulospinal tract in the spinal cord for postural reflexes; (c) to the reticular formation of the midbrain and brainstem for integration with other sensory information; (d) to the oculomotor nuclei (cranial nerve III) via the medial longitudinal fasciculus (MLF) and abducens nuclei (cranial nerve VI) for control of horizontal eye move-ments which compensate for head turn (angular acceler-ation); (e) to the temporal lobe of the cortex for awareness of the head motion; and (f) to the vestibular sense organs

Table II   Central Vestibular Vertigo[a]

Diagnosis	Duration	Characteristics	Cause
Multiple sclerosis	Days to months	Positional vertigo and disturbance of equilibrium	Sclerotic patches in brain and spinal cord
Tumors fossa posterior	Minutes	Central positional vertigo, moderated	Pressure on brainstem
Apoplexia cerebelli	Weeks	Very acute, serious vertigo, accompanied by symptoms of cerebellar paralysis	Lesion arteria cerebelli
Acute vermis syndrome	Minutes to hours	Paroxysmal vertigo, vegetative symptoms, neurological disorders	Pressure on arteria vertebralis
Wallenberg's syndrome	Days to weeks	Acute rotary vertigo with vegetative symptoms, homolateral paralysis of the palate, trigeminus paralysis, contralateral sensibility disturbance	Ischemia arteria cerebelli posterior inferior
Arteria cerebelli superior syndrome	Weeks	Acute vertigo, vegetative symptoms, cerebellar hemiataxia, hemiataxia, hypotonia, intentional tremor, disturbances in speech	Obstruction arteria cerebelli superior
Cerebral sclerosis	Long-lasting	Giddiness, unsteadiness, sway movements	Diminished cerebral blood flow
Arachnoiditis pontocerebellaris (Barany syndrome)	Hours	Attacks of rotary vertigo, occipital headache, vegetative symptoms, lesions of the n. vestibularis, n. cochlearis, n. trigeminus, n. abducens, n. facialis, and cerebellum	Arachnoiditis fossa posterior
Migraine equivalent	Hours	Vertigo by unilateral headache, vegetative symptoms	Migraine
Intoxication			
Barbiturates		Positional vertigo and positional nystagmus	Disinhibition
Alcohol		Positional vertigo and positional nystagmus	
Opiates		Vertical spontaneous nystagmus	

[a] From Oosterveld (1982) with permission.

Table III   Peripheral Vestibular Vertigo[a]

Diagnosis	Duration	Characteristics	Cause
Meniere's disease	Minutes to days	Irregular attacks of vertigo with tinnitus, hearing disorder, and vegetative symptoms	Endolymphatic hydrops
Labyrinthine vascular accident	Weeks	Sudden vertigo, with or without hearing disorder	Ischemia labyrinthii
Acute labyrinthitis	Days to weeks	Acute vertigo, vegetative symptoms, hearing impairment, and tinnitus	Otitis media
Serous labyrinthitis	Chronic	Rotary vertigo	Chronic otitis media sometimes fistula horizontal canal
Neuronitis vestibularis	Days to weeks	Acute rotary vertigo, vegetative symptoms	Viral infection nervus vestibularis
Neuritis vestibularis	Days to weeks	Acute rotary vertigo, vegetative symptoms, hearing disorder	Viral infection nervus octavus
Vestibular encephalitis	Days	Acute rotary vertigo, vegetative symptoms, eye muscle disorders, pyramidal track disorders	Viral infection
Herpes zoster oticus	Weeks	Rotary vertigo, vegetative symptoms, earache, vesicular eruptions external ear canal and concha, sometimes paresis n. facialis	Viral infection
Paroxysmal positional vertigo	Less than 30 seconds	Positional vertigo	Disorder canal system
Childhood vertigo	Minutes	Paroxysmal vertigo in children up to 12 years, no vegetative symptoms, no hearing disorder	Unknown
Motion sickness	Days to weeks	Rotary vertigo and vegetative symptoms	Linear accelerations, Coriolis effects

[a] From Oosterveld (1982) with permission.

Table IV Epileptic Vertigo[a]

Diagnosis	Duration	Characteristics	Cause
Temporal lobe epilepsy	Seconds	Acute attacks of vertigo, gastric aura, followed by diminished consciousness or unconsciousness	Focus temporal lobe
Vestibular epilepsy	Seconds	Absences, dizziness spells, no vestibular symptoms, EEG disturbances, nonprovokable	Focus gyrus temporalis superior
Vestibulogenic epilepsy	Minutes	Unconsciousness, dizziness spells, vestibular symptoms, no EEG disturbances, provokable	Low epileptic stimulation threshold

[a] From Oosterveld (1982) with permission.

via the efferent vestibular pathway for control of input to the vestibular nuclei (Clark, 1986). In ENG testing, the peripheral vestibular system includes the vestibular division of the eighth cranial nerve and the labyrinthine vestibular end organ. The central vestibular system includes the central vestibular nuclei and the medial longitudinal fasciculus.

II. SYSTEMS WHICH CONTROL HORIZONTAL EYE MOVEMENTS

A. *VESTIBULO-OCULAR REFLEX*

The vestibulo-ocular reflex is the basis for the caloric test in the ENG battery. During the caloric test, the patient lies

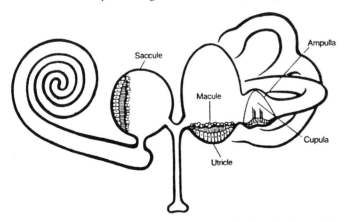

Figure 1 Diagram of the membranous inner ear showing the crista of the lateral semicircular canal and the macule of the saccule and utricle. From Frenzel (1982) with permission.

supine with the head elevated 30° above the horizontal so the horizontal canal is in the vertical position, which is optimal for convection current formation. Since the superior and posterior canals are essentially noncontributory in the response to caloric testing, the vestibulo-ocular reflex for only horizontal movements, that is, head turn to the right or left, will be described.

When the head is stationary and upright, there is a spontaneous resting electrical discharge generated from the crista ampullaris of one horizontal canal which is equal to that from the other horizontal canal. When the head is turned, for example, to the right, the endolymph in both horizontal canals moves in the opposite direction, that is, to the left, because of inertia. Therefore, the endolymph will move toward the utricle in the right horizontal canal (imagine that the utricle is situated near the midline of the head), and away from the utricle in the left horizontal canal. As a result of the endolymph movement in the right horizontal canal toward the utricle, the kinocilium in that canal will also be bent toward the utricle, that is, show utriculopetal deviation. Thus, head movement to the right is associated with utriculopetal deviation of the kinocilium in the right horizontal canal. The reader should recall that utriculopetal deviation of the horizontal canal results in increased electrical discharge from that canal. As a result of the endolymph movement in the left horizontal canal away from the utricle, the kinocilium of that canal will also be bent away from the utricle, that is, show utriculofugal deviation. Thus, head movement to the right is associated with utriculofugal deviation of the kinocilium in the left horizontal canal. The reader should recall that utriculofugal deviation of the horizontal canal is associated with decreased electrical discharge from that canal.

The increased electrical discharge from the right horizontal canal is transmitted through the vestibular nerve to the right superior, lateral, medial, and inferior vestibular nuclei in the upper medulla oblongata of the brainstem. Figure 3 shows a schematic of the primary three neuronal pathways from the horizontal canal to the central nervous system. Although there are six neuronal pathways from the vestibular nuclei to the central nervous system, we will discuss the following three major pathways.

1. First Pathway

In the first pathway, information from the right vestibular nucleus (in the case of head turn to the right) is transmitted through the contralateral (left) pontine paramedian reticular formation (PPRF), and then to the left abducens nucleus. From the abducens nucleus, information travels through the left abducens nerve to the left lateral rectus and again, through the midline, through the right medial longitudinal fasciculus to the right oculomotor nucleus; the right oculomotor nucleus gives rise to the right oculomotor (third) nerve which innervates the medial rectus of the right

HORIZONTAL
SEMICIRCULAR

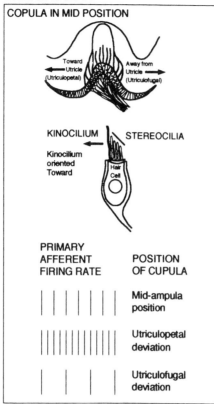

POSTERIOR & SUPERIOR
SEMICIRCULAR CANAL

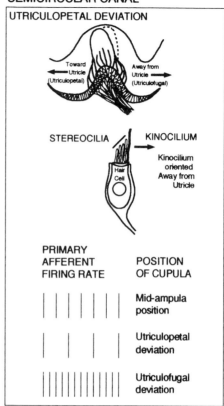

Figure 2 Kinocilium orientation in the semicircular canals. From McGee (1986) with permission.

eye. Thus, when the head is turned to the right, there is excitation of the left lateral rectus and right medial rectus eye muscles so the eyes are turned to the left. This phenomenon in response to head turn (angular acceleration) is the vestibulo-ocular reflex. Since there is decreased electrical discharge from the left horizontal canal at the same time there is increased electrical discharge from the right horizontal canal, there is inhibition of the left medial rectus and right lateral rectus, which facilitates the leftward eye movement during head turn to the right. The compensatory slow eye movements in response to the head movements keep the visual target on the fovea (central vision area) during head movement. When the head is turned so there is a compensatory slow eye deviation of more than 40° from the midline, then a central mechanism intervenes which causes an involuntary rapid eye movement back to the midline. The neuronal mechanism of this central mechanism for the fast phase following the vestibulo-ocular reflex is the same as that for saccades and the fast component of optokinetic eye movements, which will be described in greater detail later.

A vestibulo-ocular reflex (slow eye movement with angu-

lar acceleration) followed by a rapid eye movement back to midline is vestibular nystagmus. The slow phase (vestibulo-ocular reflex) and fast phase of vestibular (jerk or rhythmic) nystagmus is illustrated in Figure 4. The direction of the nystagmus is defined by the direction of the fast phase.

2. SECOND PATHWAY

The second pathway, composed of the vestibulospinal tracts, is shown in Figure 3. The vestibulospinal tracts play a major role in vestibular reflex reactions initiated by head movements. The vestibulospinal tracts include the lateral vestibulospinal and medial vestibulospinal tracts, although the former are more predominant in the vestibular reflex reaction in the neck muscles that helps to stabilize the position of the head. Basically, input from the lateral vestibular nucleus is transmitted through the ipsilateral lateral vestibulospinal tract, which extends for the entire length of the spinal cord and branches to the flexor and extensor muscles, primarily in the neck region in the vestibular reflex reaction. Because the vestibulospinal tract has connections with the autonomic nervous system, disorders of the vestibular end organs, vestibular nerve, or vestibular nuclei may

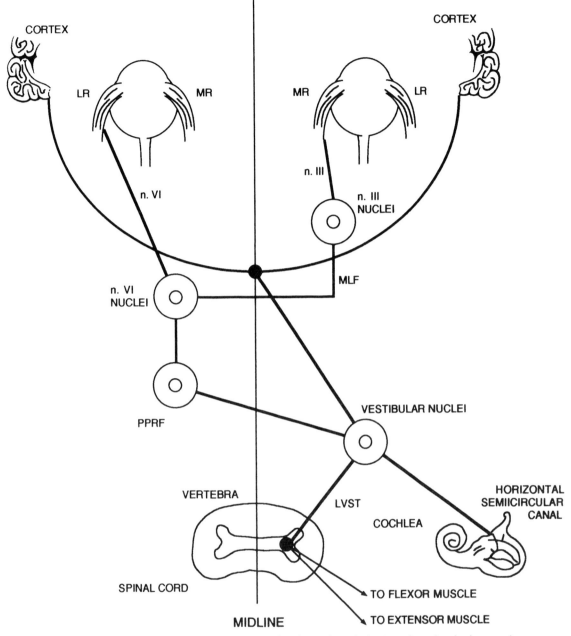

Figure 3 A schematic of the primary three neuronal pathways from the horizontal canal to the the central nervous system. The first pathway is the vestibulo-ocular reflex. The second pathway involves the vestibulospinal tract. The third pathway involves the temporal lobe of the cortex. LR, lateral rectus muscle; MR, medial rectus muscle; MLF, medial longitudinal fasciculus; PPRF, pontine paramedial reticular formation; VN, vestibular nucleus; LVST, lateral vestibulospinal tract; n. VI, abducens nucleus; n. III, oculomotor nucleus. Adapted, in part, from Pappas (1985).

be associated with vegetative symptoms, for example, nausea, vomiting, and sweating.

3. Third Pathway

The third pathway involving the cortex is illustrated in Figure 3. This pathway serves to provide awareness of head turn (angular acceleration).

4. Vestibular Nystagmus Induced by Stimulation Other Than Head Turn
a. Peripheral Vestibular Pathology

Pathology of the peripheral vestibular system will result in decreased electrical activity on the pathological side compared with the resting spontaneous electrical activity on the unaffected side. For example, a left labyrinthectomy will

Slow Phase

A

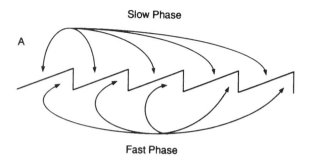

Fast Phase

Slow Phase

B

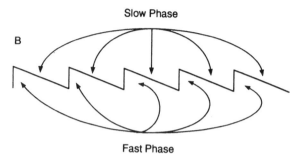

Fast Phase

Figure 4 (A) Schematic representation of left-beating nystagmus. The slow phase is indicated by the diagonal lines and the fast phase is indicated by the vertical lines. The direction of the nystagmus can be identified quickly by observing whether the slow component is on the right or left side of the fast component. In this example, the slow component is on the left side of the fast component so it is left-beating. (B) A schematic of right-beating nystagmus (the slow component is on the right of the fast component).

result in elimination of electrical activity in the left vestibular system compared with the resting spontaneous electrical activity in the right vestibular system. The greater electrical activity on the right will elicit a vestibulo-ocular reflex similar to that induced by head turn to the right followed by a fast saccadic eye movement back to the midline. Therefore, excitation of the left lateral rectus and right medial rectus extrinsic eye muscles will occur so the slow phase is to the left (affected side). The fast phase will be to the right (unaffected side). Thus, vestibular nystagmus resulting from peripheral vestibular pathology will "beat," that is, will be in the direction of the unaffected side. The greater electrical activity on the right side with respect to the absent electrical activity on the left side will be perceived by the temporal cortex as head turn to the right, accounting for the sensation of vertigo (hallucination of motion). Along with the imagined head turn, there is activation of the vestibulospinal pathway so corrective muscular movements such as a false step and fall and vegetative symptoms may occur. If the disorder is chronic and stable (or is very slowly progressive), there is a restoration of the sense of equilibrium, that is, disappearance of vertigo and related symptoms by a process of central nervous system compensation.

b. Caloric Stimulation

Unequal electrical discharges in the vestibular system can also be induced with caloric stimulation, that is, irrigation of the ear canal with warm or cool air or water (above or below the normal resting body temperature). With a warm stimulus, the endolymph is heated and expands, thereby becoming less dense. As a result, the endolymph in the horizontal canal stimulated rises toward the utricle (near the midline). Thus, warm stimulation will result in utriculopetal deviation in the ear stimulated, similar to the response induced by a head turn. For example, irrigation of the right ear with warm water will induce utriculopetal deviation in the right ear followed by a left vestibulo-ocular reflex (slow phase) and then a right fast phase. Thus, warm caloric irrigation of the right ear induces a vestibular reaction similar to that induced by head turn to the right. The warm caloric-induced nystagmus will beat in the direction of the ear stimulated.

With a cool stimulus, the endolymph is cooled and shrinks, thereby becoming more dense than normal. As a result, the endolymph in the horizontal canal stimulated will be pulled down by the force of gravity away from the utricle. Thus, cool stimulation of the ear canal will result in utriculofugal deviation in the ear stimulated, similar to the response induced by a head turn. For example, irrigation of the right ear with cool water will induce utriculofugal deviation in the right ear followed by a right vestibulo-ocular reflex (slow phase) and then a left fast phase eye movement. Thus, cool caloric irrigation of the right ear induces a vestibular reaction similar to that induced by head movement to the left. The cool caloric-induced nystagmus will beat in the direction opposite the ear stimulated.

c. Rotary Stimulation

Unequal electrical discharges in the vestibular system can also be induced in normal persons through rotary stimulation, for example, when sitting in a chair rotating about its vertical axis in the clockwise then counterclockwise then clockwise direction, and so forth. Under this condition, the head moves sinusoidally about its vertical axis. Unequal electrical discharges result only if there is angular acceleration. That is, the chair must rotate in a circle with ever increasing velocity until a predetermined peak velocity is reached. A constant velocity will not result in unequal electrical discharges from the vestibular labyrinths.

With rotation in one direction, utriculopetal movement of the endolymph in the horizontal canal on that side and utriculofugal movement of the endolymph in the opposite horizontal canal occur. For example, clockwise rotation results in utriculopetal deviation in the right horizontal canal and utriculofugal deviation in the left horizontal canal. The utriculopetal deviation on the right side will be followed by a left vestibulo-ocular reflex (slow phase) and then a right involuntary fast phase eye movement. Thus, clockwise rotary stimulation induces a vestibular reaction similar to that induced by head turn to the right. The clockwise rotary-induced nystagmus will beat to the right.

Counterclockwise rotation results in utriculopetal deviation in the left horizontal canal and utriculofugal deviation in the right horizontal canal. The utriculopetal deviation on the left side will be followed by a right vestibulo-ocular reflex (slow phase) and then a left involuntary fast phase eye movement. Thus, counterclockwise rotary stimulation induces a vestibular reaction similar to that induced by head turn to the left. The counterclockwise rotary-induced nystagmus will beat to the left.

B. SACCADIC EYE MOVEMENT

Saccades, refixations, are very rapid voluntary eye movements from target to target, occurring with a velocity of at least 90°/s but not more than 900°/s (Kileny, 1982). Saccades also maintain the image of fast-moving objects (velocity exceeding 90°/s) on the fovea (central vision area) of the retina.

According to Daroff, Troost, and Leigh (1990), saccades originate in the frontal eyefield of the cortex (Brodmann's area 8) which projects to the contralateral PPRF. Input from that PPRF is fed to the abducens nucleus on the same side which controls the lateral rectus muscle, also on the same side, and across the midline to the oculomotor nucleus, which controls the medial rectus of the other eye. The saccadic system is illustrated in Figure 5. Thus, a right saccadic eye movement is controlled by the left frontal

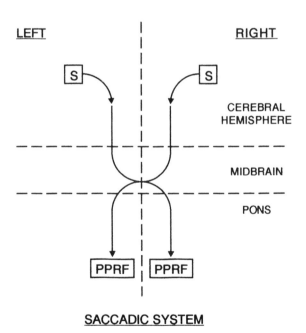

SACCADIC SYSTEM

Figure 5 A schematic of the saccadic system. S indicates initiation of saccades in the cerebral hemisphere. The pathways decussate in the lower midbrain and upper pons, to terminate in the contralateral pontine paramedia reticular formation (PPRF). From Daroff, Troost, & Leigh (1990) with permission.

eyefield, the right PPRF, right abducens nucleus, and right lateral rectus muscle, and the left oculomotor nucleus and left medial rectus. The theory that the frontal lobes are the origin of saccadic eye movements appears to be supported by the clinical finding of saccadic palsy in patients with unilateral hemispheric lesions (Daroff *et al.*, 1987). Research suggests that the PPRF has a predominant role in the generation of saccadic eye movements. (Bender & Shanzer, 1964; Daroff & Hoyt, 1971; Daroff *et al.*, 1987; Sharpe, Rosenberg, Hoyt, & Daroff, 1974; Yee, Baloh, Honrubia, & Jenkins, 1982).

C. SMOOTH PURSUIT EYE MOVEMENTS

The smooth pursuit system (also called the slow pursuit system) enables tracking of a slowly and smoothly moving object. It keeps the image of the object on the fovea despite movement of the object. The origin of smooth pursuit eye movements is the parieto-occipital visual association area of the cerebral cortex ipsilateral to the direction of the moving target. Thus, a target slowly moving to the right is controlled by the right hemisphere and a target slowly moving to the left is controlled by the left hemisphere. This theory is supported by clinical evidence that a deep parieto-occipital lesion on one side causes a defect in pursuit on the same side (Daroff *et al.*, 1987). For example, with a deep parieto-occipital visual association area lesion on the right side, there is a defect in tracking objects moving to the right. Input from the parieto-occipital visual association area is transmitted through a pathway to the ipsilateral PPRF. The output from the PPRF is fed to the ipsilateral abducens nucleus controlling the lateral rectus of the ipsilateral eye and the medial rectus of the contralateral eye. The smooth pursuit system is illustrated in Figure 6.

D. OPTOKINETIC EYE MOVEMENTS

The optokinetic eye movement system is involved when persons attempt to follow repetitive visual targets moving across the visual field, such as a display of vertical stripes moving toward the right or left (Kavanagh & Babin, 1986). If a person attempts to follow an individual target from one side to the other, the slow component of the optokinetic system is hypothesized to be the same as that described for smooth pursuit eye movements (Yee, *et al.*, 1982). If the person simply stares at the moving display of vertical stripes, the slow component of the optokinetic system is hypothesized to be primarily a smooth pursuit eye movement with some subsidiary contributions from a subcortical optikinetic pathway (Yee *et al.*, 1982). The fast component of the optokinetic system is an involuntary, rapid eye movement (regardless of whether one stares at the display or attempts to track individual stripes). For example, with a display of stripes moving to the right, input from the right parieto-occipital visual association area is fed to the right

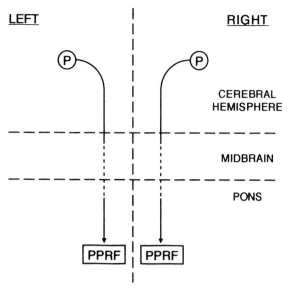

LEFT   **RIGHT**

CEREBRAL
HEMISPHERE

MIDBRAIN

PONS

PURSUIT SYSTEM

Figure 6 Pursuit (P) pathway. This pathway either undergoes a double decussation or remains ipsilateral (dotted lines), terminating in the ipsilateral PPRF. From Daroff and Troost (1978), with permission.

PPRF, the right abducens nucleus, and right lateral rectus, and the left oculomotor nucleus and left medial rectus so the slow component (smooth pursuit eye movement) is to the right. Then the fast component to the left will originate from the right frontal eye field which projects to the left PPRF which controls the left lateral rectus via the left abducens nucleus and the right medial rectus via the right oculomotor nucleus.

III. PRINCIPLES UNDERLYING ELECTRONYSTAGMOGRAPHY RECORDINGS

The eyes have an electrical potential, the corneoretinal potential, in which the cornea (front of the eye) has a positive electrical charge (+) and the retina (back of the eye) has a negative electrical charge (−). The corneoretinal potential is a DC (constant) electrical potential of approximately 1 mV. Because of the electrical potential difference between the positive cornea and the negative retina, the eye acts as a dipole (molecule having two equal and opposite charges).

When horizontal eye movements are recorded, the noninverting electrode is placed at the outer canthus of the right eye and the inverting electrode is placed at the outer canthus of the left eye with the ground electrode placed in the middle of the forehead. The effect of changes in the orientation of the corneoretinal potential resulting from eye movement on the voltage between the recording electrodes and the graphic representation of these voltage changes are shown in Figure 7. When the eyes move to the right, the

inverting electrode (labeled "+" in Figure 7) detects a large positive charge and the inverting electrode (labeled "−" in Figure 7) detects a smaller positive charge (because of dipole movement) which is inverted to become a small negative charge. The differential amplifier adds the charge from the noninverting electrode to the charge from the inverting electrode. (The reader should recall the principle underlying differential amplifiers discussed in the Chapter 7.) The resultant charge is positive. Thus, eye movement to the right is associated with a positive charge and, by convention, there is an upward deflection of the recording pen (see Figure 7).

When the eyes move to the left, the noninverting electrode detects a small positive charge (because of dipole movement) and the inverting electrode detects a large positive charge. The differential amplifier adds the small positive charge from the noninverting electrode to the large negative charge (the large positive charge is inverted) from the inverting electrode. The resultant charge is negative. Thus, eye movement to the left is associated with a negative charge, and, by convention, there is a downward deflection of the recording pen (see Figure 7).

When vertical eye movements are recorded, the noninverting electrode is placed above one eye and the inverting electrode is placed below one eye. When the eye moves upward, a large positive charge is detected at the noninverting electrode and a small positive charge is detected at the inverting electrode. The large positive charge is added to the small negative charge (the small positive charge is inverted). The resultant charge is positive, and by convention, is associated with an upward deflection of the recording pen. When the eye moves downward, the noninverting electrode detects a small positive charge and the inverting electrode detects a large positive charge. The small positive charge is added to the large negative charge (the large positive charge is inverted). The resultant charge is positive and, by convention, is associated with a downward deflection of the recording pen. Since blind patients with nonfunctioning retinas have no corneoretinal potential, ENG recordings usually cannot be obtained from them.

The standard electrode placement procedure just described contains a bitemporal pair of electrodes sensitive to horizontal eye movements, a vertical pair of electrodes sensitive to vertical eye movements, and a ground electrode. With this procedure, it is assumed that there is conjugate movement of the eyes, that is, the eyes move together in the same direction. To detect disconjugate eye movement (eyes moving in different directions), a different electrode placement must be employed. If only a two-channel nystagmograph is available, the clinician must determine whether to record horizontal or vertical eye movements from each eye. To record horizontal eye movements from each eye, electrodes should be placed on the outer canthus of each eye, on the forehead, and on the bridge of the nose. If a patient with a single blind eye is encountered, a single-eye

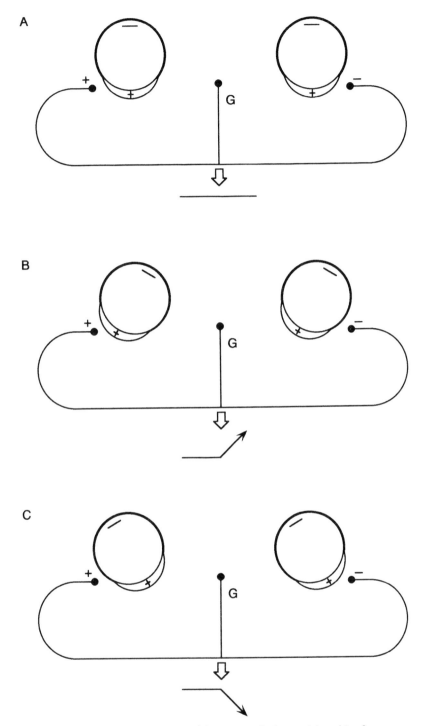

Figure 7 Effect of changes in the orientation of the corneoretinal potential resulting from eye movement on the voltage between the recording electrodes and the graphic representation of these voltage changes. (A) Eyes are centered and the recording is a straight, horizontal line. (B) Eyes are turned to the right so the recording shows the slow component going upwards (upwards deflection of the pen). (C) Eyes are turned to the left so the recording shows the slow component going downwards (downwards deflection of the pen).

recording may be preferred. In such cases, vertical and horizontal eye movements can be recorded with electrodes placed on the outer canthus of the good eye, the good-eye side of the bridge of the nose, above and below the good eye, and on the forehead.

IV. MEASUREMENT OF NYSTAGMUS STRENGTH

The duration (the time period between the first beat and the last beat) of the nystagmus was employed by early investigators as a measure of the nystagmus strength (Fitzgerald & Hallpike, 1942; Jongkees, 1948; Lundberg, 1940). The velocity of the slow component and the frequency (number of beats per unit time) represented measures of nystagmus strength not commonly used until ENG was introduced. Other measures of nystagmus strength that have been used include latency (time from the onset of irrigation to the first sequential beat) and amplitude (total degrees of eye deflection). The velocity (slope) of the slow phase is now the most commonly used measure of nystagmus strength. Henriksson (1956) compared the velocity of the slow phase and duration of nystagmus measures of nystagmus strength and found the former measure to be more sensitive than the latter measure to vestibular excitation. The slow-phase velocity corresponds best to alterations in firing rate of the vestibular neurons (Henriksson, 1956).

Theoretically, a complete rotation of the eyeball around its axis encompasses an arc of 360°. During the slow phase of the nystagmus, the eyes cover part of this arc. The size of this arc in degrees is the slow-phase velocity of the nystagmus. Since the magnitude of the slow-phase velocity of the nystagmus has diagnostic import, a calibration is necessary to equate the degrees of eye movement with the number of mm of pen deflection on the strip-chart recorder. This calibration procedure will be more fully described later.

Figure 8 shows the procedure for measuring the slow-phase velocity of nystagmus. To identify the slow-component, look for a diagonal line. If the diagonal line slopes downward on the right of the vertical line, the nystagmus is right-beating; if the diagonal slopes downward on the left of the vertical line, the nystagmus is left-beating on the horizontal recording. On the vertical recordings, a diagonal line sloping downwards on the right of the vertical line signifies an up-beating nystagmus and a diagonal line sloping downwards on the left of the vertical line signifies a down-beating nystagmus. With a ruler, draw a line through the diagonal (slow-phase component) which projects beyond the diagonal. Draw a horizontal line (10 mm) to the right or left of the extended diagonal line at either the top or the bottom, respectively. (This can be done starting at any point along the diagonal line.) Now draw a vertical line from the horizontal line so that it intersects with the diagonal line. Note that if the horizontal line is drawn in the wrong direction, the vertical line will never intersect with the diagonal line. Measure the height of the vertical line from the horizontal line to the intersection with the diagonal line in mm. This height, in mm, represents the slow-phase velocity of that individual beat. The slow-phase velocity is 23°/s in Figure 8A and 15°/s in Figure 8B.

V. ENG PROCEDURE

The patient should be instructed against ingestion of anti-vertigenous or central nervous system medications for 24–36 hr prior to the ENG. The patient should also be

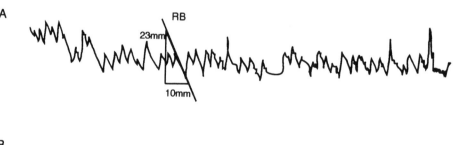

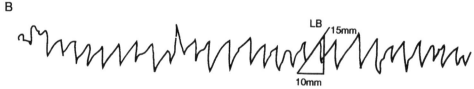

Figure 8 Illustration of the procedure for measuring the SPV of nystagmus. A diagonal line is drawn through the slow-phase component. A horizontal line of 10 mm is drawn below the tracing to the left of the diagonal line for right-beating nystagmus and to the right of the diagonal line for left-beating nystagmus. The height of the vertical line from the horizontal line to the intersection with the diagonal line yields the nystagmus speed in deg/s. (A) Right-beating nystagmus of 23°/s. (B) Left-beating nystagmus of 15°/s.

instructed against ingestion of alcohol for 36 hr prior to the ENG test, and food, beverages, and smoking 2–4 hr prior to the ENG examination.

A. CALIBRATION

1. DETERMINING THE DISTANCE BETWEEN A FIXATION POINT AND THE MIDPOINT OF THE CALIBRATION LIGHT BAR

There should be a 20° angle between fixation points, that is, each fixation point should be 10° from the midline. According to Coats (1986), the distance from the patient to the midpoint of the calibration light bar should be at least 3 ft to minimize convergence, the fixation points should be easily visible but not too large, and vertical as well as horizontal fixation points should be used if vertical recordings are made. The distance between a fixation point and the midline of the calibration light bar is equivalent to the distance from the patient's forehead to the midline of the calibration light bar times a constant associated with the desired angle between the fixation points. Figure 9 illustrates this concept. For example, if the angle between fixation points is 20° (the angle employed for calibration), then

the distance between the fixation point and the midline of the calibration light bar is equivalent to the distance from the patient's forehead to the midline of the calibration light bar times 0.1763. If the distance from the patient's forehead to the midline of the calibration light bar is 100 in, then the distance between each fixation point to the midline is 17.63 in. That is, there will be a distance of 35.26 in. between the two fixation points which subtend an angle of 20°.

For gaze testing, fixation points are placed at 20° and 30° angles from the midline of the calibration light bar. Therefore, the distance from a fixation point located 20° from the midline of the calibration light bar to the midline of the calibration light bar is equivalent to the distance from the patient's forehead to the midline of the calibration light bar times 0.3640. The value of the constant is 0.5774 for fixation points located 30° from the midline of the calibration light bar. Therefore, if the distance from the patient's forehead to the midline of the calibration light bar is 100 in, the distance from a fixation point located 20° from the midline of the calibration bar to the midline of the calibration light bar is 36.40 in (72.80 in between fixation points). If the distance from the patient's forehead to the midline of the calibration light bar is 100 in, the distance from a fixation point located 30° from the midline of the calibration bar to the midline of the calibration light bar is 57.74 in (105.48 in between fixation points).

2. SKIN PREPARATION AND ELECTRODE ATTACHMENT

If single-channel recordings are used to record horizontal eye movements, an electrode is placed at the outer canthus of each eye and in the middle of the forehead. Two-channel recordings are preferred so that vertical eye movements can be recorded. Vertical recordings may have diagnostic significance and are helpful in ruling out eyeblinks. If vertical recordings are obtained in addition to horizontal recordings, electrodes should also be placed above and below one eye in the plane of the pupil with the patient gazing straight ahead. Electrode placements for single-channel and dual-channel recordings are shown in Figure 10.

Single-eye recordings may be preferable to the standard bitemporal electrode placement in patients with one blind eye or disconjugate oculomotor abnormalities. With single-eye recordings, electrodes are placed at the outer canthus of one eye (the good eye), on the other side of the eye just medial to the bridge of the nose, and on the forehead. If single-eye recordings are to be employed in patients with disconjugate eye movements, two-channel recordings are necessary so the horizontal movements of one eye can be recorded in one channel and the horizontal movements of the other eye can be recorded in the second channel.

Gold, silver, or silver–silver chloride cupped electrodes are commonly employed. Gold electrodes are more stable

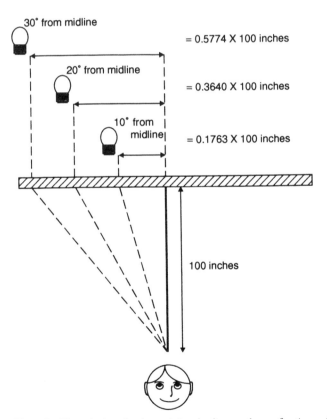

30° from midline

= 0.5774 X 100 inches

20° from midline

= 0.3640 X 100 inches

10° from midline

= 0.1763 X 100 inches

100 inches

Figure 9   The technique for determining the distance from a fixation point to the midline of the calibration light bar is illustrated. In this example, the distance from the patient's forehead to the midline of the calibration light bar is 100 inches. The constants by which this distance is multiplied for fixation points 10, 20, and 30° from the midline are shown.

A

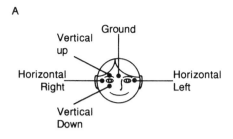

B

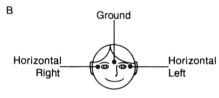

Figure 10 (A) Electrode placement for recording horizontal and vertical eye movements with a two-channel recorder. (B) Electrode placement for recording horizontal eye movements with a single-channel recorder.

and the lower limit of their frequency response extends to DC. The lower limit of the frequency response of silver electrodes also extends to DC but silver electrodes are not as stable as gold electrodes. Silver–silver chloride electrodes are relatively inexpensive and relatively stable if the surface coating is not damaged. The electrodes should be kept clean and not indiscriminately mixed or exchanged, otherwise an impedance imbalance will be seen at the amplifier, resulting in DC drift or increased noise in the recordings (Teter, 1983).

Electrode sites should be cleaned, first with a cotton ball or gauze pad soaked in alcohol so all traces of make-up and oil are removed and then with an abrasive agent such as Omni-prep. A small amount of a coupling agent which is highly conductive, containing sodium chloride or calcium chloride, and pastelike, to support electrode placement, should be spread over the electrode site. The area on which electrode paste is applied should be kept small to prevent artifacts. Put a generous dab of electrode paste in the cupped disk of the electrode, taking care not to put so much that secure attachment of the electrode to the skin is prevented. Place a cotton ball on top of the electrode and then tape the cotton ball and electrode sandwich to the skin. Electrode impedance should be checked with an impedance meter; some commercially available ENG devices contain an impedance meter. Optimal electrode impedance is below 5000 ohms but the impedance should not exceed 8000 ohms. Electrode impedance is reduced through careful skin preparation, the use of clean electrodes, and firm attachment of the electrodes to the skin. To prevent pulling on the electrodes, the electrode leads should be taped to the patient's shoulder.

3. PROCEDURE

Prior to doing calibration, the examiner should visually inspect the patient's eyes for abnormalities of extraocular muscle function (disconjugate eye movements, paresis), and spontaneous and gaze nystagmus. (Spontaneous and gaze nystagmus will be described later in this chapter.) The examiner should also inspect the ear canals to ascertain their shape, and the presence of any obstructions or tympanic membrane perforations.

Light adaptation has a substantial effect on the magnitude of the corneoretinal potential. Therefore, following Coats (1975), we recommend doing the entire ENG test in a dimly lit room to minimize the effects of light adaptation on the corneoretinal potential resulting from opening and closing the eyes.

The examiner should select the type of recording filter desired, that is, high-pass (AC) or low-pass (DC) filter. With DC coupling, the pen accurately follows eye movement. If the eye movement causes the pen to move off the chart, the pen will remain off the chart for as long as the eyes remain in that position. The pen can be brought back on the chart by using the offset control or reducing the gain. The use of DC coupling is not recommended in patients with extraneous eye movements. The advantage of DC coupling is that information is provided regarding the precise position of the eyes. We recommend that, if DC coupling is employed, it should be employed only by experienced ENG examiners. With AC coupling, the extraneous low-frequency potentials that sometimes develop across the recording electrodes are not seen. The advantage of AC coupling is that the pen is centered regardless of eye position. Thus, if the eye movement drives the pen to the edge of the chart, the pen will drift back to midline while the eyes remain in the position which drove the pen to the edge of the chart. The disadvantage of AC coupling is that there is loss of information regarding the precise position of the eyes.

The patient should be sitting and looking straight ahead. The examiner should check for the presence of spontaneous nystagmus (nystagmus obtained in this position) with the recorder on 1/4 gain (Teter, 1983). The patient is instructed to look back and forth (without moving the head) between two fixation points placed horizontally at 10° angles on both sides of the midline of the calibration light bar. The fixation points are commonly spots on the wall or a crossbar with flashing lights which can be rotated for vertical calibration and gaze testing. The gain of the recorder should be adjusted so that 20° of eye movement is associated with a pen deflection of 20 mm. Coats (1986) suggests that, since it is difficult to obtain 10, exactly 20-mm consecutive excursions (5 in each direction), the examiner should adjust the gain so approximately half the eye movements produce pen deflections exceeding 20 mm and the other half produce pen deflections less than 20 mm. If vertical recordings are obtained, this procedure should be repeated with fixation points placed above and below the midline of the calibration light bar.

From these 10 pen deflection, the correction factor can be calculated. The slow-phase velocity (SPV) of the nystagmus is multiplied by the correction factor. The heights (in mm) of the 10 deflections should theoretically total 200, that is, 20° of eye rotation should produce a 20 mm pen deflection so for 10 excursions, there would be a 200 mm total. The examiner should sum the heights of the 10 excursions. Then, 200 is divided by the examiner's obtained total height (200/obtained total). Figure 11 shows the height in mm for each of the 10 deflections. In this figure, the sum of the 10 pen deflections is 214.5 mm. The ratio 200/214.5 is 0.93. Thus, 0.93 represents the number of degrees equivalent to 1 mm of pen deflection. The average SPV obtained for any ENG subtest is multiplied by 0.93, the correction factor in this case.

The fixations to the right and left during calibration involve saccadic eye movements. Thus, the saccadic system is evaluated during calibration.

B. GAZE TESTING

The patient should be sitting with head erect. The examiner should instruct the patient to look straight ahead (at the midline of the calibration light bar) for 20–30 s. Recordings should then be obtained with the patient in this position but with the eyes closed. When the eyes are closed, a concentration task of appropriate difficulty should be done aloud by the patient, for example, counting by 1s, 2s, 3s, and so forth. This procedure enables the examiner to evaluate any latent spontaneous nystagmus.

Recordings should then be obtained with the patient sitting, head erect, under the following conditions: (a) eyes fixated upon a fixation point 30° to the right of the midline of the calibration light bar for 30 s; (b) eyes straight ahead for 3 s; (c) eyes fixated upon a fixation point 30° to the left of the midline of the calibration light bar for 30 s; and (d) eyes straight ahead for 3 s; and if vertical recordings are

obtained, (e) eyes fixated upon a fixation point 30° above the midline of the calibration light bar for 30 s; (f) eyes straight ahead for 3 s; (g) eyes fixated upon a fixation point 30° below the midline of the calibration light bar for 30 s; and (h) eyes centered for 3 s; then (i) eyes closed for 30 s with a concentration task performed aloud by the patient. Some examiners also perform gaze testing at fixation points located 20° from the midline of the calibration light bar (Coats, 1975, 1986). According to Stockwell (1983), fixations at 20° from the midline of the calibration light bar do not provide any additional diagnostic information. Stockwell (1983) suggests that if nystagmus is present with eyes open on lateral gaze, DC recordings are desirable so that it can be more easily determined whether the SPV is increasing exponentially, decreasing exponentially, or is constant during the nystagmus beat.

C. PENDULAR TRACKING

The patient should be sitting with the head erect. A sinusoidal pattern is created with a small swinging ball on a string suspended from the wall, a moving spot of light projected on a screen, an array of light-emitting diodes which are lit up sequentially, a fingertip or pentip swinging back and forth, or a fixation point placed on the arm of a metronome or the end of a metronome. Those methods which automatically generate sinusoidal patterns are preferred to those methods which manually generate sinusoidal patterns since the former control for target speed. The examiner instructs the patient to fixate on the sinusoidally moving target without moving the head. The peak-to-peak excursions of the sinusoidally moving target should be approximately 30°. Tracking should be obtained at a slow speed of approximately 10°/s and at a fast speed of approximately 25°/s. If there is a vertical channel, tracking should be done in the vertical as well as horizontal direction. Pendular (sinusoidal) tracking enables the evaluation of the smooth pursuit (also called the slow pursuit) eye movement system.

D. OPTOKINETIC TESTING

The patient should be sitting with the head erect. A pattern of vertical black stripes alternating with white stripes moving horizontally is generated by a hand-operated drum, a rotating cylinder lowered over the patient's head, or an optokinetic projector. An optokinetic stimulus can also be generated with an array of light-emitting diodes which are lit automatically, available in some commercial devices. The optokinetic drum can be turned so that a vertically moving as well as horizontally moving pattern can be generated. With the rotation cylinder over the patient's head, the pattern fills all of the visual field but a vertically moving pattern cannot be generated. With the optokinetic projector, the stimulus pattern fills most of the visual field

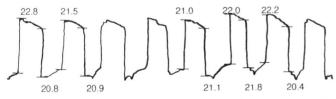

Figure 11 Tracing for horizontal calibration and the procedure for obtaining the correction factor to be applied to the average SPV calculated for ENG test. The heights of 10 pen deflections are shown. The total of these heights is equal to 214.5 mm. Therefore, the calibration factor is 200/214.5 or 0.93.

and can be turned to provide a vertically moving pattern. Furthermore, the stimulus pattern can be changed. The array of light-emitting diodes generates a pattern filling most of the visual field, and a vertically as well as horizontally moving pattern can be generated. According to Coats (1986), an effective optokinetic stimulus is one that fills at least 30% of the visual field.

The patient should be instructed to watch or focus on the stripes without moving the head. With this instruction, the "stare" nystagmus is obtained (Honrubia, Downey, Mitchell, & Ward, 1968) and the slow component of the nystagmus reflects smooth pursuit eye movements with some contributions from a subcortical optokinetic pathway. If the patient is told to track the individual stripes, the "look" nystagmus is obtained (Honrubia *et al.*, 1968) and the slow component of the nystagmus reflects only smooth pursuit eye movements. It is preferable to attempt to elicit the stare nystagmus for the evaluation of the optokinetic eye movement system. The pattern should be moving at a slow rate of approximately 20°/s and at a fast rate of approximately 40°/s. Recordings of the eye movements should be obtained under the conditions of (a) moving left to right at the slow speed, (b) moving right to left at the slow speed, (c) moving left to right at the fast speed, (d) moving right to left at the fast speed, (e) moving down to up at the slow speed (if the vertical channel is used), and (f) moving up to down at the slow speed (if the vertical channel is used). For each condition, a 20-s recording should be obtained. Coats (1986) recommends repeating recordings at the slow speed in each direction.

E. POSITIONAL TESTING

The positional tests identify the presence of nystagmus elicited by certain head positions which do not involve head movement. Recordings should be obtained first with eyes closed for 30 s in each of the following positions: (a) sitting; (b) supine, head level with the chest; (c) supine, head turned so right ear is down; (d) supine, head turned so the left ear is down; and (e) supine with head hanging over the end of the examining table. If nystagmus is present during any of these positions, then recordings should be obtained with eyes open for 30 s in the head position which yielded the nystagmus with the eyes closed. Stockwell (1983) recommended that, if nystagmus is present with the head right or the head left (eyes closed), then recordings should be obtained (eyes closed) with the whole body turned to the right or left to determine if neck rotation was the cause of the nystagmus. The patient should be moved slowly into each test position in order to ensure that any nystagmus recorded is the result of a stationary head position rather than any movement. When the eyes are closed, the patient should perform a concentration test of appropriate difficulty aloud.

F. DIX–HALLPIKE TEST

This test is designed to determine if any nystagmus can be elicited with a specific rapid body maneuver. With the Dix–Hallpike maneuver, the posterior semicircular canal rather than the horizontal canal is maximally stimulated. A nystagmus elicited with this maneuver is considered paroxysmal nystagmus, which is predominantly rotary but contains sufficient horizontal and/or vertical components to be recordable. Coats (1986) suggests that if the nystagmus is recorded with ENG, two-channel recordings (horizontal and vertical) must be obtained. If two-channel recordings are not available, then the test should be done under visual observation only and not with ENG.

If the test is recorded with ENG, the following procedure should be employed. The patient should be sitting with the head turned (slowly) 45° to the right with eyes closed and the examiner standing behind the patient. One hand should be grasping the top of the patient's head and the other hand should be against the back. The examiner should rapidly pull the patient backward keeping the neck in the turned position until the patient is lying supine with the head hanging over the end of the examining table to the right. The patient should be kept in this position for at least 30 s during which a recording is obtained. The examiner should inquire whether the patient is dizzy and, if so, the nature of the dizziness to determine if the dizziness reproduces the symptomatology. Then the patient should be instructed to open the eyes and fixate on a point such as the nose. A recording should be obtained for 20 s with the eyes open. The patient then brought back to the sitting position for at least 15 s. If nystagmus is obtained, the procedure should be repeated to determine if the response is fatigable. This entire procedure should then be repeated with the head turned to the left (after the patient is brought back to the sitting position for at least 15 s).

If the test is done without ENG, the patient should be instructed to keep the eyes open throughout the procedure. Some examiners move the patient backward and then turn the head to the right during the maneuver. Stockwell (1983) contends that this alternative procedure is less effective in eliciting nystagmus and can elicit neck rotation effects which complicate the interpretation of the nystagmus.

G. CALORIC TESTING

Standard alternate binaural bithermal caloric testing employs the open-loop system in which water is injected directly into the ear canal. Cool water is injected first into one ear and then into the other ear. The procedure is then repeated with warm water. With the air-calorics modification of this test, air rather than water is delivered into the ear canal. The closed loop system is similar to the open-loop system except that the water enters an expandable, silastic balloon in the ear canal.

The advantages of air-calorics testing over open-loop water calorics testing are (a) feasibility in cases of tympanic membrane perforation or mastoid cavity, which are at risk of infection from open-water irrigation; (b) risk of electric shock is eliminated; (c) testing involves less mess; and (d) less time is required for air to reach the desired temperature (Wetmore, 1986). The disadvantages of air-calorics testing compared with the open-loop water calorics testing include (a) excessive noise levels, (b) a feeling of burning in the ear canal, (c) a feeling of ear pain, (d) the response is more greatly affected by room temperature and location of the irrigating tip in the ear canal since air has a reduced heat-carrying capacity compared with water, and (e) the occurrence of the inverted response in cases of tympanic-membrane perforations and mastoid cavities, in which the nystagmus initially beats away from the stimulated side and then beats toward the stimulated side because of the dryness of the air, regardless of how moist the ear canal is (the inverted response can be avoided if the air is saturated with water vapor) (Wetmore, 1986).

The advantages of closed-loop water system are (a) feasibility in cases of tympanic-membrane perforations and mastoid cavities, and (b) the testing involves less mess. This method involves lower noise levels than those involved during air-calorics testing (Wetmore, 1986). The disadvantages of the closed-loop water calorics test are (a) risk of tympanic-membrane perforation if the balloon explodes in the canal, and (b) improper propagation of the temperature if the irrigating tip is improperly positioned so that there is a large air bubble between the irrigating tip and the tympanic membrane (Kileny & Kemink, 1986).

The simultaneous binaural bithermal calorics test represents another modification of the open-loop water calorics test employed by Brookler (1976). In this procedure, both ears are irrigated simultaneously with cool water. Then both ears are irrigated simultaneously with warm water. Little research has been done to substantiate Brookler's findings with the simultaneous binaural bithermal calorics test. Also, the false-positive rate of this modification is unknown.

We recommend that the open-loop calorics alternate binaural bithermal calorics test be used generally with water-calorics; in cases of tympanic-membrane perforations or mastoid cavities, alternate binaural bithermal calorics testing should be done with open-loop air calorics or closed-loop water calorics.

The alternate binaural bithermal open-loop calorics test procedure follows. Water temperature of 31°C is used for the cool irrigation and water of 43°C is used for the warm irrigation. The patient should be supine with the head ventroflexed by 30° to bring the horizontal canals into the vertical position so they will be optimally stimulated by the irrigations. A special ENG table can be used to achieve this elevation of the head or a headrest, sandbag, or folded pillows can be placed under the patient's head. Fixation points should be placed so they can be easily seen by the patient without head movement. Calibration should be repeated so that a new correction factor can be obtained prior to each irrigation since the calibration changes as the test proceeds (Coats, 1986). According to Coats (1986), rest periods between irrigations prevents the nystagmus induced in one irrigation from influencing the response in the next irrigation. To further reduce the possibility of a response from one irrigation influencing the response from another irrigation, the following order of irrigations are chosen so successive responses beat in opposite directions: (a) calibration, (b) right-ear cool irrigation for 40 s with eyes closed, (c) recording with eyes closed and mental tasking done aloud for approximately 90 s following onset of irrigation, (d) fixation test, that is, recording with eyes open and fixated on a finger or point on the wall for 10 s, (e) 5-min rest period, (f) calibration, (g) left-ear cool irrigation for 40 s with the eyes closed, (h) recording with the eyes closed and mental tasking done aloud for approximately 90 s following onset of irrigation, (i) fixation test, that is, recording with eyes open and fixated on a finger or point on the wall for 10 s, (j) 10-min rest, (k) calibration, (l) left-ear warm irrigation for 40 s with the eyes closed, (m) recording with eyes closed and mental tasking done aloud for approximately 90 s following the onset of irrigation, (n) 5-min rest period, (o) calibration, (p) right-ear warm irrigation for 40 s with eyes closed, and (q) recording with the eyes closed and mental tasking done aloud for approximately 90 s following the onset of irrigation. The fixation test need not be done after each irrigation but should be obtained for one right-beating response and one left-beating response. The rest period, a convenient time for taking a history and calculating the SPV of the nystagmus, can be shortened if the recording shows the absence of nystagmus with eyes closed.

According to Coats (1986), the following variables should be kept constant throughout caloric testing: (a) position of the patient's head, (b) position of the irrigation tube within the canal, (c) flow rate of irrigation (which can be kept constant with the use of the same tip for all irrigations), and (d) patient's alertness, which is kept constant through the use of a mental task which is of appropriate difficulty, that is, difficult enough so that central suppression of the nystagmus will be prevented and easy enough so that excessive voluntary eye movements and muscle artifacts will not be created. Table V., from Coats (1986), lists the various concentration tasks in order of increasing difficulty. Coats (1986) stresses the importance of ensuring that the stimulus temperature remains constant throughout an

Table V Suggested Concentration Tasks for Minimizing Central Suppression of Vestibular Nystagmus[a,b]

1. Count by 1s
2. Count by 2s
3. Count by 3s
4. Subtract 1s serially, beginning with some high number (e.g., 300)
5. Subtract 2s
6. Subtract 3s
7. Subtract 4s
8. Subtract 6s
9. Subtract 7s
10. Recite the alphabet backward
11. Recite the alphabet backward, giving a person's name (male or female may be specified) beginning with each letter as it is recited

[a] From Coats (1986) with permission.
[b] Listed in order of increasing difficulty.

irrigation. The following procedures are recommended (Coats, 1986) to ensure constancy of stimulus temperature throughout an irrigation: (a) insulating the tube, leaving 1 ft at the end to provide flexibility for easy manipulation of the tube, (b) setting the thermostat a little above the desired irrigation temperature to compensate for cooling as the stimulus travels from the bath to the irrigation tip, and (c) purging into a catch basin immediately prior to irrigation.

If air-calorics are done, the temperature of the air should be 50°C for the warm irrigation and 24°C for the cool irrigation with an irrigation duration of 60 s (Stockwell, 1983). Brookler, Baker, and Grams (1979) recommended that, for closed-loop water calorics, the temperature should be 28°C for the cool irrigation and 46°C for the warm irrigation with an irrigation duration of 45 s.

Monothermal caloric tests have been employed both as a screening test to determine which patients should receive the full binaural bithermal calorics test and also as an alternative to the binaural bithermal calorics test. In the monothermal warm water screening test developed by Barber, Wright, and Demanuele (1971), one ear and then the other ear is irrigated with only warm water of 44°C. The Kobrak minimal caloric test involves irritgating first one ear and then the other ear with 5 ml of ice water (0°C). McCabe and Ryu (1979) suggest that if 5 ml does not elicit an adequate response, then the ear should be irrigated with 10 ml of ice water; if 10 ml of ice water does not elicit an adequate response, the ear is then irrigated with 20 ml of ice water. In the Torok monothermal differential caloric test (Torok, 1969), first one ear and then the other ear is irrigated with 10 ml of 20°C water for 5 s (weak stimulus) followed by 100 ml of 20°C water for 20 s (strong stimulus). If there is no response for either irrigation, the ear is then irrigated with 100 ml of ice water (0°C) for 20 s.

H. MENTAL ALERTING TASKS

Nystagmus is suppressed in "reverie" states and is maximal in intensity in "environment-oriented" states. Various mental alerting tasks performed aloud have been employed to minimize central inhibition of nystagmus during the ENG procedure. Davis and Mann (1987) investigated the effects of two active mental alerting (i.e., arithmetic problem-solving and answering of reflexive questioning such as "What is your favorite color?") and two passive listening (i.e., music such as Tchaikovsky's Nutcracker Suite and story-telling such as the Rainbow Passage) on the SPV of caloric-induced nystagmus in 40 normal young adults. Passive listening mental alerting tasks have been employed when testing infants and children and the difficult-to-test population. Davis and Mann (1986) found that the mean SPV for the active tasks was significantly greater by approximately 8% than the mean SPV for the passive listening tasks. There was a difference of only 1.5% between the two active mental alerting tasks. Slow-phase velocity values of less than or equal to 5°/s occurred in 40% of the subjects under the passive mental-alerting condition as opposed to 2.5% under the active condition. Davis and Mann (1986) concluded that, since passive mental-alerting tasks result in significant suppression of nystagmus, diagnosis of vestibular pathology from caloric testing cannot be made unless active and not passive mental-alerting tasks are employed.

VI. LOW-FREQUENCY SINUSOIDAL HARMONIC ACCELERATION TESTING

Barany (1907) developed rotational testing in which the patient was seated in a chair which was spun manually in a circle for 10 rotations over a 20-s period and then suddenly stopped. The eye movements were then observed (postrotatory nystagmus). With the Barany test, the horizontal canals are stimulated by an abrupt deceleration. The disadvantages of the Barany test are:

1. The nystagmus from only one acceleration rate is investigated.
2. Only postrotary nystagmus (nystagmus evoked after rotation) rather than perrotary nystagmus (nystagmus evoked during rotation) is evaluated.
3. The acceleration rate is affected by the patient's weight and the distribution of the patient's weight in the chair. Since the acceleration rate cannot be kept constant for each person, normative data cannot be obtained.

These disadvantages are overcome with low-frequency sinusoidal harmonic acceleration testing. In low-frequency sinusoidal harmonic acceleration testing, the standard horizontal electrode placement is employed and the patient is seated in a special chair with the head placed in the position for maximal stimulation of the horizontal semicircular canals. The chair is motorized and its movement is controlled by a computer.

The commonly employed frequencies for low-frequency sinuosoidal harmonic acceleration testing are 0.01, 0.02, 0.04, 0.08, and 0.16 Hz. Since these frequencies are multiples of the fundamental frequency (0.01 Hz), this series of frequencies in considered to be sinusoidal harmonic acceleration. The frequency is the number of times that the chair is rotated about its vertical axis in 1 s. At the frequency of 0.01 Hz, the chair makes 2.2 complete turns in each direction (clockwise and counterclockwise direction) for a total of 795° in each direction. Therefore, at the frequency of 0.01 Hz, it takes 220 s for the chair to make 2.2 turns in a given direction. At the other frequencies, the chair makes 4.4 turns in each direction for a total of 1584° in each direction. Therefore, at the frequencies of 0.02, 0.04, 0.08, and 0.16 Hz, it takes 220, 110, 55, and 27.5 s respectively, to complete 4.4 rotations in a particular direction.

At each frequency, the velocity is increased from 0 to 50°/s by the end of a single cycle. This process of increasing velocity is repeated 2.2 times at the frequency of 0.01 Hz and 4.4 times at the other frequencies. As the frequency increases, the period decreases. Therefore, as the frequency increases, the amount of time over which the velocity increases from 0 to 50°/s decreases so the acceleration increases. For example, the acceleration to peak velocity is 3°/s at the frequency of 0.01 Hz. The acceleration to peak velocity is 50°/s at the frequency of 0.16 Hz. At each frequency, the testing is done in the clockwise and then counterclockwise direction.

The computer removes the fast phase components and automatically calculates the slow-phase components of the nystagmus elicited during the rotations. The eye velocity during the slow phase as a function of time is calculated and compared with the chair velocity automatically. Several response parameters are automatically calculated by the computer. These response parameters include phase, gain, and symmetry.

The phase parameter describes the inverted eye velocity relative to the chair acceleration at the different frequencies. The computer provides a printout of the eye-velocity relative to the chair acceleration at the various frequencies. At high frequencies above 1 Hz, the inverted eye-velocity as a function of time curve is essentially identical to the chair velocity as a function of time curve. When the inverted eye-velocity curve is compared with the chair-acceleration curve, there is said to be a phase lag. The phase response parameter is the most sensitive and reliable of the rotary test response parameters.

The gain parameter is the ratio of the inverted peak eye velocity to the peak chair velocity as a function of frequency. The computer provides a printout of this ratio as a function of frequency. If rotation is done in the light with visual fixation and a stationary background, the gain is increased markedly, particularly at the low frequencies. The disadvantage of the gain response parameter is the large intersubject variability. Factors contributing to the large intersubject variability include stress, fatigue, level of mental alertness, and habituation (Ruben, 1984).

Symmetry is the difference in peak eye velocity between clockwise and counterclockwise rotation as a function of frequency. It is the directional or labyrinthine preponderance as a function of frequency and the computer automatically provides this plot. The directional preponderance is calculated automatically by the computer using the formula

$$DP = (VR - VL)/(VR + VL) \times 100$$

where DP equals direcitonal preponderance, VR is the peak slow component eye velocity to the right and VL is the peak slow component eye velocity to the left. Symmetry is the least sensitive of the rotational response parameters to chronic vestibular pathology (Hirsch, 1986).

The advantages of low-frequency sinusoidal harmonic acceleration testing over caloric testing are:

1. Low-frequency sinusoidal harmonic acceleration testing has high test–retest reliability. Thus, vestibular function can be monitored with this test over time to determine whether any pathology is worsening, improving, or is stable.

2. With low-frequency sinusoidal harmonic acceleration testing, the course of central compensation can be objectively followed over time and correlated with the subjective sensation of dizziness.

3. Multiple graded stimuli can be applied in a short period of time with low-frequency sinusoidal harmonic acceleration testing.

4. Patients can be tested with low-frequency sinusoidal harmonic acceleration testing very soon after middle- and inner-ear surgery.

5. Low-frequency sinusoidal harmonic acceleration testing is relatively comfortable for the patient since it generally does not induce nausea or vertigo, so children as young as 2 years old and other difficult-to-test patients can be evaluated.

6. The response to low-frequency sinusoidal harmonic acceleration testing is unaffected by anatomic variations in the physical structure of the external auditory meatus or temporal bone or by tympanic membrane abnormality.

7. The phase measure is unaffected by vestibular-suppressant drugs. (Hirsch, 1986; Wolfe, Engelken, & Olson, 1982).

The major disadvantages of low-frequency sinusoidal harmonic acceleration testing in comparison with caloric testing include the extremely high cost of equipment and the inability to determine which labyrinth is the pathologic one. With low-frequency sinusoidal harmonic acceleration testing, both labyrinths are stimulated simultaneously. The very high cost associated with the instrumentation for the test has been primarily responsible for the limited clinical use of this test. The findings of Wolfe *et al.* (1982) support the use of low-frequency sinusoidal harmonic acceleration testing as an adjunct to caloric testing rather than in place of it.

VII. PEDIATRIC ENG TEST MODIFICATIONS

The standard light bar can be employed for calibration and gaze testing in children at least 3.5 years of age (Cyr, 1983). Some manufacturers such as Tracoustics have developed a special pediatric light bar consisting of lamps with lampshades containing painted cartoon characters; such a device is useful for testing children between 6 months and 3.5 years of age (Cyr, 1983).

For pendular tracking, Cyr (1983) suggested that the parent can hold the infant on the lap in a rocking chair so the infant is in a horizontal position, perpendicular to the parent. The child is instructed to fixate on a lighted toy situated directly above the child. As the parent rocks, the infant's eyes move from side to side.

For optokinetic testing, a drum lowered over the child's head or a film projector can be used. For very young children, as young as 6 months of age, projected cartoon characters on the wall are an effective optokinetic stimulus (Balkany & Finkel, 1986; Cyr, 1983).

Since children can detect even small amounts of light, positional testing must be done in darkness to minimize visual suppression of any nystagmus. Therefore, positional testing should be done in a completely darkened room or with the child blindfolded (Cyr, 1983).

Closed-loop caloric irrigation is recommended for use in children since no water spillage from the ear will occur if the child moves around. Cyr (1983) suggested the use of simultaneous binaural bithermal testing rather than alternate binaural bithermal caloric testing in children since the former procedure minimizes the sensation of vertigo, reduces the number of irrigations that must be performed, and eliminates the need for calibration between irrigations since both ears are compared with the same recorder sensitivity; if no response is obtained, one ear must be irrigated to rule out bilateral absence of vestibular function. Binaural bithermal caloric testing cannot be done in children less than 4 years of age (Balkany & Finkel, 1986). Ice-water caloric testing can be done in children between 6 months

and 4 years of age (Balkany & Finkel, 1986). In order to minimize visual suppression of the nystagmus, mental tasking can be accomplished sufficiently with the playing of taped music or nursery rhymes. There is a maturational effect on caloric-induced nystagmus. From birth to 6 months, the amplitude and slow-phase velocity increase but the latency of the nystagmus decreases (Balkany & Finkel, 1986). Nystagmus with a small slow-phase velocity and extended wave forms is characteristic of very young children (Balkany & Finkel, 1986).

Low-frequency sinusoidal harmonic acceleration testing can be done in infants as young as approximately 1–3 months of age (Balkany & Finkel, 1986; Cyr, 1983). For this test, the infant is held on the parent's lap so one arm is around the infant's body and the other arm tilts the infant's head 30° forward. Most children will have the typical nystagmus with this test, although some, particularly the very young infant, may show just a sinusoidal curve (Balkany & Finkel, 1986).

VIII. ENG INTERPRETATION

A. SACCADIC TESTING

Ocular dysmetria is the production of hypermetric saccades or hypometric saccades during calibration. With hypermetric saccades, the eyes overshoot the target and additional saccades are required to bring the eyes back to the target. With hypometric saccades, the eyes undershoot the target and additional refixations are necessary for the eyes to reach the target. Ocular dysmetria is illustrated in Figure 12. Ocular dysmetria is considered present if at least 50% of the calibration excursions have overshoot or undershoot (Coats, 1975; Haring and Simmons, 1973). The presence of eyeblinks must be ruled out before diagnosing overshoots. Eyeblinks, which appear similar to overshoots, are present on both the horizontal and vertical recordings. On the vertical channel, they occur as large pen excursions. True overshoots during horizontal calibration will appear on only the horizontal but not the vertical recording. Ocular dysmetria is generally consistent with pathology outside the brainstem such as cerebellar pathology (Baloh, Konrad, & Honrubia, 1975; Selhorst, Stark, Ochs, & Hoyt, 1976; Zee, Yee, Cogan, Robinson, & Engel, 1976).

Ocular flutter differs from ocular dysmetria in that the overshoot is spiky rather than squared off in appearance. More than one spiky overshoot may be present on a saccade. The presence of ocular flutter is consistent with brainstem disorders (Steenerson, Van de Water, Sytsma, & Fox, 1986).

Internuclear ophthalmoplegia or saccadic slowing should be suspected if the velocities during saccadic eye movements are slower than normal. Figure 13 shows slower than nor-

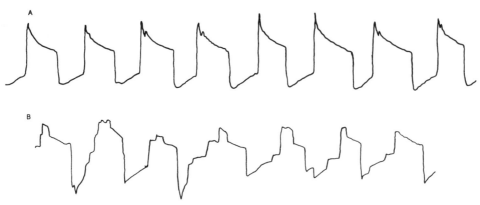

Figure 12 Ocular dysmetria on calibration testing. (A) Overshoot on saccades to the right. (B) Undershoot on saccades to the right. Courtesy of Dr. David Miller, San Diego Veterans Administration Medical Center.

mal velocities of the saccades characteristic of internuclear ophthalmoplegia or saccadic slowing; prolonged calibration must be ruled out. Slower than normal velocities of the saccades appear as a rounding of the corners on calibration testing. Differentiation between internuclear ophthalmoplegia and saccadic slowing can be made with separate-eye recordings. Separate-eye recordings show disconjugate eye movement and nystagmus during fixations in the case of internuclear ophthalmoplegia as contrasted with conjugate eye movements in the case of saccadic slowing. Internuclear ophthalmoplegia is consistent with medial longitudinal fasciculus lesions between the third and sixth nerve nuclei (Pola & Robinson, 1976). Saccadic slowing is consistent with central nervous system disorders such as brainstem lesions (Baloh, Honrubia, & Sills, 1977), diseases of the neuromuscular junction, for example, myasthenia gravis (Baloh & Keesey, 1976), spinocerebellar degeneration (Steenerson *et al.,* 1986), progressive supranuclear palsy (Steenerson *et al.,* 1986), and lesions of the oculomotor neurons and extraocular muscles (Bahill & Troost, 1979; Baloh & Honrubia, 1976).

Persons with saccadic palsy (total paralysis) or paresis (partial paralysis) caused by unilateral hemispheric lesions can make saccadic movements in one direction but these movements are impaired in the opposite direction (Daroff *et al.,* 1990). The direction of impaired saccadic movement is contralateral to the side of the lesion. For example, persons with right hemispheric lesions will have normal saccadic movements to the right but saccades to the left will be impaired.

B. SPONTANEOUS NYSTAGMUS

The presence of spontaneous nystagmus is evaluated during the gaze test procedure and also at the beginning of the positional tests when the patient is sitting with the head erect. The average slow-phase velocity (SPV) is calculated for the three strongest beats in the eyes closed (EC) and/or eyes open (EO) condition.

Horizontal spontaneous nystagmus is nystagmus present on the horizontal recording in the EC condition (of course, in the sitting position with the head erect). The average SPV is less than 7°/s. Horizontal spontaneous nystagmus is also sometimes referred to as idiopathic nystagmus. It is present in 15–30% of normal persons (Barber & Wright, 1973; Coats, 1969; Fluur & Eriksson, 1961; Lambert, 1986).

Vertical spontaneous nystagmus is nystagmus present on the vertical recording in only the EC condition. The average SPV is usually greater than 10°/s and the nystagmus is usually up-beating. It is present in approximately 80% of normal persons.

Pathological horizontal nystagmus is present on the horizontal recording in the EO and/or EC condition. The average SPV is greater than 7°/s. Pathological horizontal nystagmus may be latent or spontaneous. It is considered latent if it is present only in the EC condition (Kavanagh & Babin, 1986). A latent nystagmus may be present for many years. It is less likely to be indicative of significant (vestibular) pathology than spontaneous nystagmus.

Pathological horizontal spontaneous nystagmus is nystagmus present on the horizontal recording in both the EC

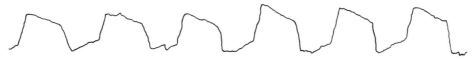

Figure 13 Slower than normal velocities of the saccades on calibration testing. Reduced velocities are shown on leftward saccades. This tracing was obtained using standard bitemporal leads. Courtesy of Dr. David Miller, San Diego Veterans Administration Medical Center.

and EO condition. In cases of chronic nonprogressive unilateral vestibular pathology, horizontal spontaneous nystagmus lasts only a few weeks, after which central compensation generally occurs and the nystagmus disappears (Kavanagh & Babin, 1986). Generally, pathological horizontal spontaneous nystagmus is a nonlocalizing finding, that is, a distinction between peripheral and central vestibular pathology cannot be made. Nevertheless, if the average SPV of the pathological horizontal spontaneous nystagmus is greater in the EC than EO condition, it tends to be indicative of peripheral vestibular pathology (Baloh & Honrubia, 1979; Coats, 1970; Dayal, Tarantino, Farkashidy, & Paradisgarten, 1974; Jung & Kornhuber, 1964). Similarly, if the average SPV of the pathological horizontal spontaneous nystagmus is greater in the EO than EC condition, it tends to be indicative of central vestibular pathology.

Vertical spontaneous nystagmus is nystagmus present on the vertical recording in the EO condition regardless of the average SPV. Down-beating vertical nystagmus is enhanced on downward gaze and is consistent with central vestibular pathology such as medullary or upper cervical spinal cord lesions (Barber & Stockwell, 1980; Gay, Newman, Keltner, & Stroud, 1974), upper brainstem lesions (Gay et al., 1974), or drug intoxication (Gay et al., 1974). Up-beating vertical nystagmus is enhanced on upward or downward gaze and is consistent with central vestibular pathology such as posterior fossa lesions or drug intoxication (Barber & Stockwell, 1980; Gay et al., 1974).

Periodic alternating nystagmus is pathological horizontal (or rotary) nystagmus present in the EC and/or EO condition. It beats first in one direction and then in the other direction in cycles. The change in beating direction occurs in regular cycles of approximately 90 s (Steenerson et al., 1986). It is consistent with cerebellomedullary region pathology (Davis & Lawton-Smith, 1971; Gay et al., 1974; Oosterveld & Rademakers, 1979; Towle & Romanul, 1970).

Square-wave jerks appear as square waves on the horizontal or vertical recording. Some normal persons demonstrate square wave jerks only in the EC condition with a peak-to-peak amplitude not exceeding 5° (Stockwell, 1983). It is pathological in the EC condition if the peak-to-peak amplitude exceeds 5° or is present in the EO condition regardless of its amplitude (Selhorst et al., 1976). Pathological square-wave jerks are consistent with cerebellar system disorders (Steenerson et al., 1986).

Congenital ocular nystagmus is horizontal or rotary nystagmus present in the EO condition and can be rhythmic or pendular. Its waveform is variable, particularly with changes in gaze direction. There is a direction of gaze, off-center gaze, called the null point where the nystagmus is greatly reduced or absent. Thus, persons with congenital ocular nystagmus often have a characteristic head tilt reflecting the null point. There is a convergence effect, that is, the reduction or disappearance of nystagmus at a point close to the face. Congenital nystagmus is present in approximately 1% of the population (Knapp, 1950).

C. GAZE NYSTAGMUS

The presence of gaze nystagmus is evaluated during the gaze test procedure. The average SPV is calculated for the three strongest consecutive beats in the EC and/or EO condition. If the average SPV exceeds 6°/s it is considered abnormal.

In normal persons, gaze nystagmus may be present at gaze deviations form midline exceeding 40°. This nystagmus is not pathological and is referred to as end-point nystagmus (Lambert, 1986). Gaze nystagmus is not present in normal persons for gaze deviations less than 40° from midline.

Horizontal unilateral gaze nystagmus appears only in one gaze direction. If the SPV is greater in the EC than EO condition, it is consistent with peripheral vestibular pathology. In such cases, the SPV is increased when the gaze direction is in the direction of the fast component of the spontaneous nystagmus (Coats, 1975). Therefore, in cases of horizontal unilateral gaze nystagmus, the presence of spontaneous vestibular nystagmus should be ruled out by asking the patient to close the eyes and observing whether there is a spontaneous nystagmus beating in the same direction as the gaze nystagmus with a SPV greater than 8°/s. Unilateral horizontal gaze nystagmus consistent with peripheral vestibular pathology is shown in Figure 14. If the SPV of the unilateral horizontal gaze nystagmus is greater in the EO than EC condition, then it is consistent with central nervous system pathology.

In cases of bilateral horizontal gaze nystagmus, the nystagmus beats to the right on right gaze and beats to the left on left gaze. Bilateral equal horizontal gaze nystagmus is

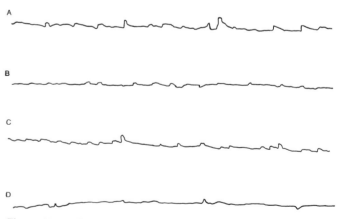

Figure 14 Unilateral right horizontal gaze nystagmus, right-beating. (A) Tracing for 20° gaze right. (B) Tracing for 20° gaze left. (C) Tracing for 30° gaze right. (D) Tracing for 30° gaze left. Courtesy of Dr. David Miller, San Diego Veterans Administration Medical Center.

present in the right and left gaze directions with an SPV that is equal in both directions. Bilateral equal horizontal gaze nystagmus is consistent with central nervous system pathology, usually brainstem pathology (Coats, 1975; Oosterveld, 1982) if drugs (barbiturates, Dilantin, alcohol) are ruled out. In cases of bilateral unequal horizontal gaze nystagmus, nystagmus is present in both gaze directions but the SPV of the nystagmus in one gaze direction differs from that in the other gaze direction. Bilateral unequal horizontal gaze nystagmus is consistent with organic central nervous system pathology (Coats, 1975). Bilateral unequal horizontal gaze nystagmus is illustrated in Figure 15.

Vertical gaze nystagmus is characterized by nystagmus in upward or downward gaze directions (on the vertical channel) and is consistent with central nervous system pathology. As mentioned previously, the nystagmus is up-beating or down-beating and may also be present in center gaze on the vertical channel. Figure 16 shows up-beating nystagmus on upward gaze. Allard and Welsh (1990) have underscored the importance of the vertical channel in gaze testing for detection of central vestibular disorders. To maximize the utility of gaze testing on the vertical channel, they recommend doing the gaze test in darkness and observing the patient's eyelids to rule out eyeblink.

D. SLOW-PURSUIT NYSTAGMUS

The presence of slow-pursuit nystagmus is evaluated during the pendular (sinusoidal) tracking procedure. In normal persons, the pursuit is smooth and uninterrupted and appears like a sinusoidal wave. Normal sinusoidal tracking is shown in Figure 17.

In cases with saccadic pursuit (also called cogwheeling), the eyes cannot keep up with the oscillating target and saccadic movements occur to allow refixation on the target. In unilateral saccadic pursuit, the superimposed corrective saccades occur only on one slope of the wave; in bilateral saccadic pursuit, the corrective saccades occur on both slopes of the wave. Saccadic pursuit is consistent with corti-

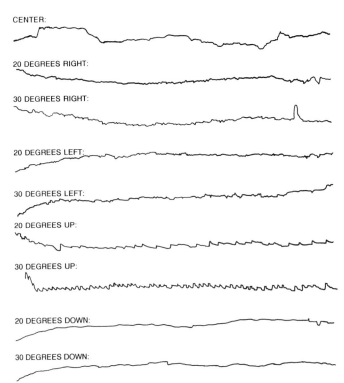

Figure 16 Up-beating vertical nystagmus on 20° and 30° upward gaze. Courtesy of Dr. David Miller, San Diego Veterans Administration Medical Center.

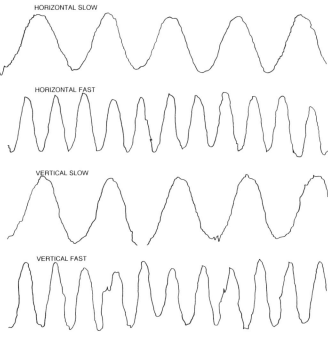

Figure 17 Normal sinusoidal tracking on the vertical and horizontal channels at fast and slow target speeds. Courtesy of Dr. David Miller, San Diego Veterans Administration Medical Center.

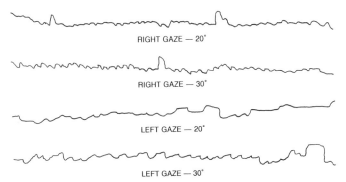

Figure 15 Bilateral unequal horizontal gaze nystagmus. Note that the nystagmus is stronger on the right than on the left gaze. Courtesy of Dr. David Miller, San Diego Veterans Administration Medical Center.

cal, brainstem, or cerebellar dysfunction (Baloh *et al.*, 1975, 1977; Baloh, Kumley, Sills, Honrubia, & Konrad, 1976; DeJong & Melvill-Jones, 1971; Jung & Kornhuber, 1964; Rodin, 1964). Unilateral saccadic pursuit may also result from an acute spontaneous nystagmus associated with an acute peripheral vestibular lesion (Baloh *et al.*, 1977; Schalen, Pyykko, Henriksson, & Wenmo, 1982). In such cases, the beating is in the direction of the defective pursuit. Since ocular defects such as paresis, lack of cooperativeness, inattentiveness, fatigue, failure to understand the task, drugs, eyeblinks, noisy recordings, and head movements as well as an acute peripheral vestibular pathology can cause saccadic pursuit, the clinician must rule out these factors before making the interpretation of central nervous system pathology (Lambert, 1986; Steenerson *et al.*, 1986). Unilateral saccadic pursuit is illustrated in Figure 18.

E. OPOTOKINETIC NYSTAGMUS

Optokinetic nystagmus is assessed during optokinetic testing. In normal persons, there is left-beating nystagmus when the stripes move to the right and right-beating nystagmus when the stripes move to the left. Symmetrical optokinetic nystagmus is shown in Figure 19. When the "look" nystagmus is elicited with the instructions to pick out the single stripes and follow them across the screen, the nystagmus is high amplitude and low frequency. When the "stare" nystagmus is elicited with the instructions to stare at the display of stripes, the nystagmus is low amplitude and high frequency.

Optokinetic nystagmus is assessed in terms of the symmetry of the pattern for the two directions (stripes moving to the right and stripes moving to the left). There is asymmetry if, in one but not the other direction, the pattern is poorly formed, with saccades interrupting the slow phase, or there is difference in the SPV of at least 10–30°/s (Barber & Stockwell, 1980). Optokinetic asymmetry is consistent with

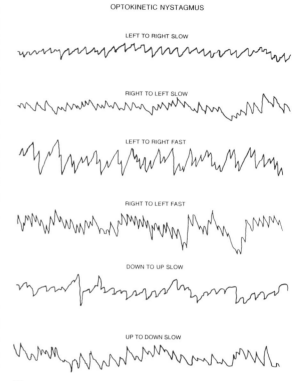

Figure 19 Normal optokinetic nystagmus. The nystagmus is symmetrical for left-to-right and right-to-left stripe movement at the slow and fast speeds and for down-to-up and up-to-down stripe movement at the slow speed. Courtesy of Dr. David Miller, San Diego Veterans Administration Medical Center.

central nervous system pathology usually involving the cerebral hemispheres (Smith & Cogan, 1960). Before the interpretation of central nervous system pathology based on optokinetic asymmetry can be made, the clinician must rule out ocular disorders (e.g., strabismus, severe extraocular muscle paresis, longstanding unilateral blindness), inattention, uncooperativeness, lack of understanding of the task, and intense peripheral vestibular spontaneous nystagmus (with an SPV exceeding 7°/s). In cases of intense peripheral vestibular spontaneous nystagmus, the optokinetic nystagmus is affected when the stimulus moves contralateral to the affected side (in the direction of the fast phase of the spontaneous nystagmus) (Baloh *et al.*, 1977; Brandt, Allum, & Dichgans, 1978; Coats, 1969). Predominantly right-beating optokinetic asymmetry is illustrated in Figure 20. Predominantly up-beating optokinetic asymmetry is illustrated in Figure 21.

If optokinetic asymmetry is present when the stripes move up or down, as evidenced by recordings on the vertical channel, there is said to be vertical optokinetic asymmetry consistent with central nervous system pathology, usually brainstem pathology (Jung & Kornhuber, 1964; Smith, 1962). A slight vertical optokinetic nystagmus is present in some normal persons so the asymmetry must be

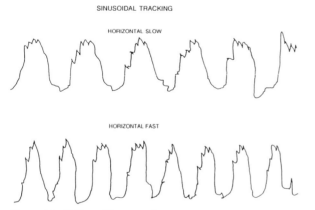

Figure 18 Unilateral horizontal saccadic pursuit which is present at both target speeds. Courtesy of Dr. David Miller, San Diego Veterans Administration Medical Center

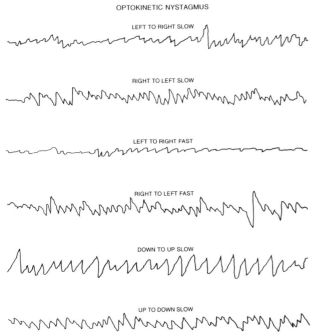

Figure 20 Asymmetrical optokinetic nystagmus, predominantly right-beating. Note that the left-to-right nystagmus is weaker than the right-to-left nystagmus at both speeds. The optokinetic nystagmus is essentially symmetrical on the vertical channel. Courtesy of Dr. David Miller, San Diego Veterans Administration Medical Center.

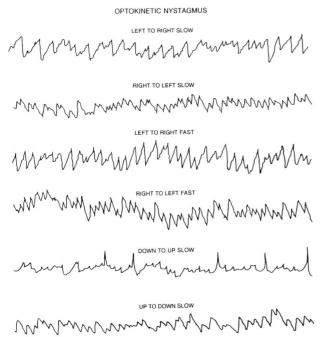

Figure 21 Asymmetrical optokinetic nystagmus, predominantly up-beating. Note that the down-to-up nystagmus is weaker than the up-to-down nystagmus. The optokinetic nystagmus is essentially symmetrical on the horizontal channel. Courtesy of Dr. David Miller, San Diego Veterans Administration Medical Center.

very large if it is present as an isolated finding that is considered abnormal (Coats, 1975). The clinician must rule out eyeblinks when vertical optokinetic asymmetry is obtained.

In cases of bilateral diminution of the optokinetic nystagmus, the SPV is reduced for both directions of stripe movement. Provided that inattention and uncooperativeness are ruled out, bilateral diminution is consistent with central nervous system pathology (Baloh, Yee, & Honrubia, 1980; Oosterveld, 1982).

The judgment of abnormal optokinetic patterns should be based on the patterns for both stimulus speeds since the faster stimulus speed should enhance the abnormality (Coats, 1975).

Resnick and Brewer (1983) reported that 31% of those with optokinetic asymmetry have gaze nystagmus and 9% of those with optokinetic asymmetry have it as an isolated ENG finding. According to Coats (1975), optokinetic abnormality present with gaze nystagmus is associated with brainstem or cerebellar pathology whereas optokinetic abnormality with normal gaze test results is associated with cerebral hemisphere dysfunction (Coats, 1970; Davidoff, Atkin, Anderson, & Bender, 1966; Jung & Kornhuber, 1964).

F. POSITIONAL NYSTAGMUS

Positional nystagmus is evaluated during positional testing. The average SPV is calculated for the three strongest consecutive beats. Positional nystagmus with an SPV less than 7°/s may occur in some normal persons in the eyes-closed but not in the eyes-open position. This nystagmus in normal persons is referred to as idiopathic positional nystagmus (Resnick & Brewer, 1983; Steenerson *et al.*, 1986; Lambert, 1986).

Positional nystagmus is considered to be pathologic if its direction changes in a single position (regardless of the SPV), if it is persistent (nystagmus continues for at least 1 min after assuming head position) in at least three head positions regardless of the SPV, if it is intermittent in at least four head positions (regardless of the SPV), or if it has an average SPV for the three strongest beats exceeding 6°/s in any single head position (Barber & Stockwell, 1980; Barber & Wright, 1973).

If positional nystagmus is present in all positions, spontaneous nystagmus must be ruled out. If it is spontaneous nystagmus, the SPV remains unchanged with position and is present in all positions. If it is positional rather than spontaneous nystagmus, the SPV will not remain constant throughout all the positions, that is, it will be modified in intensity or direction as the head position changes.

The direction of the nystagmus can be classified anatomically (right-beating or left-beating) or in relation to gravity (geotropic or ageotropic). Geotropic direction-changing nystagmus is right-beating when the right ear is down and left-beating when the left ear is down; that is, geotropic direction-changing positional nystagmus beats toward the ground. Ageotropic direction-changing nystagmus is left-beating when the right ear is down and right-beating when the left ear is down; that is, ageotropic positional nystagmus beats away from the ground.

Abnormal positional nystagmus is also classified according to whether it is direction-changing with head-position changes, direction-changing in a single head position, or direction-fixed. Direction-changing with head-position changes refers to positional nystagmus which beats in one direction in one head position and beats in the opposite direction in another head position. Direction-changing within a head position refers to positional nystagmus which beats in one direction for a single head position and then beats in the opposite direction while the head is kept in the same position. Direction-fixed refers to positional nystagmus which beats in the same direction regardless of the head position.

Direction-fixed positional nystagmus which has an SPV greater in the eyes-closed than eyes-open condition is usually consistent with peripheral vestibular pathology (Barber & Stockwell, 1980). Left-beating, direction-fixed po-

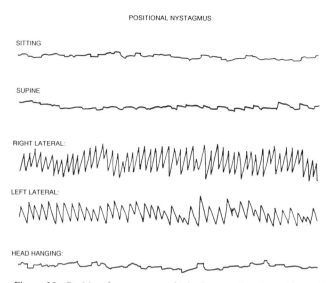

Figure 23 Positional nystagmus which changes direction with position changes. Note that the nystagmus is left-beating in the right lateral position and right-beating in the left lateral position. Courtesy of Dr. David Miller, San Diego Veterans Administration Medical Center.

sitional nystagmus under the eyes-closed condition is illustrated in Figure 22.

Positional nystagmus which is direction-changing with head-position changes and has an SPV which is greater in the eyes closed than eyes open condition is a nonlocalizing finding (Coats, 1975; Steenerson *et al.*, 1986; Stockwell, 1983). Figure 23 illustrates positional nystagmus in the eyes-closed condition which is direction-changing with changes in head position.

Positional nystagmus which is direction-changing in a single head position in the eyes-closed or eyes-open condition is a strong sign of central vestibular pathology (Oosterveld, 1982; Steenerson *et al.*, 1986). Direction-changing nystagmus within a single position in the eyes-closed condition is shown in Figure 24.

When positional nystagmus which is direction-changing

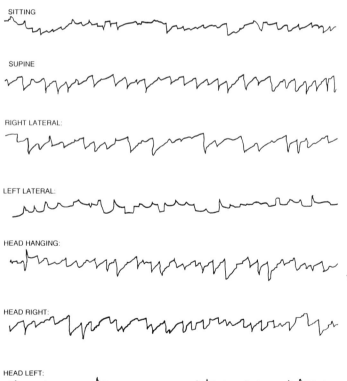

Figure 22 Direction-fixed positional nystagmus. Note that left-beating nystagmus is present in all positions except head left. Courtesy of Dr. David Miller, San Diego Veterans Administration Medical Center.

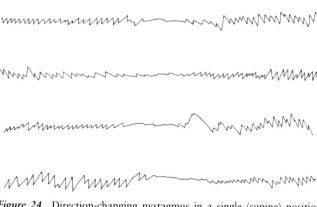

Figure 24 Direction-changing nystagmus in a single (supine) position under the eyes-closed condition. Courtsey of Dr. David Miller, San Diego Veterans Administration Medical Center.

with head-position changes and which is greater in the eyes-closed than eyes-open condition is obtained, drug ingestion (alcohol, quinine, barbiturates) should be ruled out. Positional alcoholic nystagmus (PAN) I occurs approximately 30 min after alcohol ingestion, is geotropic direction-changing, and lasts for approximately 3 hr (Hill, Collins, & Schroeder, 1973). PAN II occurs approximately 5 hr after alcohol ingestion, may last up to 24 hr, and is ageotropic direction-changing (Hill *et al.*, 1973).

Positional nystagmus which has an SPV greater in the eyes-open than in the eyes-closed condition and is direction-fixed or direction-changing is generally consistent with central vestibular pathology, most commonly resulting from head injuries, vertebral basilar ischemia, and posterior fossa tumors (Harrison & Ozsahinoglu, 1972; Oosterveld, 1982, Stockwell, 1983).

The clinician should be aware that positioning nystagmus (benign paroxysmal vertigo) can be induced during positional testing by moving the patient into the head position too quickly.

G. PAROXYSMAL NYSTAGMUS

The presence of paroxysmal nystagmus is evaluated during the Dix–Hallpike maneuver. Some normal persons display a sudden burst of nystagmus whih disappears after the head position is achieved.

According to Dix and Hallpike (1952), the classical response, also called benign paroxysmal nystagmus, has the following features: (a) latency of 0.5–8.0 s after the position is achieved, (b) transient (the nystagmus builds up in intensity and then disappears in 2–10 s), (c) subjective vertigo, often violent, and (d) fatigable (the nystagmus disappears or is reduced significantly when the manuever is repeated). Coats (1975) employs all of these criteria except the latency criterion in judging whether a classical response has occurred, since recording the response to the Dix–Hallpike maneuver under the eyes-closed condition may reduce or abolish the latent period which would be observed under the eyes-open condition. According to Coats (1975), the classical response is unilateral and beats toward the downward ear (when the downward ear is the pathologic ear). Unilateral benign paroxysmal nystagmus is usually secondary to peripheral vestibular dysfunction (Dayal *et al.*, 1974). Unilateral benign paroxysmal nystagmus is often present in persons more than 55 years of age, some cases complaining of posttraumatic dizziness following head trauma, some cases of chronic middle-ear infection, some cases following stapes surgery, and some rare cases of pernicious anemia (Coats, 1975). Figure 25 illustrates a unilateral classical Dix–Hallpike response on both the horizontal and vertical channels for the down–right maneuver. Bilateral benign paroxysmal nystagmus is a nonlocalizing finding (Longridge & Barber, 1978).

If nystagmus is present but does not meet all of the criteria for a classical response (latency is not a criterion), then

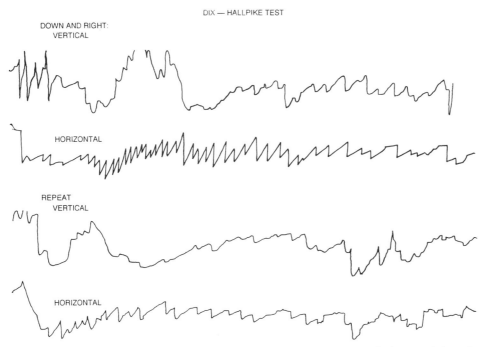

Figure 25 Classical Dix–Hallpike response. Note the left-beating nystagmus on the horizontal channel and down-beating nystagmus on the vertical channel associated with dizziness on the initial down–right maneuver. Upon repetition of the maneuver in the same direction, the nystagmus was reduced and the patient was less dizzy. Courtesy of Dr. David Miller, San Diego Veterans Administration Medical Center.

the response is considered to be nonclassical. Resnick & Brewer (1983) reported that the criterion for a classical response which is most often not satisfied is vertigo. The nonclassical response is a nonlocalizing finding; nevertheless, the nonclassical response is more likely to be associated with central vestibular than peripheral vestibular pathology (Cawthorne & Hinchcliffe, 1961; Hallpike, 1962; Harrison & Ozsahinoglu, 1975; Steenerson *et al.*, 1986). A nonclassical response to the Dix–Hallpike maneuver for the down–right side is shown in Figure 26.

The clinician should ideally employ both the vertical and horizontal channels for recording the response to the Dix–Hallpike maneuver since the response has horizontal and vertical components; in many cases, the vertical component is stronger the horizontal component. The response to the Dix–Hallpike maneuver must be differentiated from positional nystagmus. If the SPV or direction of the response to the Dix–Hallpike procedure is the same as that for the positional nystagmus, the response is merely a reflection of the positional nystagmus. If the SPV or direction of the response to the Dix–Hallpike maneuver differs from that of the positional nystagmus, it can be assumed that the response was elicited by the Dix–Hallpike maneuver and is not reflective of the positional nystagmus.

H. CALORIC NYSTAGMUS

Caloric nystagmus is evaluated during caloric testing. In normal persons, nystagmus is induced approximately 20 s after irrigation onset, increases in intensity for approximately another 40 s and thereafter declines (Stockwell, 1983). It is right-beating for right–warm and left–cool irrigations and left-beating for left–warm and right–cool irrigations. The beating direction may reverse after 120–180 sec following onset of irrigation (Stockwell, 1983). Stockwell suggests that the average SPV for each irrigation be based on the three strongest consecutive nonartifactual beats occurring during the 10-s interval in which the nystagmus is most intense. If spontaneous nystagmus is present, its average SPV is subtracted from the average SPV of caloric irrigations if it beats in the same direction as the caloric nystagmus and is added to the average SPV of the caloric irrigations if it beats in the direction opposite to the caloric nystagmus. Bithermal calorics is considered to be the strongest ENG test for the identification of peripheral vestibular pathology.

Unilateral weakness (UW), also called canal paresis, is calculated using the following formula (Coats, 1965; Jongkees & Philipszoon, 1964):

$$UW = \frac{\text{Right-ear response} - \text{left-ear response}}{\text{Total right and left,}} \times 100$$
$$\text{warm and cool responses}$$
$$= \frac{(RC + RW) - (LC + LW)}{RW + LW + RC + LC} \times 100$$

UW exceeding an absolute value of 20% is abnormal. A positive UW value means that there is a unilateral weakness on the left. A negative UW value means that there is a

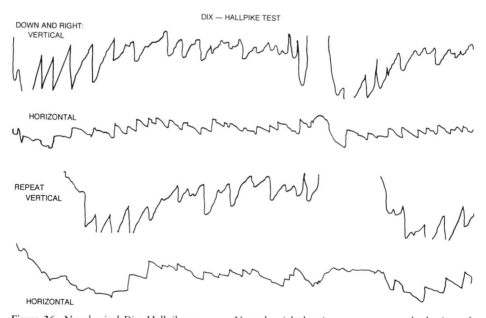

Figure 26 Nonclassical Dix–Hallpike response. Note the right-beating nystagmus on the horizontal channel and down-beating nystagmus on the vertical channel without dizziness on the initial down–right maneuver. Similar results were obtained upon repetition of the maneuver in the same direction without fatigability. Courtesy of Dr. David Miller, San Diego Veterans Administration Medical Center.

unilateral weakness on the right. The values of UW can vary between +100% and −100%.

UW is usually consistent with peripheral vestibular disorders. Nevertheless, vestibular nuclei lesions can involve vestibular nerve fibers and cause UW but such lesions nearly always produce other central findings along with UW (Coats, 1975). Therefore, an isolated UW is always a peripheral vestibular finding (Baloh & Honrubia, 1979). UW is the most common abnormal finding in cases of peripheral vestibular pathology (Resnick & Brewer, 1983). It is suggested that if the SPV based on three beats yields borderline UW values, the UW be calculated based on the average SPV of 10 consecutive beats from the period of maximum SPV caloric response or the average SPV of all the beats in the 10-s period of maximum SPV caloric responses. UW is also considered to be present if the combined SPV for the warm and cool irrigations in a given ear is less than 12–15°/s (Stockwell, 1983). Figure 27 ilustrates a left unilateral weakness on the calorics test. Figure 28 illustrates right unilateral weakness on the calorics test.

Bilateral weakness (BW) or hypoactivity is defined as total (combined) SPV for the right and warm irrigations in each ear not exceeding 12–15°/s. It is consistent with bilateral peripheral vestibular pathology resulting from, for example, ototoxic poisoning, drug ingestion, bilateral Meniere's disease, or central nervous system pathology (Simmons, 1973). BW associated with central nervous system pathology is usually present with abnormal optokinetic nystagmus. Bilateral weakness is shown in Figure 29.

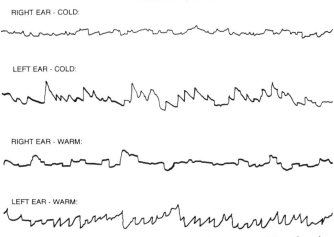

Figure 28 Right unilateral weakness on caloric testing. Note that the caloric nystagmus in the left warm and left cold conditions is markedly stronger than in the right warm and right cold conditions. Courtesy of Dr. David Miller, San Diego Veterans Administration Medical Center.

Hyperactivity is defined as an average SPV exceeding 50°/s for a cool irrigation or exceeding 80°/s for a warm irrigation (Barber & Stockwell, 1976). Hyperactivity can be unilateral or bilateral. Bilateral hyperactive vestibular responses are consistent with central vestibular and other central nervous system pathology (Torok, 1970) and may reflect loss of cerebellar inhibition (Spector, 1975; Torok, 1970). Unilateral hyperactive vestibular responses are a nonlocalizing finding (Kavanagh & Babin, 1986; Torok, 1970). When hyperactive vestibular responses are obtained, the clinician should rule out unusual caloric transfer qualities such as a mastoidectomy, tympanic membrane perforation, or an atrophic or retracted tympanic membrane (Steenerson et al., 1986).

Direction preponderance (DP) is calculated using the formula

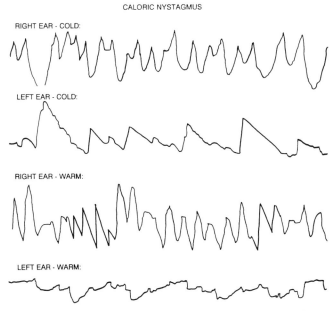

Figure 27 Left unilateral weakness on caloric testing. Note that the caloric nystagmus in the right cold and right warm conditions is markedly stronger than the left cold and left warm conditions. Courtesy of Dr. David Miller, San Diego Veterans Administration Medical Center.

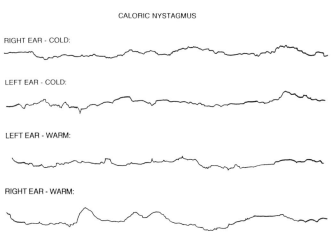

Figure 29 Bilateral weakness on caloric testing. Courtesy of Dr. David Miller, San Diego Veterans Administration Medical Center.

$$DP = \frac{(RW + LC) - (RC + LW)}{RW + LW + RC + LC} \times 100$$

DP values can vary between positive and negative infinity. DP values exceeding an absolute value of 30% are considered abnormal. A positive DP represents caloric nystagmus that is predominantly right-beating. A negative DP represents nystagmus that is predominantly left-beating. DP has traditionally been considered a nonlocalizing finding indicative of peripheral or central vestibular pathology; if it is an isolated finding, it is considered to be indicative of central vestibular pathology. The validity of DP is debatable since the value is affected by the order of caloric irrigations given. DP is also generally associated with spontaneous nystagmus. McCabe & Ryu (1979) consider DP worthless. Our clinical experience substantiates McCabe and Ryu's (1979) impression of DP.

The failure-of-fixation test should be done approximately 90 after the onset of irrigation. Alpert (1974) suggests administering the failure-of-fixation test approximately 10–20 s after the peak SPV has been reached in the eyes-closed condition. The fixation index (FI) is calculated as

FI = (SPV in EO)/(SPV in EC)

An FI exceeding 0.6–0.7 is considered pathologic (Alpert, 1974; Barber, 1978). The FI is sometimes abnormal in normal persons when the SPV of the caloric response in the eyes closed condition exceeds 60–70°/s (Glaser & Stockwell, 1979). Otherwise, an abnormal FI is considered to be consistent with central nervous system pathology, usually vestibulocerebellar pathology, primarily the flocculus and its connections (Takemori & Cohen, 1974). The clinician should rule out sedation (especially barbiturates), contact lenses (especially if they are new or uncomfortable), intense SPV for an irrigation, and peripheral ocular pathology when an abnormal FI is obtained (Coats, 1975). Normal fixation suppression is illustrated in Figure 30. Failure of fixation suppression is shown in Figure 31.

Secondary phase nystagmus, also called premature caloric reversal, is caloric nystagmus which reverses its direction prior to 140 sec following onset of irrigation and has a

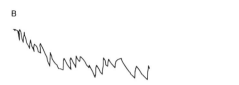

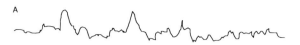

Figure 31 Failure of fixation suppression. (A) Obtained on the right, warm, eyes-closed condition. (B) Obtained on the right, warm, eyes-open condition. Courtesy of Dr. David Miller, San Diego Veterans Administration Medical Center.

SPV exceeding 7°/sec. The clinician must rule out resumption of spontaneous nystagmus. Secondary phase nystagmus is consistent with central vestibular pathology (Barber & Stockwell, 1980; Kavanagh & Babin, 1986).

Caloric inversion, in which the nystagmus beats in the direction opposite to that expected, is considered consistent with brainstem pathology (Kavanagh & Babin, 1986; Steenerson *et al.*, 1986). The clinician must rule out incorrect insertion of electrode leads before giving the interpretation of central nervous system disorder to caloric inversion (Steenerson *et al.*, 1986).

I. ROTARY NYSTAGMUS

Normal persons demonstrate a phase lag of nearly 90° (when inverted eye velocity is analyzed with reference to chair acceleration) for high-frequency rotation (0.16 Hz). The phase lag decreases in normal persons as the frequency of sinusoidal stimulation decreases, approaching 0° at 0.01 Hz. A phase lag is considered abnormal at a given frequency of stimulation if it is below 2 SD of the mean phase lag in normal persons. Abnormal phase lag is considered to be a sensitive indicator of peripheral vestibular pathology (Jenkins, 1985; Olson & Wolfe, 1981; Olson, Wolfe, & Engelken, 1981). Normal and abnormal phase lag are shown in Figure 32.

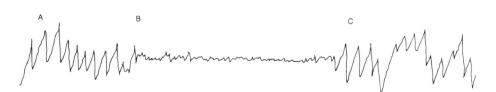

Figure 30 Normal fixation suppression during caloric testing. (A) Obtained with the eyes closed. (B) Obtained with the eyes open and fixated. (C) Obtained with the eyes closed. Courtesy of Dr. David Miller, San Diego Veterans Administration Medical Center.

In normal persons, the gain increases as the frequency of rotation increases, approaching unity at 0.16 Hz when rotational testing is performed in darkness or with the patient blindfolded. Reduced gain (less than 2 SD below the mean gain in normal persons, especially at low-frequency rotations, is consistent with peripheral vestibular pathology (Hirsch, 1986; Jenkins, 1985; Wolfe & Kos, 1977). Increased gain (greater than 2 SD above the mean gain in normal persons) is consistent with the presence of cerebellar lesions (Baloh, Jenkins, Honrubia, Yee, & Lau, 1979). Normal and abnormal gain is illustrated in Figure 33.

As previously mentioned, symmetry is reported as directional preponderance. In normal persons, the DP decreases as the frequency of rotational testing increases, approaching 0 at 0.16 Hz. DP outside the range defined by 2 SD from the mean DP (significant asymmetry) has been reported in patients with severe active Meniere's disease and labyrinthectomy (Olson & Wolfe, 1981; Wolfe, Engelken, Olson, & Kos, 1978). DP is insensitive to chronic vestibular abnormalities. It may detect an acute or complete unilateral peripheral vestibular paralysis but is often insensitive to unilateral paresis (Hirsch, 1986). DP does not provide localizing or lateralizing information (Hirsch, 1986). Normal and abnormal DP are illustrated in Figure 34.

J. PITFALLS IN ENG TESTING AND INTERPRETATION

Stimulus delivery during calorics testing can adversely affect the calorics responses (Barber & Stockwell, 1980; Kileny & Kemink, 1986). Air- and closed-loop irrigation systems are more prone than open-water irrigation systems to the blocking of the entrance to the medial ear canal by an air bubble, resulting in stimulus temperature variation leading to an erroneous unilateral weakness. Similar erroneous findings can occur if the irrigation tip is held too laterally (Kileny & Kemink, 1986). The calorics results may be affected because of interference in stimulus delivery in cases

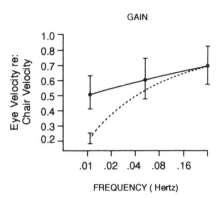

Figure 33 (—), Normal values; (— — —), bilateral vestibular paresis. From Hirsch (1986) with permission.

of natural anatomic variations or surgical distortion of the ear canal, middle-ear space, and mastoid system; cerumen impaction; external auditory canal lesions (e.g., osteomas or exostoses); or chronic suppurative otitis media leading to tympanic membrane perforation or other abnormalities (Barber & Stockwell, 1980; Kileny & Kemink, 1986). To avoid interference with stimulus delivery during calorics testing, Kileny & Kemink (1986) suggest (a) purging prior to irrigation, (b) use of a system with continuous irrigation in which the water continuously circulates between the irrigation tip and reservoir, and (c) irrigating immediately after purging.

Technical artifacts that can distort the ENG tracing may result from improper electrode contact and excessively high electrode impedance (Barber & Stockwell, 1980; Kileny & Kemink, 1986). High electrode impedance or unequal electrode impedances can cause a baseline shift and/or a 60-Hz hum in the ENG tracing as illustrated in Figure 35. A broken electrode wire, an electrode loosely attached to the

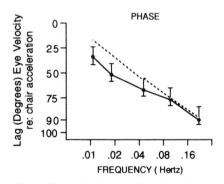

Figure 32 (—), Normal phase lag relative to acceleration; (— — —), pathologic phase lag. From Hirsch (1986) with permission.

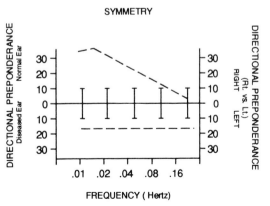

Figure 34 (—), Normal ± 1 SD; (— — —), active severe Meniere's patients; (– – –), postoperative acoustic tumor removal. From Hirsch (1986) with permission.

skin, or an electrode lead that moves can also produce technical artifacts. A broken electrode wire produces wild voltage fluctuations as shown in Figure 36. If the electrode is not firmly attached to the skin and moves, particularly when the patient squints, large voltage fluctuations can result, as shown in Figure 37. Moving electrode leads can produce a low-frequency potential as shown in Figure 38. The operation of electrical switches may produce transient high-amplitude voltages as illustrated in Figure 39. Technical electrode artifacts can be avoided by routinely checking electrodes and their leads for continuity, careful skin preparation and electrode application, and keeping electrode impedances below 10,000 ohms prior to administering the ENG test (Barber & Stockwell, 1980; Kileny & Kemink, 1986).

Physiologic artifacts can also adversely affect the ENG recordings. Eyeblinks superimposed on the calibration saccadic recordings may be mistaken for calibration overshoot consistent with cerebellar involvement (Barber & Stockwell, 1980; Kileny & Kemink, 1986). As mentioned previously, eyeblinks look like nystagmus, appear simultaneously on the recordings from the horizontal and vertical channels, and have a greater amplitude on the tracing from the vertical than the horizontal channel as illustrated in Figure 40. Muscle potentials arising from the contraction of the facial or neck muscles represent another physiologic artifact which can distort the ENG tracing. This artifact produces a very-high-frequency electrical signal in the tracing and appears as a fuzzy tracing, as shown in Figure 41. This artifact can be reduced by asking the patient to relax the face (Barber & Stockwell, 1980). Another physiologic artifact can result from head movement during ENG testing (Barber & Stockwell, 1980; Kileny & Kemink, 1986). Head movement during calibration can result in a recording which may be suggestive of overshoot consistent with cerebellar lesions (Kileny & Kemink, 1986). Poor or distorted vision can result in a physiologic artifact, especially during the sinusoidal tracking and optokinetic tests, because irregular excursions may result, suggestive of brainstem or cerebellar disease. The clinician must ensure that the head does not move during ENG testing and should ascertain the patient's visual condition prior to the ENG test; if significant correction is needed, the patient should wear the

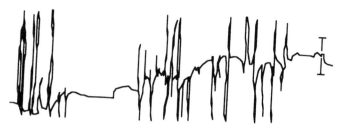

Figure 36 Broken electrode wire. From Barber and Stockwell (1980) with permission.

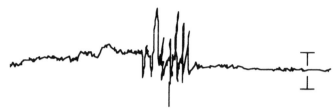

Figure 37 Electrode movement. From Barber and Stockwell (1980) with permission.

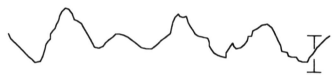

Figure 38 Electrode lead wire movement. From Barber and Stockwell (1980) with permission.

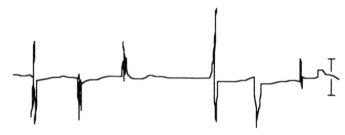

Figure 39 Voltage transients produced by an electrical switch. From Barber and Stockwell (1980) with permission.

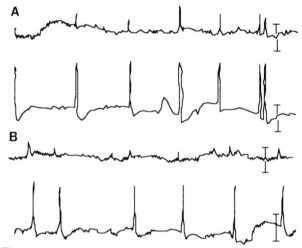

Figure 40 (A) Vigorous eye blinks with the eyes open. *Upper tracing,* bitemporal leads; *lower tracing,* vertical leads. (B) Same patient, same leads, eyes closed. From Barber and Stockwell (1980) with permission.

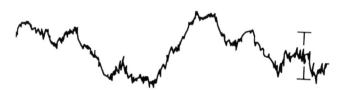

Figure 35 Baseline shift and 60-Hz "hum" usually caused by poor electrode contact. From Barber and Stockwell (1980) with permission.

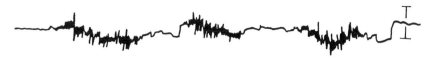

Figure 41 Muscle potentials. From Barber and Stockwell (1980) with permission.

corrective lenses during the ENG procedure (Barber & Stockwell, 1980; Kileny & Kemink, 1986).

According to Steenerson *et al.* (1986), central nervous system disorder is usually characterized by CNS signs on multiple tests in the ENG battery. A single CNS sign on just one ENG test in the ENG battery should be cautiously interpreted.

REFERENCES

Alpert, J. N. (1974). Failure of fixation suppression: A pathologic effect of vision on caloric nystagmus. *Neurol., 24,* 891–896.

Allard, B., & Welsh, T. (1990). Diagnostic value of vertical nystagmus recorded from ENG. *Ear Hear., 11,* 62–65.

Bahill, A. T., & Troost, B. T. (1979). Types of saccadic eye movements. *Neurol., 29,* 1150–1152.

Balkany, T. J., & Finkel, R. S. (1986). The dizzy child. *Ear Hear., 7,* 138–142.

Baloh, R. W., & Honrubia, V. (1976). Reaction time and accuracy of the saccadic eye movements of normal subjects in a moving-target task. *Aviat. Space Environ. Med., 47,* 1165–1167.

Baloh, R. W., & Honrubia, V. (1979). *Clinical neurophysiology of the vestibular system.* Philadelphia: Davis.

Baloh, R. W., & Keesey, J. C. (1976). Saccade fatigue and responses to edophonium for the diagnosis of myasthenia gravis. *Ann. N. Y. Acad. Sci., 274,* 631–641.

Baloh, R. W., Konrad, H. R., & Honrubia, V. (1975). Vestibulo–ocular function in patients with cerebellar atrophy *Neurol., 25,* 160–168.

Baloh, R. W., Kumley, W., Sills, A. W., Honrubia, V., & Konrad, H. (1976). Quantitative measurements of smooth pursuit eye movements. *Ann. Otol. Rhinol., Laryngol., 85,* 111–119.

Baloh, R. W., Honrubia, V., & Sills, A. (1977). Eye tracking and optokinetic nystagmus: Results of quantitative testing in patients with well-defined nervous system lesions. *Ann. Otol. Rhinol. Laryngol., 86,* 108–114.

Baloh, R. W., Jenkins, H. A., Honrubia, V., Yee, R. D., & Lau, C. G. Y. (1979). Visual–vestibular interaction and cerebellar atrophy. *Neurol., 29,* 116–119.

Baloh, R. W., Yee, R. D., & Honrubia, V. (1980). Optokinetic nystagmus and parietal lobe lesions. *Ann. Neurol., 7,* 269–276.

Barany, R. (1907). *Physiologie und Pathologie des Bogengangsapparates beim Menschen.* Vienna: Deuticke.

Barber, H. O. (1978). Current ideas on vestibular diagnosis. *Otolaryngol. Clin. N. Am., 11,* 283–300.

Barber, H. O., & Stockwell, C. W. (1976). *Manual of electronystagmography.* St. Louis: Mosby.

Barber, H. O., & Stockwell, C. W. (1980). *Manual of electronystagmography,* 2d ed. St. Louis: Mosby.

Barber, H. O., & Wright, G. (1973). Positional nystagmus in normals. *Adv. Otorhinolaryngol., 19,* 276–285.

Barber, H. O., Wright, G., & Demanuele, F. (1971). The hot caloric test as a clinical screening device. *Arch. Otolaryngol., 94,* 335–337.

Bender, M. B., & Shanzer, S. (1964). Oculomotor pathways defined by electric stimulation and lesions in the brainstem of monkey. In M. B. Bender (ed.), *The oculomotor system,* pp. 81–94. New York: Harper & Row.

Brandt, T. H., Allum, J. H. J., & Dichgans, J. (1978). Computer analysis of optokinetic nystagmus in patients with spontaneous nystagmus of peripheral vestibular origin. *Acta Otolaryngol., 86,* 115–122.

Brookler, K. H. (1976). The stimulus binaural bithermal. *Laryngoscope, 86,* 1241.

Brookler, K. H., Baker, A. H., & Grams, G. (1979). Closed loop water irrigator system. *Otolaryngol. Head Neck Surg., 87,* 364–365.

Cawthorne, T., & Hinchcliffe, R. (1961). Positional nystagmus of the central type as evidence of subtentorial metastases. *Brain, 84,* 415–426.

Clark, K. R. (1986). Torsion swing chair. *Ear Hear., 7,* 191–197.

Coats, A. C. (1965). Directional preponderance and unilateral weakness as observed in the electronystagmographic examination. *Ann. Otol. Rhinol. Laryngol., 74,* 655–668.

Coats, A. C. (1969). The diagnostic significance of spontaneous nystagmus as observed in the electronystagmographic examination. *Acta Otolaryngol., 67,* 33–42.

Coats, A. C. (1970). Central electronystagmographic abnormalities. *Arch. Otolaryngol., 92,* 43–53.

Coats, A. C. (1975). Electronystagmography. In L. J. Bradford (ed.), *Physiological measures of the audio-vestibular system,* pp. 37–85. New York: Academic Press.

Coats, A. C. (1986). ENG examination technique. *Ear Hear., 7,* 143–150.

Cyr, D. G. (1983). The vestibular system: Pediatric considerations. *Sem. Hear., 4,* 33–45.

Daroff, R. B., & Hoyt, W. F. (1971). Supranuclear disorders of ocular control systems in man: Clinical, anatomical, and physiological correlations. In P. Bach-y-Rita, C. C. Collins, & J. E. Hyde (eds.), *The control of eye movements,* pp. 175–235. New York: Academic Press.

Daroff, R. B., & Troost, B. T. (1978). Supranuclear disorders of eye movements. In J. S. Glaser (ed.), *Neuro-ophthalmology,* pp. 201–218. Hagerstown, Maryland: Harper & Row.

Daroff, R. B., Troost, B. T., & Leigh, R. J. (1990). Supranuclear disorders of eye movements. In J. S. Glaser (ed.), Neuro-ophthalmology, 2d ed, pp. 299–323. Philadelphia: J. B. Lippincott.

Davidoff, R. A., Atkin, A., Anderson, P. J., & Bender, M. (1966). Optokinetic nystagmus and cerebral disease. *Arch. Neurol., 14,* 73–81.

Davis, D. G., & Lawton-Smith, J. (1971). Periodic alternating nystagmus: A report of eight cases. *Am. J. Ophthalmol., 72,* 757–762.

Davis, R. I., & Mann, R. C. (1987). The effects of alerting tasks on caloric induced vestibular nystagmus. *Ear Hear., 8,* 58–60.

Dayal, V. S., Tarantino, L., Farkashidy, J., & Paradisgarten, A. (1974). Spontaneous and positional nystagmus: A reassessment of clinical significance. *Laryngoscope, 84,* 203–2044.

DeJong, J. D., & Melvill-Jones, G. (1971). Akinesia, hypokinesia, and bradykinesia in the oculomotor system of patients with Parkinson's disease. *Exp. Neurol., 32,* 58–68.

Dix, M. R., & Hallpike, C. S. (1952). The pathology, symptomatology, and diagnosis of certain disorders of the vestibular system. *Ann. Otol. Rhinol. Laryngol., 61,* 987–1016.

Fitzgerald, G., & Hallpike, C. S. (1942). Studies of the human vestibular function. I. Observations on the directional preponderance ("Nystagmusberetschaft") of caloric nystagmus resulting from central lesions. *Brain, 65,* 115–137.

Fluur, E., & Eriksson, L. (1961). Nystagmographic recording of vertical eye movements. *Acta Otolaryngol., 53,* 486–492.

Frenzel, H. (1982). *Spontan- und Provokations-nystagmus.* Basel: Karger.

Gay, A. J., Newman, N. M., Keltner, J. L., & Stroud, M. H. (1974). Nystagmus. In A. J. Gay, N. Newman, J. L. Keltner, & M. H. Stroud (eds.) *Eye movement disorders,* pp. 65–69. St. Louis: Mosby.

Glaser, R. G., & Stockwell, C. W. (1979). Fixation suppression: A clinical reevaluation. Paper presented at the Annual Convention of the American Speech-Language-Hearing Association, Atlanta, Georgia.

Hallpike, C. S. (1962). Vertigo of central origin. *Proc. R. Soc. Med., 55,* 364–370.

Haring, R. D., & Simmons, F. B. (1973). Cerebellar defects detectable by ENG calibration. *Otolaryngol., 98,* 14–17.

Harrison, M. S., & Ozsahinoglu, C. (1975). Positional vertigo. *Arch. Otolaryngol., 101,* 675–678.

Henriksson, N. G. (1956). Speed of slow component and duration in caloric nystagmus. *Acta Otolaryngol. Supp., 46,* 1–29.

Hill, R. J., Collins, W. E., & Schroeder, D. J. (1973). Influence of alchol on positional nystagmus over 24-hour periods. *Ann. Otol. Rhinol. Laryngol., 82,* 103–110.

Hirsch, B. E. (1986). Computed sinusoidal harmonic acceleration. *Ear Hear., 7,* 198–203.

Honrubia, V., Downey, W. L., Mitchell, D. P., & Ward, P. H. (1968). Experimental studies on optokinetic nystagmus. II. Normal humans. *Acta Otolaryngol., 65,* 441–448.

Jenkins, H. A. (1985). Long-term adaptive changes of vestibulo-ocular reflex in patients following acoustic neuroma surgery. *Laryngoscope, 95,* 1224–1234.

Jongkees, L. B. W. (1948). Value of the caloric test of the labyrinth. *Arch Otolaryngol., 48,* 402–417.

Jongkees, L. B. W., & Philipszoon, A. J. (1964). Electronystagmography. *Acta Otolaryngol. Suppl., 189,* 1–33.

Jung, R., & Kornhuber, H. H. (1964). Results of electronystagmography in man: The value of optokinetic, vestibular and spontaneous nystagmus for neurological diagnosis and research. In M. Bender (ed.), *The oculomotor system,* pp. 428–482. New York: Harper & Row.

Kavanagh, K. T., & Babin, R. W. (1986). Definitions and types of nystagmus and calculations. *Ear Hear., 7,* 157–166.

Keim, R. J. (1985). The pitfalls of limiting ENG testing to patients with vertigo. *Laryngoscope, 95,* 1208–1212.

Kileny, P. (1982). Evaluation of vestibular function. In J. Katz (ed.), *Handbook of clinical audiology,* 3d ed., pp. 585–603. Baltimore: Williams & Wilkins.

Kileny, P., & Kemink, J. L. (1986). Artifacts and errors in the electronystagmographic (ENG) evaluation of the vestibular system. *Ear Hear., 7,* 151–156.

Knapp, H. (1950). Kommt Spontannystagmus bei Gesunden vor? *Hals Nasen Ohren, 2,* 17–19.

Lambert, P. R. (1986). Nonlocalizing vestibular findings on electronystagmography. *Ear Hear., 7,* 182–185.

Longridge, N. S., & Barber, H. O. (1978). Bilateral paroxysmal positional nystagmus. *J. Otolaryngol., 7,* 395–400.

Lundberg, N. (1940). On differences in vestibular tonus. *Acta Otolaryngol., 28,* 501–504.

McCabe, B., & Ryu, J. (1979). Clinical electronystagmography. In Vestibular physiology in *understanding the dizzy patient,* pp. 51–60. Rochester, Minnesota: American Academy of Otolaryngology.

McGee, M. L. (1986). Electronystagmography in peripheral lesions. *Ear Hear., 7,* 167–175.

Olson, J. E., & Wolfe, J. W. (1981). Comparison of subjective symptomatology and responses to harmonic acceleration in patients with Meniere's disease. *Ann. Otol. Suppl. 86, 90,* 15–17.

Olson, J. E., Wolfe, J. W., & Engelken, E. J. (1981). Responses to low frequency harmonic acceleration in patients with acoustic neuromas. *Laryngoscope, 91,* 1270–1277.

Oosterveld, W. J. (1982). A report from Europe. In V. Honrubia & M. A. B. Brazier (eds.), *Nystagmus and vertigo: Clinical approaches to the patient with dizziness.* pp. 133–144. New York: Academic Press.

Oosterveld, M. J., & Rademakers, W. J. A. C. (1979). Nystagmus alternans. *Acat Otolaryngol., 87,* 404–409.

Pappas, P. G. (1985). *Diagnosis and treatment of hearing impairment in children: A clinical manual.* San Diego: College-Hill Press.

Pola, J., & Robinson, D. A. (1976). An explanation of eye movements seen in internuclear ophthalmoplegia. *Arch. Neurol., 33,* 447–452.

Resnick, D. M., & Brewer, C. C. (1983). The electronystagmography test battery: Hit or myth? *Sem. Hear., 4,* 23–32.

Rodin, E. A. (1964). Impaired ocular pursuit movements. *Arch. Neurol., 10,* 327–330.

Ruben, W. (1984). Rotational vestibular testing. *Am. J. Otol., 5,* 441–442.

Schalen, L., Pyykko I., Henriksson, N. G., & Wennmo, C. (1982). Slow eye movements in patients with neurological disorders. *Acta Otolaryngol. Suppl., 386,* 321–334.

Selhorst, J. B., Stark, L, Ochs, A. L., & Hoyt, W. F. (1976). Disorders of cerebellar ocular motor control. I. Saccadic overshoot dysmetria, an oculographic control system and clinico-anatomic analysis. *Brain, 99,* 497–508.

Sharpe, J. A., Rosenberg, Hoyt, W. F., & Daroff, R. B. (1974). Paralytic pontine exotropia. *Neurol., 24,* 1076–1082.

Simmons, F. B. (1973). Patients with bilateral loss of caloric response. *Ann. Otol. Rhinol. Laryngol., 82,* 175–178.

Smith, J. L. (1962). Vertical optokinetic nystagmus. *Neurol., 12,* 48–52.

Smith, J. L., & Cogan, D. G. (1960). Optokinetic nystagmus in cerebral disease. A report of 14 autopsied cases. *Neurol., 10,* 127–137.

Spector, M. (1975). Electronystagmographic findings in central nervous system disease. *Ann. Otol., 84,* 374–378.

Steenerson, R. L., Van de Water, S. M., Sytsma, W. H., & Fox, E. J. (1986). Central vestibular findings on electronystagmography. *Ear Hear., 7,* 176–181.

Stockwell, C. W. (1983). *ENG workbook.* Baltimore: University Park Press.

Takemori, S., & Cohen, B. (1974). Loss of visual suppression of vestibular nystagmus after flocculus lesions. *Brain Res., 72,* 213–224.

Teter, D. L. (1983). The electronystagmography test battery and interpretation. *Sem. Hear., 4,* 11–21.

Torok, N. (1969). Differential caloric stimulations in vestibular diagnosis. *Arch Otolaryngol., 90,* 78–83.

Torok, N. (1970). The hyperactive vestibular response. *Acta Otolaryngol., 70,* 153–162.

Towle, P. A., & Romanul, F. (1970). Periodic alternating nystagmus: First pathologically studied case. *Neurol., 20,* 408.

Wetmore, S. J. (1986). Extended caloric tests. *Ear Hear., 7,* 186–190

Wolfe, J. W., & Kos, C. M. (1977). Nystagmus responses of the rhesus monkey to rotational stimulation following unilateral labyrinthectomy. Final report. *Trans. Am. Acad. Ophthalmol. Otolaryngol., 84,* 38–45.

Wolfe, J. W., Engelken, E. J., & Olson, J. E. (1982). Low-frequency harmonic acceleration in the evaluation of patients with peripheral labyrinthine disorders. In V. Honrubia & M. A. B. Brazier (eds.),

Nystagmus and vertigo: Clinical approaches to the patient with dizziness, pp. 95–105. New York: Academic Press.

Wolfe, J., Engelken, E., Olson, J., & Kos, C. (1978). Vestibular responses to bithermal caloric and harmonic acceleration. *Ann. Otol. Rhinol. Laryngol., 87,* 861–867.

Yee, R. D., Baloh, R. W., Honrubia, V., & Jenkins, H. A. (1982). Patho-

physiology of optokinetic nystagmus. In V. Honrubia & M. A. B. Brazier (eds.), *Nystagmus and vertigo: Clinical approaches to the patient with dizziness,* pp. 251–275. New York: Academic Press.

Zee, D. S., Yee, R. D., Cogan, D. G., Robinson, D. A., & Engel, W. K. (1976). Ocular motor abnormalities in hereditary cerelsellar atoxia. *Brain, 99,* 207–234.

CHAPTER 9

PERSPECTIVES ON SITE-OF-LESION TESTS AND CASE STUDIES

In previous chapters, we presented the basic concepts underlying each of the tests which attempt to identify the locus of the lesion along the auditory pathway from the cochlea to the auditory cortex. Although the accuracy of each test singly in detection of pathology in the auditory pathway was discussed in earlier chapters, the contribution of a battery of tests was not discussed. In this chapter, the contribution of each test will be compared with those of other tests with respect to differentiation of the site of lesion. The concept of the site-of-lesion test battery will also be addressed in this chapter.

Jerger (1961) noted that no audiologic test was able to perfectly differentiate between retrocochlear (eighth nerve and cerebellopontine angle) and cochlear sites of pathology. He found, however, that when a battery of audiologic tests (Bekesy, SISI, and ABLB) was administered, the accuracy in detection of ears with retrocochlear pathology was 100%. Tillman (1969) contended that the likelihood of correct differentiation between cochlear and retrocochlear sites of pathology increases as the number of test results consistent with a particular site increases, expecially for cochlear site of lesion. Jerger (1962) elaborated upon the concept of the site-of-lesion test battery:

The key to the successful use of hearing tests in otologic diagnosis seems to be in the employment of multiple test batteries rather than single tests alone. While individual test results are often capricious and unreliable, the overall pattern of results obtained from a suitable two or three test battery appears to be stable and more meaningful. (p.139)

The site-of-lesion battery is most profitably employed when its purpose is to identify site rather than etiology of disorder. Thus, the results of a site-of-lesion battery will provide evidence for a cochlear, retrocochlear, or central site of auditory pathology. Although retrocochlear disorders are frequently acoustic neuromas, other etiologies of retrocochlear disorders include vascular insults, infections such as meningitis and herpes zoster, trauma, multiple sclerosis, diabetes, syphilis, and asphyxia. Similarly, etiologies

other than intracranial tumors affecting the central auditory nervous system include multiple sclerosis, meningitis, diabetes, kernicterus, syphilis, trauma, toxoplasmosis, asphyxia, and cerebrovascular disorders including atherosclerosis, hypertensive arteriosclerosis, aneurysms, and arteriovenous malformations.

Traditionally, the purpose of site-of-lesion testing was to differentiate between cochlear and retrocochlear sites of lesion in cases with unilateral or asymmetrical sensorineural hearing impairment. Central auditory testing was considered essential in cases with normal hearing with complaints of difficulty understanding speech, particularly in noisy situations. In recent years, audiologic tools such as brainstem auditory-evoked potentials testing and acoustic-reflex threshold testing have been used successfully to detect acoustic neuromas at the early stage of the disease and, in many cases, before the onset of hearing impairment. (Hearing impairment is the initial symptom in 50% of the cases.) Therefore, the primary purpose of site-of-lesion testing in cases with normal-hearing sensitivity and complaint of difficulty hearing speech is to differentiate between retrocochlear and central auditory nervous system pathology; a negative result on this testing and follow-up neurologic testing would indicate either a normal auditory system or a very subtle, subclinical retrocochlear or central auditory pathology. Of course, in cases with unilateral or asymmetrical sensorineural hearing impairment, the primary purpose of site-of-lesion testing is still to differentiate between cochlear and retrocochlear sites of lesion.

I. CRITERIA FOR EVALUATING TEST PERFORMANCE

A variety of approaches have been employed to evaluate the ability of specialized tests to predict the site of lesion. For example, Jerger and Jerger (1983) applied decision matrix analysis to the results of four site-of-lesion tests obtained from 20 patients with surgically-confirmed eighth-nerve disorders and 20 patients with cochlear disorders. In this decision matrix analysis, the results of each site-of-lesion test were classified as true positive if the test correctly identified a retrocochlear ear, false positive if the test misidentified a cochlear ear as a retrocochlear ear, true negative if the test correctly identified a cochlear ear, and false negative if the test misidentified a retrocochlear ear as a cochlear ear. Table I shows the model for decision matrix analysis as applied to the differentiation of cochlear from retrocochlear disorder. This model can be equally well applied in the differentiation between ears with and without central auditory pathology. In such cases, a result is classified as true positive if the test correctly identifies a central auditory impaired ear, false positive if the test misidentifies a normal ear as a central auditory impaired ear, true negative if the test correctly identifies a normal ear, and false negative if the test misidentifies a central auditory impaired ear as a normal ear. The sensitivity, specificity, predictive value of a positive result, predictive value of a negative result, and efficiency of a test are based on the analysis of the positive (true and false) and negative (true and false) results. These terms are well defined by Jerger & Jerger (1983) within the context of cochlear as opposed to retrocochlear pathology but they also apply within the context of the presence or absence of central auditory pathology.

Sensitivity refers to the accuracy of a test in correctly identifying patients with eighth nerve site. Sensitivity is defined as the ratio of true-positive results to the total number of patients with eighth nerve site. In contrast, specificity refers to the accuracy of a test in correctly rejecting patients with cochlear site. Specificity is defined as the ratio of true-negative results to the total number of patients with cochlear site.

Predictive value is related to the incidence of false-negative results in patients with eighth nerve site and the incidence of false-positive results in patients with coch-

lear site. The predictive value of positive results is defined as the ratio of true-positive results in patients with eighth nerve site to the total number of positive results in all patients. The predictive value of negative results is defined in the same way; the percent of all negative results that are true-negative findings.

Finally, the efficiency of a test refers to the overall accuracy of test results. Test efficiency is defined as the percent of all results that are correct, whether positive or negative. (Jerger & Jerger, 1983, p.150)

The sensitivity is also referred to as the hit rate and the specificity is also referred to as the correct-rejection rate (Turner & Nielsen, 1984). An alternative term for the false-negative rate is the miss rate. Similarly, the false-alarm rate refers to the false-positive rate. The sum of the false-alarm (false-positive) and correct-rejection (specificity) rates yields the total number of true negative (e.g., cochlear or noncentral auditory impaired ears) ears and totals 100%. The sum of the hit (sensitivity) and miss (false-negative) rates yields the total number of true positive (e.g., retrocochlear or central auditory impaired) ears and totals 100%. The sum of the hit and false-alarm rates yields the total number of ears with positive (true and false) results and the sum of the miss and correct-rejection rates yields the total number of ears with negative (true and false) results.

Turner and Nielsen (1984) demonstrated that the hit and false-alarm rates are influenced by the criterion for determining whether the test outcome is negative or positive with respect to retrocochlear pathology. By varying the criterion, the hit and false-alarm rates can be manipulated. Nevertheless, there is a trade-off between the hit and false-alarm rates. That is, increasing the hit rate will cause the false-alarm rate to also increase. The relations among false-alarm rate, hit rate, and criterion can be shown on the receiver operating characteristic (ROC) curve which shows the hit rate as a function of false-alarm rate for different criteria. The ROC curve can be plotted on linear or double-probability coordinates. An example of an ROC curve plotted on double-probability coordinates is shown in Figure 1. The ROC curve plotted on double-probability coordinates will be a straight-line function with a slope equal to +1 if the probability distribution curves (PDC; probability of obtaining a score as a function of the test score for a retrocochlear or cochlear ear) for both cochlear ears and retrocochlear ears have a normal distribution and are equal in variance. Turner and Nielsen (1984) demonstrated that the PDC based on the suprathreshold speech-recognition data reported by Owens (1971) and the PDC based on the brainstem auditory-evoked potentials interaural wave V latencies reported by Selters and Brackmann (1977) are not normal curves with equal variance since the ROC curves plotted on double-probability coordinates did not yield straight-line functions.

Table I Model Decision Matrix [Galen & Gambino, 1975] for Reporting Results of Diagnostic Audiologic Tests for Eighth Nerve versus Cochlear Sites of Disorder[a,b]

	Results		
Site	Positive	Negative	Total
Eighth nerve	true positive	false negative	*n* eighth nerve
Cochlear	false positive	true negative	*n* cochlear
Total	*n* positive	*n* negative	grand total

[a] Reprinted from Jerger and Jerger (1983) with permission.
[b] The sum of the rows yields the total number of patients with eighth nerve (*n* eighth nerve) or cochlear (*n* cochlear) disorders. The sum of the columns yields the total number of times that a test was positive (*n* positive) or negative (*n* negative). Sensitivity, positive results in eighth nerve site, (true positive)/(*n* eighth nerve). Specificity, negative results in cochlear site, (true negative)/*n* cochlear). Predictive value of positive result, (true positive)/(*n* positive). Predictive value of negative result, (true negative)/(*n* negative). Efficiency of test, (true positives + true negatives)/(grand total).

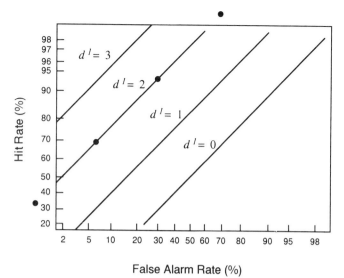

Figure 1 Receiver operating characteristic curves plotted on double probability coordinates. Values of HT or FA near 0 or 100% can cause problems when plotting on double probability coordinates because of the nonlinear characteristics of these coordinates. Four values of HT/FA from the probability distribution curves for cochlear and retrocochlear ears are plotted to form the curve labeled d' = 2. The values HT/FA = 0/0%, 100/100% could not be plotted because the double probability coordinates will never reach 0 or 100%. Two (30/1% and 99/30%) of the four values lie outside the particular axes selected. The other three curves are calculated from the probability distribution curves for cochlear and retrocochlear ears. Individual data points are not shown for these curves. From Turner and Nielsen (1984) with permission.

When the PDCs are not normal curves with equal variances, than d', a measure of the overlap between the PDCs for the cochlear and retrocochlear ears and calculated based on the hit and false-alarm rates for a particular point on the ROC curve (criterion), will vary with the criterion. When the PDCs are normal curves and have equal variances, the d' will be constant regardless of the criterion. In such cases, tests can be compared based on the d's. A single d' for one test can be compared with that for another test since the d's along each ROC curve are equivalent. The better test is the one with the larger d'. When the PDC curves are not normal curves and do not have equal variances, the interpretation of d' is not so straightforward. If all the d's calculated for each point on the ROC curve (criterion) for one test are superior to those for another test, then it is clear which test is better. Otherwise, the d' for one test at a single specified point of the ROC curve (criterion) can be compared with that for another test at a single specified point of the ROC curve (criterion) and the larger d' indicates the better test but only for the criterion evaluated. The test with the larger d' for a particular criterion may have a smaller d' with another criterion.

Posterior probabilities include the probability of a retrocochlear ear (or central auditory impaired ear) given a positive test result, the probability of a retrocochlear ear (or

central auditory impaired ear) given a negative result, the probability of a cochlear ear (or ear without central auditory impairment) given a negative result, and the probability of a cochlear ear (or ear without central auditory impairment) given a positive result. Jerger and Jerger (1983) derived the predictive value of a positive result (i.e., the probability of a retrocochlear ear given a positive result) and the predictive value of a negative result (i.e., the probability of a cochlear ear given a negative result). The formulas used by Jerger and Jerger (1983) for calculating the predictive values of positive and negative results are shown in Table I. The Jerger and Jerger (1983) predictive-value formulas did not correct for the actual prevalence of retrocochlear impairment in the suspect population. Since they used equal numbers of cochlear and retrocochlear ears in their study and their predictive-value formulas did not correct for the actual prevalence of retrocochlear impairment, the assumed prevalence was 50%. The prevalence of a disease (e.g., retrocochlear or central auditory impairment) in the suspect population depends on the criteria used to define a member of the suspect population (Turner & Nielsen, 1984). According to Hart and Davenport (1981), based on reports from centers which see large numbers of retrocochlear ears, the prevalence of retrocochlear impairment in the at-risk population is 5%. The prevalence of retrocochlear impairment is lower when considering reports from centers that see few retrocochlear impaired ears. To derive the posterior probabilities, that is, probability of a retrocochlear ear given a positive result (Pr [RE/+]), probability of a retrocochlear ear given a negative result (Pr[RE/−]), probability of a cochlear ear given a negative result (Pr[CE/−]), and probability of a cochlear ear given a positive result (Pr[CE/+]), Turner and Nielsen (1984) used the following formulas based on the prevalence of retrocochlear pathology in the suspect population:

$$\Pr[RE/+] = \frac{1}{1 + \dfrac{(FA)(1-Pd)}{(HT)(Pd)}}$$

$$\Pr[RE/-] = \frac{1}{1 + \dfrac{(1-HT)(1-Pd)}{(1-FA)(Pd)}}$$

$$\Pr[CE/-] = \frac{1}{1 + \dfrac{(1-HT)(Pd)}{(1-FA)(1-Pd)}}$$

$$\Pr[CE/+] = \frac{1}{1 + \dfrac{(HT)(Pd)}{(FA)(1-Pd)}}$$

where Pr is probability, RE is a retrocochlear ear, CE is a cochlear ear, + is a positive result, − is a negative result, HT is the hit rate, FA is the false-alarm rate, and Pd is the prevalence (also called prior probability) of retrocochlear pathology in a suspect population. These formulas can be applied to the evaluation of tests for differentiating between ears with and without central auditory impairment. If a prevalence rate of 5% is assumed for a retrocochlear disorder in the suspect population, then the probability of a retrocochlear ear given a positive result (Pr[RE/+]) does not exceed 50% even for a test having a hit rate of 95% and a false-alarm rate of 5%. In such cases, however, the probability of a cochlear ear given a negative result (Pr[CE/−]) approaches 100% (Turner & Nielsen, 1984). Thus, in such circumstances, using a highly sensitive test with a low false-alarm rate and assuming a prevalence rate of 5%, the chance that positive result represents a retrocochlear ear is, at best, only 50%. In centers where audiologists are loose in their criteria for defining the "at-risk" population, the probability that a positive result on an audiologic test represents a retrocochlear ear is even lower than 50% (assuming the false-alarm rate is 5% and the hit rate is 95%).

Predictive value of positive and negative test results depends on the prevalence of the disease. Table II, from Turner and Nielsen (1984), who reanalyzed the data from Jerger and Jerger (1983), shows the changes in the predictive value of positive and negative results as the prevalence changes. Note that when the prevalence of retrocochlear pathology is high (50%), such as when comparing two equal-sized groups of retrocochlear and cochlear ears, the Pr(RE/+) and Pr(RE/−) are relatively high. The Pr(RE/+) and Pr(RE/−) become lowered substantially when the prevalence rate is lowered to 5%. The opposite effect is observed for Pr(CE/−) when decreasing the preva-

lence rate. When the prevalence rate is 5%, the Pr(CE/−) is between 97 and 99%; the Pr(CE/−) is lowered to 67–96% when the prevalence rate is 50%. In conclusion, therefore, the audiologist working in a center where the prevalence of retrocochlear pathology is low should not be disheartened if many of the positive results turn out to be false-positive results. The prevalence of retrocochlear pathology in a large center is the same as that in small centers provided that the criteria used to define the "at-risk" population are the same. The prevalence of retrocochlear pathology at a center specializing in retrocochlear disorders will be higher than that of a typical center since the specialized center's criteria for "at-risk" persons are stricter than those of the typical center; the specialized center sees many patients who failed the audiologic-test battery at another center.

Efficiency is another criterion for assessing test performance. Test efficiency, the percentage of all test results correctly identified, was derived by Turner and Nielsen (1984) using the formula

$$EFF = HT(Pd) + (1\text{-}FA)(1\text{-}PD)$$

The test efficiency, like the posterior probabilities, is dependent on the hit and false-alarm rates and disease prevalence. When the prevalence is low, the efficiency is highest in tests with small false-alarm rates. Turner and Nielsen (1984) contend that efficiency is not a useful measure to differentiate among tests. Even if the efficiency of a test is 90%, classification of all ears as cochlear without even administering a test will yield a higher efficiency (95%) since the prevalence of cochlear pathology is 95% and the prevalence of retrocochlear pathology is only 5%. The errors made will be the retrocochlear ears.

Table II Calculations of Predictive Value, Information Content, and Efficiency for a Prevalence of Retrocochlear Disease of 50 and 5%[a,b]

Test[c]	Hit rate (%)	False alarm rate %	Predictive value (%) Positive Pr[RE/+] 50%	5%	Negative Pr[CE/−] 50%	5%	Information (%) Negative Pr[RE/−] 50%	5%	Efficiency (%) 50%	5%
ABR	97	12	89	30	96	>99	4	<1	92	88
ARC	85	30	74	13	82	99	18	1	78	71
BCL	85	30	74	13	82	99	18	1	78	71
PIPB	65	10	87	25	72	98	28	2	78	89
BEK	50	0	100	100	67	97	33	3	75	98
STAT2	45	10	82	19	62	97	38	3	68	88

[a] Reprinted from Turner and Nielsen (1984) with permission.
[b] All calculations in this table except predictive value, information content, and efficiency for prevalence of 5% are from Jerger (1983) and Jerger and Jerger (1983). Our calculations use Jerger's measures of HT/FA and a prevalence of 5%. Note that information content-positive result is equivalent to predictive value-positive result.
[c] ABR, auditory brain stem response; ARC, acoustic reflexes; BCL, Bekesy comfortable loudness; PIPB, performance-intensity function for phonetically-balanced monosyllabic words; BEK, Bekesy audiometry; STAT2, suprathreshold adaptation test (using frequencies 500, 1000, and 2000 Hz).

Table III Tests and Criteria for Interpreting a Positive Result[a]

Test	Criteria for a positive result
ABLB	Derecruitment/no recruitment
SISI	≤ 70%
SISIM	≤ 70%
BEK	Type III or IV
TDT	> 30 dB
STAT 1, 500 and 1000 Hz	C tone not heard for 60 s
STAT 2, 500, 1000, and 2000 Hz	C tone not heard for 60 s
STAT 4, 500, 1000, 2000, and 4000 Hz	C tone not heard for 60 s
SD	≤ 30%
PIPB	Rollover
ART	Elevated/absent
ARD	Magnitude decreases at least 50% in 5 or 10 s
ARC	Elevated/absent ART or reflex decay
ABR	Prolonged V, I–III, I–V, interaural V, etc.
ENGC	Unilateral weakness ≥ 25%
BCL	Comparison of interrupted and continuous signals at a comfortable loudness level
FBB	Comparison of backward continuous with forward continuous and interrupted threshold tracings

[a] Following Turner *et al.* (1984a).

Turner, Shepard, and Frazer (1984a) evaluated the hit (HT) and false-alarm (FA) rates associated with the various site-of-lesion tests. The criteria for interpretation of a positive result for the various site-of lesion tests are shown in Table III. Studies were eliminated from analysis only if the criterion employed for a particular test was markedly different from the one indicated in Table III. The HT and FA rates were calculated based on data from 170 papers published between 1968 and 1983. The average HT and FA rates, the standard deviations associated with the average HT and FA rates, and the range of HT and FA rates were obtained. In order to determine if the HT and FA rates calculated from all the studies differed from those calculated from only those studies which presented data from both retrocochlear and cochlear ears, restricted average HT and FA rates were obtained based on the data from only those studies which evaluated both cochlear and retrocochlear ears. As a check on the possibility that extreme values from some studies unduly influenced the average HT and FA rates, modified HT and FA rates based on the data from all studies except those with the highest and lowest FA and HT were obtained. Since the restricted and modified averages were in good agreement with the overall averages, the overall but not the restricted or modified averages are shown in Table IV. As Table IV shows, the tests with the highest HT rates (exceeding 80%) are the combined

Table IV Average Hit and False-Alarm Rates for the Various Audiologic Tests Based on Data Presented in Tables II and III[a,b]

Test	Sh	Nh	Rh	Dh	HTa	Sf	Nf	Rf	Df	FAa
ABLB	12	511	52–100	14	59	4	374	0–33	15	10
SISI	5	490	50–80	9	65	4	410	8–24	8	16
SISIM	5	286	50–96	17	69	4	336	9–27	14	10
BEK	15	723	15–74	17	49	8	585	0–24	8	7
BCL	3	40	85–86	1	85	3	119	0–30	17	8
FBB	4	51	57–100	19	71	4	312	0–19	9	5
TDT	16	999	17–100	20	70	8	800	4–32	9	13
STAT1	1	20	[c]	[d]	45	1	70	[c]	[d]	0
STAT2	3	46	45–83	20	54	2	95	4–10	[d]	5
STAT4	1	20	[c]	[d]	70	1	75	[c]	[d]	13
SD	12	965	15–58	13	45	5	356	0–29	11	18
PIPB	7	78	63–100	14	74	5	184	1–33	11	4
ART	17	873	40–100	17	73	9	1520	3–24	7	10
ARD	15	370	36–100	20	63	6	2159	1–27	9	4
ARC	23	1333	70–100	9	84	12	2719	5–31	10	15
ABR	22	818	81–100	7	95	10	1289	0–30	10	11
ENGC	19	955	77–94	11	85	4	413	28–53	12	33

[a] From Turner *et al.* (1984a).
[b] Sh, Number of studies used to calculate HTa; NH, number of ears used to calculate HTa; Rh, range of hit rates for each test (%); Dh, standard deviation of hit rates for each test (%); Sf, number of studies used to calculate FAa; Nf, number of ears used to calculate FAa; Rf, range of false-alarm rates for each test (%); Df, standard deviation of false-alarm rates for each test; HTa, average hit rate for each test; FAa, average false-alarm rate for each test.
[c] Not calculated; requires at least two articles for the calculation.
[d] Not calculated; requires at least three articles for the calculation.

acoustic-reflex threshold and decay, the ABR, and ENG calorics tests. The tests with the lowest FA rates (<10%) are the STAT1 tone-decay test, PI–PB test, acoustic-reflex decay test, forward–backward Bekesy test, STAT2 test, conventional Bekesy test, and Bekesy comfortable-loudness test. The speech-discrimination and the STAT1 tests had the lowest HT rates (<50%). The tests with the highest HT rates were also the tests with the relatively higher FA rates indicating the previously mentioned trade-off between HT and FA rate. The ENGC, the SD, and the ABLB tests all had FA rates exceeding 15%, and the ENGC test had the highest FA rate (33%).

Inspection of Table IV also reveals that the HT and FA rates of the modified versions of the traditional tests (SISIM, BCL, FBB, and PI–PB) are generally superior to those of their traditional counterparts. The HT and FA rates, however, were generally based upon substantially smaller numbers of ears for the modified than for the traditional tests. Turner *et al.* (1984a) noted that test performance is highest at the time the test is created; it diminishes as additional data are gathered over time. Sanders (1984a) observed that the specificity for the ABLB, SISI, and Bekesy remained substantially unchanged from the report by Jerger (1961) to the report by Sanders, Josey, and Glasscock (1974). The HT rate, however, for these tests decreased substantially from the time of the Jerger report (1961) to the Johnson report (1977). Thus, more data are needed before a definitive comparison can be made between the traditional tests and their modified counterparts.

In addition to the average HT and FA rates, Turner *et al.* (1984a) also calculated the average d' associated with the various audiologic site-of-lesion tests (based on HT and FA rates from 170 studies). The tests with the largest d's, equivalent to at least 2.0, were the BCL, FBB, PI–PB, ARD, ARC, and ABR. The test with the smallest d' was the SD.

Turner *et al.* (1984a) concluded that, based on the d', HT, and FA, the ABR test was the best audiologic test available for differentiating between cochlear and retrocochlear sites. The next best test was ARC and the worst was SD. Turner *et al.* (1984a) also applied clinical decision analysis to the various radiologic tests used to identify retrocochlear lesions. Their results revealed that posterior fossa cisternography with computed tomography and metrizamine with computed tomography had HT rates exceeding 96%, FA rates less than or equal to 2%, and d' greater than 4.0. These tests are considered definitive radiologic tests for mass lesions of retrocochlear site.

II. EVALUATION OF THE PERFORMANCE OF THE TEST BATTERY

Recently, the performance of the test-battery approach has been evaluated (Jerger & Jerger, 1983; Thomsen, Nyboe,

Borum, Tosi, & Barfoed, 1981; Turner, Frazer, & Shepard, 1984b). Jerger and Jerger (1983) observed that tests could be combined into a test battery using a lax or strict approach. With the former, the result of the test battery is positive for retrocochlear pathology if the outcome of any of the tests in the battery yields a positive outcome. On the other hand, with the strict approach, the battery is positive for retrocochlear pathology only if all of the tests within the battery yield a positive outcome.

The combination of tests can be parallel or series (Turner *et al.*, 1984b). Figure 2 shows a schematic for the combination of tests in parallel or series. With the parallel approach, the decision regarding test-battery outcome is made after all the tests are administered. With the lax (loose) parallel approach, the test battery is considered to have a positive outcome if, after all the tests are administered, any one or more of the tests had a positive result. With the strict parallel approach, the test battery is considered to have a positive outcome if, after all the tests are administered, all of the tests have a positive outcome. With the series approach, a decision is made after each test is administered. In the series-positive approach, a positive result on the first test leads to the administration of the second test; a positive result on the second test leads to the administration of the third test, and so forth, until all the tests in the battery have been administered. A negative result, however, at any point, eliminates the patient from further testing. All the tests must yield a positive outcome in order for the patient to be referred for follow-up. The series-positive approach is essentially the same as the parallel approach with a strict criterion. With the series-negative approach, the decision for follow-up is made after the administration of each test. In contrast to the series-positive approach, subsequent tests are administered

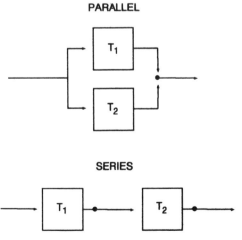

Figure 2 Two techniques for combining tests T_1 and T_2 into a protocol. At a decision point (solid dot), a decision is made about future testing or treatment. That decision is based on a single test result for a series protocol and multiple test results for a parallel protocol. From Turner, Frazer, and Shepard (1984b) with permission.

in sequence only after a negative result is obtained. Whenever a positive result occurs, further testing is eliminated and the patient is referred for follow-up. This approach is essentially the same as the parallel approach with a loose criterion. Figure 3 shows a schematic representation of the series-positive and series-negative approaches. Turner *et al.*(1984b) indicated that criteria do not have to be either loose or strict. That is, an intermediate approach can be employed; an example of an intermediate criterion is to require a positive outcome on at least 3 of 6 tests in a test battery.

Turner *et al.* (1984b) tested the assumption that the test battery is superior to (provides additional and more useful information than) a single audiologic test. They outlined the rationale for administering a test battery as follows: (a) to obtain a higher HT or lower FA than could be obtained with a single audiologic test; (b) to construct a "super" test with higher HT and lower FA rates than any of the individual tests; and (c) to screen patients to determine which will be referred for the "definitive" test which, because of financial cost, morbidity, mortality, or other reason cannot be administered to everyone. Turner *et al.* (1984b) contended that the test-battery or protocol performance could be predicted if the approach to the test combination is known (i.e., loose or strict and parallel or series), the HT and FA rates of the component tests are known, and the correlations among the tests are known.

If there is a positive correlation among two tests, then the ears identified as positive by the second test tend to be the same as those identified by the first test. If there is a negative correlation between two tests, then the ears identified as positive by the second test tend not to be those identified as positive by the first test. With zero correlation, there is the absence of a positive or negative correlation between tests. With a maximum positive correlation between two tests, all of the retrocochlear ears identified by the second test were also identified by the first test. With a maximum negative correlation between two tests, none of the ears identified as retrocochlear by the second test were identified as retrocochlear by the first test. With a zero correlation between two tests, 50% of the ears identified as retrocochlear by the second test were also identified as retrocochlear by the first test and the other 50% of the ears identified as retrocochlear by the second test were not identified as retrocochlear by the first test.

Turner *et al.* (1984b) calculated the limits of the HT and FA rates for the series-positive and series-negative test protocols under the conditions of maximum-positive, maximum-negative, and zero correlation. A series-positive protocol was considered the same as a parallel protocol with a strict criterion. A series-negative protocol was considered a parallel protocol with a loose criterion. The equations for the limiting HT and FA rates for the protocol under the maximum-positive and maximum-negative correlation conditions are:

$$
\begin{aligned}
\text{Loose/max+:} \quad & HT_p(1/+) = HT_x \\
& FA_p(1/+) = FA_x \\
\text{Strict/max+:} \quad & HT_p(x/+) = HT_n \\
& FA_p(s/+) = FA_n \\
\text{Loose/max-:} \quad & HT_p(1/-) = \text{MIN (SHT or 100)} \\
& FA_p(1/-) = \text{MIN (SFA or 100)} \\
\text{Strict/max-:} \quad & HT_p(s/-) = \text{MAX} \\
& \qquad\qquad [SHT - 100\,(N-1) \text{ or } 0] \\
& FA_p(s/-) = \text{MAX} \\
& \qquad\qquad [SFA - 100\,(N-1) \text{ or } 0]
\end{aligned}
$$

where N is the number of tests, HT_x is the maximum individual test HT rate, FA_x is the maximum individual test FA rate, HT_n is the minimum individual test HT rate, FA_n is the minimum individual test FA rate, SHT is the sum of the individual test HT rates, SFA is the sum of the individual test FA rates, MAX (A or B) is the greater (more positive) of the numbers "A" or "B", and MIN (A or B) is the smaller of the numbers "A" or "B."

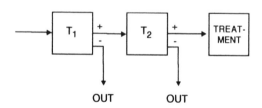

SERIES - POSITIVE

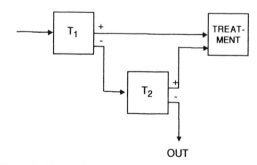

SERIES - NEGATIVE

Figure 3 Two techniques for combining tests T_1 and T_2 into a series protocol. "Out" means that the patient receives no additional testing or treatment. From Turner, Frazer, and Shepard (1984b) with permission.

$$
\begin{aligned}
\text{Strict/zero:} \quad & HT_p(s/z) = (HT_1)\,(HT_2)\ldots(HT_N) \\
& FA_p(s/z) = (FA_1)\,(FA_2)\ldots(FA_N) \\
\text{Loose/zero:} \quad & HT_p(l/z) = HT_1 + HT_2(1 - HT_1) \\
& \qquad + HT_3(1 - HT_2)\,(1 - HT_1) \\
& \qquad + \ldots HT_N[\,(1 - HT_{N-1}) \\
& \qquad (1 - HT_{N-2})\ldots(1 - HT_1)\,]
\end{aligned}
$$

$$FA_p(l/z) = FA_1 + FA_2$$
$$(1 - FA_1) + FA_3(1 - FA_2)$$
$$(1 - FA_1) + \ldots FA_N$$
$$[1 - FA_{N-1}]$$
$$(1 - FA_{N-2}) \ldots (1 - FA_1)]$$

where N is the number of tests; $HT_1, HT_2 \ldots HT_N$ is the hit rate of the first, second, . . .Nth individual test in protocol; FA_1, FA_2, FA_N is the false-alarm rate of the first, second, . . . Nth individual test in protocol.

The HT_p and FA_p both decrease as the criterion is changed from loose to strict. The HT_p and FA_p also vary with test correlation. With a loose criterion, as the test correlation decreases from maximum positive to maximum negative, the HT_p increases beyond the maximum individual test HT and the FA_p increases beyond the maximum individual test FA. With a strict criterion, as the test correlation decreases from maximum positive to maximum negative, the HT_p decreases below the minimum individual test HT and the FA_p decreases below the minimum individual test FA. The greatest difference between the protocol and individual-test performance is achieved under the maximum negative-correlation condition and the minimum difference between the protocol and individual-test performance is achieved under the maximum positive-correlation condition.

It is never possible to construct a protocol so the HT_p is higher than the best individual-test HT and the FA_p is lower than the smallest individual-test FA. Under the loose criterion, the HTp may be better than the best individual-test HT but the FA_p will never be better than the worst individual-test FA. Under the strict criterion, the HT_p will never be better than the worst individual-test HT but the FA_p may be better than the best individual-test FA.

Although the test protocol cannot yield both higher HT_p and lower FA_p rates than the best individual-test HT and FA rates, the protocol can be used to obtain either an HT_p better than the best individual-test HT or an FA_p better than the best individual-test FA.

Turner et al. (1984b) compared the Jerger and Jerger (1983) protocol performance data with their own calculations of protocol performance under the maximum-positive, zero, and maximum-negative correlation conditions based on the individual HT and FA values reported by Jerger and Jerger (1983). Comparison of the Jerger and Jerger (1983) protocol values with the Turner et al. (1984) predicted values revealed that the HT_p and FA_p rates fell between those predicted under the maximum positive-correlation condition and those predicted under the maximum negative-correlation condition. These protocol-performance data also revealed a positive correlation among the combined acoustic-reflex threshold and decay tests, PI–PB test, and BCL test. Jerger and Jerger's (1983) protocol-performance data also showed that it is possible to

create a protocol with an HT_p better than the best individual-test HT or an FA_p better than the best individual-test FA_p but not both HT_p and FA_p better than the best individual test HT and FA rates.

Turner et al. (1984b) recommended that a protocol should be used only if there is a specific rationale. Moreover, the clinician should be consistent in the use of a lax or strict and parallel or series approach toward combination of tests in protocol. According to Turner et al. (1984b), the series is preferred to the parallel approach since it results in a time saving; with a parallel approach, all tests need to be administered before a protocol outcome is determined. Turner et al. (1984b) recommended that clinical data regarding protocol performance (at least the limits on protocol performance) be calculated. Turner et al. (1984b) suggested that the optimum protocol be determined not only on the basis of the HT, FA, d', and so on, but also on considerations of financial cost, morbidity, mortality, and so forth. The latter considerations represent a cost-benefit analysis approach. Turner et al. (1984b) concluded that several radiologic techniques can be considered definitive ultimate tests but their "cost" is too great to be used on every patient. They recommended that the brainstem auditory-evoked potentials test be used as a screening protocol to determine which patient gets the definitive test using the definitive series-positive approach. That is, if the brainstem auditory-evoked potentials test is positive, the patient is referred for a definitive radiologic test. If the brainstem auditory-evoked potentials test is negative, on the other hand, the patient does not get referred for a definitive radiologic test. The use of this protocol is supported by the recent findings of Mair, Okstad, Laukli, and Anke (1988).

Turner (1988) predicted protocol performance for a variety of commonly employed protocols based on protocol design, knowledge of individual-test performance, and test correlation. Turner (1988) derived the individual-test performance (HT and FA) from the Turner et al. (1984a) report. Turner (1988) assumed that test correlation for audiologic tests, based on limited research, is mid-positive, that is, midway between maximum-positive and zero correlation. The protocol HT and FA rates [$HT_p(m)$ and $FA_p(m)$] for a mid-positive correlation was defined as:

$$HT_p(m) = \frac{HT_p(z) + HT_p(+)}{2}$$
$$FA_p(m) = \frac{FA_p(z) + FA_p(+)}{2}$$

where $HT_p(m)$ is the HT rate for the protocol under the mid-positive correlation condition, $FA_p(m)$ is the FA rate for the protocol under the mid-positive correlation condition, $HT_p(z)$ is the HT rate for the protocol under the zero correlation, $FA_p(z)$ is the FA rate for the protocol under the zero correlation, $HT_p(+)$ is the HT rate for the protocol under the maximum-positive correlation, and $FA_p(+)$ is the FA rate for the protocol under the maximum-positive correlation. A prevalence rate of 5% with respect to retrocochlear disease was assumed.

In protocol one (P_1), the screening protocol consists of the brainstem auditory-evoked potentials test combined with the definitive test [e.g., magnetic resonance imaging (MRI)] in series positive. That is, a positive result on the brainstem auditory-evoked potentials test leads to administration of the definitive test. If a negative result on the brainstem auditory-evoked potentials test is obtained, the patient exits at that point and does not receive the definitive test. Here, the brainstem auditory-evoked potentials test is the screening protocol and the combination of the brainstem auditory-evoked potentials test and definitive test is the total protocol.

In protocol 2 (P_2), the combined acoustic-reflex threshold and decay (ARC) screening tests are combined in series positive with the brainstem auditory-evoked potentials screening test which is combined in series positive with the definitive test (MRI). With this protocol, a positive result must be obtained on both the ARC and the BAEP test before the patient is referred for the definitive test. If a negative result is obtained on the ARC, the patient exits and does not go for the BAEP or MRI test. If a positive result is obtained on the ARC, the BAEP test is administered; if a negative result is obtained, the patient exits and does not take the definitive test.

In protocol 3 (P_3), the ABLB, ARC, PI–PB, SISI, and tone-decay tests are combined in parallel with a loose criterion. This block of parallel tests with a loose criterion is combined in series positive with the definitive test. Thus, a positive result on any one or more of the screening tests (ABLB, ARC, PI–PB, SISI, TDT) sends the patient for the definitive test. If a negative result is obtained on all of the screening tests, the patient exits and does not receive the definitive test. The total protocol consists of the screening tests and the definitive test.

In protocol 4 (P_4), a block of tests (ABLB, ARC, PI–PB, SISI, and TDT) are administered in parallel with a loose criterion. This block of tests is combined in series positive with the brainstem auditory-evoked potentials test which is combined in series positive with the definitive test. If any of the block of parallel tests with a loose criterion yields a positive result, the patient is referred for BAEP testing. The BAEP test must be positive for the patient to be referred for the definitive test. Thus, a positive result must be obtained on the block of tests combined in parallel with a loose criterion and on the BAEP test in order for the patient to be referred for the definitive test. If a negative result is obtained on all of the tests in a block combined in parallel with a loose criterion, the patient "exits and does not receive the BAEP test or the definitive test. If the patient obtains a positive result on the block of tests combined in parallel with a loose criterion but a negative result on the BAEP test, the patient exits and does not receive the definitive test. The screening protocol consists of the block of tests combined in parallel with a loose criterion (ABLB, ARC, PI–PB, SISI, and TDT) and the BAEP test. The total protocol consists of the block of tests combined in parallel with a loose criterion, the BAEP test, and the definitive test.

In protocol 5 (P_5), the combined acoustic-reflex threshold and decay tests are combined in series negative with the BAEP test; the series-negative tests are combined in series positive with the definitive test. With this protocol, a positive result on the ARC test leads to referral for the definitive test. A negative result on the ARC test leads to administration of the BAEP test; a positive result on the BAEP test leads to administration of the definitive test whereas a negative result causes the patient to exit and not receive the definitive test. The screening protocol consists of the combined acoustic-reflex threshold and decay tests and the BAEP test. The total protocol consists of the combined acoustic-reflex threshold and decay test, BAEP test, and the definitive test.

Table V shows the predicted HT, FA, predictive value for

Table V Comparison of Predicted Performance for Selected Audiologic Protocols[a]

Protocol	HTs/HTp (%)	FAs/FAp (%)	[+]s/[+]p (%)	[−]s/[−]p (%)	EFs/EFp (%)
P1 − ABR + DEF	95/95	11/0	31.3/100	99.7/99.7	89.3/99.8
P2 − ARC + ABR + DEF	82/82	6/0	40.5/100	99.0/99.1	93.1/99.1
P3 − ABLB * ARC * PIPB * SISI * TDT + DEF	92/92	31/0	13.4/100	99.4/99.6	70.0/99.6
P4R − ABLB * ARC * PIPB * SISI * TDT + ABR + DEF	89/89	8/0	36.9/100	99.4/99.4	91.8/99.5
P5 − [ARC − ABR] + DEF	97/97	20/0	20.6/100	99.8/99.8	81.1/99.9

[a] Reprinted from Turner (1988) with permission. DEF indicates the definitive test. A "+" between tests indicates series-positive; "−" between tests indicates series-negative; "*" between tests indicates tests in parallel with a loose criterion; tests enclosed by "[ ]" means that all patients who test positive on enclosed screening protocol receive the definitive test. HTs/HTp, hit rate of screening/total protocol; FAs/FAp, false alarm of screening/total protocol; [+]s/[+]p, posterior probability of being correct with a positive test result for screening/total protocol; [−]s/[−]p, posterior probability of being correct with a negative test result for screening/total protocol; EFs/EFp, efficiency of screening/total protocol.

a positive result, predictive value for a negative result, and efficiency rates for the screening and total protocols for P_1, P_2, P_3, P_4, and P_5 based on a prevalence rate of 5%, a mid-positive correlation, and the individual HT and FA rates as provided by Turner *et al.* (1984a). Note that the HT rate of the total protocol is the same as and does not exceed the HT rate of the screening protocol since patients who are negative on the screening protocol are not referred for the definitive test. According to this table, the highest screening-protocol HT rate is achieved by P_5, the lowest screening-protocol FA rate is achieved by P_2, the highest screening-protocol predictive value of a positive result is achieved by P_2, the highest screening-protocol predictive value of a negative result is achieved by P_5, and the highest screening-protocol efficiency rate is achieved by P_2. P_1, the most popular protocol, has a slightly lower HT rate than P_5 but P_5 has a higher FA rate than P_1. This conclusion regarding the superiority of P_1 to P_5 with respect to the FA rate is based on the 15% FA rate of the ARC reported by Turner *et al.* (1984a).

III. APPLICATION OF COST–BENEFIT ANALYSIS TO AUDIOLOGIC TESTS

Dobie (1985) expanded upon the concept of cost–benefit analysis. He discussed the cost of false-positive (FP) and false-negative (FN) results with respect to audiologic testing. An FP result, according to Dobie (1985), could lead to a CT scan with air contrast which involves financial expenditure, loss of time, inconvenience, and possibly a severe headache. (At present, however, an FP result is more likely to lead to high-resolution CT scan with contrast or magnetic resonance imaging; these tests are associated with financial expenditure, loss of time, and, in the former case, may be associated with an allergic reaction. The MRI test is contraindicated in persons with lead stitches or pacemakers.) An FN result may cost the patient his or her life or result in surgical complications if the disease is identified later as a result of the progression of the lesion. The consequence of an FN result, therefore, is greater than that of an FP result. Dobie (1985) suggested selecting a ratio of cost associated with an FN (CFN) to the cost associated with an FP result (CFP). A CFN/CFP ratio equivalent to 5 indicates that, for every FN result, there may be 5 FP results incurred with the test. With this approach, the clinician must determine an acceptable CFN/CFP ratio. Dobie (1985) noted that although classifying all suspect ears as cochlear leads to a 5% FN rate (the FN rate associated with "no test"), the fact that BAEP testing results in mostly FP errors which are less costly than FN errors makes it preferable to administer BAEP testing than not to administer any test. Dobie (1985) calculated the cost of errors associated with the BAEP test having an HT rate of 97% and an FP rate of

12% when the prevalence of retrocochlear disease is 5% in a population of 2000. If the prevalence of acoustic neuroma is 5%, then 100 patients will have acoustic neuroma and 1900 patients will not have acoustic neuroma. The cost associated with BAEP testing would be equivalent to the cost incurred by the resultant number of false positives plus the cost incurred by the number of resultant false negatives.

The cost of BAEP testing can be restated, since the relative cost ratio of the false negatives to the false positives is 5, as equivalent to the cost incurred by the number of false positives plus the cost of the false-positive equivalent of the false negatives (number of false negatives multiplied by the relative cost ratio). If the FP rate is 12%, the FN rate is 3%, 100 patients have acoustic tumor, and 1900 patients do not have acoustic tumor, then the cost associated with BAEP testing is equivalent to the number of false positives (12% of 1900 which is 228) plus the number of false negatives times the relative cost ratio (3% of 100 multiplied by 5 which yields 15). Thus, the cost of BAEP testing is the cost associated with 228 + 15 false positives or 243 false positives.

If no audiologic testing is done, this means that all suspect ears are classified as cochlear. Doing no testing means that the FP rate is 0% and the FN rate is 100%. The cost of doing no testing would be equivalent to the cost of the number of false positives (0) plus the following: the cost of 100% × 100 patients with acoustic neuroma multiplied by 5 which yields 500 false-positive equivalents. Thus, the cost associated with classifying all ears as cochlear is equivalent to the cost of 500 false positives. Therefore, the cost of doing no testing is approximately twice the cost of doing BAEP testing, which makes the BAEP test, with a cost of 243 false positives, superior to no testing at all, which is associated with a cost of 500 false positives.

Cost–benefit analysis using Dobie's (1985) approach can be applied to other audiologic tests such as the PI–PB test. Let us assume that the false-negative rate of the PI–PB test is 26% (Turner *et al.*, 1984a), the false-positive rate is 4% (Turner *et al.*, 1984a), and the prevalence of acoustic neuroma is 5% in a population of 2000, yielding 100 patients with acoustic neuroma and 1900 patients without acoustic neuroma. The cost associated with the PI–PB test would be equivalent to the number of false positives (4% of 1900 which is 76) plus the number of false negatives times the relative cost ratio (26% of 100 multiplied by 5 which yields 130). The cost of PI–PB testing is the cost associated with 76 + 130 false positives or 206 false positives. Thus, application of the cost–benefit model (Dobie, 1985) to the PI–PB and BAEP tests reveals that the cost of PI–PB testing is lower than that of BAEP testing. It appears that the cost–benefit approach (Dobie, 1985) is biased toward tests with low false-positive rates and is relatively insensitive to the HT rate of the test.

IV. PROPOSED PROTOCOL FOR DETECTION OF RETROCOCHLEAR AND CENTRAL PATHOLOGY

A. RETROCOCHLEAR

Kusakari, Okitsu, Kobayashi, et al. (1981) reported that only 1.4% of 2307 patients referred to an otoneurology clinic had cerebellopontine-angle tumors. The prevalence of cerebellopontine-angle tumors in the high-risk population (unilateral sensorineural hearing impairment, unilateral tinnitus, and/or dizziness) is higher than in the no-risk population, as evidenced by the reports of Caparosa (1979) who found cerebellopontine-angle tumors in 3.1% of 4200 high-risk patients over an 11-year period. The prevalence of acoustic tumors can be exceedingly small in some clinics, as evidenced by the report of Alberti, Symons, and Hyde (1979), who identified only a single case of acoustic tumor in 1873 patients seen in an occupational hearing-conservation program; interestingly, this acoustic-tumor patient had a symmetrical audiometric configuration. Because the occurrence of acoustic tumors is rare, Mair et al. (1988) recommended that a screening test for retrocochlear pathology be a test with the highest sensitivity and specificity.

Based on the evaluation of test performance, Mair et al. (1988), Cohen and Prasher (1988), and Antonelli, Bellotto, and Grandori (1987) supported Turner et al.'s (1984a) conclusion that the best screening test for retrocochlear pathology is the BAEP test. Turner (1988) found that, not only was the BAEP test by itself superior to the other audiologic tests for screening for retrocochlear pathology, it was also by itself superior to any audiologic test battery. Recall from Turner et al. (1984b) that because of the positive correlation between audiologic tests, adding other audiologic tests to the BAEP screening test for retrocochlear pathology increases either the sensitivity or specificity but not both the sensitivity and specificity of the protocol. Turner et al.'s (1984b) analysis of Owens' (1971) data bear out this conclusion.

Turner (1988) recommended the use of the P_1 or P_5 retrocochlear screening protocol. Recall that the P_5 consists of the ARC and BAEP tests combined in series negative. Turner (1988) determined the HT and FA rates for P_5 based on a mid-positive correlation between tests to be 97 and 20%, respectively. In calculating the HT and FA rate of the P_5 protocol, Turner (1988) assumed that the HT and FA rates for the BAEP test were 95 and 11%, respectively, and that the HT and FA rates for the ARC test were 84 and 15%, respectively, based on the data from Turner et al. (1984a). The criterion for the acoustic-reflex threshold test underlying the HT and FA rates for the ARC as reported by Turner et al. (1984a) did not consider the effect of magnitude of hearing impairment.

Recall from Chapter 3 that the acoustic-reflex threshold is dependent upon the magnitude of the hearing impairment. Also recall from Chapter 3 that Silman and Gelfand (1981) developed the 90th percentiles for the acoustic-reflex thresholds based upon the magnitude of the hearing impairment; acoustic-reflex threshold levels exceeding the 90th percentiles for the 500-, 1000-, and/or 2000-Hz tonal activators were assumed to be consistent with retrocochlear pathology. As mentioned previously in Chapter 3, the results of the study by Olsen, Bauch, and Harner (1983) on 30 cochlear-impaired ears and 30 ears with surgically confirmed cerebellopontine-angle tumors matched for hearing impairment revealed that the HT and FA rates of the combined acoustic-reflex threshold [based on the Silman & Gelfand (1981) 90th percentiles] and decay test were 83 and 10%, respectively. The results of the study by Sanders (1984b) on 100 cochlear-impaired ears and 129 confirmed acoustic-tumor ears revealed that the HT and FA rates of the acoustic-reflex threshold [based on the Silman & Gelfand (1981) 90th percentiles] and decay test were 85 and 11%, respectively. A weighted average of the HT and FA rates of the combined acoustic-reflex threshold and decay test reveals an HT rate of approximately 84.5% and an FA rate of approximately 11%.

The results of recent research suggest that the correlation between the acoustic-reflex threshold and BAEP tests is a maximum-positive rather than mid-positive one (Bauch et al., 1983; Cohen & Prasher, 1988). For example, Bauch et al., (1983) reported that, of the 25 ears with acoustic tumor detected by the ARC test, only 1 of these 25 ears did not show abnormal BAEP results. Cohen and Prasher (1988) reported that all of the ears with confirmed cerebellopontine-angle tumors who showed abnormal acoustic-reflex results also showed abnormal BAEP results.

If the weighted HT and FA rates of the ARC based on the results of Sanders (1984b) and Olsen et al. (1983) are employed in the P_5 series-negative (or parallel-loose) protocol, and if a maximum-positive correlation between the ARC and BAEP tests is assumed, then the P_5 protocol from Turner (1988) will have an HT rate of 95% and an FA rate of 11%. [According to Turner (1988), the HT rate of a series-negative protocol with a maximum-positive correlation is equivalent to the largest HT rate of the individual tests and the FA rate of a series-negative protocol with a maximum-positive correlation is equivalent to the largest FA rate of the individual tests.] The HT and FA rates of this P_5 protocol using the weighted average data calculated from Olsen et al. (1983) and Sanders (1984b) for the ARC are the same as those reported for Turner's (1988) P_1 protocol consisting of only the BAEP audiologic screening test. Although the benefits of the revised P_5 and P_1 will be the same, the cost of P_1 will exceed that of P_5 because the BAEP test is more expensive and time-consuming to administer than the ARC test, which is a routine part of the audiologic test battery. Thus, we recommend the use of the P_5 protocol based on a maximum-positive correlation and the use of the 90th percentiles for the ARC test.

If a mid-positive correlation between the ARC and BAEP tests is assumed (as assumed by Turner, 1988), and the weighted average data calculated from Olsen *et al.* (1983) and Sanders (1984b) are used for the HT and FA rates of the ARC (i.e., HT rate of 85% and FA rate of 11%), then the HT and FA rates of the P_5 series-negative protocol will be 97 and 16%, respectively. This protocol (P_5 based on mid-positive and the 90th percentiles for the ARC) would be clearly superior to all protocols except for P_1 with an HT of 95% and an FA of 11%. Again, deciding between P_1 and P_5 would depend on cost–benefit analysis. Certainly, this P_5 (mid-positive correlation) HT and FA rate based on an ARC using the 90th percentiles criterion is superior to the P_5 (mid-positive correlation) HT and FA rate (97 and 20%, respectively) based on an ARC which does not use the 90th percentiles criterion.

Recall that the P_5 based on a maximum-positive correlation (suggested by recent literature) and an ARC with the 90th percentiles criterion has an HT and FA of 95 and 11%; these HT and FA rates are superior to those for P_2, P_3, and P_4 and are equal to those for P_1 (ARC is not based on the 90th percentiles) for a mid-positive correlation. Although the HT and FA rates for the P_5 based on a maximum-positive correlation and the use of the 90th-percentile levels as a criterion for the ARC are equal to the P_1 based on a mid-positive correlation and an ARC which does not employ the 90th-percentiles criterion, the cost-benefit analysis for the former is better than that of the latter.

If a prevalence of 5% for retrocochlear pathology is assumed, and if the weighted HT and FA rates based on the use of the 90th-percentile levels for the acoustic-reflex threshold (Olsen *et al.*, 1983; Sanders, 1984) are employed for the ARC test, then the predictive value of a positive result [Pr (RE/+)] is equivalent to 29% as compared with the 22% reported by Turner *et al.* (1984a). This predictive value is very close to that reported for the BAEP test by Turner *et al.* (1984a)(31%).

We recommend giving the ARC test (the first component of the P_5) to everyone, not just to the at-risk, since the ARC test is a part of the routine audiologic battery; the BAEP test (second component of the P_5) would be given only to those who are at-risk and who yield negative results on the ARC test. Persons should be considered at risk if they have any one or more of the following characteristics: (a) (abnormal rollover index (PI–PB function to be performed whenever there is asymmetry in suprathreshold speech-recognition scores outside the 95% confidence limits; or the suprathreshold speech-recognition score at the estimated PB_{max} level is less than 80% for a pure-tone average less than or equal to 30 dB HI); (b) asymmetrical or unilateral sensorineural

hearing impairment; (c) asymmetrical tinnitus; (d) dizziness; (e) ataxia; or (f) facial paralysis or numbness of the face. Thus, we recommend that the P_5 be given under these conditions. All those who are at-risk as just defined should receive protocol testing. All persons receiving audiologic evaluations should receive complete acoustic-immittance testing including acoustic-reflex threshold and decay testing. Those who obtain positive results which are repeatable (see Chapter 3), even at just a single activating frequency, on the ARC test should also be referred for the definitive medical test regardless of whether or not they are at risk for retrocochlear pathology. All persons who obtain negative results on the ARC test but who are at-risk as just defined should receive BAEP testing. Persons who obtain positive results on the BAEP test should be referred for the definitive test such as MRI. Thus, persons referred for the definitive medical test are those at risk who fail the modified P_5 and those not at risk who obtain positive ARC results.

EFFECT OF MAGNITUDE OF HEARING IMPAIRMENT ON THE ACOUSTIC-REFLEX THRESHOLD AND DECAY TESTS AND BAEP TEST

Silman and Galfand (1981) found that the 90th-percentile levels for the acoustic-reflex thresholds in persons with cochlear hearing impairment of 80 dB HL or more were essentially 125 dB HL for all tonal activators. Therefore, when the magnitude of the hearing impairment is 80 dB HL or more, the presence of acoustic reflexes is negative for retrocochlear pathology. In such cases, however, when the acoustic reflexes are absent, differentiation cannot be made between cochlear and retrocochlear pathology.

Silman and Gelfand (1981) reported that the frequency of occurrence of absent acoustic reflexes increases directly with the magnitude of the hearing impairment. For the 2000-Hz activator, the frequency of occurrence of absent acoustic reflexes increases from 0% for magnitudes between 0 and 25 dB HL (inclusive), to 30% for magnitudes between 80 and 85 dB HL, and to 58% for magnitudes between 90 and 110 dB HL. For the 1000-Hz activator, the frequency of occurrence of absent acoustic reflexes increases from 0% for magnitudes between 0 and 25 dB HL (inclusive), to 22% for magnitudes between 80 and 85 dB HL, and to 40% for magnitudes between 90 and 110 dB HL. For the 500-Hz activator, the frequency of occurrence of absent acoustic reflexes increases from 0% for magnitudes between 0 and 35 dB HL (inclusive), to 15% for magnitudes between 80 and 85 dB HL, and to 56% for magnitudes between 90 and 110 dB HL. Figure 4 shows the relation between magnitude of the hearing impairment and frequency of occurrence of absent reflexes for the 500-, 1000-, and 2000-Hz tonal activators. Similar findings were obtained by Gelfand and Piper (1984). These results show that the acoustic reflex is absent in a substantial proportion

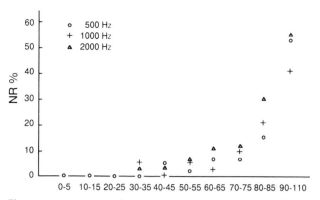

Figure 4 Proportions of absence of acoustic reflexes as a function of hearing loss. From Silman and Gelfand (1981) with permission.

of ears with cochlear hearing impairment when the magnitude of the hearing impairment exceeds 80 dB HL. Acoustic-reflex decay testing is precluded by absent acoustic reflexes. Thus, differentiation between cochlear and retrocochlear pathology cannot be done in cases of absent acoustic reflexes, which are especially frequent when the magnitude of the hearing impairment exceeds 80 dB HL. Nevertheless, an absent acoustic reflex at one frequency does not imply a similar absence at another frequency. In many cases, especially in cases of sloping sensorineural hearing impairment, although the acoustic reflex is absent at the higher frequencies, it is present at the lower frequencies; in such cases, differentiation between cochlear and retrocochlear pathology can be made on the basis of the acoustic-reflex threshold and decay tests administered using the lower frequency tonal activators (provided the magnitude of the hearing impairment does not exceed 80 dB HL at these lower frequencies).

As for the acoustic reflexes, the likelihood of absent BAEPs and distorted waveform morphology increases as the magnitude of hearing impairment associated with cochlear pathology increases. Mair *et al.* (1988) concluded that differentiation between cochlear and retrocochlear pathology cannot be made when the pure-tone threshold exceeds 80 dB HL at 4000 Hz. Our clinical experience suggests that differentiation between cochlear and retrocochlear lesions based on the BAEPs can be made even when the hearing impairment exceeds 80 dB HL at 4000 Hz if better hearing sensitivity is present at 2000 Hz. Thus, when the two-frequency pure-tone average based on 2000 and 4000 Hz exceeds 80 dB HL, the BAEP test should be eliminated from the recommended protocol.

For the ARC and BAEP tests, the problem of differentiation between cochlear and retrocochlear pathology is increased when the magnitude of the hearing impairment exceeds 80 dB HL. Whether the hearing impairment exceeds or is less than 80 dB HL, the acoustic-reflex threshold test is performed as part of the routine audiologic evalu-

ation to identify conductive or facial-nerve pathology and to assist in detection of functional hearing impairment.

If the hearing impairment exceeds 80 dB HL, and the patient is not at risk for retrocochlear pathology, we recommend that the ARC test be performed but the patient not be referred for definitive testing, regardless of whether thresholds beyond the 90th-percentile levels (i.e., absent) are obtained, because the prevalence of absent acoustic reflexes is high in persons with cochlear hearing impairment when the magnitude of the hearing impairment exceeds 80 dB HL. Thus, the patient is not referred for definitive testing regardless of whether the acoustic reflexes are present or absent when the hearing impairment exceeds 80 dB HL and the patient is not at risk for retrocochlear pathology.

The question then arises of whether the acoustic-reflex thresholds should be interpreted with respect to differentiation between cochlear and retrocochlear pathology, since the patient will not be referred for the definitive test regardless of the acoustic-reflex threshold result. We suggest that the acoustic-reflex thresholds in such cases not be examined for the purpose of differentiating between cochlear and retrocochlear pathology except when there is a change (i.e., from present to absent) in the acoustic-reflex thresholds from test to test unaccompanied by change in the hearing-threshold levels. The acoustic-reflex decay test should be performed in persons with hearing impairment exceeding 80 dB HL who are not at risk for retrocochlear pathology, and whose acoustic-reflex results permit this testing. If the acoustic-reflex decay results are negative, the patient should not be referred for the definitive test. If the acoustic-reflex decay results are positive, the patient should be referred for the definitive test. In summary, when the magnitude of the hearing impairment exceeds 80 dB HL and the patient is not at risk for retrocochlear pathology, the patient is not referred for the definitive test unless there is positive acoustic-reflex decay or unless there is a change in the acoustic-reflex thresholds from test to test unaccompanied by a change in the hearing-threshold levels.

If the magnitude of the hearing impairment exceeds 80 dB HL, and the patient is at risk for retrocochlear pathology, we recommend that acoustic-reflex threshold testing be done, just as it is done for persons with no more than 80 dB HL hearing impairment, for the purpose of identifying conductive hearing impairment or facial-nerve pathology and to assist in identifying functional hearing impairment. Again, as for the no-risk persons with hearing impairment exceeding 80 dB HL, the question arises of whether the acoustic-reflex thresholds should be interpreted with respect to differentiation between cochlear and retrocochlear pathology in persons with hearing impairment exceeding 80 dB HL who are at risk for retrocochlear pathology. If, in such cases, the acoustic reflexes are present (i.e., negative results are obtained), the patient is referred for the definitive test. Because of the high likelihood of absent or distorted waveforms, BAEP testing, in such cases, will not contribute to the differential diagnosis. If, in such cases, the acoustic reflexes are absent (i.e., differentiation cannot be made between cochlear and retrocochlear pathology), the patient should still be referred for the definitive test since the BAEP test is not useful in these cases. Thus, regardless of whether present or absent acoustic reflexes are obtained, persons with hearing impairment exceeding 80 dB HL who are at risk for retrocochlear pathology should be referred for the definitive test. Therefore, the acoustic-reflex thresholds should not be interpreted with respect to the differentiation between cochlear and retrocochlear pathology in persons with hearing impairment exceeding 80 dB HL at 500, 1000, and 2000 Hz and who are at risk for retrocochlear pathology; these cases will be referred for the definitive test regardless of the acoustic-reflex threshold. Since patients having hearing impairment exceeding 80 dB HL who are at risk will be referred for the definitive test regardless of the acoustic-reflex thresholds, acoustic-reflex decay testing in such cases is noncontributory.

In summary, when the hearing impairment exceeds 80 dB HL, acoustic-reflex threshold testing is done as part of the routine audiologic test (i.e., identification of conductive/facial-nerve/functional hearing impairment). If the patient is not at risk, acoustic-reflex decay testing should be done. These no-risk patients should be referred for the definitive test only when positive acoustic-reflex decay results are obtained or when there is a change in the acoustic-reflex threshold levels between one test and another, unaccounted for by a change in the hearing-threshold levels or conductive pathology. If the patient is at risk for retrocochlear pathology, acoustic-reflex decay testing is noncontributory. All at-risk patients will be referred for the definitive test regardless of the acoustic-reflex threshold and decay results.

B. CENTRAL

Sparse data are available which have reported the sensitivity and specificity of the central speech tests to auditory intra-axial brainstem and temporal-lobe pathology. Antonelli et al. (1987) evaluated 25 patients with intra-axial brainstem lesions (metastases, gliomas, hemorrhages, cysts, unidentified masses, and pinealomas) and 16 patients with temporal-lobe lesions (hemorrhages, spongioblastomas, astrocytomas, oligodendroglioma, temporal lobectomy for temporal-lobe epilepsy). The central tests evaluated included the Italian version of the Bocca and Calearo (1963) monaural low-pass filtered sentences, monaural time-compressed sentences, binaural alternating sentences, and the Italian version of the Jerger and Jerger (1975) SSI–ICM and SSI–CCM tests. Since the filtered speech tests and time-compressed speech tests were assumed to be reduced by both intra-axial brainstem and temporal-lobe lesions,

only the sensitivity and not the specificity was reported for these tests. According to Jerger and Jerger (1975), the SSI–ICM is particularly affected by intra-axial brainstem lesions whereas the SSI–CCM is particularly affected by temporal-lobe lesions.

The sensitivity and specificity of these tests, as reported by Antonelli et al. (1987) are shown in Table VI. Note that the sensitivity for the Bocca and Calearo (1963) sensitized tests and Jerger SSI–ICM are low (less than 80%). On the other hand, the SSI–CCM test, has a sensitivity of 80% and specificity of 83.3%, indicating that is is sensitive to temporal-lobe lesions and insensitive to intra-axial brainstem lesions. In Chapter 6, it was noted that the SSI test had the highest sensitivity to cortical lesions compared with the other central speech tests. The slow vertex potentials, which are affected by factors such as attention, have not proven useful in the detection of cortical lesions (Parving, Elberling, & Salomon, 1981). Therefore, the only audiologic test for detection of temporal-lobe lesions which has relatively high sensitivity and specificity is the SSI–CCM test. As mentioned previously in Chapter 6, the sensitivity of the SSI–CCM test is not high enough to warrant its use as a screening tool for temporal-lobe pathology. Nevertheless, the use of the SSI–CCM in normal-hearing patients who complain of difficulty hearing in noisy or group situations and who have negative results on P_5 will strengthen the basis of referral for neurologic follow-up. (Of course, normal-hearing persons with normal SSI–CCM findings and normal P_5 findings, who complain of difficulty in noisy or group situations, should also be referred for neurologic follow-up.)

Table VI also reveals that none of these central speech tests is sensitive to intra-axial brainstem lesions. That is, none of the central speech tests has a sensitivity to intra-axial brainstem lesions exceeding 75%. The ARC test has a sensitivity of only 70% to intra-axial brainstem lesions

Table VI Speech Audiometry: "Central" Test Outcome[a]

Test[b]	Sensitivity (%)		Specificity (%)	
	BS[c]	TL[d]	BS	TL
DS and T-CS	62.5	75	—	—
B-SS	56.25	6.25	93.75	—
SSI-ICM	75	50	—	—
SSI-CCM	16.7	80	—	83.3

[a] Reproduced from Antonelli et al. (1987).
[b] DS, sentences low-pass filtered with a cut-off frequency of 5000 Hz and a slope of 16 dB/octave; T-CS, sentences subjected to a temporal compression of 60%; B-SS, alternating sentences switched between ears at switching rates from 1–20/s; SSI-ICM, synthetic sentence index under the ipsilateral competing message condition; SSI-CCM, synthetic sentence index under the competing message condition.
[c] BS, brainstem.
[d] TL, temporal lobe.

(Cohan & Prasher, 1988), which is not surprising since the most rostral part of the brainstem tapped by the ARC is the superior olivary complex, which is in the low brainstem. Cohen and Prasher reported that the BAEP test had a 90% sensitivity to intraxial brainstem lesions including vertebro-basilar ischemia, glioma (brainstem tumors are relatively rare), multiple sclerosis, degenerative disorders, and brainstem infarcts and unknown lesions. Thus, the BAEP test is the best audiologic screening test for detection of intra-axial brainstem pathology. Recall from Chapter 7 that a prolonged I–III interpeak latency is characteristic of retrocochlear or low intra-axial brainstem pathology whereas a prolonged III–V interpeak latency is characteristic of intra-axial brainstem (lower and upper) pathology. Antonelli *et al.* (1987), who used electrocochleography to obtain wave I if wave I was absent from the conventional BAEP waveform, reported that, with respect to detection of lower pontine or upper pontine–midbrain sites, a prolonged I–III interpeak interval had a sensitivity of 85.7% and a specificity of 80%. Of course, wave I is often difficult to detect without the aid of electrocochleography in cases where hearing impairment is present. (See Chapter 7 to review techniques for enhancing wave I.) When wave I is absent, the I–III interpeak interval cannot be used to differentiate between retrocochlear or lower pontine and upper pontine–midbrain pathology.

V. CONCEPT OF COMBINED COCHLEAR AND RETROCOCHLEAR SITES AND THE TRADITIONAL SITE-OF-LESION TEST RESULTS

Administration of the traditional site-of-lesion test battery (e.g., SISI, tone-decay, and ABLB tests) (see Chapter 5) to patients at risk for retrocochlear pathology has yielded inconsistent results in many cases, that is, cochlear and retrocochlear signs. Newby and Popelka (1985) stated:

> It must be kept in mind that some sensorineural impairments are truly combined sensory and neural involvements, and it should be expected that in such cases tests designed to identify the site of lesion would yield equivocal results. (p. 241)

Miller (1985) noted that inconsistent or mixed audiologic patterns are often present in persons with small acoustic tumors because of secondary tumor pressure on the cochlear blood supply or a coexisting, unrelated cochlear disorder. We concur with this hypothesis in some cases with inconsistent results. Nevertheless, we feel that the majority of "inconsistent" cases reflect the fact that the traditional site-of-lesion tests have differential sensitivity to acoustic tumors. The findings of Turner and his colleagues support this implication.

Dix and Hood (1953) reported that in several cases with early acoustic tumors, complete loudness recruitment was present prior to tumor removal and absent following the tumor removal. Simonton (1956) obtained similar findings. Dix and Hood (1953) suggested that the complete recruitment resulted from the disruption of the cochlear blood supply by pressure from the eighth-nerve tumor. The histological findings by Suga and Lindsay (1976) supported the hypothesis of Dix and Hood (1953). We do not dispute that, in such cases, there were combined cochlear and retrocochlear sites of pathology. We hypothesize, however, that the presence of recruitment in these cases reflected the lack of sensitivity of the ABLB test to the eighth-nerve tumor (with absence of recruitment or derecruitment being the measures of eighth-nerve pathology); the absence of recruitment following tumor removal probably reflects additional damage to the eighth nerve from the surgery. That is, when the magnitude of damage to the eighth nerve is sufficient, the ABLB test may show absence of recruitment.

VI. CASE ILLUSTRATIONS

A. CASE 1

Case 1 is a 46-year-old male with a 20-year history of military and industrial noise exposure.

For case 1, Figure 5A shows the pure-tone air- and bone-conduction thresholds, SRTs, speech-recognition scores, tympanograms, static-acoustic middle-ear admittance, contralateral acoustic-reflex thresholds, and contralateral acoustic-reflex decay results. Figure 5B shows the Carhart tone-decay results, ABLB, and SISI results. Figure 5C shows the caloric tracings. Figure 5D shows the summary for the BAEP peak and interpeak latencies. Figure 5E shows the single-channel brainstem auditory-evoked potentials for rarefaction clicks presented at 85 dBnHL.

Using the classification system in Chapter 2, the pure-tone air- and bone-conduction thresholds are consistent with normal hearing-threshold levels in the low–mid and high frequencies in the right ear. In the left ear, the pure-tone air- and bone-conduction thresholds are consistent with a moderately severe sensorineural hearing impairment in the low–mid frequencies and a severe sensorineural hearing impairment in the high frequencies. The audiometric configuration in the left ear is a precipitously sloping one (see Chapter 2). The SRT corroborates the two-frequency pure-tone average in the left ear and the three-frequency pure-tone average in the right ear (see Chapter 2). The speech-recognition scores exceed the Thornton and Raffin (1978) 95% critical-differences limits; the left-ear score is significantly poorer than the right-ear score at 30 dB SL relative to the SRT. Since the suprathreshold speech-recognition scores for the two ears were asymmetrical, a

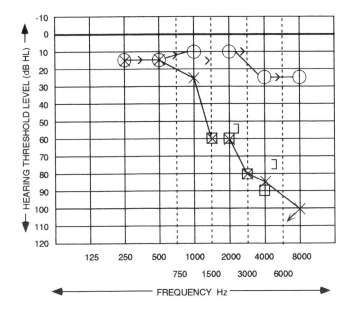

PURE TONE AVERAGE (500-2000 Hz) in dB			
	Right	Left	Best din. avg.
Two freq.	10	20	
Three freq.	12	28	

	UNAIDED				UNAIDED			
	Right	HL	Left	HL	Right	HL	Left	HL
SAT		dB		dB		dB		dB
SRT	15	dB	25	dB		dB		dB
WORD RECOG	88 % at 45	dB	38 % at 55	dB	% at	dB	% at	dB
	% at	dB	58 % at 65	dB	% at	dB	% at	dB
	% at	dB	50 % at 75	dB	% at	dB	% at	dB
	% at	dB	48 % at 85	dB	% at	dB	% at	dB
MCL		dB		dB		dB		dB
UCL		dB		dB		dB		dB
MATERIALS								

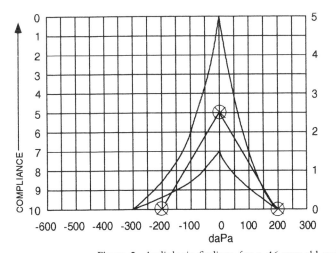

ACOUSTIC REFLEX

STIMULUS RIGHT   (CONTRALATERAL)   STIMULUS LEFT

% decay in 10 sec	THRESHOLD dB		Hz	THRESHOLD dB		% decay in 10 sec
	SL	HL		HL	SL	
neg		90	500	85		neg
neg		90	1000	80		neg
		95	2000	95		
			4000			

(IPSILATERAL)

			500			
			1000			
			2000			

STATIC COMPLIANCE $C = C_2 - C_1$

RIGHT			LEFT		
1.6 C_2	1.1 C_1	0.5 C	1.5 C_2	1.0 C_1	0.5 C

Figure 5 Audiologic findings for a 46-year-old male. (A) *Top*, Pure-tone air- and bone-conduction thresholds, bilaterally. Middle, SRTs and suprathreshold speech-recognition scores for PB words, bilaterally. *Bottom*, Tympanograms for the two ears (*left side*) and the contralateral acoustic-reflex threshold and decay results and static-acoustic admittance (*right side*), bilaterally.

TONE DECAY (Carhart-STAT-Rosenberg-Circle One)

	Right								Left					
	250	500	1K	2K	4K	8K			250	500	1K	2K	4K	8K
Decay (dB)		0	0	0						0	0	0		
Decay (dB)														
Decay (dB)														

TONE DECAY (Owens Test)

Ear	Freq.	SL dB	Decay in Seconds		Ear	Freq.	SL dB	Decay in Seconds		Ear	Freq.	SL dB	Decay in Seconds
		5					5					5	
		10					10					10	
		15					15					15	
		20					20					20	

LOUDNESS BALANCE (ABLB-MLB-CIRCLE ONE)

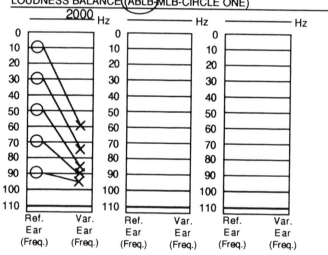

BEKESY SUMMARY

Right Ear:

Bekesy

Left Ear:

Bekesy

SISI (Standard-High Level-Circle One)

	Right								Left					
	250	500	1K	2K	4K	8K			250	500	1K	2K	4K	8K
% Correct				35								95		
Presentation Level (dB SL)				20								20		
dB Masking														

Figure 5 (continued)   (B) *Top,* Carhart tone-decay results at 500, 1000, and 2000 Hz. *Middle,* ABLB results at 2000 Hz. *Bottom,* SISI results (standard presentation level) at 2000 Hz, bilaterally.

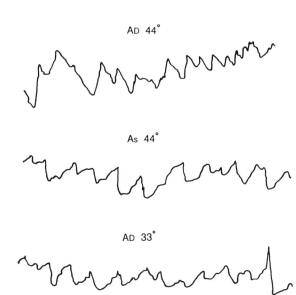

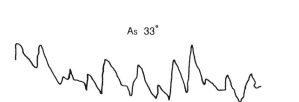

Figure 5 (continued) (C) Caloric tracings for the right (A_D) and left (A_S) ears under the warm (44°C) and cool (33°C) conditions.

PEAK AND INTERPEAK LATENCY (ms)

INTENSITY	I	II	III	IV	V	VI	VII	I-V	III-V	I-III	REP. RATE (per s)
RE											
	1.52	2.60	3.76	4.72	5.56			4.04	1.80	2.24	11.4
85	1.48	2.64	3.84	4.76	5.56			4.08	1.72	2.36	

PEAK AND INTERPEAK LATENCY (ms)

INTENSITY	I	II	III	IV	V	VI	VII	I-V	III-V	I-III	REP. RATE (per s)
LE											
85		3.50	5.80		7.48				1.68		11.4
		3.48	5.80		7.32				1.52		

Figure 5 (continued) (D) Summary of the BAEP peak and interpeak latencies for single-channel BAEP recordings obtained for rarefaction clicks at 85 dBnHL at a repetition rate of 11.4/s, bilaterally.

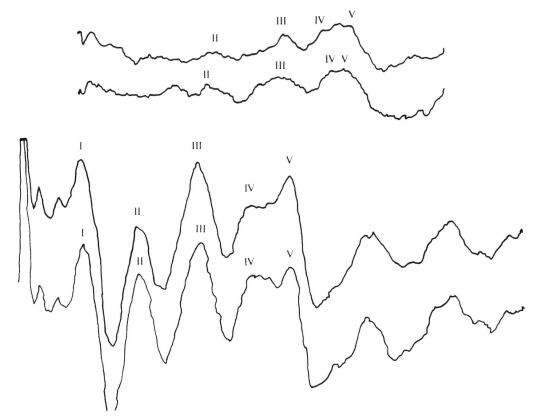

Figure 5 (continued) (E) Test–retest BAEP tracings for the left ear (*top*) and the right ear (*bottom*).

PI–PB function was obtained for the left ear. The rollover index for the left ear was 0.17, which is negative with respect to retrocochlear pathology.

The static-acoustic middle-ear admittance and tympanometric results were consistent with normal middle-ear function, bilaterally (see Chapter 3). The contralateral acoustic-reflex threshold did not exceed Silman and Gelfand (1981) 90th percentile levels, bilaterally (see Chapter 3). Contralateral acoustic-reflex decay was negative with respect to retrocochlear pathology, bilaterally (see Chapter 3).

The ABLB results at 2000 Hz reveal complete recruitment, consistent with left cochlear pathology (see Chapter 5). The Carhart tone-decay results at 500, 1000, and 2000 Hz are negative, bilaterally (see Chapter 5). The SISI scores were consistent with cochlear pathology in the left ear and normal-hearing in the right ear (see Chapter 5).

The brainstem auditory evoked potentials, recorded at 85 dBnHL, revealed normal peak and interpeak latencies for the right ear, consistent with normal auditory nervous system function on the right side to the level of the lateral lemniscus (see Chapter 7). In the left ear, the III–V interpeak latency is normal, consistent with normal high brainstem function, bilaterally (see Chapter 7). Even when 0.35 ms is subtracted from the absolute latency for wave V (0.1 ms for every 10 dB loss beyond 50 dB HL at 4000 Hz), the absolute wave V latency for the left ear is prolonged, consistent with retrocochlear pathology in the left ear (see Chapter 7). The interaural wave V difference exceeds 0.3 msec, even when the absolute latency of wave V is corrected for hearing loss in the left ear (see Chapter 7). The BAEP indicators of retrocochlear pathology in the left ear were the prolonged absolute latency of wave V and the prolonged interaural wave V latency. The caloric tracings are symmetrical for the right and left ear under the cool and warm conditions, consistent with normal vestibular function, bilaterally (see Chapter 8). High-resolution CAT scan with contrast was negative, bilaterally.

The absence of a false-positive ARC finding combined with the presence of a false-positive BAEP illustrates the lower false-positive rate for the ARC than for the BAEP test and the increased false-positive rate for the BAEP test in cases of significant high-frequency hearing impairment. If the modified P_5 protocol had been followed (which it was), the patient would have been referred for BAEP testing although the ARC test results were negative because the patient was at-risk for retrocochlear pathology; of course, the patient would then be referred for the definitive medical test after obtaining positive BAEP results.

B. CASE 2

Case 2 is a 61-year-old male who presented with hearing impairment of gradual onset over a 15-year period, high-pitched tinnitus in the right ear, and occasional mild ataxia to the right. For Case 2, Figure 6A shows the pure-tone air- and bone-conduction thresholds, SRTs, suprathreshold speech-recognition scores, static-acoustic middle-ear admittance, tympanograms, contralateral acoustic-reflex thresholds, and contralateral acoustic-reflex decay results. Figure 6B shows the Carhart tone-decay results, ABLB results, and SISI results. Figure 6C shows the summary BAEP peak and interpeak latencies. Figure 6D shows the one-channel BAEP recordings to rarefaction clicks at 70 dBnHL with a repetition rate of 11.4/s. Figure 6E shows the caloric tracings under the warm and cool conditions.

The pure-tone air- and bone-conduction thresholds are consistent with a moderate sensorineural hearing impairment in the low–mid frequencies and a severe sensorineural hearing impairment in the high frequencies (see Chapter 2). In the left ear, the pure-tone air- and bone-conduction thresholds are consistent with normal hearing-threshold levels in the low and mid frequencies and a mild sensorineural hearing impairment in the high frequencies (see Chapter 2). The audiometric configuration is gradually sloping, bilaterally. The SRT corroborates the two-frequency pure-tone average, bilaterally (see Chapter 2). Although the right and left suprathreshold speech-recognition scores at 30 dB SL relative to the SRT did not exceed the Thornton and Raffin (1978) 95% critical-differences limits (see Chapter 5), a PI–PB function was obtained for the right ear. The rollover index for the right ear was 0, which is negative with respect to retrocochlear pathology (see Chapter 5). The Carhart tone-decay results were negative, bilaterally at 500, 1000, and 2000 Hz (see Chapter 5). The SISI results were consistent with cochlear pathology in the right ear and normal-hearing in the left ear.

The static-acoustic middle-ear admittance and tympanometric results for the 220-Hz probe tone were consistent with normal middle-ear function, bilaterally (see Chapter 3). The contralateral acoustic-reflex thresholds for the right ear (probe left) were absent for the right ear and present at levels not exceeding the Silman and Gelfand (1981) 90th percentile levels for the left ear (probe right)

Figure 6 Audiologic findings for a 61-year-old male. (A) *Top*, Pure-tone air- and bone-conduction thresholds, bilaterally. *Middle*, SRTs and suprathreshold speech-recognition scores for PB words. *Bottom*, Tympanograms (*left side*) and contralateral acoustic-reflex threshold and decay results and static acoustic middle-ear admittance (*right side*), bilaterally.

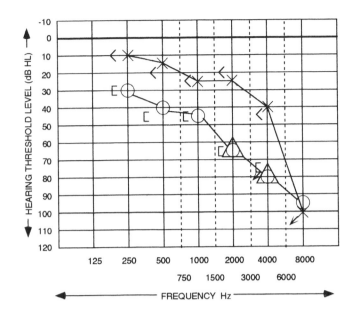

LEGEND

			Right (Solid)	Left (Dashed)
Air	Unmasked			
	Unmasked NR			
	Masked			
	Masked NR			
	Soundfield			
	Soundfield NR			
Mastoid Bone:	Unmasked			
	Unmasked NR			
	Masked			
	Masked NR			
Forehead Bone:	Unmasked			
	Unmasked NR			
	Masked			
	Masked NR			

Response consistency: good moderate poor

Validity: acceptable questionable

PURE TONE AVERAGE (500-2000 Hz) in dB

	Right	Left	Best din. avg.
Two freq.	43	20	
Three freq.	50	22	

	UNAIDED				UNAIDED			
	Right	HL	Left	HL	Right	HL	Left	HL
SAT		dB		dB		dB		dB
SRT	35	dB	15	dB		dB		dB
WORD RECOG	76 % at 65	dB	88 % at 45	dB	% at	dB	% at	dB
	84 % at 75	dB	% at	dB	% at	dB	% at	dB
	84 % at 85	dB	% at	dB	% at	dB	% at	dB
	% at	dB	% at	dB	% at	dB	% at	dB
MCL		dB		dB		dB		dB
UCL		dB		dB		dB		dB
MATERIALS								

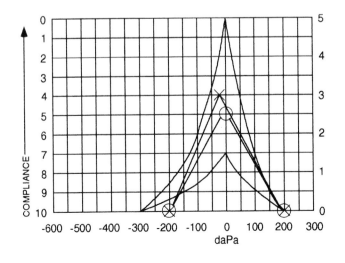

ACOUSTIC REFLEX

(CONTRALATERAL)

STIMULUS RIGHT				STIMULUS LEFT			
% decay in 10 sec	THRESHOLD dB		Hz	THRESHOLD dB		% decay in 10 sec
	SL	HL		HL	SL	
		Abs	500	85		neg
		Abs	1000	80		neg
		Abs	2000	95		
			4000			

(IPSILATERAL)

			500			
			1000			
			2000			

STATIC COMPLIANCE $C = C_2 - C_1$

RIGHT			LEFT		
1.4 C_2	0.8 C_1	0.6 C	1.5 C_2	0.8 C_1	0.7 C

TONE DECAY (Carhart-STAT-Rosenberg-Circle One)

Right

	250	500	1K	2K	4K	8K
Decay (dB)		5	5	10		
Decay (dB)						
Decay (dB)						

Left

	250	500	1K	2K	4K	8K
Decay (dB)		5	5	5		
Decay (dB)						
Decay (dB)						

TONE DECAY (Owens Test)

Ear	Freq.	SL dB	Decay in Seconds
		5	
		10	
		15	
		20	

Ear	Freq.	SL dB	Decay in Seconds
		5	
		10	
		15	
		20	

Ear	Freq.	SL dB	Decay in Seconds
		5	
		10	
		15	
		20	

LOUDNESS BALANCE (ABLB-MLB-CIRCLE ONE)

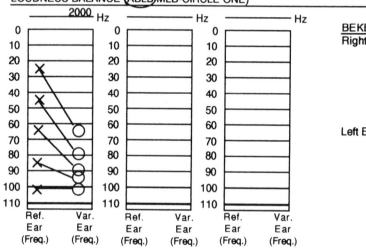

BEKESY SUMMARY

Right Ear:

BEKESY

Left Ear:

BEKESY

SISI (Standard-High Level-Circle One)

Right

	250	500	1K	2K	4K	8K
% Correct				85		
Presentation Level (dB SL)				20		
dB Masking						

Left

	250	500	1K	2K	4K	8K
% Correct				25		
Presentation Level (dB SL)				20		
dB Masking						

Figure 6 (continued) (B) *Top,* Carhart tone-decay results at 500, 1000, and 2000 Hz. *Middle,* ABLB results at 2000 Hz. *Bottom,* SISI results (standard presentation level at 2000 Hz, bilaterally.

PEAK AND INTERPEAK LATENCY (ms)

AD

INTENSITY	I	II	III	IV	V	VI	VII	I-V	III-V	I-III	REP. RATE (per s)
70					7.16						11.4
					7.14						

AS PEAK AND INTERPEAK LATENCY (ms)

INTENSITY	I	II	III	IV	V	VI	VII	I-V	III-V	I-III	REP. RATE (per s)
70	2.20	3.24	4.36	5.72	6.08			3.88	1.66	2.16	11.4
	2.08	3.24	4.36	5.60	6.12			4.04	1.76	2.28	

(Left axis labels: (dB) SPL (HL) SL)

Figure 6 (continued) (C) *Top*, Absolute BAEP latencies for the right ear, and *bottom*, Absolute and interpeak BAEP latencies for the left ear, for rarefaction clicks presented at 70 dBnHL at a repetition rate of 11.4/s.

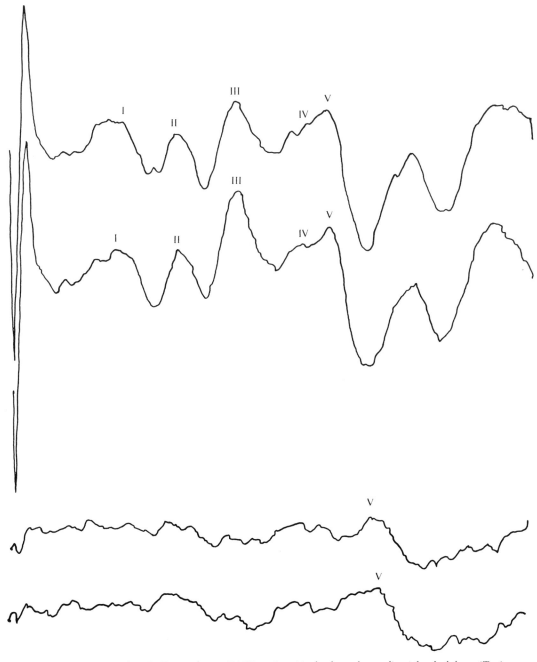

Figure 6 (continued) (D) Test and retest BAEP tracings (single-channel recordings) for the left ear (*Top*) and right ear (*Bottom*).

354

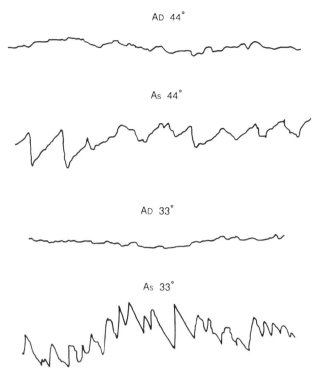

Figure 6 (continued) (E) Caloric tracings for A$_D$ and A$_S$ under the warm (44°C) and cool (33°C) conditions.

(see Chapter 3). These contralateral right-ear acoustic-reflexes were consistent with right retrocochlear pathology (see Chapter 3). The contralateral acoustic-reflex decay was negative for the left ear (see Chapter 3).

The BAEPs, obtained at 70 dBnHL, revealed normal peak and interpeak latencies for the left ear consistent with normal left auditory nervous system in the brainstem to the level of the lateral lemniscus (see Chapter 7). In the right ear, however, the BAEPs, obtained at the same intensity, revealed distorted waveform morphology and a prolonged absolute latency for wave V (see Chapter 7). The absolute latency for wave V remains significantly prolonged, even after subtracting 0.3 ms from the value (for 30 dB correction beyond 50 dB HL at 4000 Hz) (see Chapter 7). Even after absolute wave V latency is corrected for hearing loss, the interaural wave V latency is significantly prolonged, consistent with retrocochlear pathology (see Chapter 7). The caloric tracings reveal essentially no response from the right ear under the warm and cool conditions and normal responses from the left ear under the warm and cool conditions. The caloric results indicated right unilateral weakness, consistent with right peripheral vestibular pathology (see chapter 8). A surgically confirmed right cerebello-pontine-angle tumor was present.

In this case, the traditional site-of-lesion results represented false-negative findings whereas the BAEPs and ARC results represented true-positive findings. Although the ENG results revealed the presence of peripheral vestibular

pathology, it did not differentiate between cochlear and eighth-nerve vestibular pathology. If the modified P$_5$ protocol had been used, the patient would have been referred directly for the definitive medical test after the positive ARC findings were obtained, obviating the need for BAEP and ENG testing. Note that Cases 1 and 2 had essentially unilateral sensorineural hearing impairment and positive BAEP findings. In Case 1, the ARC results were true-negative results in contrast with the false-positive BAEP results whereas, in Case 2, the ARC and BAEP results were both true-positive ones.

C. CASE 3

Case 3 is a 53-year-old female who presented with a right-ear hearing impairment following an upper respiratory infection. Subsequent to the right-ear hearing impairment, an intermittent right-ear high-pitched tinnitus and pressure developed. After the onset of tinnitus and aural pressure, the patient noticed a marked increase in right-ear difficulty. Ten years prior to the hearing impairment, the patient experienced slight imbalance which was short-lasting.

The pure-tone air- and bone-conduction thresholds, SRTs, suprathreshold speech-recognition scores, static-acoustic admittance, 220-Hz tympanograms, contralateral acoustic-reflex thresholds, and contralateral acoustic-reflex decay results are shown in Figure 7A. Figure 7B shows the summary of the BAEP peak and interpeak latencies. Single-channel recordings obtained for rarefaction clicks presented at a repetition rate of 31/s are shown in Figure 7C. The complete two-channel ENG results are shown in Figure 7D and 7E.

The pure-tone air- and bone-conduction thresholds are consistent with essentially normal hearing thresholds in the low–mid frequencies and severe sensorineural hearing impairment in the high frequencies with a notch at 4000 Hz in the right ear (see Chapter 2). In the left ear, the pure-tone air- and bone-conduction thresholds are consistent with normal-hearing threshold levels in the low–mid and high frequencies (see Chapter 2). The SRT corroborates the three-frequency pure-tone average, bilaterally (see Chapter 2).

The 220-Hz tympanometric results and static acoustic middle-ear admittance are consistent with normal middle-ear function, bilaterally (see Chapter 3). Note that the static acoustic outer-ear admittance values are consistent with the presence of intact tympanic membranes, bilaterally (see Chapter 3). The right contralateral (probe left) acoustic reflexes were questionable at 120 dB HL for the 500-Hz and 1000-Hz activators and absent for the 2000-Hz activator. Thus, the right contralateral acoustic-reflex thresholds exceed the Silman and Gelfand (1978) 90th percentile levels, consistent with right retrocochlear pathology (see Chapter 3). The left contralateral acoustic-reflex thresholds did not exceed the Silman and Gelfand (1978) 90th percentile lev-

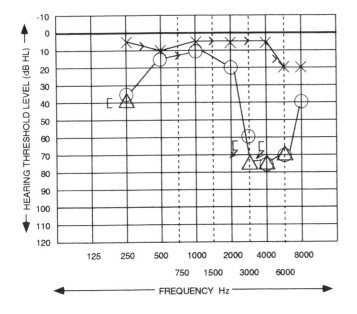

PURE TONE AVERAGE (500-2000 Hz) in dB			
	Right	Left	Best din. avg.
Two freq.	13	5	
Three freq.	15	7	

	UNAIDED				UNAIDED			
	Right	HL	Left	HL	Right	HL	Left	HL
SAT		dB		dB		dB		dB
SRT	15	dB	10	dB		dB		dB
WORD RECOG	72 % at 45	dB	100 % at 45	dB	% at	dB	% at	dB
	% at	dB	% at	dB	% at	dB	% at	dB
	% at	dB	% at	dB	% at	dB	% at	dB
	% at	dB	% at	dB	% at	dB	% at	dB
MCL		dB		dB		dB		dB
UCL		dB		dB		dB		dB
MATERIALS								

ACOUSTIC REFLEX

(CONTRALATERAL)

STIMULUS RIGHT					STIMULUS LEFT		
% decay in 10 sec	THRESHOLD dB		Hz	THRESHOLD dB		% decay in 10 sec
	SL	HL		HL	SL	
		120 ?	500	85		neg
		120 ?	1000	80		neg
		Abs	2000	95		neg
			4000			

(IPSILATERAL)

			Hz			
			500			
			1000			
			2000			

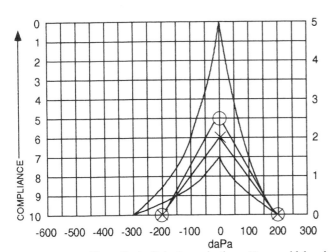

STATIC COMPLIANCE $C = C_2 - C_1$

RIGHT			LEFT		
1.55 C_2	1.10 C_1	0.45 C	1.50 C_2	1.10 C_1	0.40 C

Figure 7 Audiologic results for a 53-year-old female. (A) *Top*, right and left pure-tone air- and bone-conduction thresholds. *Middle*, SRTs and the suprathreshold PB word-recognition scores, bilaterally. *Bottom*, Tympanograms (*left side*) and the contralateral acoustic-reflex thresholds, bilaterally, left contralateral acoustic-reflex decay results, and static-acoustic middle-ear admittance, bilaterally (*right side*).

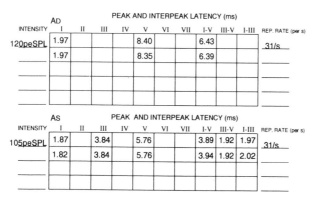

INTENSITY	AD PEAK AND INTERPEAK LATENCY (ms)										REP. RATE (per s)
	I	II	III	IV	V	VI	VII	I-V	III-V	I-III	
120peSPL	1.97				8.40			6.43			31/s
	1.97				8.35			6.39			

INTENSITY	AS PEAK AND INTERPEAK LATENCY (ms)										REP. RATE (per s)
	I	II	III	IV	V	VI	VII	I-V	III-V	I-III	
105peSPL	1.87		3.84		5.76			3.89	1.92	1.97	31/s
	1.82		3.84		5.76			3.94	1.92	2.02	

Figure 7 (continued) (B) *Top*, Absolute and interpeak BAEP latencies when clicks were presented at 120 dBpeSPL in the right ear and *bottom*, at 105 dBpeSPL in the left ear, at a repetition rate of 31/s.

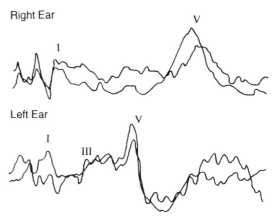

Figure 7 (continued) (C) Test and retest single-channel BAEP recordings for the left ear (*bottom*) and right ear (*top*).

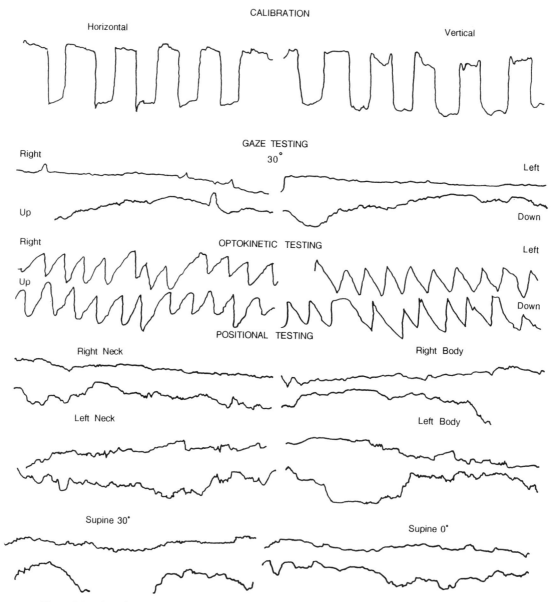

Figure 7 (continued) (D) ENG tracings for calibration, 30° gaze left and right and up and down, optokinetic testing, positional testing (right neck, right body, left neck, left body, supine at 30°, supine at 0°.

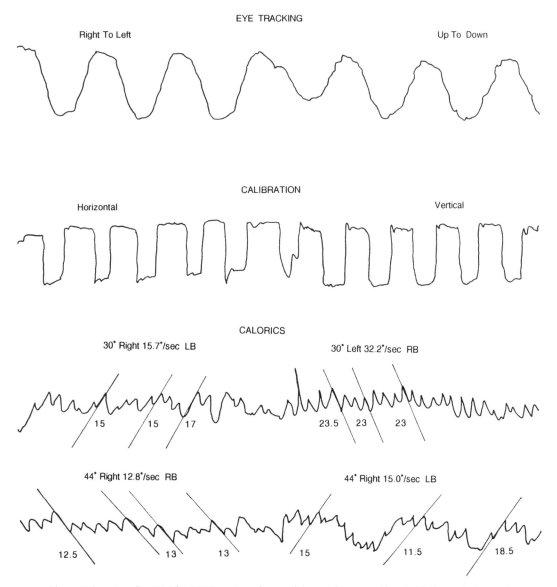

Figure 7 (continued) (E) The ENG tracings for pendular tracking, recalibration before calorics, and alternate binaural bithermal calorics under the warm (44°C) and cool (30°C) conditions. This case was contributed by Drs. John Jakimetz and Kevin O'Flaherty of Manhattan Audiological Services, New York.

els, consistent with the absence of left-ear retrocochlear pathology (see Chapter 3). The left contralateral acoustic-reflex decay results were negative with respect to retro-cochlear pathology (see Chapter 3).

The left BAEP results, obtained at 105 dBpeSPL, reveal normal absolute and interpeak latencies, consistent with normal auditory nervous system function on the left side to the level of the lateral lemniscus (see Chapter 7). The right BAEP results, obtained at 120 dBpeSPL, reveal a prolonged absolute latency of wave V and a prolonged I–V interpeak latency, consistent with right retrocochlear pathology. Interestingly, in contrast with the BAEPs for Cases 1 and 2, wave I is present. The presence of wave I in this case may be related to the relatively low hearing-threshold levels at

2000 and 8000 Hz compared with the high hearing-threshold levels at these frequencies in Cases 1 and 2. The ENG results revealed normal saccadic tracings, normal gaze results, normal optokinetic results, normal positional tracings, normal pendular tracking, and normal caloric findings, bilaterally (see Chapter 8). CAT scan revealed a 1-cm right intracanicular acoustic tumor confirmed surgically.

In this case, the BAEP and ARC results revealed true-positive findings whereas false-negative ENG results were obtained. Similar to Case 2, if the modified P_5 protocol had been employed, the patient would have been referred directly for the definitive medical test after the ARC test, obviating the need for BAEP and ENG testing.

D. CASE 4

Case 4 is a female in her early 30s who was in a car accident which resulted in right-sided hemiplegia. As a result of the accident, this patient was in a coma for 10 days. This patient reported left-ear tinnitus, difficulty hearing in the left ear, distortion in the quality of speech in the left ear, some left-ear fullness and pressure, all of which subsided after 1 year following the accident.

Figure 8A shows the pure-tone air-conduction thresholds, SRTs, suprathreshold speech-recognition scores, left-ear PI–PB function results, static-acoustic middle-ear admittance, tympanograms, contralateral acoustic-reflex thresholds, and the results of contralateral acoustic-reflex decay testing. Figure 8B shows the summary of the BAEP peak and interpeak latencies. Figure 8C illustrates the single-channel recordings of BAEPs elicited with rarefaction clicks presented at repetition rates of 15.2/s and 55.2/s at 60 and 80 dB HL. In Figure 8D, the rapidly alternating speech perception (Willeford) scores, binaural-fusion (Willeford) scores, SSW scores under the competing condition, dichotic-digits (Musiek, 1983), competing-sentences (Willeford) scores, and monaural low-pass filtered-speech test (Willeford) scores.

Although the bone-conduction thresholds are not shown, the pure-tone air-conduction thresholds are consistent with normal hearing-threshold levels in the low–mid and high frequencies, bilaterally (see Chapter 2). The SRT corroborates the three-frequency pure-tone average, bilaterally (see Chapter 2). The right- and left-ear suprathreshold speech-recognition scores do not exceed the Thornton and Raffin (1978) 95% critical-differences limits (see Chapter 5). The rollover index for the left ear is 0, which is negative with respect to retrocochlear pathology on the left side (see Chapter 5).

The tympanometric and static-acoustic middle-ear admittance results were consistent with normal middle-ear function, bilaterally (see chapter 3). The right contralateral acoustic-reflex threshold levels did not exceed the Silman and Gelfand (1981) 90th percentiles, consistent with the absence of retrocochlear pathology on the right side (see chapter 3). The left contralateral acoustic reflexes were absent for all tonal activators and therefore exceeded the Silman and Gelfand (1981) 90th percentiles, consistent with left retrocochlear pathology on the right side (see Chapter 3). The left contralateral acoustic reflexes were absent for all tonal activators and therefore exceeded the Silman and Gelfand (1981) 90th percentiles, consistent with left retrocochlear pathology (see Chapter 3). The right contralateral acoustic-reflex decay results were negative at 500 Hz but borderline (50% decay) at 1000 Hz (see Chapter 3).

The RASP score was reduced, consistent with brainstem dysfunction (see Chapter 6). The binaural-fusion score was normal, consistent with normal brainstem function (see

Chapter 6). The SSW score in the competing condition was normal for the right ear and reduced for the left ear, consistent with a brainstem or cortical dysfunction (laterality unknown) (see Chapter 6). The dichotic-digits scores were reduced, bilaterally, with a greater reduction for the left ear, consistent with brainstem or cortical dysfunction (laterality unknown) (see Chapter 6). The competing-sentences score was depressed maximally in the left ear and was within normal limits in the right ear, consistent with brainstem or cortical dysfunction (see Chapter 6). The low-pass filtered-speech scores were markedly reduced for the left ear and within normal limits for the right ear, consistent with a cortical lesion on the right side (contralateral-ear effect) or a brainstem lesion (laterality unknown) (see Chapter 6).

The BAEPs for the right ear revealed normal peak and interpeak latencies, consistent with normal right auditory nervous system function to the level of the lateral lemniscus (see Chapter 7). The BAEPs for the left ear at 80 dB HL reveal distorted waveform morphology for waves after peak III compared with the BAEPs for the right ear. Note that no responses are present in the left ear at 60 dB HL, despite the presence of normal hearing in that ear, in contrast with the clearly defined BAEP for the right ear at that intensity. These left-ear BAEPs are consistent with left high-brainstem pathology (see Chapter 7). Neurologic follow-up revealed left pontine contusion, particularly in the mid pons region.

The absent left contralateral acoustic reflexes combined with the normal waves I–III of the BAEPs from the left suggest that the damage is in the low pons rostral to the cochlear nuclei, in the vicinity of the acoustic-reflex arc, on the left side. The borderline right contralateral acoustic-reflex decay represents a false-positive finding. In this case, all of the central auditory test results, except for the binaural-fusion test, were true-positive ones; left-ear deficits were apparent.

E. CASE 5

Case 5 is a right-handed, 59-year-old female.

The pure-tone air-conduction thresholds, SRTs, and suprathreshold speech-recognition scores are shown in Figure 9A. The rapidly alternating speech perception score (Willeford), binaural-fusion (Willeford) score, corrected SSW scores under the competing condition, dichotic-digits scores (Musiek, 1983), competing-sentences (Willeford) scores, and low-pass filtered-speech (Willeford) scores are shown in Figure 9B.

Although the bone-conduction thresholds are not shown, the air-conduction thresholds are consistent with essentially normal hearing-threshold levels in the low–mid and high frequencies, bilaterally. The SRT corroborates the three-frequency pure-tone average, bilaterally (see Chapter 2). The right and left suprathreshold speech-recognition scores

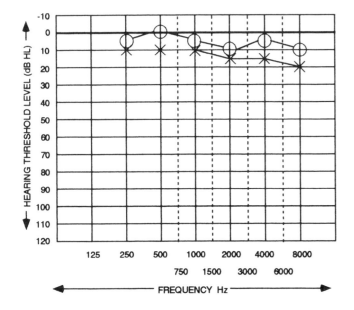

LEGEND

		Right (Solid)	Left (Dashed)
Air	Unmasked		
	Unmasked NR		
	Masked		
	Masked NR		
	Soundfield		
	Soundfield NR		
Mastoid Bone:	Unmasked		
	Unmasked NR		
	Masked		
	Masked NR		
Forehead Bone:	Unmasked		
	Unmasked NR		
	Masked		
	Masked NR		

Response consistency: good moderate poor

Validity: acceptable questionable

PURE TONE AVERAGE (500–2000 Hz) in dB			
	Right	Left	Best din. avg.
Two freq.			
Three freq.	5	12	

	UNAIDED				UNAIDED			
	Right	HL	Left	HL	Right	HL	Left	HL
SAT		dB		dB		dB		dB
SRT	5	dB	5	dB		dB		dB
WORD RECOG	100 % at 35	dB	88 % at 35	dB	% at	dB	% at	dB
	% at	dB	88 % at 85	dB	% at	dB	% at	dB
	% at	dB	% at	dB	% at	dB	% at	dB
	% at	dB	% at	dB	% at	dB	% at	dB
MCL		dB		dB		dB		dB
UCL		dB		dB		dB		dB
MATERIALS								

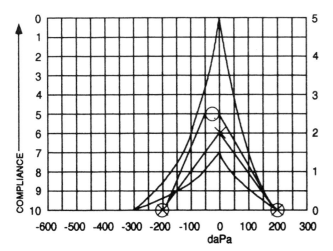

ACOUSTIC REFLEX

STIMULUS RIGHT   (CONTRALATERAL)   STIMULUS LEFT

% decay in 10 sec	THRESHOLD dB SL	THRESHOLD dB HL	Hz	THRESHOLD dB HL	THRESHOLD dB SL	% decay in 10 sec
neg		90	500	Abs		
neg		90	1000	Abs		
		85	2000	Abs		
			4000			

(IPSILATERAL)

			500			
			1000			
			2000			

STATIC COMPLIANCE $C = C_2 - C_1$

RIGHT			LEFT		
C_2	C_1	2.0 C	C_2	C_1	1.3 C

Figure 8 Audiologic findings of a female in her early 30s. (A) *Top*, pure-tone air-conduction thresholds, bilaterally. *Middle*, SRTs and suprathreshold PB word-recognition scores, bilaterally. *Bottom*, Tympanograms (*left side*) and the contralateral acoustic-reflex thresholds, bilaterally, right contralateral acoustic-reflex decay results, and static-acoustic middle-ear admittance, bilaterally (*right side*).

PEAK AND INTERPEAK LATENCY (ms)

AD

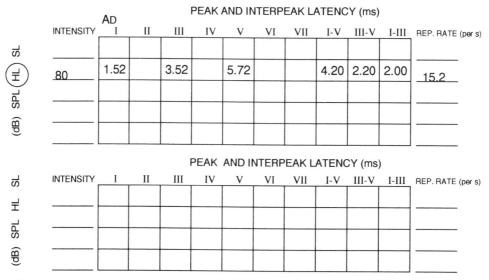

INTENSITY	I	II	III	IV	V	VI	VII	I-V	III-V	I-III	REP. RATE (per s)
80	1.52		3.52		5.72			4.20	2.20	2.00	15.2

PEAK AND INTERPEAK LATENCY (ms)

INTENSITY	I	II	III	IV	V	VI	VII	I-V	III-V	I-III	REP. RATE (per s)

Figure 8 (continued) (B) Absolute and interpeak BAEP latencies for rarefaction clicks presented at a repetition rate of 15.2/s for the right ear.

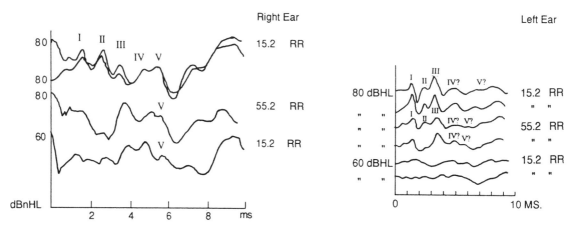

Figure 8 (continued) (C) *Left,* Right ear. Single-channel test–retest BAEP tracings at 80 dBnHL at a repetition rate of 15.2/s, the test BAEP tracings at 80 dB nHL at a repetition rate of 55.2/s, and the test BAEP tracings at 60 dBnHL at a repetition rate of 15.2/s. *Right,* Left ear. Single-channel test--retest BAEP tracings at 80 dBnHL at a repetition rate of 15.2/s, at 80 dBnHL at a repetition rate of 55.2/s, and at 60 dBnHL at a repetition rate of 15.2/s. (The right side of Figure 8C is reprinted from Musiek & Geurkink, 1982, with permission.)

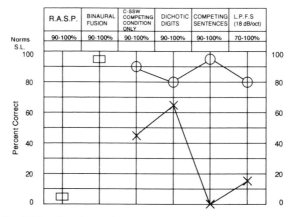

Figure 8 (continued) (D) Results of central auditory testing (RASP, binaural-fusion test, SSW-corrected score under the competing condition, dichotic-digits test, competing-sentences test, and low-pass filtered-speech test). This case was contributed by Dr. Frank E. Musiek of the Hitchcock Clinic, Hanover, New Hampshire.

A

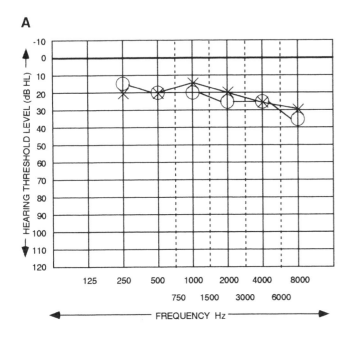

LEGEND

		Right (Solid)	Left (Dashed)
Air	Unmasked		
	Unmasked NR		
	Masked		
	Masked NR		
	Soundfield		
	Soundfield NR		
Mastoid Bone:	Unmasked		
	Unmasked NR		
	Masked		
	Masked NR		
Forehead Bone:	Unmasked		
	Unmasked NR		
	Masked		
	Masked NR		

Response consistency: good moderate poor

Validity: acceptable questionable

PURE TONE AVERAGE (500-2000 Hz) in dB			
	Right	Left	Best din. avg.
Two freq.			
Three freq.	22	18	

	UNAIDED				UNAIDED			
	Right	HL	Left	HL	Right	HL	Left	HL
SAT		dB		dB		dB		dB
SRT	15	dB	17	dB		dB		dB
WORD RECOG	90 % at 45	dB	90 % at 47	dB	% at	dB	% at	dB
	% at	dB	% at	dB	% at	dB	% at	dB
	% at	dB	% at	dB	% at	dB	% at	dB
	% at	dB	% at	dB	% at	dB	% at	dB
MCL		dB		dB		dB		dB
UCL		dB		dB		dB		dB
MATERIALS								

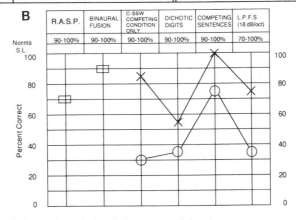

Figure 9 Audiologic findings of a right-handed, 59-year-old female. (A) *Top,* Pure-tone air-conduction thresholds, bilaterally. *Bottom,* SRTs and suprathreshold PB speech-recognition scores, bilaterally. (B) Results of central auditory testing (RASP, binaural-fusion test, SSW-corrected score under the competing condition, dichotic-digits test, competing-sentences test, and low-pass filtered-speech test). This case was contributed by Dr. Frank E. Musiek of the Hitchcock Clinic, Hanover, New Hampshire.

do not exceed the Thornton and Raffin (1978) 95% critical-differences limits (see Chapter 5).

The RASP score is reduced, consistent with brainstem dysfunction (see Chapter 6). The binaural-fusion test score was within normal limits (see Chapter 6). The SSW scores under the competing condition were abnormal, bilaterally with a greater depression in the right ear, consistent with brainstem or cortical dysfunction (laterality unknown) (see Chapter 6). The dichotic-digits scores are reduced, bilaterally, consistent with a cortical or brainstem lesion (laterality unknown) (see Chapter 6). The competing-sentences score is normal for the left ear but abnormal for the right ear, consistent with a brainstem or cortical lesion (laterality unknown) (see Chapter 6). The low-pass filtered-speech scores were normal for the left ear and abnormal for the right ear, consistent with a cortical or brainstem lesion (laterality unknown) (see Chapter 6). Neurologic follow-up revealed a left temporal-lobe tumor.

Note that the RASP results were consistent with a brainstem rather than temporal-lobe lesion. Note that contralateral-ear effects were present for all the central auditory tests, consistent with the classical concept of contralateral-ear effects in cases of cortical lesions (see Chapter 6). Also note that the ipsilateral-ear score was slightly depressed in the SSW test, consistent with the classical concept of slight ipsilateral-ear effects in cases of cortical lesions (see Chapter 6).

F. CASE 6

Case 6 is a 39-year-old female. The patient complained of difficulty hearing in noise after head trauma in a car accident.

The pure-tone air- and bone-conduction thresholds, SRTs, and suprathreshold speech-recognition scores are shown in Figure 10A. Figure 10B shows the corrected SSW scores under the competing condition, dichotic-digits scores, competing-sentences (Willeford) scores, and low-pass filtered-speech (Willeford) scores.

The pure-tone air- and bone-conduction thresholds are consistent with normal hearing-thresholds levels in the low–mid and high frequencies, bilaterally (see Chapter 2). The SRT corroborates the three-frequency pure-tone average, in the left ear and the two-frequency pure-tone average in the right ear (see Chapter 2). The right and left speech-recognition scores do not exceed the Thornton and Raffin (1978) 95% critical-differences limits (see Chapter 5).

The SSW score is abnormal for the left ear and normal for the right ear, consistent with brainstem or cortical dysfunction (laterality unknown) (see Chapter 6). The dichotic-digits score is also abnormal for the left ear and within normal limits for the right ear, consistent with a brainstem or cortical dysfunction (laterality unknown) (see Chapter 6). The competing-sentences scores are normal, bilaterally

consistent with normal cortical function (see Chapter 6). The low-pass filtered-speech score is normal, bilaterally consistent with normal cortical function (see Chapter 6). Neurologic follow-up revealed the presence of a right temporal-lobe hematoma.

Note that abnormal scores were obtained for the left ear on both the dichotic-digits and SSW tests; these results, under the classical concept, are consistent with a cortical lesion on the contralateral (right) side (see Chapter 6). Also note that the contralateral-ear effect seen in this case is less marked than that seen in Case 5, consistent with the classical concept that left temporal-lobe lesions have greater contralateral-ear effects than right temporal-lobe lesions (see Chapter 6). Although Cases 5 and 6 both had temporal-lobe lesions, the competing-sentences and low-pass filtered-speech test results were normal in Case 6 but abnormal in Case 5, underscoring the conclusion in Chapter 6 that the site, magnitude, and etiology of the lesion may account for the inconsistent findings reported for central lesions in the literature for a given central auditory test. Although one might conclude, based on Cases 5 and 6, that a battery of central auditory tests is needed to detect central auditory pathology, the reader is cautioned that a battery of tests increases the false-positive rate compared with a single test.

G. CASE 7

Case 7 is a right-handed 71-year-old male with ataxia who was referred from neurology.

The pure-tone air- and bone-conduction thresholds, SRTs, and suprathreshold speech-recognition scores are shown in Figure 11A. The BAEPs for rarefaction clicks presented at 80 dB HL at a repetition rate of 15.7/s are shown in Figure 11B. Figure 11C shows the summary BAEP peak and interpeak latencies. Illustrated in Figure 11D are the rapidly alternating speech perception (Willeford) score, SSW scores in the competing condition, time-compressed (60%) NU-6s, dichotic-digits (Musiek, 1983), and competing-sentences (Willeford) scores.

The pure-tone air- and bone-conduction thresholds are consistent with normal hearing threshold levels through 2000 Hz with a moderate sensorineural hearing impairment at 4000 Hz, bilaterally. The SRT corroborates the three-frequency pure-tone average in the right ear and two-frequency pure-tone average in the left ear (see Chapter 2). The right and left suprathreshold speech-recognition scores do not exceed the Thornton and Raffin (1978) 95% critical-differences limits (see Chapter 5).

Inspection of the BAEPs reveals normal waveform morphology for the right ear and distorted waveform morphology for the left ear. Note that only wave I is clearly present in the left ear. These results are consistent with normal right auditory nervous system function to the level of the lateral

A

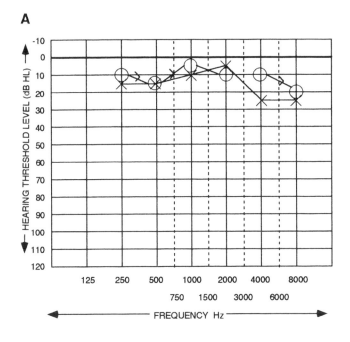

LEGEND

		Right (Solid)	Left (Dashed)
Air	Unmasked Unmasked NR Masked Masked NR Soundfield Soundfield NR		
Mastoid Bone:	Unmasked Unmasked NR Masked Masked NR		
Forehead Bone:	Unmasked Unmasked NR Masked Masked NR		

Response consistency: good moderate poor

Validity: acceptable questionable

PURE TONE AVERAGE (500-2000 Hz) in dB			
	Right	Left	Best din. avg.
Two freq.	8	8	
Three freq.	10	10	

	UNAIDED				UNAIDED			
	Right	HL	Left	HL	Right	HL	Left	HL
SAT		dB		dB		dB		dB
SRT	8	dB	10	dB		dB		dB
WORD RECOG	100 % at 43	dB	96 % at 45	dB	% at	dB	% at	dB
	% at	dB	% at	dB	% at	dB	% at	dB
	% at	dB	% at	dB	% at	dB	% at	dB
	% at	dB	% at	dB	% at	dB	% at	dB
MCL		dB		dB		dB		dB
UCL		dB		dB		dB		dB
MATERIALS								

B

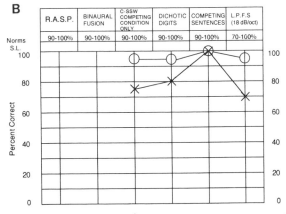

	R.A.S.P.	BINAURAL FUSION	C-SSW COMPETING CONDITION ONLY	DICHOTIC DIGITS	COMPETING SENTENCES	L.P.F.S (18 dB/oct)
Norms S.L.	90-100%	90-100%	90-100%	90-100%	90-100%	70-100%

Figure 10 Audiologic results of a 39-year-old female. (A) *Top,* Pure-tone air- and bone-conduction thresholds, bilaterally. *Bottom,* SRTs and suprathreshold PB word-recognition scores, bilaterally. (B) Results of central auditory testing (SSW-corrected score under the competing condition, dichotic-digits test, competing-sentences test, and low-pass filtered-speech test). This case was contributed by Dr. Frank E. Musiek of the Hitchcock Clinic, Hanover, New Hampshire.

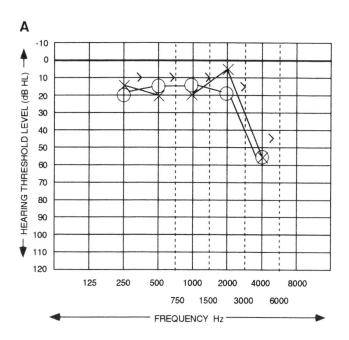

A

LEGEND

		Right (Solid)	Left (Dashed)
Air	Unmasked Unmasked NR Masked Masked NR Soundfield Soundfield NR		
Mastoid Bone:	Unmasked Unmasked NR Masked Masked NR		
Forehead Bone:	Unmasked Unmasked NR Masked Masked NR		

Response consistency: good moderate poor

Validity: acceptable questionable

PURE TONE AVERAGE (500-2000 Hz) in dB			
	Right	Left	Best din. avg.
Two freq.	15	13	
Three freq.	17	15	

	UNAIDED				UNAIDED			
	Right	HL	Left	HL	Right	HL	Left	HL
SAT		dB		dB		dB		dB
SRT	20	dB	16	dB		dB		dB
WORD RECOG	92 % at 55	dB	100 % at 51	dB	% at	dB	% at	dB
	% at	dB	% at	dB	% at	dB	% at	dB
	% at	dB	% at	dB	% at	dB	% at	dB
	% at	dB	% at	dB	% at	dB	% at	dB
MCL		dB		dB		dB		dB
UCL		dB		dB		dB		dB
MATERIALS								

Figure 11 Audiologic findings of a right-handed 71-year-old male. (A) *Top*, pure-tone air- and bone-conduction thresholds, bilaterally. *Bottom*, SRTs and suprathreshold PB word-recognition scores, bilaterally.

B   Right Ear

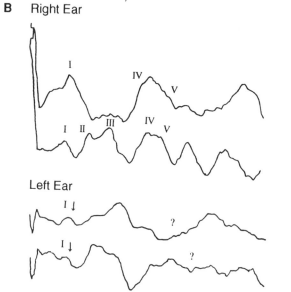

Figure 11 (continued) (B) Test–retest single-channel BAEP tracings for clicks presented at 80 dBnHL at a repetition rate of 15.7/s for the right ear (*top*) and left ear (*bottom*).

C

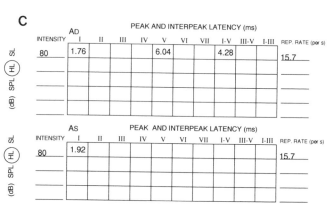

Figure 11 (continued) (C) *Top*, Absolute peak and interpeak BAEP latencies for the right ear. *Bottom*, Absolute BAEP wave I latency for the left ear.

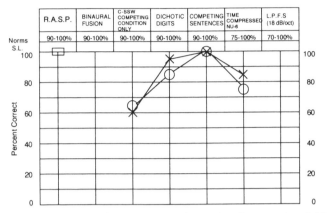

Figure 11 (continued) (D) Results of central auditory testing (RASP, SSW-corrected score under the competing condition, dichotic-digits test, competing-sentences test, and time-compressed NU-6 test). This case was contributed by Dr. Frank E. Musiek of the Hitchcock Clinic, Hanover, New Hampshire.

lemniscus and abnormal left brainstem function (see Chapter 7).

The rapidly alternating speech perception score is within normal limits, consistent with normal brainstem function (see Chapter 6). The SSW scores are bilaterally reduced, consistent with brainstem or cortical dysfunction (laterality unknown) (see Chapter 6). The dichotic-digits score is normal for the left ear but slightly abnormal for the right ear, consistent with brainstem or cortical dysfunction (laterality unknown) (see Chapter 6). The competing-sentences scores are within normal limits consistent with normal cortical function (see Chapter 6). The time-compressed speech score is within normal limits bilaterally. Neurologic follow-up revealed a large tumor in the left thalamus (upper brainstem) and left hemisphere of the cerebellum.

In contrast with Case 4 (left brainstem pathology), the RASP score was normal rather than abnormal, the SSW scores were reduced bilaterally rather than unilaterally, and the competing-sentences scores were normal rather than abnormal unilaterally. This case also shows the variability in central test scores for a given site of pathology. On the other hand, the BAEP results for Cases 4 and 7 correctly revealed the site and laterality of the brainstem lesion.

H. CASE 8

Case 8 is a 28-year-old female with vertigo and "buzzing" tinnitus in the right ear of 4 months duration.

The pure-tone air-conduction thresholds, SRTs, PB (NU-6) and SSI (0 MCR) speech-recognition scores, static-acoustic middle-ear admittance, tympanograms, contralateral acoustic-reflex thresholds, and the results of contralateral acoustic-reflex decay testing are shown in Figure

12A. Figure 12B shows the contralateral acoustic-reflex decay tracings. Figure 12C shows the Carhart, Olsen–Noffsinger, and STAT tone-decay results and the Bekesy comfortable-loudness results. Figures 12D and 12E show the Bekesy comfortable-loudness tracings. Figure 12F shows the single-channel BAEP recordings obtained for alternating clicks presented at 85 dBnHL at a repetition rate of 21.1/s. Figure 12G illustrates the summary BAEP peak and interpeak latencies. Figures 12H–J shows the ENG (horizontal channel) results. Figure 12K shows the summary of the ENG results.

The pure-tone air-conduction thresholds are consistent with normal-hearing thresholds in the low-mid and high frequencies, bilaterally. The SRT corroborates the three-frequency pure-tone average, bilaterally (see Chapter 2).

The static-acoustic middle-ear admittance and tympanometric results were consistent with normal middle-ear function, bilaterally. The right contralateral acoustic-reflex thresholds exceed the Silman and Gelfand (1981) 90th percentile levels at 500 Hz, consistent with right retrocochlear pathology (see Chapter 3). The left contralateral acoustic-reflex threshold levels do not exceed the Silman and Gelfand 90th percentile levels at any activating frequency and are consistent with the absence of left retrocochlear pathology (see Chapter 3). The right contralateral acoustic-reflex decay results are positive for the right ear at 1000 Hz but negative at 500 Hz; note that at least 50% decay occurs within the first 5 s at 1000 Hz (see Chapter 3). The left contralateral acoustic-reflex decay results are negative at 500 and 1000 Hz (see Chapter 3).

The rollover index is 0.6 (positive) for the SSI for the right ear, consistent with right retrocochlear pathology (see Chapter 5). The NU-6 rollover index, on the other hand, was negative (0.17). No rollover in SSI or NU-6 scores was present for the left ear, consistent with the absence of left retrocochlear pathology (see Chapter 5).

The results of STAT tone-decay testing are positive for the right ear at all frequencies, consistent with right retrocochlear pathology, and negative at 500 and 4000 Hz in the left ear, consistent with the absence of left retrocochlear pathology (see Chapter 5). Similarly, positive results were obtained for the Olsen–Noffsinger tone-decay test at all frequencies in the right ear and negative results were obtained at all frequencies in the left ear (see Chapter 5). Carhart tone-decay testing (with the starting level modified to be 20 dB SL) revealed, in the right ear, 85 dB of tone decay at 500 Hz, 25 dB of tone decay at 1000 Hz, and more than 80 dB of tone decay at 2000 Hz, also consistent with right retrocochlear pathology (see Chapter 5). Note that all of the tone-decay tests revealed similar findings.

In the right ear, a Type P1 Bekesy comfortable-loudness tracing was obtained, consistent with right retrocochlear pathology (see Chapter 5). In the left ear, a Type N1 Bekesy

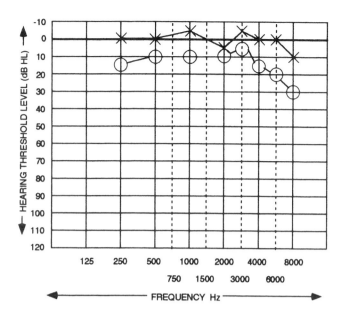

PURE TONE AVERAGE (500-2000 Hz) in dB			
	Right	Left	Best din. avg.
Two freq.			
Three freq.	10	0	

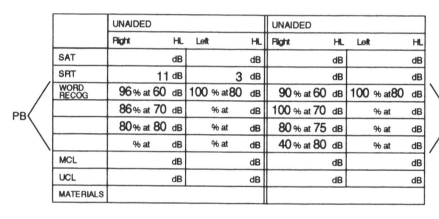

	UNAIDED				UNAIDED			
	Right	HL	Left	HL	Right	HL	Left	HL
SAT		dB		dB		dB		dB
SRT	11	dB	3	dB		dB		dB
WORD RECOG	96 % at 60	dB	100 % at 80	dB	90 % at 60	dB	100 % at 80	dB
	86 % at 70	dB	% at	dB	100 % at 70	dB	% at	dB
	80 % at 80	dB	% at	dB	80 % at 75	dB	% at	dB
	% at	dB	% at	dB	40 % at 80	dB	% at	dB
MCL		dB		dB		dB		dB
UCL		dB		dB		dB		dB
MATERIALS								

PB ⟨ ... ⟩ SSI

ACOUSTIC REFLEX

STIMULUS RIGHT (CONTRALATERAL) STIMULUS LEFT

% decay in 10 sec	THRESHOLD dB		Hz	THRESHOLD dB		% decay in 10 sec
	SL	HL		HL	SL	
neg		105	500	85		neg
pos		100	1000	90		neg
		100	2000	90		
			4000			

(IPSILATERAL)

			500			
			1000			
			2000			

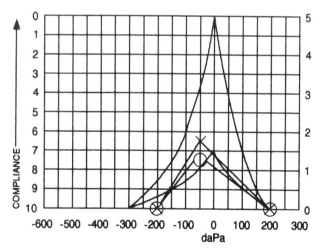

STATIC COMPLIANCE $C = C_2 - C_1$

RIGHT			LEFT		
C_2	C_1	0.35 C	C_2	C_1	0.55 C

Figure 12 Audiologic findings for a 28-year-old female. (A) *Top*, Right and left pure-tone air-conduction thresholds. *Middle*, SRTs and SSI and suprathreshold PB-word speech-recognition scores, bilaterally. *Bottom*, Tympanograms, bilaterally (*left side*) and the contralateral acoustic-reflex threshold and decay results and static-acoustic middle-ear admittance, bilaterally (*right side*).

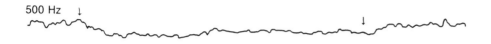

Left Crossed Acoustic Reflex Decay at 10 dB above the ART

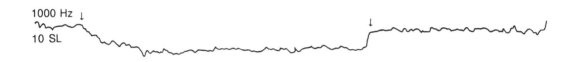

500 Hz

1000 Hz

10 SL

Right Crossed Acoustic Reflex Decay at 10 dB above the ART

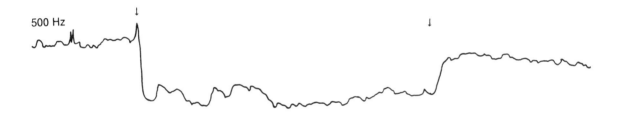

500 Hz

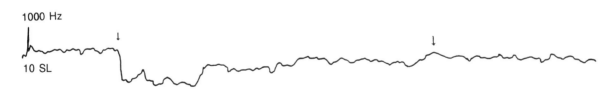

1000 Hz

10 SL

Figure 12 (continued) (B) Contralateral acoustic-reflex decay tracings at 500 and 1000 Hz for the left ear (*top*) and right ear (*bottom*).

TONE DECAY ((Carhart) STAT) Rosenberg-Circle One)   (Olsen-Noffsinger)

		Right								Left					
		250	500	1K	2K	4K	8K		250	500	1K	2K	4K	8K
Carhart	Decay (dB)		85	25	80+									
O-N	Decay (dB)		>10	>10	>10						0	0	0	
STAT	Decay (dB)		POS	POS	POS	POS				NEG	DNT	DNT	NEG	

TONE DECAY (Owens Test)

Ear	Freq.	SL dB	Decay in Seconds
		5	
		10	
		15	
		20	

Ear	Freq.	SL dB	Decay in Seconds
		5	
		10	
		15	
		20	

Ear	Freq.	SL dB	Decay in Seconds
		5	
		10	
		15	
		20	

LOUDNESS BALANCE (ABLB-MLB-CIRCLE ONE)

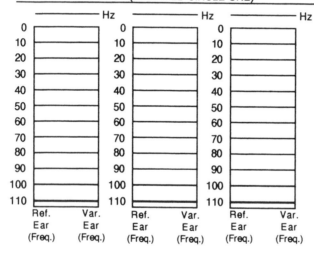

BEKESY SUMMARY Comfortable Loudness
Right Ear:

Type P1

Left Ear:

Type N1

SISI (Standard-High Level-Circle One)

	Right							Left					
	250	500	1K	2K	4K	8K		250	500	1K	2K	4K	8K
% Correct													
Presentation Level (dB SL)													
dB Masking													

Figure 12 (continued) (C) *Top*, Carhart, Olsen–Noffsinger, and STAT tone-decay results at 500, 1000, and 2000 Hz. *Middle*, Classification of the Bekesy Comfortable Loudness tracings.

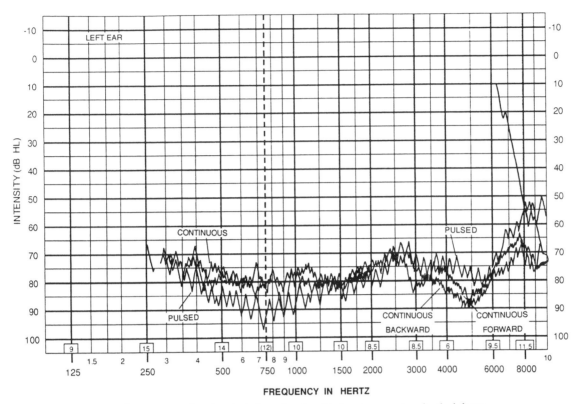

Figure 12 (continued) (D) Bekesy Comfortable Loudness tracings for the left ear.

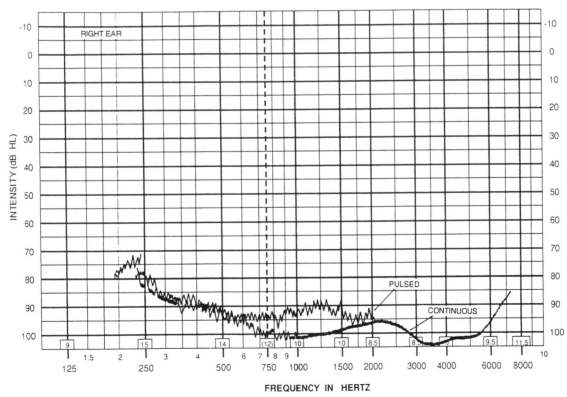

Figure 12 (continued) (E) Bekesy Comfortable Loudness tracings for the right ear.

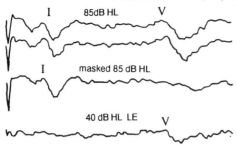

RIGHT EAR

CROSSOVER TO LE (delayed)

I   85dB HL   V

I   masked 85 dB HL

40 dB HL LE   V

LEFT EAR

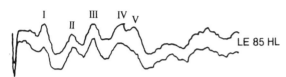

I   III   IV V
II

LE 85 HL

Figure 12 (continued) (F) Single-channel BAEP recordings obtained for alternating clicks presented at 85 dBnHL at a repetition rate of 21.1/s for the right ear (*top*) and left ear (*bottom*).

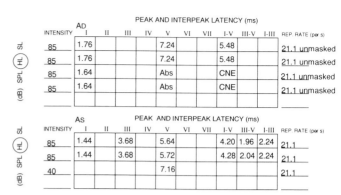

	AD							PEAK AND INTERPEAK LATENCY (ms)				
INTENSITY	I	II	III	IV	V	VI	VII	I-V	III-V	I-III	REP. RATE (per s)
85	1.76				7.24			5.48			21.1 unmasked
85	1.76				7.24			5.48			21.1 unmasked
85	1.64				Abs			CNE			21.1 unmasked
85	1.64				Abs			CNE			21.1 unmasked

SL (dB) SPL (HL)

	AS							PEAK AND INTERPEAK LATENCY (ms)				
INTENSITY	I	II	III	IV	V	VI	VII	I-V	III-V	I-III	REP. RATE (per s)
85	1.44		3.68		5.64			4.20	1.96	2.24	21.1
85	1.44		3.68		5.72			4.28	2.04	2.24	21.1
40					7.16						21.1

SL (dB) SPL (HL)

Figure 12 (continued) (G) Summary of the BAEP peak and interpeak latencies for the right ear (*top*) in the masked and unmasked conditions and for the left ear (*bottom*).

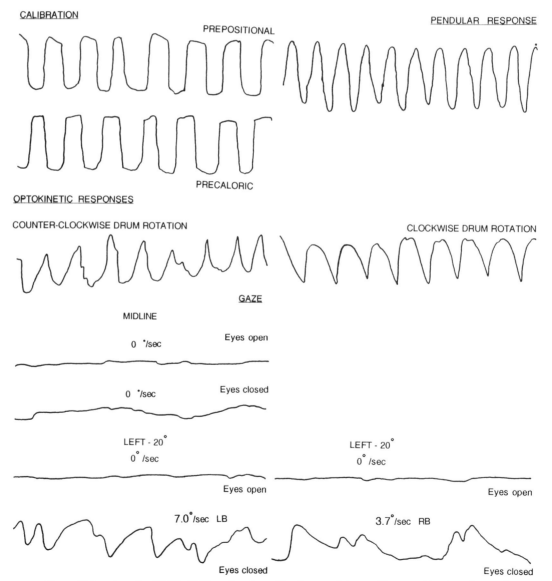

CALIBRATION

PREPOSITIONAL

PENDULAR RESPONSE

PRECALORIC

OPTOKINETIC RESPONSES

COUNTER-CLOCKWISE DRUM ROTATION

CLOCKWISE DRUM ROTATION

GAZE

MIDLINE

0 °/sec   Eyes open

0 °/sec   Eyes closed

LEFT - 20°
0° /sec

LEFT - 20°
0° /sec

Eyes open

Eyes open

7.0°/sec LB

3.7°/sec RB

Eyes closed

Eyes closed

Figure 12 (continued) (H) The ENG tracings for calibration, pendular tracking, optokinetic testing, and 20° and midline gaze testing.

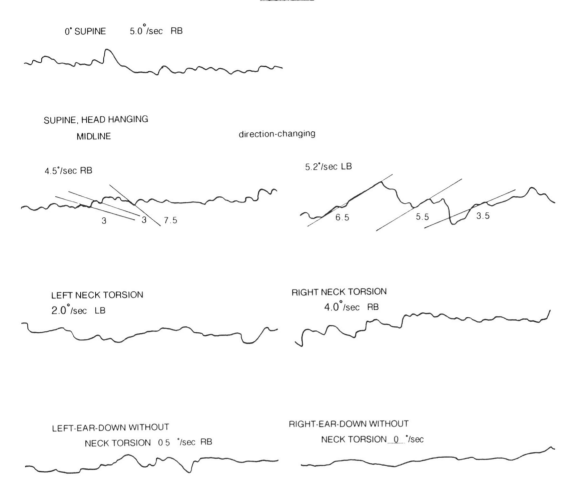

POSITIONAL

0° SUPINE   5.0°/sec RB

SUPINE, HEAD HANGING

MIDLINE   direction-changing

4.5°/sec RB   5.2°/sec LB

3   3   7.5   6.5   5.5   3.5

LEFT NECK TORSION   RIGHT NECK TORSION
2.0°/sec LB   4.0°/sec RB

LEFT-EAR-DOWN WITHOUT   RIGHT-EAR-DOWN WITHOUT
NECK TORSION 0.5 °/sec RB   NECK TORSION 0 °/sec

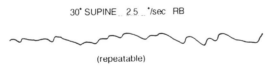

30° SUPINE 2.5 °/sec RB

(repeatable)

Figure 12 (continued) (I) The ENG tracings for positional testing (0° supine, head-hanging, left neck, right neck, left body, right body, and 30° supine).

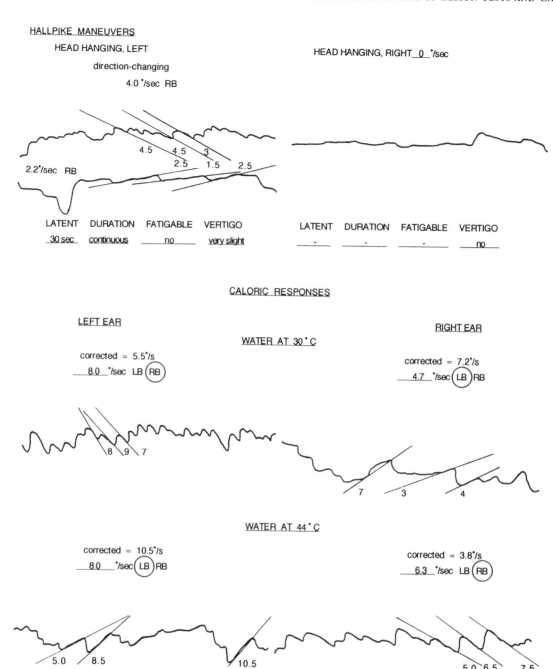

Figure 12 (continued)   (J) The ENG tracings for the Dix–Hallpike maneuver and caloric testing.

ELECTRONYSTAGMOGRAPHY

CALIBRATION SACCADES
NORMAL_____√_____

DYSMETRIC_____

TRACKING RESPONSE
SINUSOIDAL___√___

OTHER_____

SPONTANEOUS, 30° SUPINE
_____2.5_____ °/s LB (RB)

OPTOKINETIC RESPONSES
SYMMETRIC___grossly___

ASYMMETRIC_____

POSITIONAL
LEFT LATERAL___0.5___ °/s LB (RB)

RIGHT LATERAL___0___ °/s LB (RB)

HEAD HANGING RB 4.5 LB 5.2 °/s LB RB

MIDLINE *Direction changing*
0° Supine=5.0°/s RB
Left neck 2.0°/s LB
Right neck 5.0°/s RB

GAZE
MIDLINE_____0_____ °/s LB RB

LEFT_____0_____ °/s LB RB

RIGHT_____0_____ °/s LB RB

HALLPIKE MANEUVERS
HEAD HANGING, LEFT___4.0___ / 2.2°/s LB °/s LB (RB)

HEAD HANGING, RIGHT___0___ °/s LB RB

LATENT DURATION FATIGABLE VERTIGO
30 sec   continuous   no   very slight
—   —   —   *no*

CALORIC RESPONSES
LEFT: °C___5.5___ °/s LB (RB)

°C___10.5___ °/s (LB) RB

°C___DNT___ °/s LB RB

RIGHT: 30°C___7.2___ °/s (LB) RB

44°C___3.8___ °/s LB (RB)

0°C___DNT___ °/s LB RB

_____ LEFT   ___√___ RIGHT

___√___ LEFT   _____ RIGHT

___√___ PRESENT   _____ ABSENT

REDUCED VESTIBULAR RESPONSE:___19___%
Corrected for 30° supine

DIRECTIONAL PREPONDERANCE:___31___%
Corrected for 30° supine

OCULAR FIXATION SUPPRESSION:

COMMENTS: *no meds/alcohol prior to testing*

Figure 12 (continued) (K) The summary of the ENG results. This case was contributed by Dr. Daniel Schwartz and Kristine Olson of the Hospital of the University of Pennsylvania, Philadelphia.

comfortable-loudness tracing was obtained, consistent with the absence of left retrocochlear pathology (see Chapter 5).

The results of BAEP testing at 85 dBnHL reveal normal absolute and interpeak latencies and normal waveform morphology for the left ear, consistent with a normal left auditory nervous system to the level of the lateral lemniscus (see Chapter 7). In the right ear, unmasked and masked BAEP recordings were obtained at 85 dBnHL. Note that when masking was added, wave V disappears, leaving only wave I in the right ear, suggesting that the presence of wave V in the unmasked recording reflects crossover to the left ear. This assumption is substantiated by the waveform morphology and wave V latency in the left-ear BAEP recording at 40 dB HL (expected crossover level). These results underscore the importance of masking during BAEP testing. The right-ear BAEP results, showing absence of waves II–V, are consistent with right retrocochlear pathology somewhere between the auditory nerve and lateral lemniscus (see Chapter 7).

Saccadic tracking was normal, consistent with a normal saccadic system (see Chapter 8). Sinusoidal tracking was also normal, consistent with a normal pursuit system (see

Chapter 8). Spontaneous nystagmus was absent in the eyes-open and eyes-closed conditions (see Chapter 8). Optokinetic nystagmus was symmetrical, consistent with a normal optokinetic pathway (see Chapter 8). Although gaze nystagmus exceeding 6°/s was present, the nystagmus occurred only with the eyes closed and was present in both directions; although this can occur in normal persons, this finding is abnormal since it is not an isolated abnormal finding in the ENG (Barber & Stockwell, 1980). During positional testing, nystagmus was present in the right and left neck torsion but not in the right and left whole body positions, indicating that the nystagmus was elicited by neck torsion rather than by position (see Chapter 8). Persistent nystagmus was present in the 0° supine, 30° supine, and head-hanging positions, consistent with pathological nonlocalizing vestibular pathology (see Chapter 8). Direction-changing nystagmus in a single position (head-hanging) was present, consistent with central nervous system disorder (see Chapter 8). The response elicited with the Dix–Hallpike maneuver was similar in magnitude and direction to the positional response during the head-hanging position. Therefore, the response during the Dix–Hallpike maneuver may be a positional rather than paroxysmal nystagmus.

The results of caloric testing reveal the absence of significant unilateral weakness. Directional preponderance was left-beating and significant although the significance of directional preponderance is controversial (see Chapter 8). Fixation suppression was present. The clearly abnormal findings on this ENG were the positional nystagmus (nonlocalizing finding) and the direction-changing nystagmus in a single position (consistent with central nervous system disorder).

A surgically-confirmed right acoustic neuroma was present.

Although the classical site-of-lesion tests (tone decay, PI–SSI, Bekesy comfortable-loudness, and ENG) yielded true positive findings, the positive finding on the ARC test indicates that if the modified P_5 protocol (mentioned earlier in this chapter) were used, the patient would have been appropriately referred for the definitive medical test. The consistency among the classical site-of-lesion tests (including ENG, ARC, and BAEP tests) supports the theory of the presence of a positive correlation among audiologic tests mentioned earlier in this chapter.

I. CASE 9

Case 9 is a 19-year-old male college student who complained only of interaural difference in the quality of sound under headphones (e.g., SONY Walkman); the right-ear quality was worse than the left-ear quality.

Figure 13A shows the air- and bone-conduction threshold levels, performance-intensity functions for the NU-6 and SSI materials, static-acoustic middle-ear admittance,

tympanograms, contralateral acoustic-reflex thresholds, and contralateral acoustic-reflex decay results. Figure 13B shows the contralateral acoustic-reflex decay tracings. Figure 13C shows the high-level SISI results, the Carhart, Olsen–Noffsinger, and STAT tone-decay results, and the conventional Bekesy results.

Figures 13D and 13E show the Bekesy sweep-frequency tracings. Figure 13F shows the single-channel BAEP recordings obtained for alternating clicks presented at 85 dBnHL (and at 95 dBnHL in the right ear) at a repetition rate of 21.1/s. Figure 13G shows the summary of the BAEP peak and interpeak latencies. Figures 13H–J show the ENG tracings. Figure 13K shows the summary ENG results.

The pure-tone air-conduction thresholds are consistent with the presence of a mild sensorineural hearing impairment in the low–mid frequencies and normal hearing-threshold levels at the high frequencies in the right ear (see Chapter 2). In the left ear, the pure-tone air-conduction thresholds are consistent with normal hearing-threshold levels at the low–mid and high frequencies (see Chapter 2).

The rollover index was positive (0.59 for the NU-6 and 0.55 for the SSI) in the right ear, consistent with right retrocochlear pathology (see Chapter 5). No rollover was present for the left ear for either speech material, consistent with the absence of left retrocochlear pathology (see Chapter 5).

The contralateral acoustic-reflex thresholds for the right ear exceed the Silman and Gelfand (1981) 90th percentile levels at all activating frequencies, consistent with the presence of right retrocochlear pathology (see Chapter 3). The left contralateral acoustic-reflex thresholds do not exceed the Silman and Gelfand (1981) 90th percentile levels at any activating frequency, consistent with the absence of left retrocochlear pathology (see Chapter 3). The contralateral acoustic-reflex decay results were positive for the right ear at 500 Hz and negative at 500 and 1000 Hz for the left ear.

The high-level (75 dB HL) SISI results are positive at 4000 Hz for the right ear and negative for the left ear (see Chapter 5). The Olsen–Noffsinger tone-decay results are positive for the right ear and negative for the left ear. Carhart tone-decay testing (starting level modified to 20 dB SL) revealed positive tone decay of at least 35 dB at all frequencies in the right ear. On the other hand, negative STAT results were obtained bilaterally.

The sweep-frequency Bekesy pattern was Type II, consistent with cochlear pathology, for the right ear and Type I, consistent with normal hearing-threshold levels, for the left ear (see Chapter 5).

The BAEP results reveal normal peak and interpeak latencies, and normal waveform morphology in the left ear; thus, negative results were obtained for the left ear (see Chapter 7). The BAEPs were absent at 85 and 95 dB HL in the right ear, positive for pathology in the right auditory nervous system somewhere between the auditory nerve and lateral lemniscus (see Chapter 7).

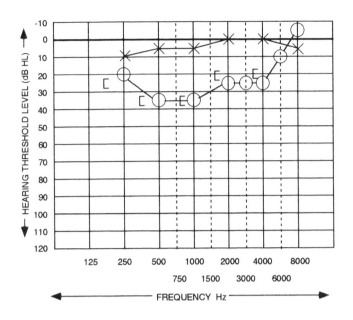

LEGEND

		Right (Solid)	Left (Dashed)
Air	Unmasked		
	Unmasked NR		
	Masked		
	Masked NR		
	Soundfield		
	Soundfield NR		
Mastoid Bone:	Unmasked		
	Unmasked NR		
	Masked		
	Masked NR		
Forehead Bone:	Unmasked		
	Unmasked NR		
	Masked		
	Masked NR		

Response consistency: good moderate poor

Validity: acceptable questionable

PURE TONE AVERAGE (500-2000 Hz) in dB			
	Right	Left	Best din. avg.
Two freq.	30	3	
Three freq.	32	3	

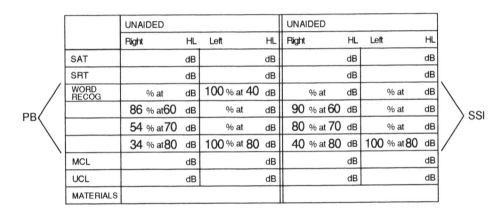

	UNAIDED				UNAIDED			
	Right	HL	Left	HL	Right	HL	Left	HL
SAT		dB		dB		dB		dB
SRT		dB		dB		dB		dB
WORD RECOG	% at	dB	100 % at 40	dB	% at	dB	% at	dB
	86 % at 60	dB	% at	dB	90 % at 60	dB	% at	dB
	54 % at 70	dB	% at	dB	80 % at 70	dB	% at	dB
	34 % at 80	dB	100 % at 80	dB	40 % at 80	dB	100 % at 80	dB
MCL		dB		dB		dB		dB
UCL		dB		dB		dB		dB
MATERIALS								

PB — SSI

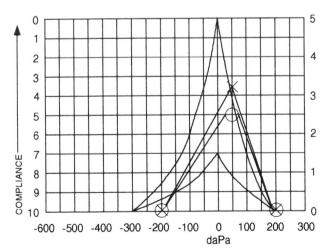

ACOUSTIC REFLEX

(CONTRALATERAL)

STIMULUS RIGHT				STIMULUS LEFT		
% decay in 10 sec	THRESHOLD dB SL	THRESHOLD dB HL	Hz	THRESHOLD dB HL	SL	% decay in 10 sec
pos		115	500	95		neg
DNT		120	1000	100		neg
		120 ?	2000	95		
			4000			

(IPSILATERAL)

		500		
		1000		
		2000		

STATIC COMPLIANCE $C = C_2 - C_1$

RIGHT			LEFT		
C_2	C_1	0.8 C	C_2	C_1	0.7 C

Figure 13 Audiologic results for a 19-year-old male college student. (A) *Top*, The pure-tone air- and bone-conduction thresholds, bilaterally. *Middle*, The PB and SSI suprathreshold speech-recognition scores, bilaterally. *Bottom*, The tympanograms, bilaterally (*left side*) and the contralateral acoustic-reflex thresholds and decay results and static-acoustic middle-ear admittance, bilaterally (*right side*).

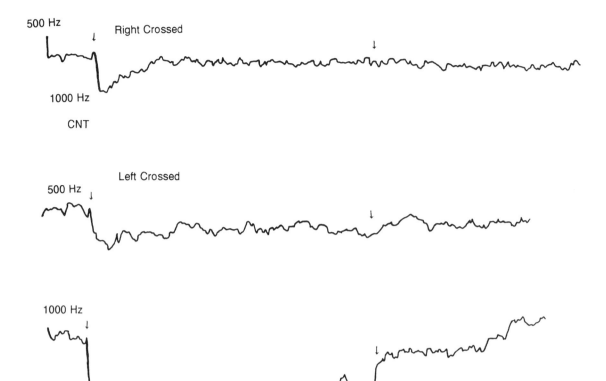

Figure 13 (continued)   (B) The contralateral acoustic-reflex decay results at 500 and 1000 Hz for the right ear (*top*) and left ear (*bottom*).

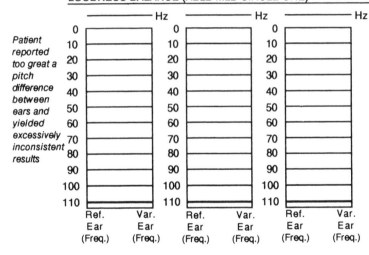

TONE DECAY ((Carhart) STAT Rosenberg-Circle One) (Olsen-Noffsinger)

		Right 250	500	1K	2K	4K	8K		Left 250	500	1K	2K	4K	8K
Carhart	Decay (dB)		55	65	65					DNT	DNT	DNT		
O-N	Decay (dB)		10+	10+	10+					0	0	0		
STAT	Decay (dB)		NEG	NEG	NEG					NEG	NEG	NEG		

TONE DECAY (Owens Test)

Ear	Freq.	SL dB	Decay in Seconds
		5	
		10	
		15	
		20	

Ear	Freq.	SL dB	Decay in Seconds
		5	
		10	
		15	
		20	

Ear	Freq.	SL dB	Decay in Seconds
		5	
		10	
		15	
		20	

LOUDNESS BALANCE (ABLB-MLB-CIRCLE ONE)

Patient reported too great a pitch difference between ears and yielded excessively inconsistent results

BEKESY SUMMARY **Conventional**

Right Ear:

Type II

Left Ear:

Type I

SISI (Standard-High Level) Circle One)

	Right 250	500	1K	2K	4K	8K		Left 250	500	1K	2K	4K	8K
% Correct					60							100	
Presentation Level (dB SL)					75							75	
dB Masking													

Figure 13 (continued) (C) The Carhart, Olsen–Noffsinger, and STAT tone-decay results for the right ear and the Olsen–Noffsinger and STAT tone-decay results for the left ear at 500, 1000, and 2000 Hz (*top*), classification of the conventional Bekesy sweep-frequency tracings, bilaterally (*middle*), and SISI scores (high-level presentation) at 4000 Hz (*bottom*), bilaterally.

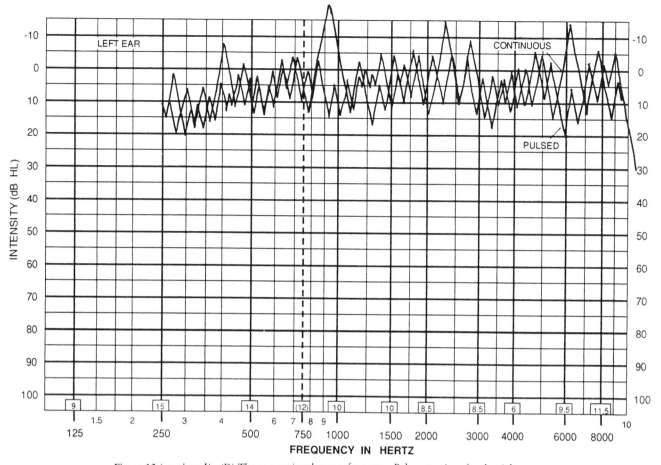

Figure 13 (continued) (D) The conventional sweep-frequency Bekesy tracings for the right ear.

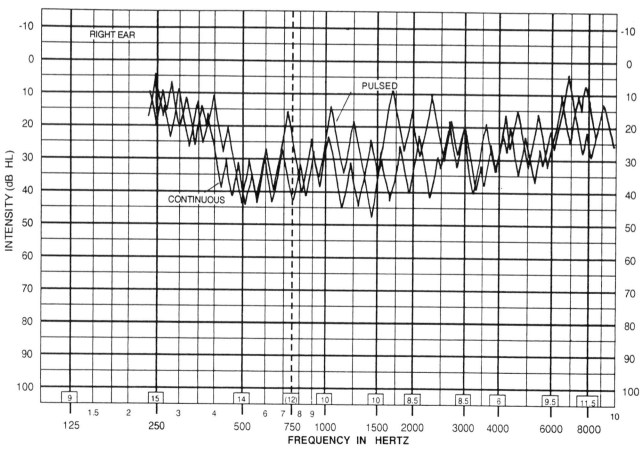

Figure 13 (continued) (E) The conventional sweep-frequency Bekesy tracings for the left ear.

Left Ear

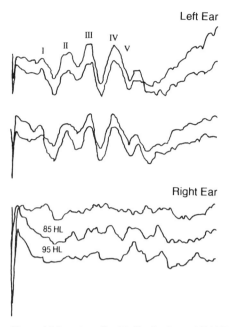

Right Ear

85 HL

95 HL

PEAK AND INTERPEAK LATENCY (ms)

AD

INTENSITY	I	II	III	IV	V	VI	VII	I-V	III-V	I-III	REP. RATE (per s)
85											21.1
95											21.1
				No Response							

SL / SPL (HL) (dB)

PEAK AND INTERPEAK LATENCY (ms)

AS

INTENSITY	I	II	III	IV	V	VI	VII	I-V	III-V	I-III	REP. RATE (per s)
85	1.48		3.84		5.40			3.92	1.56	2.36	21.1
	1.48		3.92		5.40			3.92	1.48	2.44	21.1

SL / SPL (HL) (dB)

Figure 13 (continued) (G) Summary of the BAEP peak and interpeak latencies, bilaterally.

Figure 13 (continued) (F) Single-channel BAEP recordings obtained for alternating clicks presented at 85dBnHL in the left ear (*top*) and at 85 and 95 dBnHL in the right ear (*bottom*) at a repetition rate of 21.1/s; a baseline recording in the absence of stimulation for the right ear is also shown.

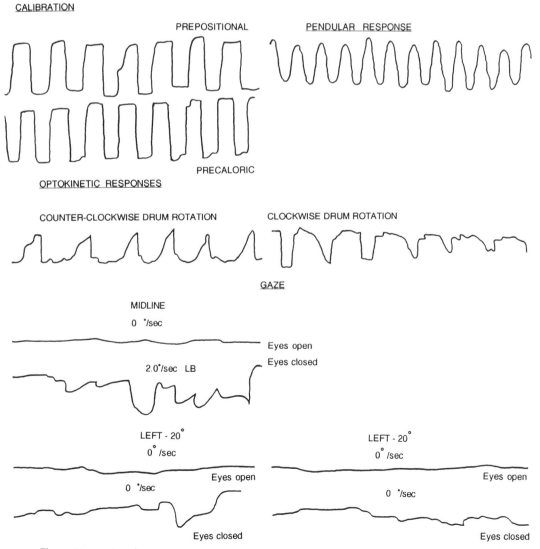

Figure 13 (continued) (H) ENG tracings for calibration, pendular tracking, optokinetic testing, and midline and 20° gaze.

379

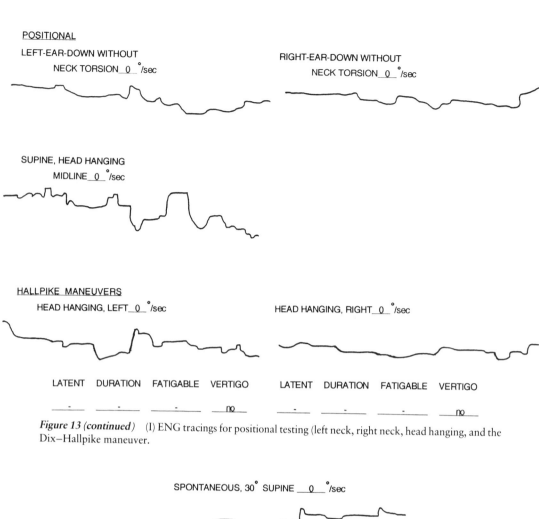

POSITIONAL

LEFT-EAR-DOWN WITHOUT NECK TORSION _0_ °/sec

RIGHT-EAR-DOWN WITHOUT NECK TORSION _0_ °/sec

SUPINE, HEAD HANGING MIDLINE _0_ °/sec

HALLPIKE MANEUVERS

HEAD HANGING, LEFT _0_ °/sec

HEAD HANGING, RIGHT _0_ °/sec

LATENT	DURATION	FATIGABLE	VERTIGO		LATENT	DURATION	FATIGABLE	VERTIGO
-	-	-	no		-	-	-	no

Figure 13 (continued) (I) ENG tracings for positional testing (left neck, right neck, head hanging, and the Dix–Hallpike maneuver.

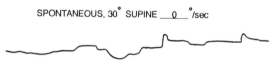

SPONTANEOUS, 30° SUPINE ___0___ °/sec

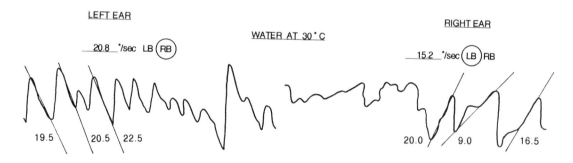

CALORIC RESPONSES

LEFT EAR

WATER AT 30°C

RIGHT EAR

_20.8_ °/sec LB (RB)

_15.2_ °/sec (LB) RB

19.5   20.5   22.5

20.0   9.0   16.5

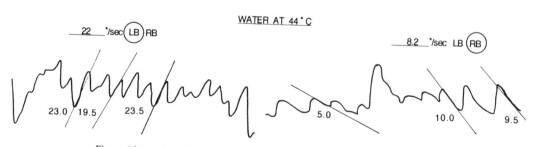

WATER AT 44°C

_22_ °/sec (LB) RB

_8.2_ °/sec LB (RB)

23.0 19.5 23.5

5.0   10.0   9.5

Figure 13 (continued) (J) ENG tracings for 30° supine and caloric testing.

ELECTRONYSTAGMOGRAPHY RESULTS

<u>CALIBRATION SACCADES</u>

NORMAL _____√_____

DYSMETRIC_____

<u>TRACKING RESPONSE</u>

SINUSOIDAL __√__

OTHER _____

<u>SPONTANEOUS, 30° SUPINE</u>

_____0_____°/s LB RB

<u>OPTOKINETIC RESPONSES</u>

SYMMETRIC_____√_____

ASYMMETRIC_____

<u>POSITIONAL</u>

LEFT LATERAL_____0_____°/s LB RB

RIGHT LATERAL_____0_____°/s LB RB

HEAD HANGING_____0_____°/s LB RB

<u>GAZE</u>   *eyes closed 2.0°/s LB*

MIDLINE_____0_____°/s LB RB

LEFT_____0_____°/s LB RB

RIGHT_____0_____°/s LB RB

<u>HALLPIKE MANEUVERS</u>

HEAD HANGING, LEFT____0____°/s LB RB

HEAD HANGING, RIGHT ___0____°/s LB RB

LATENT DURATION FATIGABLE VERTIGO

___—___ ____—____ ____—____ ___*no*___

__—__ ___—___ ___—___ ___*no*___

<u>CALORIC RESPONSES</u>

LEFT: 30°C___20.8___°/s LB (RB)

44°C___20.0___°/s (LB) RB

0°C___*DNT*___°/s LB RB

RIGHT: 30°C___15.2___°/s (LB) RB

44°C___8.2___°/s LB (RB)

0°C___*DNT*___°/s LB RB

REDUCED VESTIBULAR RESPONSE: _-29.3_ %   _____ LEFT   ___√___ RIGHT

DIRECTIONAL PREPONDERANCE: _-12.4_ %   ___√___ LEFT   _____ RIGHT

OCULAR FIXATION SUPPRESSION: __√__ PRESENT   _____ ABSENT

COMMENTS:

Figure 13 (continued)   (K) Summary of the ENG results. This case was contributed by Dr. Daniel Schwartz and Kristine Olson of the Hospital of the University of Pennsylvania, Philadelphia.

Saccadic tracking was normal, consistent with a normal saccadic system (see Chapter 8). Sinusoidal tracing was normal, consistent with a normal pursuit system (see Chapter 8). Spontaneous nystagmus was absent. Symmetrical optokinetic responses were obtained, consistent with a normal optokinetic system (see Chapter 8). The results of gaze, positional, and Dix–Hallpike maneuvers were also negative. The results of caloric testing revealed right unilateral weakness, consistent with right peripheral vestibular pathology (vestibular end organ or nerve). Significant directional preponderance was absent and there was no failure of fixation suppression.

The patient had a surgically confirmed right acoustic tumor. The following tests yielded true-positive findings for the right ear: performance intensity functions for the SSI and NU-6 materials, contralateral acoustic-reflex threshold

and decay, high-level SISI, Olsen–Noffsinger and Carhart tone-decay testing, BAEP testing, and ENG. Although the ENG test was positive, it failed to differentiate between vestibular end-organ and vestibular nerve pathology. Interestingly, unlike Case 8 who complained of vertigo and had normal caloric findings, this patient did not complain of vertigo (or even tinnitus), yet had unilateral weakness. Negative findings were obtained on the Bekesy and STAT tone-decay tests. This case illustrates the higher sensitivity of the Carhart and Olsen-Noffsinger tone-decay tests compared with the STAT test. As for Case 8, if the modified P_5 protocol had been employed for Case 9, this patient would have been referred directly for the definitive medical test after the positive ARC findings were obtained, obviating the need for the classical site-of-lesion and even the BAEP test.

J. CASE 10

Case 10 is a 24-year-old female with a 5-year history of right-ear tinnitus, progressive hearing impairment in the right ear, and momentary positional dizziness on quick turning.

Figure 14A shows the pure-tone air- and bone-conduction thresholds, SRTs, suprathreshold speech-recognition scores for monosyllabic PB words at a signal-to-noise ratio of +10 dB, performance-intensity function for the SSI (0 MCR), static-acoustic middle-ear admittance, and contralateral and ipsilateral acoustic-reflex thresholds. Figure 14B shows the admittance tympanograms (220-Hz probe tone). Figure 14C shows the interpretation of the conventional Bekesy test results. Figures 14D and 14E show the sweep-frequency conventional Bekesy tracings. Figures 14F and 14G show the single-channel recordings for the BAEPs elicited using rarefaction and condensation clicks in the left ear and rarefaction clicks in the right ear, with a repetition rate of 8/s at 115 dB SPL. Figure 14H shows the summary of the BAEP peak and interpeak latencies. Figure 14I shows the caloric ENG tracings.

The pure-tone air- and bone-conduction thresholds are consistent with normal hearing-threshold levels in the low-mid and high frequencies in the left ear (see Chapter 2). In the right ear, the pure-tone air- and bone-conduction thresholds are consistent with normal hearing-thresholds in the low-mid frequencies and a moderately severe sensorineural hearing impairment in the high frequencies (see Chapter 2). The SRT corroborates the three-frequency pure-tone average in the left ear and the two-frequency pure-tone average in the right ear (see Chapter 2). The speech-recognition scores for the right and left ears did not exceed the Thornton and Raffin (1978) 95% critical-differences limits. The SSI rollover index was negative, bilaterally (0.1 for the right ear and 0 for the left ear) (see Chapter 5).

The admittance-pressure function and static-acoustic middle-ear admittance were consistent with normal middle-ear function, bilaterally (see Chapter 3). The contralateral acoustic-reflex thresholds exceed the Silman and Gelfand 90th percentile levels for the right ear at all activating frequencies and for the left ear at 500 and 1000 but not 2000 Hz (see Chapter 3). The ipsilateral reflex thresholds are positive for the right ear and negative for the left ear (see Chapter 3).

The Bekesy tracings reveal a Type II pattern for the right ear, consistent with a right cochlear pathology, and a Type I pattern for the left ear, consistent with normal hearing thresholds (see Chapter 5).

The BAEP waveform and peak and interpeak latencies (compared with the clinic normative limits) are normal for the left ear (see Chapter 7). The right BAEP is absent, consistent with right auditory nervous system pathology

somewhere between the auditory nerve and lateral lemniscus.

Although not shown, the gaze and positional test results were within normal limits and spontaneous nystagmus was absent. The caloric tracings were normal, consistent with a normal vestibular system.

The patient had a very large right cerebellopontine angle tumor with extension both anteriorly and superiorly toward the tentorial notch. The tumor originated in the cerebellopontine angle outside the internal auditory meatus.

True positive results were obtained on the right and left contralateral and right ipsilateral acoustic-reflex thresholds and BAEPs. False-negative findings were obtained on the suprathreshold speech-recognition scores (with reference to the 95% critical-differences limits), PI–SSI, conventional Bekesy, and ENG tests. In contrast to Cases 8 and 9, the rollover on the SSI was negative in this case of retrocochlear pathology. This case also illustrates that the classical site-of-lesion tests have a lower sensitivity than the acoustic-reflex and BAEP tests. It is hypothesized that the elevated left acoustic-reflex thresholds reflect tumor pressure in the vicinity of the right facial nuclei. If the modified P_5 protocol mentioned earlier in this chapter had been employed, the patient would have been referred for the definitive medical test after the positive acoustic-reflex threshold findings.

K. CASE 11

Case 11 is a 47-year-old male who attributed his hearing difficulty to noise exposure.

Figure 15A shows the pure-tone air- and bone-conduction thresholds, SRTs, performance-intensity functions for PI–PB words (based on 50 items per level), static-acoustic middle-ear admittance, tympanograms (220-Hz probe tone), contralateral acoustic-reflex thresholds, and contralateral acoustic-reflex decay results. Figure 15B shows the ABLB laddergrams at 500, 1000, and 2000 Hz, Olsen–Noffsinger tone-decay results at 500, 1000, and 2000 Hz, and standard SISI scores at 500, 1000, and 2000 Hz.

The pure-tone air- and bone-conduction thresholds are consistent with a moderate sensorineural hearing impairment in the low–mid frequencies and a severe sensorineural hearing impairment in the high frequencies in the right ear. In the left ear, the pure-tone air- and bone-conduction thresholds are consistent with normal hearing-threshold levels in the low–mid frequencies and a mild sensorineural hearing impairment in the high frequencies (see Chapter 2). The SRT corroborates the pure-tone average, bilaterally (see Chapter 2). The suprathreshold speech-recognition scores for the right and left ears at 30 dB SL exceeded the 95% critical-differences limits, consistent with right retrocochlear pathology. Because of this significant difference in suprathreshold speech-recognition scores between ears, PI–PB functions were obtained (see Chapter 5). The roll-

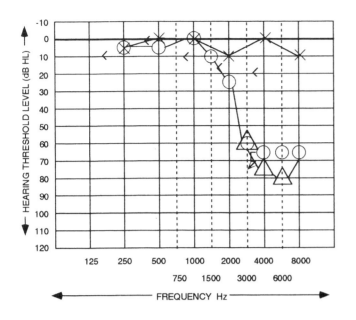

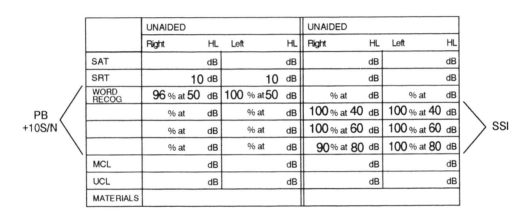

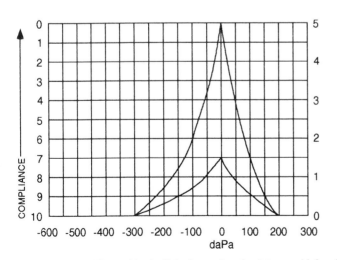

Figure 14 Audiologic results of a 24-year-old female. (A) *Top*, pure-tone air- and bone-conduction thresholds, bilaterally. *Middle*, SRTs and PB (+10 S/N ratio) and SSI suprathreshold speech-recognition scores, bilaterally. *Bottom*, Contralateral and ipsilateral acoustic-reflex decay results and static acoustic middle-ear admittance (*right side*), bilaterally.

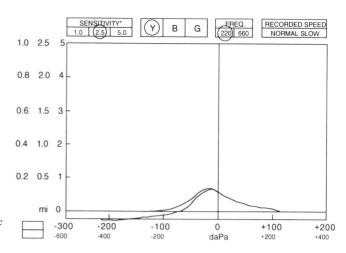

Figure 14 (continued) (B) Admittance tympanograms (220-Hz probe tone), bilaterally.

TONE DECAY (Carhart-STAT-Rosenberg-Circle One)

	Right								Left					
	250	500	1K	2K	4K	8K			250	500	1K	2K	4K	8K
Decay (dB)														
Decay (dB)														
Decay (dB)														

TONE DECAY (Owens Test)

Ear	Freq.	SL dB	Decay in Seconds
		5	
		10	
		15	
		20	

Ear	Freq.	SL dB	Decay in Seconds
		5	
		10	
		15	
		20	

Ear	Freq.	SL dB	Decay in Seconds
		5	
		10	
		15	
		20	

LOUDNESS BALANCE (ABLB-MLB-CIRCLE ONE)

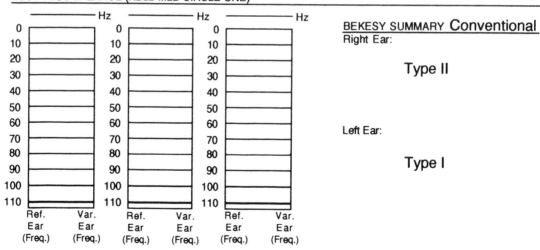

BEKESY SUMMARY Conventional

Right Ear:

Type II

Left Ear:

Type I

SISI (Standard-High Level-Circle One)

	Right								Left					
	250	500	1K	2K	4K	8K			250	500	1K	2K	4K	8K
% Correct														
Presentation Level (dB-SL)														
dB Masking														

Figure 14 (continued) (C) Classification of the conventional sweep-frequency Bekesy tracings (*middle*).

384

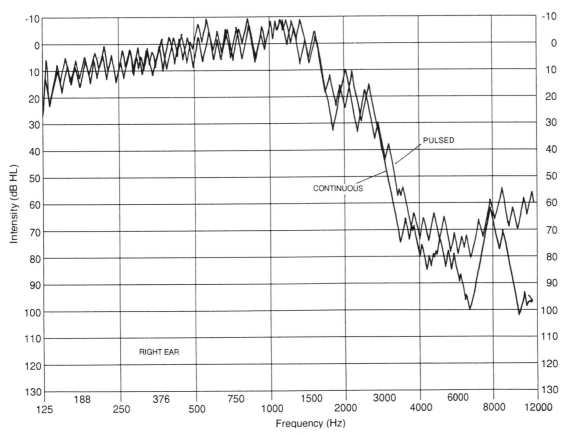

Figure 14 (continued) (D) Conventional sweep-frequency Bekesy tracings for the right ear.

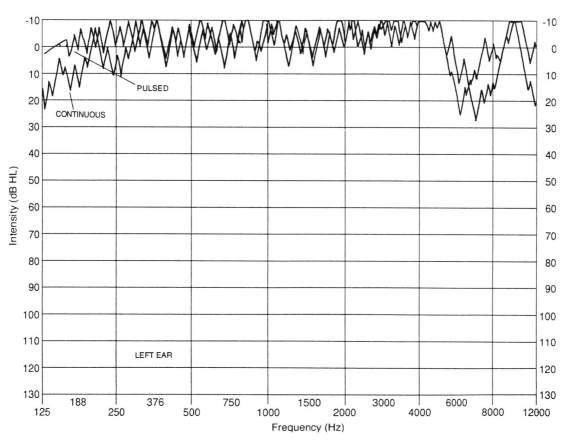

Figure 14 (continued) (E) Conventional sweep-frequency Bekesy tracings for the left ear.

385

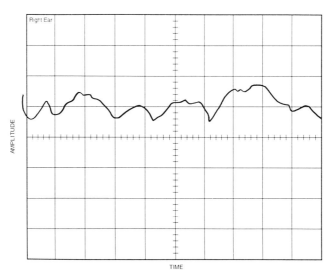

Figure 14 (continued) (F) Single-channel BAEP recording obtained for rarefaction clicks at a repetition rate of 8/s and at 115 dBpeSPL in the right ear.

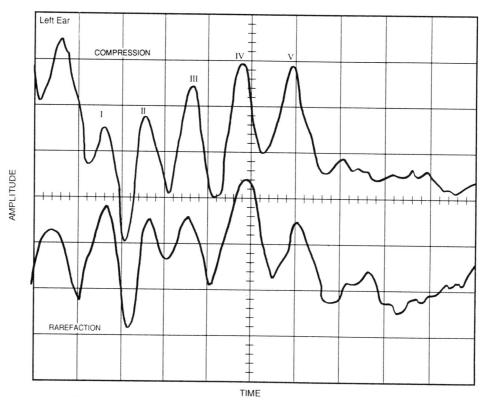

Figure 14 (continued) (G) Single-channel BAEP recordings for compression and rarefaction clicks presented at a repetition rate of 8/s and at 115 dBpeSPL in the left ear.

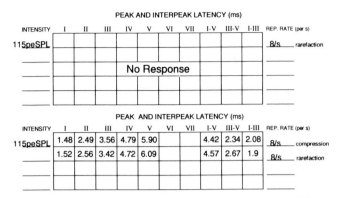

PEAK AND INTERPEAK LATENCY (ms)

INTENSITY	I	II	III	IV	V	VI	VII	I-V	III-V	I-III	REP. RATE (per s)	
115peSPL											8/s	rarefaction
				No Response								

PEAK AND INTERPEAK LATENCY (ms)

INTENSITY	I	II	III	IV	V	VI	VII	I-V	III-V	I-III	REP. RATE (per s)	
115peSPL	1.48	2.49	3.56	4.79	5.90			4.42	2.34	2.08	8/s	compression
	1.52	2.56	3.42	4.72	6.09			4.57	2.67	1.9	8/s	rarefaction

Figure 14 (continued) (H) Summary of the BAEP peak and interpeak latencies.

CALORIC TESTING

RIGHT COLD   LEFT COLD

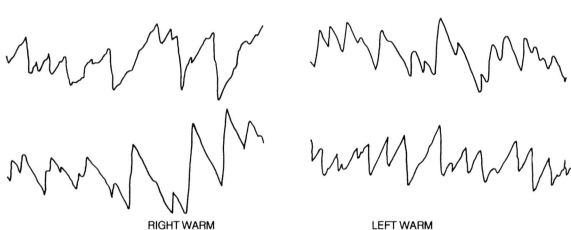

RIGHT WARM   LEFT WARM

Figure 14 (continued) (I) Caloric tracings. This case was contributed by Dr. F. Roohi of the Neurology Department and Dr. D. L. Kisiel of the Otolaryngology Department of Long Island College Hospital, Brooklyn, New York.

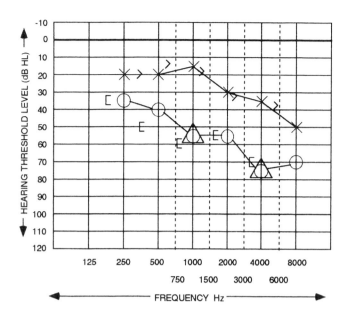

		Right (Solid)	Left (Dashed)
Air	Unmasked		
	Unmasked NR		
	Masked		
	Masked NR		
	Soundfield		
	Soundfield NR		
Mastoid Bone:	Unmasked		
	Unmasked NR		
	Masked		
	Masked NR		
Forehead Bone:	Unmasked		
	Unmasked NR		
	Masked		
	Masked NR		

Response consistency: good moderate poor

Validity: acceptable questionable

PURE TONE AVERAGE (500-2000 Hz) in dB			
	Right	Left	Best din. avg.
Two freq.	48	18	
Three freq.	50	22	

	UNAIDED				UNAIDED			
	Right	HL	Left	HL	Right	HL	Left	HL
SAT		dB		dB		dB		dB
SRT	55	dB	20	dB		dB		dB
WORD RECOG	72 % at 85	dB	90 % at 50	dB	% at	dB	% at	dB
	16 % at 95	dB	96 % at 60	dB	% at	dB	% at	dB
	0 % at 105	dB	92 % at 70	dB	% at	dB	% at	dB
	% at	dB	% at	dB	% at	dB	% at	dB
MCL		dB		dB		dB		dB
UCL		dB		dB		dB		dB
MATERIALS								

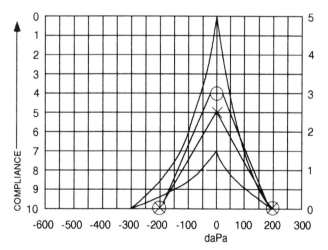

ACOUSTIC REFLEX

(CONTRALATERAL)

STIMULUS RIGHT   STIMULUS LEFT

% decay in 10 sec	THRESHOLD dB		Hz	THRESHOLD dB		% decay in 10 sec
	SL	HL		HL	SL	
pos		100	500	90		neg
neg		115	1000	95		neg
		Abs	2000	100		
			4000			

(IPSILATERAL)

			500			
			1000			
			2000			

STATIC COMPLIANCE $C = C_2 - C_1$

RIGHT			LEFT		
C_2	C_1	1.0 C	C_2	C_1	1.0 C

Figure 15 Audiologic findings for a 47-year-old male. (A) (*Top,*) Right and left pure-tone air- and bone-conduction thresholds. *Middle,* SRTs and suprathreshold speech-recognition scores for PB words, bilaterally. *Bottom,* Tympanograms, bilaterally (*left side*) and the contralateral acoustic-reflex threshold and decay results and static-acoustic middle-ear admittance, bilaterally (*right side*).

TONE DECAY (Carhart-STAT-Rosenberg-Circle One) (Olsen-Noffsinger)

		Right								Left				
	250	500	1K	2K	4K	8K		250	500	1K	2K	4K	8K
Decay (dB)		0	0	10+					0	0	0		
Decay (dB)													
Decay (dB)													

TONE DECAY (Owens Test)

Ear	Freq.	SL dB	Decay in Seconds		Ear	Freq.	SL dB	Decay in Seconds		Ear	Freq.	SL dB	Decay in Seconds
		5					5					5	
		10					10					10	
		15					15					15	
		20					20					20	

LOUDNESS BALANCE (ABLB-MLB-CIRCLE ONE)

BEKESY SUMMARY
Right Ear:

Bekesy

Left Ear:

Bekesy

SISI (Standard) High Level-Circle One)

		Right								Left				
	250	500	1K	2K	4K	8K		250	500	1K	2K	4K	8K
% Correct		85	100	90					25	30	40		
Presentation Level (dB SL)		20	20	20					20	20	20		
dB Masking													

Figure 15 (continued)   (B) Top, Olsen-Noffsinger tone-decay results at 500, 1000, and 2000 Hz, bilaterally. Middle, ABLB results at 500, 1000, and 2000 Hz. Bottom, SISI (standard presentation level) results at 500, 1000, and 2000 Hz, bilaterally.

over index was positive (1.0) for the right ear, consistent with right retrocochlear pathology and negative (0.04) for the left ear (see Chapter 5).

The static-acoustic middle-ear admittance and tympanometric results were consistent with normal middle-ear function, bilaterally (see Chapter 3). The contralateral acoustic-reflex thresholds exceed the Silman and Gelfand (1981) 90th percentile levels only in the right ear at 1000 and 2000 Hz, consistent with right retrocochlear pathology (see Chapter 3). The contralateral acoustic-reflex decay results were positive in the right ear (stimulus ear) only, at

500 Hz, also consistent with right retrocochlear pathology (see Chapter 3).

The ABLB results revealed complete recruitment, consistent with cochlear pathology at 500 and 1000 Hz, but no recruitment at 2000 Hz, consistent with retrocochlear pathology in the right ear (see Chapter 5). The Olsen–Noffsinger tone-decay results were negative for the left ear, consistent with the absence of left retrocochlear pathology, and positive for the right ear at 2000 Hz, consistent with right retrocochlear pathology (see Chapter 5). The 20-dB SL SISI scores are high for the right ear, consistent with the presence of right cochlear pathology; in the left ear, the SISI scores are low at 500 and 1000 Hz, consistent with normal-hearing sensitivity and are inconclusive at 2000 Hz.

The results of CAT scans indicated a right acoustic tumor (2 cm in size) that was surgically confirmed.

True positive results were obtained on the ARC test, ABLB, suprathreshold speech-recognition scores (with reference to the 95% critical-differences limits), PI–PB roll-over index, and tone-decay tests. False-negative findings were obtained on the SISI test. If the modified P_5 protocol mentioned earlier in this chapter had been employed, this patient would have been referred for the definitive medical test after the positive ARC findings.

ACKNOWLEDGMENT

The form used to summarize the traditional site-of-lesion test results, appearing in Figures 5B, 6B, 12C, 13C, 14C, and 15B, was adapted from the figure on page 127 from Kaplan, H. (1984), Cochlear/retrocochlear central test battery. In H. Kaplan, V. S. Gladstone, & J. Katz (eds.), *Site of lesion testing: Audiometric interpretation.* Vol. II. Baltimore: University Park Press.

REFERENCES

Alberti, P. W., Symons, F., & Hyde, M. L. (1979). Occupational hearing loss. *Acta Otolaryngol.*, 87, 255–263.

Antonelli, A. R., Bellotto, R., & Grandori, F. (1987). Audiologic diagnosis of central versus eighth nerve and cochlear auditory impairment. *Audiology.*, 26, 209–226.

Barber, H. O., & Stockwell, C. W. (1980) *Manual of electronystagmography.* 2d ed. St. Louis: Mosby.

Bauch, C. D., Olsen, W. O., & Harner, S. G. (1983). Auditory brain-stem response and acoustic reflex test: Results for patients with and without tumor matched for hearing loss. *Arch. Otolaryngol.*, 109, 522–525.

Bocca, E., & Calearo, C. (1963). Central hearing processes. In J. Jerger (ed.), *Modern developments in audiology*, pp. 337–370. New York: Academic Press.

Caparosa, R. J. (1979). Cost-benefit ratio in our search for cerebellopontine angle tumors. *Laryngoscope*, 89, 410–418.

Cohen, M., & Prasher, D. (1988). The value of combining auditory brainstem responses and acoustic reflex threshold measurements in neuro-otological diagnosis. *Scand. Audiol.*, 17, 153–162.

Dix, M. R., & Hood, J. D. (1953). Modern developments in pure tone audiometry and their application to the clinical diagnosis of end-organ deafness. *J. Laryngol.*, 67, 343–357.

Dobie, R. A. (1985). The use of relative cost ratios in choosing a diagnostic test. *Ear Hear.*, 6, 113–116.

Galen, R., & Gambino, S. (1975). *Beyond normality: The predictive value and efficiency of medical diagnosis.* New York: Wiley.

Gelfand, S. A., & Piper, N. (1984). Acoustic reflex thresholds: Variability and distribution effects. *Ear Hear.*, 5, 228–234.

Hart, R. G., & Davenport, J. (1981). Diagnosis of acoustic neuroma. *Neurosurg.*, 9, 450–463.

Jerger, J. F. (1961). Recruitment and allied phenomena in differential diagnosis. *J. Aud. Res.*, 1, 145–151.

Jerger, J. (1962). Hearing tests in otologic diagnosis. *Asha*, 4, 139–145.

Jerger, J., & Jerger, S. (1975). Clinical validity of central auditory tests. *Scand. Audiol.*, 4, 147–163.

Jerger, S. (1983). Decision matrix and information theory analysis in the evaluation of neuro-audiologic tests. *Sem. Hear.*, 4, 121–132.

Jerger, S., & Jerger, J. (1983). Evaluation of diagnostic audiometric tests. *Audiology.*, 22, 144–161.

Johnson, E. W. (1977). Auditory test results in 500 cases of acoustic neuroma. *Arch. Otolaryngol.*, 103, 152–158.

Kusakari, J., Okitsu, T., Kobayashi, T., *et al.* (1981). ABR audiometry in the diagnosis of cerebellopontine angle tumors. *Oto.-Rhino.-Laryngol.*, 43, 336–344.

Mair, I. W. S., Okstad, S., Laukli, E., & Anke, I. M. (1988). Screening for retrocochlear pathology. *Scand. Audiol.*, 17, 163–169.

Miller, M. H. (1985). The integration of audiologic findings. In J. Katz (ed.), *Handbook of clinical audiology*, 3d ed. pp. 259–272. Baltimore: Williams & Wilkins.

Musiek, F. E. (1983). Assessment of central auditory dysfunction: The dichotic digit test revented. *Ear Hear.*, 4, 79–83.

Musiek, F. E., & Geurkink, N. A. (1982). Auditory brain stem response and central auditory test findings for patients with brain stem lesions: A preliminary report. *Laryngoscope*, 92, 891–900.

Newby, H. A., & Popelka, G. R. (1985). *Audiology*, 5th ed. Englewood Cliffs, New Jersey: Prentice-Hall.

Olsen, W. O., Bauch, C. D., & Harner, S. G. (1983). Application of Silman and Gelfand (1981) 90th percentile levels for acoustic reflex thresholds. *J. Speech Hear. Dis.*, 48, 330–332.

Owens, E. (1971). Audiologic evaluation in cochlear versus retrocochlear lesions. *Acta Otolaryngol. Suppl.*, 283, 1–45.

Parving, A., Elberling, C., & Salomon, G. (1981). Slow cortical responses and the diagnosis of central hearing loss in infants and young children. *Audiology.*, 20, 465–479.

Sanders, J. W. (1984a). Diagnostic audiology. In J. L. Northern (ed.), *Hearing disorders*, 2d ed., pp. 25–40. Boston: Little, Brown.

Sanders, J. W. (1984b). Evaluation of the 90th percentile levels for acoustic reflex thresholds. Paper presented at the Annual Convention of the American Speech–Language–Hearing Association, San Francisco.

Sanders, J. W., Josey, A. F., & Glasscock, M. E. (1974). Audiologic evaluation in cochlear and eighth nerve disorders. *Arch. Otolaryngol.*, 100, 283–293.

Selters, W. A., & Brackman, D. E. (1977). Acoustic tumor detection with brain stem electric response audiometry. *Arch. Otolaryngol.*, 103, 181–187.

Silman, S., & Gelfand, S. A. (1981). The relationship between magnitude of hearing loss and acoustic reflex threshold levels. *J. Speech Hear. Dis.*, 46, 312–316.

Simonton, K. M. (1956). End-organ deafness. *Arch. Otolaryngol.*, 63, 262–269.

Suga, F., & Lindsay, J. R. (1976). Histopathological observations of presbycusis. *Ann. Otol. Rhinol. Laryngol.*, 85, 169–184.

Thomsen, J., Nyboe, P., Borum, P., Tos, M., & Barfoed, C. (1981). Acoustic neuromas: Diagnostic efficiency of various test combinations. *Arch. Otolaryngol.*, 107, 601–607.

Thornton, A., & Raffin, M. J. M. (1978). Speech discrimination scores modeled as a benomial variable: *J. Speech Hear. Res.*, 21, 507–518.

Tillman, T. W. (1969). Special hearing tests in otoneurologic diagnosis. *Arch. Otolaryngol.*, 89, 51–56.

Turner, R. G. (1988). Techniques to determine test protocol performance. *Ear Hear.*, 9, 177–189.

Turner, R. G., & Nielsen, D. W. (1984). Application of clinical decision analysis to audiological tests. *Ear Hear.*, 5, 125–133.

Turner, R. G., Shepard, N. T., & Frazer, C. J. (1984a). Clinical performance of audiological and related diagnostic tests. *Ear Hear.*, 5, 187–194.

Turner, R. G., Frazer, G. J., & Shepard, N. T. (1984b). Formulating and evaluating audiologic test protocols. *Ear Hear.*, 5, 321–330.

STIMULUS CALIBRATION

I. BRAINSTEM AUDITORY-EVOKED POTENTIALS CALIBRATION

A. INTENSITY

1. CLICK

Intensity in dB SPL is usually determined using the formula

$$dB\ SPL = 20 \log P_1/P_2$$

where P_1 is the SPL in micropascal (μPa) of the stimulus to be measured, and P_2 is the reference SPL (20 μPa). To obtain P_1, the root-mean-square (rms) for the instantaneous amplitudes of several sinusoidal waveforms is calculated. The formula for the rms value of amplitude is

$$rms = \{\Sigma(P^2)/N\}^{1/2}$$

where P is the instantaneous pressure amplitude and N is the number of observations (number of instantaneous amplitudes).

The rms value of intensity represents the average sound pressure over time. Generally, when the fast mode of the sound-level meter (SLM) is employed, the time period for the rms average is usually 250 ms. The rms for a click is not an accurate representation of its average SPL since the average over a 250-ms period is calculated over the silent off-times as well as the on-times (Burkard, 1984). Therefore, other methods of quantification of the click intensity must be employed.

One method of click-intensity determination involves the calculation of instantaneous peak SPL (pSPL). The formula used to calculate the pSPL is:

$$pSPL = 20 \log (P_{max}/P_{ref})$$

where P_{max} is equivalent to the maximum instantaneous pressure in μPa and P_{ref} is equivalent to 20 μPa. Certain SLMs have the capacity to measure pSPL based on this formula. These instruments have special amplifiers with peak detectors which indicate P_{max} for brief sounds having durations as small as 50 μs and have a peak-hold capability (Burkard, 1984). In our clinic, the pSPL is measured with the Quest SLM that has a peak detector and peak-hold capacity.

When an SLM with a peak detector and peak-hold capacity is unavailable, click intensity can be quantified by calculating the peak equivalent SPL (peSPL). With this approach, a click from the BAEP generator is routed through an earphone coupled to 6-cm^3 coupler and through an SLM. The AC output of an SLM is directed to an oscilloscope. The peak-to-peak (p–p) or baseline-to-peak (b–p) voltage of the click is measured. A pure tone instead of a click is then delivered through the same earphone, coupler, SLM, and oscilloscope. The amplitude of the pure tone is adjusted until it is equivalent to that of the click (peak-to-peak or baseline-to-peak). The rms intensity value of the pure tone in dB SPL can be read from the SLM. This rms value is the peSPL of the click.

An alternative to the physical measurement of the click intensity is the commonly used behavioral approach. In this approach, the behavioral threshold for the click stimulus for a group of 10 normal-hearing young adults (pure-tone thresholds not exceeding 20 dB HL) is established. The mean of the behavioral thresholds is 0 dBnHL for BAEP audiometry. For example, if the BAEP is elicited at an intensity which is 30 dB above the mean behavioral threshold, then the click intensity is 30 dBnHL. The behavioral thresholds should be measured in an audiometric booth which meets ANSI S3.1-1977 standards. For measurement of the behavioral threshold of the click, Gorga, Abbas, and Worthington (1985) recommended a click repetition rate of 50/s. They felt that this click rate was a compromise between low repetition rates needed to obtain a clear BAEP waveform and high repetition rates needed to obtain a low behavioral click threshold.

Since click intensity is commonly specified in dBnHL, we recommend that the initial calibration of click intensity be made using the behavioral method and using pSPL method if an SLM with a peak detector and peak-hold capacity is available. Follow-up calibrations at periodic intervals can be made using the pSPL method, the results of which are compared with those of the initial calibration. If an SLM with a peak detector and peak-hold capacity is unavailable, then the clinically feasible method of physical measurement suggested by Weber, Seitz, and McCutcheon (1981) should be employed at the initial and follow-up calibrations. The Weber *et al.* method involves routing the click train to an earphone coupled to a conventional SLM. The click rate is increased until a stable acoustic signal can be read on the SLM. If the physical measurements on follow-up calibrations reveal changes, the reference intensity for 0 dBnHL should be adjusted accordingly.

2. TONEBURST/TONEPIP

Gorga *et al.* (1985) recommended increasing the duration of the toneburst/tonepip until it is long relative to the response time of the SLM, so that a relativelay stable reading can be made on the SLM. In this procedure, the toneburst/tonepip is routed from the BAEP generator to the earphone coupled to a 6-cm³ coupler and an SLM. The intensity of the toneburst/tonepip is specified in terms of dB SPL relative to 20 μPa.

B. ACOUSTIC WAVEFORM

An acoustic waveform shows amplitude as a function of time for an acoustic stimulus. The acoustic stimulus for calibrating the acoustic waveform should be the same as that used in brainstem auditory-evoked potentials assessment. For example, if clicks are used in brainstem auditory-evoked potentials assessment, then the acoustic waveform of the click should be obtained.

Acoustic waveforms can be obtained by routing the stimulus from the signal generator of the brainstem auditory-evoked potentials system through an earphone coupled to a 6-cm³ coupler which, in turn, is coupled to a sound-level meter (with the filter in the off position). The AC output from the sound-level meter is then routed to an oscilloscope. The oscilloscope would show the acoustic waveform of the stimulus.

Another way of obtaining the acoustic waveform is, instead of routing the AC output of the sound-level meter to the oscilloscope, routing the AC output to the differential amplifier of the averager of the brainstem auditory-evoked potentials device. In this case, the sound-level meter is like a patient in terms of the hook-up. The stimulus from the signal generator of the brainstem auditory-evoked potentials device is used to trigger the averager. The time window should be 2 rather than 10 ms. The sensitivity should be maximal or near maximal; the clinician should experiment with the sensitivity to derive the sensitivity yielding the optimal waveform on the monitor. We have found that 16–20 samples and an intensity of 80–90 dBnHL yield the optimal waveform on the monitor. The waveform of the acoustic stimulus should be stored for comparisons in fu-

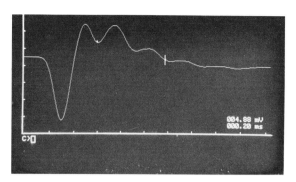

Figure 1 An example of an acoustic waveform for a click presented through TDH-49 earphones. The acoustic waveform was obtained by routing the stimulus from the signal generator of the brainstem auditory-evoked potentials device to the differential amplifier of the averager of the brainstem auditory-evoked potentials device.

ture calibration. An example of the acoustic waveform for a click presented through TDH-49 earphones obtained using this method is shown in Figure 1.

Alteration of the acoustic waveform can occur if the acoustic spectrum of the stimulus changes. Changes in the acoustic spectrum of the stimulus can result from physical damage to the earphones (e.g., dropping the earphones). Therefore, periodic calibration of the acoustic waveform of the stimulus should be made, particularly when the earphones are dropped.

C. ACOUSTIC SPECTRUM

Although the acoustic waveform grossly indicates whether the acoustic characteristics of the earphone change following physical damage of the earphones, it cannot indicate the frequency characteristics of the acoustic stimulus delivered to the ear through the earphone.

The frequency response of the earphone affects the acoustic spectrum as well as the acoustic waveform of a stimulus. Different earphones, even those of the same model, may have different frequency responses. Figure 2A shows the click spectra of three earphones which differ in frequency response. Figure 2B shows the brainstem auditory-evoked potentials elicited with a click for each of the spectra shown in Figure 2A. Figure 2 reveals that earphones with different frequency responses yield brainstem auditory-evoked potentials which differ in latencies. The clinician should be knowledgeable regarding the frequency responses of the two earphones as evidenced by the acoustic spectra for a given headset so that interaural latency differencies can be interpreted appropriately. If the earphones need to be changed, the clinician should select replacement earphones which have acoustic spectra similar to those of

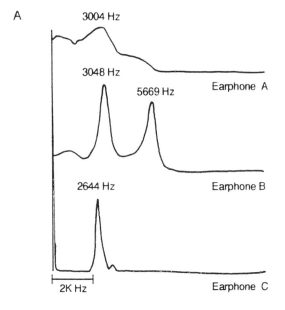

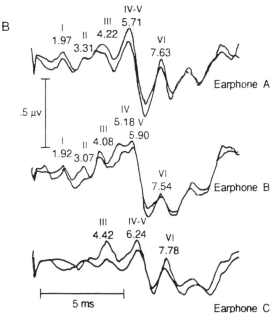

Figure 2 (A) Click spectra recorded from 3 earphones. (B) ABRs from the 3 earphones in (A). Rarefaction clicks at 60 dB SL were presented at a rate of 13/s. To produce the same polarity clicks, a negative electrical pulse was fed to earphones A and C, and a positive electrical pulse was fed to earphone B. Reprinted with permission from Weber *et al.* (1981).

the old earphones so that new normative brainstem auditory-evoked potential data do not need to be obtained.

If a real-time spectral analyzer is available, the acoustic spectrum of the stimulus can be measured with the AC output routed from the sound-level meter to the input of the real-time spectral analyzer. If a real-time spectral analyzer is unavailable, the clinician should obtain the acoustic spectrum of the earphone from the manufacturer.

D. POLARITY

The polarity of the acoustic stimulus at the output of the earphones should be evaluated. It cannot be assumed, for example, that selecting condensation clicks on the brainstem auditory-evoked potentials device will actually yield condensation pulses.

According to Gorga *et al.* (1985), the DC output of the sound-level meter is routed to the oscilloscope. Before introducing any stimulus, the oscilloscope should show a flat line. To generate a positive pulse from the earphone, gently press the back of the earphone and observe on the oscilloscope whether a positive or negative deflection is observed. Ideally, a positive deflection occurs when you press on the back of the earphone. Nevertheless, the polarity is positive when you press against the back of the earphone regardless of the direction of the deflection. The DC output from the sound-level meter should now be disconnected. Instead, the AC output from the sound-level meter should be routed to the oscilloscope. A click should be presented. If the deflection is in the same direction as that observed when you pressed on the back of the earphone, then it can be assumed that the polarity was positive (condensation). If the deflection is in the opposite direction to that observed when you pressed on the back of the earphone, it can be assumed that the polarity was negative.

If an oscilloscope is unavailable, the polarity can be evaluated by routing the stimulus from the output of the sound-level meter to the differential amplifier of the averager of the brainstem auditory-evoked potentials device. 16–20 sweeps are needed (see the procedure for calibrating the acoustic waveform of a stimulus using the differential amplifier of the averager of the brainstem auditory-evoked potentials device) for this technique the polarity of the earphone, the cords, and the plug of the earphone must be matched.

E. REPETITION RATE

To calibrate the repetition rate using the oscilloscope, the AC output from the sound-level meter is routed to the oscilloscope. (The signal is routed to the sound-level meter in the manner described for calibration of the acoustic waveform.) The oscilloscope should have a time window of 300–400 ms. Present clicks at the desired repetition rate. Measure the time interval between two successive clicks on the oscilloscope. The repetition rate is equal to 1000 ms divided by the time interval (in ms). For example, if the time interval between two clicks is 100 ms, then the repetition rate is 1000 ms divided by 100 ms that is, 10 clicks/s.

If an oscilloscope is unavailable, an alternative method can be used that involves routing the AC output from the sound-level meter to the differential amplifier of the averager of the brainstem auditory-evoked potentials device. In this method, 16–20 samples are used, the time window is 300–400 ms, and the intensity is 80–90 dBnHL. Again, the sensitivity should be at or near maximum (whichever yields the optimal waveform). Obtain the average of the 16–20 click-elicited samples. Using the cursors, calculate the interval in ms between two clicks on the monitor of the brainstem auditory-evoked potentials monitor. The repetition rate is equivalent to 1000 ms divided by the duration of the measured time interval. Figure 3 shows the determination of the interval between two clicks on the monitor of the brainstem auditory-evoked potentials device.

II. ACOUSTIC-IMMITTANCE CALIBRATION

The acoustic admittance of a volume of air enclosed in a cavity can be determined if the volume of the cavity and the atmospheric conditions are known. The acoustic admittance of a volume of air enclosed in a hard-walled cavity is specified in polar notation by the formula

$$YA = fV/k$$

where f is the probe-tone frequency, V is the volume of the hard-walled cavity, and k is a constant obtained from the formula

$$k = (\rho c^2)/2\pi$$

where ρ is the ambient density of the air in kg/m^3 and c is the velocity of sound in m/s. The k value under standard atmospheric conditions (P_o of 776.0 mm Hg., temperature of 22°C, and relative humidity of 50%) is 227,840.858. Table I gives the k values for different cities (which differ in P). Using the formula $YA = fV/k$, the acoustic admittance of 1 cm^3 of air (air in a hard-walled cavity has no conductance so the admittance is composed only of susceptance) is equivalent to 1 acoustic mmho for the 226-Hz probe tone and 3 mmhos for the 678-Hz probe tone. Therefore, when the acoustic-admittance device is calibrated with a hard-

Table I The k Values for Washington, D.C., Syracuse, New York, Iowa City, Iowa, and Denver, Colorado[a]

City	Elevation[b] (m)	Temperature[b] (°C)	Relative humidity[b] (%)	k value[c]
Washington, D.C.	34	22	50	225,076
Syracuse	182	22	50	220,608
Iowa City	224	20	50	219,812
Denver	1613	22	50	184,750

[a] Adapted from Lilly (1970).
[b] The elevation (m), temperature (°C), and relative humidity (%) are shown for these cities.
[c] Converted for cgs units.

walled cavity, 1 cm^3 of air should be equivalent to 1 acoustic mmho. Similarly, the commonly used 2-cm^3 hard-walled cavity should yield an acoustic admittance or susceptance of 2 acoustic mmho and acoustic conductance of 0 mmho.

For calibration of the sensitivity scale for acoustic-reflex measurement, see Silman (1984).

III. AUDIOMETRIC CALIBRATION

A. AIR CONDUCTION

For calibration of air-conduction signals, a sound-level meter with a third-octave band analyzer and condenser microphone, 6-cm^3 coupler (NBS 9-A), 500-gm weight, frequency counter, oscilloscope, and voltmeter are required. For calibration of air-conduction thresholds, the earphone is placed on an NBS-9A coupler and the 500-gm weight is placed on the earphone. The output is read from the sound-level meter in dB SPL relative to 20 μPa. For pure-tone and narrow-band noise calibration, the sound-level meter is set on the linear scale, the weighting filter is on, and the third-octave band is set to the frequency tested. For speech-noise and broad-band noise calibration, the weighting filter is off.

The S3.6–1989 standard reference equivalent threshold sound-pressure levels for different earphones are shown in Table II. The tolerance for sound-pressure level accuracy is ± 3 dB through 4000 Hz and ± 5 dB at 6000 and 8000 Hz. The interim reference equivalent threshold sound-pressure levels (ANSI S3.6–1989) for the Etymotic ER-3A insert earphones are shown in Table III. To measure the sound-pressure level of broad-band noise, the output of the sound-level meter is measured at each third-octave band from 250 to 4000 Hz. The input to the sound-level meter (from the output of the audiometer) is the broad-band noise, but the weighting filter is on. The output sound-pressure level at each third-octave band should be within ± 5 dB of the output sound-pressure level at 1000 Hz. The accuracy of

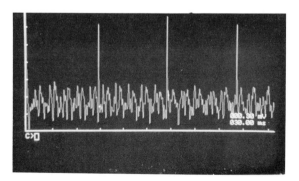

Figure 3 The interval between two clicks as seen on the monitor of a Nicolet Compact Auditory System.

Table II Standard Reference Equivalent Sound-Pressure Levels Relative to 20 μPa for Different Earphones[a]

Earphone	Frequency (Hz)										
	125	250	500	750	1000	1500	2000	3000	4000	6000	8000
WE[b] 705	45.5	24.5	11.0	7.5	6.5	6.5	8.5	7.5	9.0	8.0	9.5
TDH[c]-39, TDH-39P	45.0	25.5	11.5	8.0	7.0	6.5	9.0	10.0	9.5	15.5	13.0
TDH-49, TDH-49P, TDH-50, TDH-50P	47.5	26.5	13.5	8.5	7.5	7.5	11.0	9.5	10.5	13.5	13.0
T[d] 1470A	47.0	27.5	13.0	8.5	6.5	5.0	8.0	7.5	9.0	17.5	17.5

[a] Adapted from ANSI S3.6–1989.
[b] Western Electric.
[c] Telephonics.
[d] Telex.

the sound-pressure level for narrow-band noise and pure tones is measured the same way, except that the tolerance is ± 5 dB of the standard reference equivalent threshold sound-pressure levels shown in Table II through 4000 Hz. For speech noise, ANSI S3.6–1989 specifies the measurement of sound-pressure spectrum density. The standard specifies that the energy per Hz should be constant from 250 to 1000 Hz and should fall off at a rate of 12 dB/octave from 1000 to 4000 Hz. The speech-noise output from the audiometer should be routed to a real-time spectral analyzer which will show decibels as a function of frequency. From this graph, lack of uniformity through 1000 Hz and fall-off rate above 1000 Hz can be determined.

Harmonic distortion of the acoustic signal can be reported as a percentage of the output of the fundamental frequency or in dB SPL. Table IV shows the maximum permissible harmonic distortion, expressed in percentage (ANSI S3.6–1989). Harmonic distortion is measured at the hearing levels listed in Table IV or at the maximum output level for the audiometer, whichever is lower. When the harmonic distortion is expressed in dB SPL, the level of any

harmonic must be at least 30 dB below the output of the fundamental frequency.

With respect to the rise characteristics of the signal, the rise time from 50 dB to 1 dB below the peak intensity should not exceed 200 ms and the rise time from 20 to 1 dB below the peak intensity shall be at least 20 ms. With respect to the fall characteristics of the signal, the fall time from peak intensity to 50 dB below the peak intensity shall not exceed 200 ms and the fall time from 1 dB below the peak intensity to 20 dB below the peak intensity shall be at least 20 ms. The rise and fall characteristics can be measured after routing the signal from the audiometer to the oscilloscope.

Attenuator linearity can be checked electronically or acoustically. Electronically, it is checked by connecting the wire from the earphone cord to the voltmeter that is connected to the output of the audiometer; this is done without disconnecting the earphone cord from the audiometer. For proper loading, the earphone is placed on the NBS-9A coupler. Acoustically, the earphone is coupled to the NBS-9A coupler and sound-level meter. Electronically, at a single

Table III Interim Reference Equivalent Threshold Sound-Pressure Levels Relative to 20 μPa for the Etymotic ER-3A Insert Earphone[a]

Frequency (Hz)	HA-1 coupler SPL	Conversion HA-1 to ear simulator
125	27.5	2.5
250	15.5	3.5
500	8.5	3.5
1000	3.5	5.5
2000	6.5	8.5
3000	5.5	10.0
4000	1.5	11.5
6000	−1.5	14.5
8000	−4.0	18.0

[a] Adapted from ANSI S3.6–1989.

Table IV Maximum Permissible Harmonic Distortion as a Function of Frequency for Air-Conducted Signals[a]

Frequency (Hz)	Hearing level (dB HL)	Harmonics				
		2nd	3rd	4th+	All subharmonics	Total harmonics
125	75	2.0	2.0	0.3	—	3.0
250	90	2.0	2.0	0.3	0.3	3.0
500	110	2.0	2.0	0.3	0.3	3.0
1000	110	2.0	2.0	0.3	0.3	3.0
2000	110	2.0	2.0	0.3	0.3	3.0
3000	110	2.0	2.0	0.3	0.3	3.0
4000	110	2.0	2.0	0.3	0.3	3.0
6000	90	2.0	—	—	0.3	3.0
8000	90	2.0	—	—	0.3	3.0

[a] Adapted from ANSI S3.6–1989.

frequency such as 1000 Hz, the voltage output is recorded at maximum to minimum attenuator settings, in 5-dB increments. Acoustically, the sound-pressure level output is recorded at attenuator settings exceeding 70 dB HL. Acoustic check of attenuator linearity is done in addition to electronic check of attenuator linearity in order to detect any nonlinearity of the earphone. According to the ANSI S3.6–1989 standard, the difference in output between any two output levels should not differ from the nominal difference by more than 3/10 of the increment or 1 dB, whichever is smaller. Since the smallest increment is 5 dB, the difference between 2 outputs should never exceed 1 dB. For example, the difference in output between the 5-dB and 10-dB attenuator settings cannot exceed 1 dB.

According to the ANSI S3.6–1989 standard, each frequency (of a diagnostic audiometer) must be within 3% of the nominal frequency. The accuracy of the frequency of the test tone can be measured using an electronic frequency counter or oscilloscope. In the former case, the earphone lead is disconnected from the output of the audiometer and the output of the audiometer is routed to the electronic frequency counter. In the latter case, the earphone lead is disconnected from the output of the audiometer and the output of the audiometer is routed to an oscilloscope. At a given attenuator setting, such as 70 dB HL, the electronic frequency counter will give a direct readout of the frequency. With an oscilloscope, the frequency is calculated by measuring the period of a sine wave and then using that value in the formula $f = 1/t$ where t is the period and f is the frequency. Recently, a new portable calibration unit that is easy to operate became available. With such a unit a comprehensive calibration could be accomplished within a few minutes.

B. BONE CONDUCTION

For calibration of bone-conduction signals from a Type B-71 bone-vibrator having a circular tip area of 175 ±25mm² attached to a headband exerting a static force of 5.4 ±0.5 N, a Type 4930 artificial mastoid is needed (ANSI

Table V Mastoid Reference Equivalent Threshold Force Levels for Audiometric Bone Vibrators[a,b]

Frequency (Hz)							
250	500	750	1000	1500	2000	3000	4000
61	59	47[c]	39	35[c]	32.5	28	31

[a] From ANSI S3.6–1989 and ANSI S3.26–1981.
[b] Force levels expressed in dB relative to 1μN. To obtain force levels relative to 1 dyne, subtract 20 dB from the values in the table.
[c] Value obtained by interpolation.

Table VI Constants to Be Added to the Values in Table V to Yield the Forehead Reference Equivalent Threshold Force Level Calibration Values for Audiometric Bone Vibrators[a]

Frequency (Hz)							
250	500	750	1000	1500	2000	3000	4000
13.5	15.0	12.5	10.0	9.0	8.5	7.5	6.5

[a] From ANSI S3.6–1989 and ANSI S3.26–1981.

S3.6–1989). The mastoid reference equivalent threshold force level calibration values for the zero setting of the audiometer hearing-level dial are shown in Table V. The constants to be added to the values in Table V to derive the forehead reference equivalent threshold force level calibration values for the zero setting of the audiometer hearing-level dial are shown in Table VI. The need to add to the mastoid values to obtain the forehead values illustrates the lower sensitivity of the forehead compared with the mastoid site for bone-conduction testing. Figure 4 illustrates the calibration apparatus arrangement for the artificial mastoid.

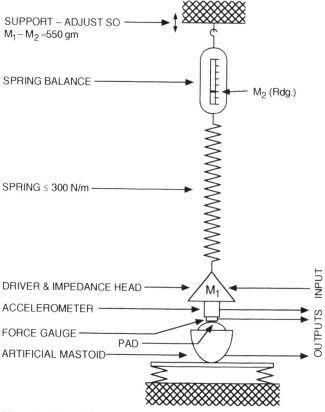

Figure 4 The calibration apparatus arrangement for the artificial mastoid. Adapted from ANSI S3.26–1981.

C. SPEECH

A speech recording should have a calibrated signal tone for calibrating the speech channel. When recorded speech is routed through the recorded speech channel of the audiometer at a given attenuator setting with the deflection of the volume level indicator meter set to zero, the output of the recorded calibrated 1000-Hz tone preceding the speech should be 12.5 dB greater than the standard reference equivalent sound-pressure level for a given earphone reported in Table II. If the output does not yield the desired value when the volume level indicator meter is set to zero, then the volume level indicator meter should be adjusted to yield this desired value; the scale of the volume level indicator meter should reflect the new 0 value.

According to ANSI S3.6–1989, the live-voice channel of an audiometer must have the following frequency response. The inputs to a microphone in the free sound field (anechoic chamber) are pure tones in the speech spectrum having constant sound-pressure levels; these inputs to the microphone are routed through the live-voice channel of the audiometer and earphone. The outputs of the earphone, as measured in the artificial ear, between 250 and 4000 Hz, should not differ by more than ±5 dB from the output at 1000 Hz; the output below 250 Hz or above 4000 Hz should not exceed by more than 10 dB, the output at 1000 Hz. As an alternative to the anechoic chamber, Konkle and Townsend (1983) place the microphone in a commercially available hearing-aid test box.

According to ANSI S3.6–1989, the frequency response of a recorded speech channel has the same characteristics as a live-voice channel except that recorded sine-wave inputs are used, the inputs are routed through the recorded speech channel, and the output sound-pressure levels should be approximately 100 dB relative to 20 μPa.

For measurement of overall distortion of the speech channel, pure tones which do not have total harmonic distortion exceeding 1% such as those from the pure-tone channel of an audiometer or oscillator, are routed to the input of the speech channel of the audiometer. The output of the speech channel is routed through an earphone coupled to an artificial ear and sound-level meter having a third-octave band filter or sound-level meter connected to a distortion analyzer. The volume level indicator meter is first set to the setting yielding the standard reference level (i.e., 12.5 dB above the standard reference level at 1000 Hz) and the attenuator setting is adjusted to yield an output sound-pressure level of 120 dB or is adjusted to the maximum, whichever yields the lower sound-pressure level output. Then the volume level indicator meter is adjusted to yield a deflection of 9 ± 1 dB more than the standard reference level. The total harmonic distortion is recorded at this volume level indicator meter setting. The total harmonic distortion of the output (of the speech channel) for 250-, 500-, 1000-, 2000-, and 4000-Hz inputs shall not exceed 3% (ANSI S3.6–1989).

D. SOUNDFIELD

Two types of environments exist for soundfield testing—free field and reverberant field. In a free-field environment, the reflections of sound waves on surfaces are insignificant. An anechoic chamber is essentially a free field. Reverberant fields are those environments other than anechoic chambers. In reverberant fields, the reflections of sound waves on surfaces are significant. Commercially available prefabricated or custom built audiometric suites are reverberant fields. Soundfield testing within an audiometric suite (reverberant field) involves presentation of stimuli through a loudspeaker.

No ANSI specifications have been developed for calibration of soundfield testing. Nevertheless, Appendix A of ANSI S3.6–1989 provides suggestions for soundfield speech testing. The ambient noise inside the audiometric suite should not exceed the levels specified in ANSI S3.1–1977 (R1986). (See Chapter 2 for the ANSI specifications of maximum ambient noise levels during audiometric testing.) The output of the loudspeaker at the approximate position of the subject's head (subject should not be present during the calibration) at 250 to 4000 Hz should be within 10 dB of the output at 1000 Hz. The output sound-pressure levels below 250 Hz and above 4000 Hz should not exceed by more than 15 dB the output at 1000 Hz. The type of stimulus input is not specified in Appendix A of the ANSI S3.6–1989 standard. We recommend the use of narrow-band noise input.

Appendix A of ANSI S3.6–1989 suggests that the reference sound-pressure level for soundfield testing be 13 dB with the loudspeakers placed at 40° to 60° azimuth. (At 0° azimuth, the loudspeaker is placed directly in front of one's face; at 90° azimuth, the loudspeaker is placed directly opposite one's ear; at 270° azimuth, the loudspeaker is on the side opposite the test ear.) The input to the loudspeaker is speech noise and the condenser microphone of the sound-level meter should be placed at the approximate position that a subject's head would be (without actually having the subject there). The sound-level meter should be set in the "A" weighting position. If the desired output sound-pressure level is not obtained, the position of the subject's head should be moved until the desired value is obtained.

Wilber (1985) recommended checking the amplifier hum or internal noise of the loudspeaker system. The attenuator dial is set near maximum (80–90 dB) and a condenser microphone is placed at the approximate location of the subject's head during the test; the output of the loudspeaker with the tone interruptor switch in the off position is measured with the condenser microphone of the sound-level meter at the test position. The measured output should be at least 50 dB less than the attenuator setting.

REFERENCES

American National Standards Institute (1977). *American National Standard criteria for permissible ambient noise during audiometric testing* (ANSI S3.1–1977(R1986)). New York: American National Standards Institute.

American National Standards Institute (1981). *American National Standard reference equivalent threshold force levels for audiometric bone vibrators* (ANSI S3.26–1981). New York: American National Standards Institute.

American National Standards Institute (1989). *American National Standard specification for audiometers* (ANSI S3.6–1989). New York: American National Standards Institute.

Burkard, R. (1984). Sound pressure level measurement and spectral analysis of brief acoustic transients. *Electroencephalogr. Clin. Neurophysiol.*, 57, 83–91.

Gorga, M. P., Abbas, P. J., & Worthington, D. W. (1985). Stimulus calibration in ABR measurements. In J. T. Jacobson (ed.), *The auditory brainstem response* pp.49–62. San Diego: College-Hill Press.

Konkle, D. R., & Townsend, T. H. (1983). Calibration measurements for speech audiometers. In D. F. Konkle & W. F. Rintelmann (eds.), *Principles of speech audiometry*, pp. 55–78. Baltimore: University Park Press.

Lilly, D. J. (1970). Acoustic impedance at the tympanic membrane: An overview of clinical applications. In D. Rose & L. Keating (eds.), *Mayo foundation impedance symposium*, pp. 74–82. Rochester, Minnesota: Mayo Clinic.

Silman, S. (1984). Magnitude and growth of the acoustic reflex. In S. Silman (ed.), *The acoustic reflex: Basic principles and clinical applications*, pp. 225–274. New York: Academic Press.

Weber, B. A., Seitz, M., & McCutcheon, M. J. (1981). Quantifying click stimuli in auditory brainstem response audiometry. *Ear Hear.*, 2, 15–19.

Wilber, L. A. (1985). Calibration: Puretone, speech, and noise signals. In J. Katz (ed.), *Handbook of clinical audiology*, 3d ed., pp. 116–150. Baltimore: Williams & Wilkins.

INDEX

Abbas, P. J., 391
Abraham, F., 56
Abrams, S., 245
Accuracy, SISI tests, 198
Achor, L., 158, 262, 264, 265, 266, 283
Acoustic immittance testing
    acoustic-reflex testing, 103, 105–120
    calibration, 394
    concept, 71–79
    conductive pathologies, 49
    infants, 120–124
    middle-ear function, 129–132
    otoscopy, 124–125
    pressure, 84–88
    static, 80–84
    static middle-ear and tympanometry, 102–103
Acoustic radiation, 23–24
Acoustic-reflex testing
    acoustic immittance, 103, 105–120
    infants, 122–124
    sensitivity to retrocochlear pathology, 71
    thresholds, 150, 190, 343–345
Acoustic schwannomas, 61–62
Acoustic spectrum, 392–393
Acoustic waveform, 392
Adaptation
    acoustic-reflex, 114–118
    Bekesy tracings and loudness recruitment, 207
    tests of auditory, 172–178
Admittance, concept of immittance, 77
Adults
    acoustic-immittance testing and middle-ear function, 131
    functional hearing loss, 137–138
Adventitious hearing impairment, 57–62
Aging
    acoustic-reflex threshold, 110
    adventitious hearing impairment, 59–60
    BAEP and subject parameters, 263
    rollover effect, 170
    vascular brainstem compression, 62–63
Air-conduction measurement
    audiometric interpretation, 44, 46–48
    basic audiologic testing, 10
    bone-conduction compared, 18–19
    calibration, 394–396
    clinical masking and interaural attenuation, 38–39
    conventional pure-tone thresholds, 11–13

discrete-frequency or sweep-frequency testing by automatic
        audiometry, 13–14
    high-frequency audiometry, 18
    initial masking, 41
    limitations, 71
    masking requirements, 40
    pediatric testing, 16–18
    rationale for frequency range used in audiometric testing, 14–15
    soundfield testing, 16
    variables affecting pure-tone, 27–29
Alberti, P., 88, 138, 140, 149, 152, 342
Albinism, 56
Alcohol
    effect on acoustic-reflex threshold, 110
    effect on BAEP, 263
Alcorn, S. R., 142
Allard, B., 319
Alpert, J. N., 326
Alternate binaural loudness balance test, 178–189
Altissimi, G., 263
Altshuler, M. W., 144, 146
American National Standards Institute (ANSI), 11, 21
American Speech and Hearing Association (ASHA)
    acoustic immittance and middle-ear effusion, 125, 126–128
    BAEP screening of infants, 290
    manual pure-tone threshold audiometry, 12–13
    SRT and pediatric population, 36
    SRT procedure, 34–36
American Speech-Language-Hearing Association, 93
Aminoglycoside antibiotics, 58
Amplifiers, BAEP, 253
Amplitude
    acoustic immittance and tympanometric peak, 88–89, 91–95,
        96–102
    BAEP ratio, 265–266, 282
Anderson, H., 39, 42, 108, 115, 158
Anthony, L., 80
Anticipation, subject, 11–12
Antonelli, A.
    BAEP and retrocochlear pathology, 342
    central auditory pathology detection, 345, 347
    hit rates and Bekesy audiometry, 207
    peripheral hearing impairment, 242
    rapidly alternating speech perception test, 238–239
    synthetic sentence identification test, 237
    time-compressed speech test and brainstem pathology, 217
Aperiodic signal, 1

Arndal, P., 196
Arnst, D. J., 226, 230
Arslan, E., 252
Artificial mastoid, 21
Ataxia, 350, 354, 362
Atresia, 52, 110
Audibility, auditory adaptation, 175–176
Audiometers, commercial and NBN bandwidths, 5–6
Auditory-evoked potentials, 151–153
Auditory system, described, 10
Auerbach, E., 56
Aural-palpebral reflex, 138
Aural pressure, 354, 357
Azzi, A., 146

Baker, A. H., 314
Bambini, M., 263
Bandwidth, 4, 5
Baran, J. A., 216, 221, 232
Barany, E., 19
Barany, R., 314
Barber, H. O., 314
Barbiturates, 110
Barelli, P. A., 138
Barr, B., 108, 115, 158
Barrett, L. S., 140
Bartels, D., 195
Bartholomeus, B., 196
Bauch, C. D.
    BAEP testing, 277, 279, 280, 282
    cochlear impaired ears, 107, 342
    speech-recognition scores and eighth-nerve pathology, 168
Beagley, H. A., 263
Beardsley, J. V., 265, 268, 271
Bearne, R. C., 31
Beasley, D. S., 165, 217, 241, 244
Beattie, R. C., 33, 169–170, 258–259
Beauchaine, K. A., 274–275, 288
Beck, W. G., 217
Beery, Q. C., 88
Beguwala, F. E., 258–259
Behavioral observation audiometry (BOA), 16–17
Behavior, functional hearing loss, 138, 142–150
Behnke, C. R., 147
Bekesy ascending/descending gap evaluation (BADGE), 148
Bekesy (automatic) audiometry, 147–148
Bekesy Comfortable Loudness (LCL) tracings, 206–207, 208
Bekesy, G.
    air- and bone-conduction stimulation, 19
    Bekesy audiometry, 200
    crossover during air-conduction testing, 38
    development of Bekesy audiometer, 158
    loudness recruitment, 207
    sweep frequency, 13
Bekesy sweep-frequency audiogram, 192–193, 200–208
Bell, J., 24
Bellotto, R., 207, 237, 342
Bell's palsy, 118
Bennett, M. J., 120, 122
Benson, R., 30, 162
Berger, K., 138, 139
Bergman, M., 153
Berk, R. L., 138
Berlin, C. I., 222, 224, 258

Berlin, H., 224
Bess, F. H., 167, 168, 169, 217
Betsworth, A., 169
Bickford, J. L., 252
Billger, J. M., 244–245
Billings, B. L., 21, 22, 23, 148, 149
Binaural fusion, 234–235
Binaural stimulation, 261
Bingea, R. L., 224–225
Binomial distribution model, 163–164
Bjorkman, G., 263, 281
Black, J. W., 149
Blair, R. L., 280
Blegvad, B., 196, 204
Block, M. G., 91
Bloom, M. J., 291
Bluestone, C. D., 88, 128, 129
Bocca, E., 216, 238, 242, 345
Boezeman, E., 267–268
Bone-conduction measurement
    acoustic radiation, 23–24
    artificial mastoid, 21
    audiometric calibration, 396
    audiometric interpretation, 44, 46–48
    basic audiologic testing, 18–19
    bone vibrator, 21–22, 23
    brainstem auditory-evoked potentials, 267–268
    clinical masking and interaural attenuation, 36–38
    functional hearing loss, 139
    high-frequency, 26
    initial masking, 41
    limitations, 71
    masking requirements, 39–40
    mechanism, 19–21
    middle-ear pathology, 24–25
    procedure, 26
    reference levels, 22–23
    tactile, 26
    tuning-fork tests, 26–27
    variables affecting pure-tone, 27–29
Bone vibrator, 21–22, 23
Bower, D., 169
Bowling, L. S., 31, 165
Boyd, R. L., 258–259
Boyle, W. F., 27
Brackmann, D., 279–280, 282, 283, 285, 333
Brainstem auditory-evoked potentials (BAEP)
    absent, 267
    auditory-evoked potentials, 151–152, 249–252
    bone-conducted signals, 267–268
    calibration, 391–394
    comatose population, 290–291
    cost of testing, 341
    defined, 249
    infants, 287–290
    instrumentation and signal processing, 252–255
    interpretation, 286–287
    magnitude of hearing impairment, 343–345
    normative data, 264–266
    pathology, 271–277, 279–286
    prediction of hearing threshold level, 266–267
    subject parameters, 262–264
    surgery and monitoring, 291–292
    technical parameters, 255–262

Brainstem disorders
  defined, 10
  lesions and low-pass filtered speech tests, 216
  vascular compression, 62–63
Brand, S., 198
Brandy, W. T., 164
Brenman, A. K., 124
Brewer, C. C., 321, 324
Brief-tone audiometry, 205
Britt, R. H., 240
Broad-band noise (BBN), 3–4, 6
Brookler, K. H., 313, 314
Brooks, D. N., 80, 82, 86, 87, 92
Brooks, E. B., 283
Bryan, S., 197
Buckard, R., 7–8
Burchfield, S. A., 165
Burgess, J., 237
Burkard, R., 260, 268
Burke, K. S., 147
Burney, P., 118
Burton, M., 148
Buus, S., 194, 196, 197, 198, 199
Byrne, D. C., 22

Cafarelli, D. L., 241
Cairns, H., 187
Calearo, C., 153, 216, 217, 238, 345
Calibration
  acoustic-immittance, 394
  audiometric, 394–398
  BAEP, 391–394
  electronystagmography, 309–311
Caloric testing, 312–314, 316
Campanelli, P. A., 138
Campbell, R., 140, 148
Caparosa, R. J., 342
Carhart-Jerger Modified Hughson-Westlake Method, 12
Carhart notch, 24
Carhart, R.
  auditory adaptation, 173
  Bekesy audiometry, 147, 207
  clinical tone-decay test, 158
  CNC lists, 164
  functional hearing loss, 139, 140
  NU-6s, 165
  otosclerosis and bone conduction threshold, 24–25
  revision of Hughson-Westlake method, 12
  SRT and pure-tone average, 32
Carhart-threshold tone-decay test, 173–174
Carrier phrase, 33
Carter, C. W., 162
Carterette, E. C., 170
Carver, W. F., 167, 186
Case histories
  illustrations, 346, 350, 354, 357–358, 362, 365, 373–374, 381–382, 389–390
  preparation for audiologic testing, 63–65
Cashman, M., 280
Cassinari, V., 216
Causey, G. D., 165
Central auditory pathology
  defined, 10

etiology, 62–63
  proposed protocol for detection, 345–346
Central auditory nervous system (CANS)
  central auditory dysfunction, 215–216
  disorders and acoustic-reflex thresholds, 109–110
Cerumen, 52, 84
Chaiklin, J. B.
  collapsed ear canals, 27
  crossover and air-conducted stimuli, 38–39
  Doerfler-Stewart test, 143
  functional hearing loss, 137, 139, 140, 141, 153
  SRT and SDT, 33
  SRT procedure, 34, 35
  SRT-PTA agreement, 32
  Stenger test, 145, 146
Cherry, R. S., 238, 245
Chiappa, K. H., 256, 260, 263, 264, 266, 283
Children
  acoustic-immittance testing, 124, 129–131, 132
  BAEP assessment, 249
  foreign bodies in external auditory meatus, 52–53
  functional hearing loss, 138
  middle-ear effusion, 124–127
  recorded versus live voice, 33
  serous otitis media, 53
  standing waves, 27
  tympanometric peak-pressure points, 87
  see also Pediatric testing
Chmiel, R. A., 237
Cholesteatoma, 54–55
Chun, T. H., 178
CID W–22
  reliability of PI function, 169–170
  speech-recognition testing, 159, 162–163
Cioce, C., 176
Citron, E., III, 147, 149
Clark, J. G., 243–244
Clark, K. T., 259
Clemis, J. D.
  BAEP testing, 272–273, 277, 279, 282, 285
  speech-recognition scores at MCL, 167
Clicks
  BAEP and rate, 256
  short-duration stimuli employed in audiologic tests, 6
Clinical masking
  central, 42
  initial resulting in overmasking, 43–44
  insert earphones, 44
  interaural attenuation, 36–39
  maximum, 42
  occlusion effect, 40–41
  technique, 42–43
Clinician, variables affecting pure-tone thresholds, 29
Coats, A. C.
  cochlear hearing impairment, 274
  Dix-Hallpike test, 323
  ENG procedure, 309, 310–311, 312, 313–314
  retrocochlear hearing impairment, 276, 277, 280, 281
Cochlear hearing impairment
  acoustic-reflex testing, 107, 114–117
  BAEPs, 273–276
  etiology, 176–177
  site-of-lesion test battery, 332
Cody, T., 54–55, 252

Coen, R. W., 258
Cohen, M., 342, 346
Coles, R. R. A., 39, 184, 197
Collapsed ear canals, 27, 110
Collard, M., 221–222, 223, 232, 241
Coma, 290–291, 358
Committee on Hearing, Bioacoustics, and Biomechanics (CHABA), 289
Common mode rejection ratio, 253–254
Competing sentences, 232–234
Compressional mode, bone conduction, 19
Conductive hearing impairment
    acoustic-reflex thresholds, 109
    audiometric interpretation, 49
    auditory adaptation tests, 177
    BAEPs, 271–273
    defined, 10
    etiology, 52–55
Coe, B., 260
Congenital hearing impairment, 55–57
Conn, M., 33, 140
Consonant-vowel (CV) syllables, 222–225
Contralateral ear effects, 218–220
Cooper, J. C., Jr., 195
Cooper, W. A., Jr., 148–149
Corliss, E., 21
Cortical evoked response testing, 152
Cost-benefit analysis, 341
Counseling, functional hearing loss, 153–154
Cox, B. P., 31
Crabtree, J. A., 202
Crandell, C. C., 22, 24
Creten, W. L., 76, 89, 91
Crista ampullaris, 299
Critical band, 5
Crosshearing, 37, 186–187
Crossover, 37
Crouzon's disease, 57
Crump, B., 118
Cullen, J. K., 240
Curry, E. T., 31
Cyr, D. G., 316
Cytomegalovirus (CMV), 55
Czuba, I., 138

Daddario, C., 252
Dadson, R. S., 21
Dahm, M., 21
Dallos, P. J., 205
Dancer, J., 33
Danhauer, J. L., 226
Daroff, R. B., 305
Data base, BAEP and size of normative, 263–264
Davenport, J., 334
Davis, H.
    absent BAEPs, 267
    auditory-evoked potentials, 252
    logons, 8
    PB lists, 162
    Speech-recognition threshold test, 30, 33, 35
    terminology, 10
Davis, R. I., 314
Dawson, G. J., 241–242
Decay tests, 343–345
Decker, R. L., 176, 178

Decraemer, W. F., 91
Delayed auditory feedback test, 148–150
Delle, J. H., 32
Demanuele, F., 314
Dempsey, C., 83
Denes-Naunton method, 192
Denes, P., 189–190, 191, 192–193, 207
Dennis, M. J., 291
deQuiros, J., 217
Dewey, G., 159, 162
Diabetes mellitus, 60
Dichotic speech tests, 217–226, 230–235
Diercks, K. J., 239
Difference-limen tests, 189–190
Digits, dichotic speech tests, 220–222
Dinner, D. S., 221–222
Diplacusis, 146
Dirks, D. D.
    artificial masttoid, 21
    bone conduction reference levels, 22
    digitalized speech recordings, 170
    loudness-discomfort level test, 190
    presbycusis, 177
    rollover effect, 169, 170
    SRT and pure-tone average, 32
    SRT procedure, 34
    SSI test reliability, 166–167
    vibrator placement, 23
Discrete-frequency testing, 13–14
Diuretics, 58
Dix, M. R.
    ABLB tests, 158, 202
    acoustic tumors, 346
    Bekesy tracings, 207
    loudness recruitment, 179–182
    paroxysmal nystagmus, 323
    SISI and accuracy, 198
Dix-Hallpike test, 312, 323–324
Dixon, F. F., 138
Dixon, R. F., 34, 188
Dizziness, 298, 382
Djupesland, G., 120
Dobie, R. A., 258, 341
Doehring, D. G., 196
Doerfler, L. G., 138, 143
Doerfler-Stewart test, 143–144
Donnelly, K., 152
Downs, M. P., 55
Down syndrome, 53, 56
Doyle, P. C., 226, 230
Doyle, W. J., 287, 288
Drugs
    acoustic-reflex threshold, 110
    BAEP and sedation of infants, 288–289
    BAEP and subject parameters, 262–263
    hearing impairment, 58
Dubno, J. R., 166–167
Dudley, J. G., 196

Earphones
    case illustration, 374
    insert and clinical masking, 44
    reference threshold levels, 15–16
Ear wax. See Cerumen

Edgerton, B. J., 31, 33
Effective masking level (EML), 6, 41
Efron, R., 220
Egan, J., 33, 142, 159, 163
Eggermont, J. J., 197, 279, 280, 281, 282, 283
Ehrlich, C. H., 202–203
Eighth-nerve pathology, 116–117, 167–168, 177, 181
Elderly
    bone-conduction thresholds, 28
    rollover effect, 170
    synthetic sentence identification test, 237–238
Elders, E., 30
Eldert, F., 162
Electric shock, 150–151
Electroacoustic-immittance device, 106
Electroacoustic method, 6
Electrocochleography, 153
Electrodermal audiometry, 150–151
Electrodes
    impedance and BAEP, 258
    skin preparation and ENG, 309–310
Electronystagmography
    interpretation, 316–329
    pediatric modifications, 316
    principles, 306, 308
    procedure, 308–314
Electrophysiologic tests, 150–153
Elidan, J., 282
Elpern, B. S., 31, 163
End-organ pathology, 181
Energy, calculation per cycle of BBN signal, 4
Engelberg, M. W., 140
Environment, aging and hearing impairment, 60
Epstein, A., 143
Eruklat, S., 197
Ethanol, 110
Eustachian tube
    acoustic immittance, 127–129
    air pressure, 85
Evaluation, site-of-lesion test performance, 332–341
Evans, E., 197
Everitt, W. L., 216–217
Exostoses, 53
External auditory meatus, 52–53
External-canal mode, 19–20
External ear, 52
External otitis, 53
Eye, systems controlling horizontal, 301–306

Fairbanks, G., 216–217
Falconer, G., 153
Fall time, 1
False-alarm rates, 119, 140, 207–208, 333
Farrer, S., 244
Feinmesser, M., 249
Feldman, A. S., 88, 97, 138, 140, 150
Fernandez, C., 25
Ferre, J. M., 244, 245
Fiellau-Nikolajsen, M., 92, 125, 128, 130
Filtered noise, stimuli employed in audiologic tests, 1, 3
Filters, BAEP, 253, 255, 257–258
Finitzo-Hieber, T., 260
Fior, R., 198
Fletcher, H., 5, 30, 32

Florentine, M., 194, 196
Flottorp, G., 120
Flynn, P. A., 226
Folsom, R. C., 269
Font, J., 34
Foreign bodies, 52
Formby, C., 8
Forward-backward Bekesy testing, 208
Forward-backward sweep tracings, 205–206
Fournier, M. S., 195
Fowler, E. P., 158, 178, 179
Frank, T., 22, 24, 26, 36
Frazer, G. J., 178, 336–337
French, N. R., 162
Frequency
    acoustic-reflex threshold, 107–108
    domain, 1
    range, 14–15, 268–271
Fria, T. J., 287, 288
Frishkopf, L. S., 252
Fritze, W., 186
Fulton, R. T., 195, 197
Functional hearing loss
    adults and prevalence, 137–138
    audiologic configuration, 141–142
    behavior, 138, 142–150
    bone-conduction thresholds, 139
    children and prevalence, 138
    clinical indicators, 154
    counseling, 153
    electrophysiologic tests, 150–153
    error responses during SRT and monosyllabic PB-word
        speech-recognition assessment, 140
    false-alarming, 140
    interaural attenuation, 139
    SRT-PTA discrepancy, 140–141
    SRT with monosyllabic PB words, 141
    terminology, 137
    test-retest reliability, 138–139
Fusion Inferred Test (FIT), 153

Gafni, M., 282
Galambos, R., 249, 252, 264, 267, 273, 275
Gang, R. P., 170
Garber, S. F., 142
Garner, W. R., 205
Garvey, W. D., 216
Gaze testing, 311
Geisler, C. D., 252
Gelfand, S. A.
    acoustic-reflex thresholds, 118, 150, 342, 343
    audiologic configuration of functional hearing loss, 141
    cochlear-impaired ears and acoustic-reflex threshold, 107, 108
    cortical pathology, 109
    Miskolczy-Fodor ABLB test, 186
    Owens tone decay test, 178
Genchur-Lukas, J., 231
Gender, BAEP subject parameters, 262, 263
Generator sites, BAEP, 266
Gerber, S. E., 226
Gerkin, K. P., 55
Geschwind, N., 218
Geurkink, N. A., 235, 238, 239, 252, 283, 285

Gilroy, J.
    binaural fusion test, 235
    dichotic CV tests, 216, 221
    masking level difference test, 241
    peripheral hearing impairment, 241
    rapidly alternating speech perception test, 238
    staggered spondaic word test, 231, 232
Gjaevenes, K., 176, 177
Gladstone, K. J., 256
Glasscock, M. E., 169, 176, 258, 279, 282, 285
Glattke, T. J., 267
Glomus jugulare, 54–55
Glomus tympaicum tumors, 55
Glorig, A., 32
Goetzinger, C. P., 177
Goldbaum, D., 27
Gold, S., 141
Goldstein, B. A., 40, 41
Goldstein, R., 137, 147, 216
Gollegly, K. M., 280, 282
Goller, M. C., 226
Goodglass, H., 218
Goodman, A., 158, 190
Gorga, M. P.
    BAEP and bone-conducted signals, 268, 269
    BAEP calibration, 391, 392, 393
    BAEP in infants, 288
    cochlear hearing impairment, 274–275
Gradenigo, G., 172
Graham, J. T., 32
Grams, G., 314
Grandori, F., 207, 237, 342
Gray, B. B., 217, 241
Green, D. S., 175–176
Green, K. W., 110
Greer, J., 54–55
Greville, K. A., 275–276
Grieg, R. G. P., 21
Griffing, T., 195
Grimes, A. M., 217, 241

Habituation, 11–12
Hagerman, B., 171
Hahn, J. F., 221–222
Haines, L., 32
Hallbrock, K., 192
Hallen, O., 88
Hall, J., 177, 262, 263, 290
Hallpike, C. S.
    ABLB tests, 158, 202
    Bekesy tracings, 207
    Hood method, 183
    loudness recruitment, 180, 181–182, 183, 187–188
    SISI and accuracy, 198
    tests of auditory adaptation, 172
Hamilton, L., 128
Hammernik, R. P., 188
Hanley, C. N., 149, 196
Harbert, F.
    Bekesy audiogram and excursion size, 193
    Bekesy audiogram modifications, 204, 205
    Bekesy tracings and loudness recruitment, 207
    eighth nerve lesions and tone decay, 173, 177

high-level SISI, 195
    SISI and increment size, 195–196
    SISI scores and presentation level, 194, 195
    tonality versus audibility, 176
Harford, E., 88, 140, 142, 147, 150, 183, 192
Harner, S. G., 107, 168, 277, 279, 280, 342
Harris, D. A., 139, 143
Harris, J. D., 32, 192, 197
Harrison, J. L., 283
Harris, R., 244
Hart, R. G., 334
Hattler, K. W., 143, 146, 147
Hawkins, J., 30
Hawkins, R. R., 143–144
Hayes, D., 237
Head injury, 57–58, 358, 362
Hearing Aid Industry Conference (HAIC), 22
Hearing impairment
    acoustic-reflex threshold and prediction, 118–119
    case illustration of progressive, 382
    magnitude and acoustic-reflex threshold, decay tests, and BAEP, 343–345
    magnitude and audiometric interpretation, 51–52
    type of and audiometric interpretation, 48–49
    see also specific type
Hecox, K.
    BAEP and amplitude ratio, 282
    BAEP and cochlear hearing impairments, 273, 275
    BAEP and contralateral masking, 260
    BAEP and infants, 249
    BAEP and normative data, 264
    BAEP and recording montage placement, 258
    BAEP and replicability, 266
Hedner, M., 281
Heller, J. W., 93
Hellman, R., 190
Henderson, D., 188
Henriksson, N. G., 308
Herer, G., 147
Hermanson, C. L., 165
Herpes simplex virus, 55–56
Herzog, H., 19
High-frequency audiometry, 18
Himmelfarb, M. Z., 121
Hirsch, I.
    absent BAEPs, 267
    auditory-evoked potentials, 252
    Bekesy audiograms and excursion size, 193
    Bekesy tracings and loudness recruitment, 207
    CID-W22, 162
    Denes-Naunton method, 192
    difference-limen tests, 190
    frequency range, 14
Hirsch, L., 30, 34
Hirsch, S. K., 8
Hit rates, 119, 333
Holmes, A., 24
Holm-Jensen, S., 87
Holmquist, J., 86, 128
Hood, J. D.
    ABLB test, 158
    acoustic tumors, 346
    Bekesy tracings, 207
    clinical masking, 43

loudness-discomfort level test, 190
    loudness recruitment, 180, 182–183, 187–188
    recruitment test methodology, 183–186
    tests of auditory adaptation, 172–173, 176, 177
Hood, L. J., 165
Hood tone-decay test, 174–175
Hood, W. H., 148
Hopkinson, N. T., 147, 202, 204
Hosford-Dunn, H., 170–171
House, W. F., 202, 283
Hudgins, C., 30, 34
Huff, S. J., 35
Hughes, R., 162, 196, 198, 202, 204, 205
Hughson-Westlake method, 12
Huizing, E. H., 25
Hulka, J., 25
Humes, L. E., 169, 260–261
Hunter's syndrome, 56
Huntington, D. A., 163
Hurler's syndrome, 56
Hutton, C. L., 148
Hyde, M. L., 280, 342
Hypothermia, 263, 290–291
Hypothyroidism, 60

Impacted tympanic membrane, 15
Impedance, concept of immittance, 71–77
Industry, functional hearing loss, 138
Inertial-ossicular mode, 19
Infants
    acoustic-immittance testing, 120–124, 129, 132
    BAEP assessment, 249, 287–290
    behavioral observation audiometry (BOA), 16–17
    low-frequency sinusoidal harmonic acceleration testing, 316
Infections, sensorineural hearing impairment, 60–61
Instructions, Bekesy audiograms, 204
Instrumentation
    acoustic immittance, 77–79
    BAEP, 252–255
Intensity
    acoustic-reflex threshold calibration, 106, 112
    BAEP calibration, 391–392
    normative data and BAEP, 264–265
    reference and BAEP, 261
Intensity difference limen (DL), 190–193
Interaural attenuation, 36–39, 44, 139
International Electrotechnical Commission, 21
Internuclear ophthalmoplegia, 316–317
Interpeak latency, infants and BAEP, 288
Interpretation, audiometric
    BAEP testing, 286–287
    Bekesy audiograms, 202
    configuration, 49, 51
    electronystagmography, 316–329
    hypothetical cases for masking by air- and bone-conduction, 44, 46–48
    ipsilateral acoustic-reflex threshold, 113–114
    magnitude of hearing impairment, 51–52
    peak-pressure points, 88
    staggered spondaic word test, 231
    type of hearing loss, 48–49
Ipsilateral ear effects, 218–220
Istre, C. O., 148
Ivey, R. G., 235

Jacobson, J. L., 252, 269
Jacobson, J. T., 230, 232, 237
Jaeger, R. P., 216–217
Jannetta, P. J., 240, 266
Jauhiainen, C., 188–189
Jeffress, L. A., 239
Jepsen, O., 150
Jerger, J. F.
    acoustic immittance, 80, 82, 83–84, 129
    acoustic-reflex threshold, 107, 110, 118
    auditory adaptation tests, 173, 177, 204–205
    BAEP testing, 262, 263, 267, 268, 273, 279
    Bekesy audiometry, 147, 158, 200–201, 202, 205–207, 208
    central auditory processing disorders, 245
    conductive pathology, 109
    contralateral brainstem lesions, 221
    cortical pathology, 109
    functional hearing loss, 139
    loudness recruitment, 183
    low-pass filtered word lists, 216
    Luscher-Zwislocki test, 191, 192
    middle-ear pressure and effusion, 130
    performance-intensity functions, 168
    recruitment test methodology, 183–186
    revised Hughson-Westlake method, 12
    rollover effect, 169, 170
    sensorineural acuity level test, 142
    SISI tests, 193, 195, 196
    site-of-lesion testing, 158-159, 332, 333, 334, 337, 339
    speech delayed auditory feedback, 150
    SRT and practice effect, 33
    SSI test, 166
    suprathreshold adaptation test, 175
    synthetic sentence identification test, 235–238
    terminology, 10
    tympanometric peak-pressure points, 87, 88
Jerger, S.
    acoustic immittance, 80
    Bekesy audiograms, 204–205, 206–207, 208
    central auditory processing disorders, 245
    cochlear hearing impairment and acoustic-reflex testing, 107
    contralateral brainstem lesions, 221
    cortical pathology, 109
    performance-intensity functions, 168
    rollover effect, 169, 170
    site-of-lesion testing, 332, 333, 334, 337, 339
    suprathreshold adaptation test, 175
    synthetic sentence identification test, 236–237
Jesteadt, W., 288
Jetty, A. J., 165
Jewett, D., 158, 249
Jirsa, R. E., 195
Johns, D. F., 242
Johnson, E. W., 167, 189, 202, 204
Johnson, G. D., 280
Johnson, K. O., 137, 146, 153
Johnston, K., 244, 263
Jokinen, K., 235
Joseph, M., 14
Josey, A. F.
    BAEP testing, 279, 280, 282, 285
    brief-tone audiometry, 205
    rollover and retrocochlear pathology, 169
    tone decay testing, 176, 177

Kahana, E., 282
Kahn, A. R., 268
Kall, A., 263
Kaminski, J. R., 288
Kamm, C., 169, 170, 190
Kankkunen, A., 17
Kapteyn, T., 267–268
Karja, J., 205, 208
Karjalainen, S., 208
Karlin, J., 30
Kasden, S. D., 149
Katz, J., 225, 230
Kavanagh, S. T., 259, 265, 268, 271
Keaster, J., 36
Keim, R. J., 298
Keith, R., 236, 244, 290, 291
Keith, W. J., 275–276
Kemink, J. L., 327
Kemker, F. J., 205
Kevanishvili, Z., 258, 281
Kiang, N. Y. S., 268
Kibbe-Michal, K., 285
Kileny, P., 117, 252, 327
Killion, M. C., 15–16
Kimura, D., 218
Kinstler, D. B., 146
Klippel-Feil syndrome, 56
Knox, A. W., 150, 177
Kobayashi, T., 342
Koch, L. J., 195
Koenig, W., 162
Koidan, D., 21
Konig, E., 191, 192
Konkle, D., 217, 397
Korsan-Bengtsen, M., 241
Kos, C., 158, 200, 207
Krainz, W., 19
Kraus, N., 267
Kruger, B., 15–16, 245
Kuhl, P., 219
Kurdziel, S. A., 10, 176–177, 178, 206, 217, 241
Kurman, B., 18
Kusakari, J., 342

Labyrinthitis, 60
Laitakari, K., 60
L'amore, P. J. J., 198–199
Lankford, J. E., 147
Larkins, D. A., 241
Lassman, J., 207
Latency-intensity function, 265
Lavender, R. W., 146
Lazenby, P. B., 151
Lazzaroni, A., 217
Lee, B., 149
Lee, F. F., 217
Lehiste, I., 164
Leigh, R. J., 305
Leiser, R. P., 241
Lengthened off-time, 147–148
Lentz, W. E., 152
Leshin, G. J., 138
Lesner, S. A., 252
Lesser, R. P., 221–222

Liden, G.
    central masking, 42
    contralateral acoustic-reflex adaptation, 114
    initial masking, 41
    intensity difference limen, 191
    interaural attenuation values for air-conduction, 39
    normal middle-ear pressure, 86–87
    tympanometric amplitude and shape, 88–89
    visual reinforcement audiometry, 17
Lilly, D. J., 80, 81, 175, 178
Linden, A., 234
Lindsay, J. R., 182, 346
Lindstrom, B., 263
Listening check, 28–29
Logon, 8
Loiselle, L., 245
Lombard, E., 142
Lombard test, 142–143
Lorente de No, R., 179, 187
Loudness-discomfort level test, 190
Loudness recruitment, 179–183, 187–188, 207
Low-frequency sinusoidal harmonic acceleration testing, 314–316
Low-pass filtered word lists, 216
Lowy, K., 19
Lubinsky, R., 141
Luders, H., 221–222
Lukas, R. A., 231
Lundborg, T., 200, 263
Lund-Iverson, L., 191–192
Lurie, M. H., 187
Luscher, E., 190–191, 192
Luscher-Zwislocki method, 190–192
Luterman, D. M., 241
Lutolf, J., 118, 178
Lybarger, S. F., 21, 22, 23
Lynn, D. J., 118
Lynn, G. E.
    binaural fusion test, 235
    dichotic speech tests, 216, 221
    competing sentences, 233–234
    masking level difference test, 240, 241
    peripheral hearing impairment, 241
    rapidly alternating speech perception test, 238
    staggered spondaic words, 231, 232
Lynn, J. M., 252

McCabe, B., 314, 326
McCandless, G. A., 152, 237–238, 263
McCoy, G., 137
McCutcheon, M. J., 392
McGee, T., 272–273, 277, 279, 282, 285
McLennan, R. O., 141
McMillan, P. M., 122, 123
Maculae, 299
Mair, I. W. S., 342, 344
Makeig, S., 252
Maki, J., 244
Malingering, 137
Malmquist, C. W., 23
Mangham, C. A., 117
Manning, W., 244
Mann, R. C., 314
Marchant, C. D., 122

Margolis, R. H.
  absolute acoustic-immittance devices, 89, 91, 92
  concept of mechanical impedance, 71
  ear as "acoustico-mechanical" system, 76
  infants and acoustic-immittance testing, 122
  ipsilateral acoustic-reflex measurement, 110
  ossicular discontinuity and tympanometric patterns, 96
  SRT-PTA relationship, 32
  static acoustic immittance, 80
  suprathreshold speech-recognition testing, 159
  tympanometric gradient, 93
Markin, N. D., 35
Marshall, L., 27
Martinez, C. D., 240
Martinez, S., 27
Martin, F. N.
  Bekesy test, 147
  binaural fusion test, 243–244
  bone-conduction thresholds, 26
  delayed auditory feedback test, 149
  Doerfler-Stewart test, 143–144
  functional hearing loss, 137, 141
  initial masking formula, 41
  masking technique, 43
  overmasking, 42
  SISI and contralateral masking, 197
  SISI scoring criteria, 194
  speech-recognition threshold, 40
  SSI test reliability, 167
  Stenger test, 146
  swinging story test, 153
Martony, J., 197–198
Masking
  Bekesy audiograms, 204
  contralateral and BAEP, 196–197, 260–261
  initial, 41
  ipsilateral and BAEP, 260
  overmasking, 41–42
  speech signals, 9
  stimuli employed in audiologic tests, 5–6
  suprathreshold speech-recognition assessment, 171–172
  suprathreshold tonal tests, 208–209
  see also Clinical masking; Effective masking level;
      Minimum effective masking
Masking level diffference test, 239–241
Mastoid abnormalities, 28
Mastoidectomy, 25
Mast, T. E., 252
Matzker, J., 234
Mauldin, L.
  acoustic immittance, 80
  acoustic-reflex threshold, 107, 118
  BAEPs elicited with bone-conducted signals, 267, 268, 273
  retrocochlear impairment and prolonged wave V latency, 279
Maurizi, M., 263
Maximum masking (MM), 42
Maxon, E. C., 268
Melnick, W., 147
Melrose, J., 241
Mendez-Kurtz, L., 119
Meniere's disease
  air-conduction testing, 14
  auditory adaptation tests, 176
  etiology, 57
  loudness recruitment, 180
Meningitis, 60
Mental alerting tasks, 314
Mental retardation, 17
Menzel, O. J., 143
Merin, S., 56
Method of Adjustment, 13
Method of Limits, 11–12
Metz, D., 107
Metz, O., 109, 158, 190
Meyer, D. H., 169, 170
Meyer, E., 281
Meyers, D. K., 35
Mickey, M. R., 190
Middle-ear
  acoustic immittance and functioning, 129–132
  air pressure, 85–88
  effusion, 122, 124–128
  medical referral and suspected pathology, 132
  pathology, 24–25, 53–55
  static acoustic immittance, 80–83, 102–103
Middle-latency auditory-evoked potential, 152–153
Migliavacca, F., 216
Miller, G. A., 204, 205
Miller, J., 14, 86
Miller, M. H., 158–159, 346
Mills, D. M., 258–259
Miltenberger, G. E., 241–242
Minimum effective masking (MEM), 6, 41
Mishler, E. T., 169, 170
Miskolczy-Fodor, F., 186
Mixed hearing impairment, 48–49
Moller, A. R., 240, 266, 280, 281, 284
Moller, M. B., 240, 280, 281, 284
Monaural loudness balance test, 189
Monaural low-redundancy speech tests, 216–217
Monosyllabic phonetically balanced (PB) words, 9, 141
Monro, D. A., 141, 146, 147, 149
Morales-Garcia, C., 173, 176, 177
Morgan, D., 32, 34, 170
Morgan, P. P., 138
Morris, H. M., 221–222
Mosher, N. A., 165
Mosher, R. A., 165
Most comfortable loudness (MCL), 167
Mouney, D., 224
Moushegian, G., 264, 266
Mucopolysaccharidosis, 56
Mueller, H. G., 217
Multiple sclerosis, 63
Munson, W. A., 5
Musiek, F. E.
  auditory-evoked potentials, 152, 252
  BAEP testing, 279, 280, 281, 282, 283, 285
  binaural fusion test, 235
  central auditory disorders, 62
  Competing Sentences Test, 234
  dichotic-digits test, 221
  low-pass filtered speech test, 216
  rapidly alternating speech perception test, 238
  staggered spondaic words, 231–232
Mussell, S. A., 167

Myasthenia gravis, 109
Myers, C. K., 32

Narrow-band noise (NBN), 4–5, 6
Naunton, R. F., 25, 189–190, 191, 192–193, 198, 207
Neely, S. T., 288
Nelson, P., 197
Nerbonne, M. S., 35
Neuberger, F., 191
Neuromuscular diseases, 117
Newby, H., 10, 138, 139, 346
Newman, C. W., 40, 41
Nickel, B., 218
Nielsen, D. W., 333, 334–335
Niemeyer, W., 118
Nilsson, G., 39, 42, 191
Nober, E. H., 26
Nodar, R. H., 241
Noffsinger, D. W.
    auditory adaptation tests, 174, 176, 177, 178
    brief-tone audiometry, 205
    masking level difference test, 239–240
    peripheral hearing impairment, 242
    time compressed speech, 217
Noffsinger, P. D., 10
Noise
    ambient and audiometric measurement, 29
    case history illustrations, 346, 350, 382
    hazardous levels and hearing impairment, 58–59
Normal-hearing persons, 177
Northern, J. L., 55
NU-6s, 164–165
Nystagmus
    caloric stimulation, 304
    dizziness associated with vestibular disorders, 298
    ENG interpretation, 317–327
    measurement of strength, 308
    mental alertness, 314
    peripheral vestibular pathology, 303–304
    rotary stimulation, 304–305

Occlusion effect, 40–41
Occupational Safety and Health Act of 1970, 138
Ochs, M. G., 260–261
Ocular dysmetria, 316
Ocular flutter, 316
Odenthal, D. W., 197
Ogiba, Y., 17
Okitsu, T., 342
Oliver, T. A., 237
Olsen, W. O.
    acoustic-reflex adaptation, , 116, 117
    artificial mastoid, 21
    auditory adaptation tests, 176–177, 178
    brief-tone audiometry, 205
    Carhart threshold tone-decay test, 174
    cochlear-impaired ears, 107, 342
    dichotic CV test, 222–223, 224
    eighth-nerve pathology, 167, 168, 178
    forward-backward sweep-frequency tracings, 206
    masking level difference test, 239-240
    normal-hearing bone-conduction threshold, 22, 23
    peripheral hearing impairment, 242
    retrocochlear-impaired subjects and acoustic-reflex threshold, 108

speaker effect on SRT, 164
    SRT procedure, 34, 35
    staggered spondaic word test, 232
    time compressed speech, 217
Optokinetic eye movements, 305–306
Optokinetic testing, 311–312
Orchik, D., 237, 244
Orientation reflex (COR) audiometry, 17
Oscilloscope, 112
Ossicular discontinuity
    acoustic immittance, 83, 96
    acoustic-reflex threshold, 109
    conductive hearing impairment, 55
    frequency range, 15
Ossicular fixation, 24–25
Osterhammel, D., 110
Osterhammel, P., 110, 196, 258, 263
Otitis media
    air-conduction testing, 14
    bone conduction thresholds, 25
    etiology, 53–54
    infants, 122
Otoscelerosis
    acoustic immittance, 83, 96
    air-conduction testing, 14
    bone conduction thresholds, 24–25
    etiology, 54
Otoscopy, 124–125
Ototoxicity, 58
Ottaviani, F., 263
Otto, W. C., 237–238, 263
Overmasking
    clinical masking, 41–42
    initial resulting in, 43–44
    suprathreshold speech-recognition testing, 171
    suprathreshold tonal tests, 209
Oviatt, D. L., 91, 118
Owen, J. H., 195
Owens, E.
    Bekesy audiograms, 202, 203, 204, 207, 208
    eighth-nerve pathology, 177, 178
    Hood tone-decay test, 174–175
    Owens tone-decay procedure and cochlear impairment, 176
    SISI testing, 196, 197
    suprathreshold speech-recognition data, 333
Ozdamar, O., 267

Paludetti, G., 263
Palva, A., 205, 208, 235
Palva, T., 188–189, 190, 205, 207
Paradise, J. L., 88, 92
Parker, W., 176, 178
Pashley, N. R. T.
Pathology
    acoustic immittance and ranges for various groups, 83–84
    acoustic immittance and tympanometric patterns, 93–94, 96–102
    effect on SISI, 194
    masking level difference test, 240–241
    staggered spondaic word test, 231
    synthetic sentence identification test, 237–238
    see also specific type
Peak latency, infants and BAEP, 287–288
Peak pressure point, 85–88
Pedersen, C. B., 205

Pedersen, K., 263
Pediatric testing
    air-conduction measurement, 16–18
    central processing disorders, 243–245
    ENG test modifications, 316
    SISI testing, 197–198
    SRT considerations, 36
    SRT performance, 171
    see also Children; Infants
Peek, B. F., 261
Pendular tracking, 311
Penley, E. D., 165
Pennington, C. D., 194
Penrod, J., 164
Perez-Abalb, M., 269
Perforated tympanic membrane, 84
Perilymphatic fistula, 57
Perinatal infection, 55
Periodic complex signal, 1
Peripheral hearing loss, 167, 241–242
Pestalozza, G., 176
Peters, J. F., 265, 267
Peterson, G. E., 164
Peterson, J. L., 86
Phelan, J. G., 146
Phonetic balance (PB), 159
Pick, H., Jr., 142
Picton, T. W., 269
Pinsker, O. T., 10
PI-PB test, 341
Piper, N., 150, 343
Play audiometry, 17–18
Podraza, B., 219
Polarity, BAEP test, 256–257, 393
Pollack, I., 204
Poole, J. P., 190
Popelka, G. R., 8, 80, 118, 121, 346
Porter, T. A., 86
Positional testing, 312
Posner, J., 167
Prasher, D., 342, 346
Presbycusis, 59–60, 177
Price, L. L., 147, 242
Priede, M., 39, 184, 197
Prosser, S., 252
Proud, G., 177
Psychogenic hearing loss, 137
Pure-tone
    average and SRT, 32–33
    conventional thresholds, 11–13
    defined, 1
    delayed auditory feedback, 148–149
    functional hearing loss and SRT, 140–141
    masking noise, 6
    variables affecting air- and bone-conduction thresholds, 27–29

Quiggle, R. R., 32

Raffin, M. J. M., 163, 165, 169–170, 171, 224–225
Ragland, A. E., 26
Raica, A. N., 241–242
Randolph, L., 27
Rapidly alternating speech perception test (RASP), 238–239
Read, D., 269

Recklinghausen's disease, 169
Recording
    infants and BAEP, 288–289
    montage placement and BAEP, 258–259
    two-channel and BAEP, 259–260
Recruitment tests, 178–190
Reddell, R. C., 147, 149
Redden, R. B., 194, 196
Reed, N., 267
Reeves, A. G., 216
Reflex modulation, 120
Reger, S. N., 12–13, 158, 200, 207
Reiland, J. K., 274–275
Rejection rate, 1, 3, 5
Renal disease, 60
Renvall, U., 86–87
Repetition rate, 282–283, 393–394
Replicability, BAEP testing, 266, 282
Resnick, D. M., 147, 235, 321, 324
Retinitis pigmentosa, 56
Retrocochlear hearing impairment
    acoustic-reflex threshold, 108–109
    BAEP testing, 276–277, 279–286
    proposed protocol for detection, 342–345
    pure-tone air- and bone-conduction measurement, 28
    site-of-lesion test battery, 332
    terminology, 10
Reynolds, E., 14, 30, 162
Richards, L. A., 22
Richards, W. D., 22
Richter, W. D., 26
Riedel, C. L., 128, 129
Riesz, R., 190
Rinne test, 26–27
Rintelmann, W. F.
    acquired sensorineural hearing impairment, 241
    functional hearing loss, 137–138
    NU-6s, 165
    SAL test, 142
    soundfield testing, 16
    Stenger test, 147
Rise time, 1
Rivera, V. M., 237
Robinson, D. W., 21
Robinson, K., 283
Robinson, M., 149
Rodenburg, M., 198–199
Roeser, R. J., 242
Rollover effect, 168–170
Romano, M. N., 249
Rose, D. E., 205, 206, 277, 279, 280
Rosenberg, P., 174, 198
Rosenberg tone-decay test, 174
Rosenblith, W. A., 204, 252
Rosenhall, U., 263, 281, 282
Rosenhamer, H. J., 263
Rossi, G. T., 240
Ross, M., 139, 163
Rossman, R., 280
Rothner, A. D., 221–222
Roush, J., 244
Rowe, M. J., 263
Rubella (German measles), 55
Rubens, A. B., 219

Ruder, L., 138
Ruhm, H. B., 148–149
Rudge, P., 283
Runge, C. A., 170
Rupp, R. R., 195
Ruth, R. A., 258
Ryu, J., 314, 326

Saccadic eye movement, 305
Saccidic testing, 316–317
Sachs, E., Jr., 283
Salicylates, 58
Salvi, R. J., 188
Sammeth, C. A., 261
Sanders, J. W.
   acoustic-reflex adaptation, 115, 116, 117
   acoustic tumors and acoustic-reflex thresholds, 108
   brainstem auditory-evoked potentials, 151
   brief-tone audiometry, 205
   cochlear-impaired ears and acoustic-reflex thresholds, 107
   electroacoustic method and effective masking levels (EML), 6
   false-alarm rates, 207
   high-level SISI, 195
   increment size modification of SISI, 196
   recruitment tests, 185–186, 188, 189
   site-of-lesion test evaluation, 337
   tone decay tests, 176, 177
Sandridge, S. A., 252
Schaefer, A. B., 240
Schafer, D., 165
Scharf, B., 190
Schlaman, M., 27
Schmidt, D., 281
Schow, R., 27
Schubert, K., 158, 172
Schuchman, G. I., 143, 146, 147
Schuknecht, H. F., 59, 158
Schulman-Galambos, C., 267
Schumaier, D. R., 165
Schwartz, D. M., 279, 283, 291, 346
Scoring
   criteria for SISI, 194
   staggered spondaic words, 226, 230–231
Scott-Nielsen, S., 80
Screening, infants and BAEP, 289–290
Seitz, M., 392
Selters, W., 279–280, 282, 283, 285, 333
Sensorineural acuity level (SAL), 142
Sensorineural hearing impairment
   audiometric interpretation, 48
   bone-conduction measurement, 18
   defined, 10
   etiology, 55–62
Sesterhenn, G., 118
Sex, subject parameters
   acoustic-reflex threshold, 110
   BAEP, 262, 263
   presbycusis, 60
Shahar, A., 141
Shanks, J. E.
   absolute acoustic-immittance devices, 89, 91, 92
   contralateral acoustic-reflex adaptation, 115
   infants and acoustic-immittance testing, 120–121

ossicular discontinuity and tympanometric patterns, 96
   small ear-canal volumes and tympanograms, 103
   static acoustic immittance, 80
   water and tympanograms, 102
Shanks, W. L., 76, 81
Shanon, E., 121
Shape, acoustic immittance and tympanometric peak, 88–89, 91–95, 96–102
Shapiro, I., 198
Sharbrough, F. W., 283
Shea, S. L., 252
Shedd, J., 192
Sheldrake, J. B., 263
Shepard, N. T., 178, 336–337
Sheperd, D. C., 147
Shimizu, H., 196
Shipp, D. B., 146, 149
Shipton, M. S., 24
Short increment sensitivity index (SISI), 190–199
Shrapnell's membrane, 87
Shurin, P., 122
Sidetone-amplification effect, 142–143
Siedentop, K., 128
Siegell, G. M., 142
Siegenthaler, B. M., 32
Signal averager, 254–255
Signal processing, BAEP, 252–255
Silman, S.
   acoustic immittance and middle-ear effusion, 125–126, 127
   acoustic-reflex thresholds, 107, 118, 119, 150, 342, 343
   audiologic configuration and functional hearing loss, 141
   cortical pathology, 109
   Owens tone decay test, 178
Silverman, C. A., 110, 118, 125–126, 127, 150
Silverman, S. R., 10, 30, 33, 162
Simmons, F., 57, 188
Simonton, K. M., 182, 346
Simpson, M., 196
Site-of-lesion tests
   cochlear and retrocochlear pathology, 332, 346
   development, 158
   sensitivity rates, 71
   speech-recognition testing, 159, 162–172
   test performance evaluation, 332–341
Sjoblom, J., 188–189
Skinner, M., 14
Sklare, D. A., 263
Smith, A., 269
Smith, B. B., 235
Smith, C. G., 92
Smooth pursuit system, 305
Snel, A., 267–268
Sohmer, H., 249, 282
Sohoel, T. H., 176, 177
Sorensen, H., 87, 174, 176, 177, 204
Sorri, M., 208
Soundfield testing, 16, 397–398
Sound-pressure level (SPL), 4
Sparks, R., 218, 219, 220–221
Speaker, effect on SRT, 164
Speaks, C.
   dichotic speech tests, 218, 219, 220
   peripheral hearing impairment, 241, 242
   synthetic sentence identification test, 166, 235–238

Speech
- audiometric calibration, 397
- delayed auditory feedback, 149–150
- digitalized recordings, 170
- frequency range used in audiometric testing, 14
- short-duration stimuli employed in audiologic tests, 8–9
- Stenger test, 146

Speech-recognition threshold (SRT)
- average and pure-tone, 32–33
- basic audiology testing, 29–30
- carrier phrase, 33
- familarization and practice, 33
- functional hearing loss and error responses, 140
- functional hearing loss and monosyllabic PB words, 141
- history of development, 30–31
- initial masking formula, 41
- masking requirements, 40
- pediatric population, 36
- procedure, 34–36
- recorded and live-voice, 33
- response mode, 33
- site-of-lesion tests, 159, 162–172
- terminology, 30

Spondaic words, 30
Spondee-error index (SERI), 140
Spondee threshold. *See* Speech-recognition threshold, 30
Spradlin, J., 195, 197
Sprague, B. H., 121, 122, 123
Staab, W. J., 16
Stach, B. A., 238
Staggered spondiac words, 225–226, 230–232
Standing waves, 27–28
Stangerup, S. E., 87
Stapedius muscle, 103
Stapells, D. R., 267, 269, 270, 288, 290
Stark, E. W., 147, 202
Starr, A., 158, 262, 264, 265, 266, 283
Steenerson, R. L., 329
Steinberg, J. C., 30
Stein, L., 138, 146, 267
Stenger, P., 144–146
Stenger phenomenon, 27
Stenger test, 144–146
Stephens, M., 205
Stevens, S., 30
Sticht, T. J., 217, 241
Stisen, B., 21
Stockard, J. E., 258, 283, 287
Stockard, J. J.
- BAEP and normative data, 262, 263
- BAEP and repetition rate, 283
- BAEP and stimulus polarity, 257
- BAEP and subject parameters, 262
- BAEP in infants, 287, 288
- I-V interpeak latency, 281–282
- latency-intensity function, 264
- recording montage placement, 258

Stockwell, C. W., 312, 325
Stokinger, T. E., 148, 149
Strand, R., 32
Studebaker, G. A., 23, 197
Sturzebecher, E., 281
Subjects, effect on BAEP, 262–264
Suga, F., 182, 346

Summerfield, A. B., 32
Sung, S. S., 177
Supra-aural earphones, 15
Suprathreshold adaptation test, 175
Suprathreshold tonal tests, 208–209
Surgery, BAEP and monitoring, 291–292
Suzuki, T., 17
Svihovec, D. V., 31, 33
Sweep-frequency testing. *See* Discrete-frequency testing
Swimmer's ear. *See* external otitis
Swinging story test, 153
Swisher, L., 196, 197
Switched speech test, 153
Swogger, J. R., 123
Symons, F., 342
Synthetic sentence identification (SSI) test, 166–167, 235–238
Syphilis, 56, 57

Tait, C. A., 244
Talmachoff, P. J., 252
Tangible reinforcement operant conditioning audiometry (TROCA), 17
Tardy, M., 128
Taylor, P. C., 238, 241
Temperature
- BAEP and subject parameters, 263
- variables affecting pure-tone thresholds, 29

Terkildsen, K., 80, 150, 196, 258, 263
Thelin, J., 166
Thompson, G., 17, 195, 240
Thomsen, J., 263
Thorndike, E. L., 162
Thornton, A. R., 163, 171, 268
Threshold, reference levels, 15–16
Thurlow, W. R., 33
Tickle response, 18
Tiffany, W. R., 149
Tillman, T. J.
- auditory adaptation tests, 176
- CNC lists, 164
- eighth-nerve pathology, 177
- NU-6s, 165
- recruitment tests, 188, 189
- sensoneural acuity level (SAL) test, 142
- speech-recognition threshold, 33, 164

Tillman, T. W., 34, 205, 207, 332
Time compressed speech, 216–217
Time domain, 1
Tinnitus, case illustrations, 350, 354, 357, 358, 365, 382
Tobey, E., 224
Tobin, H., 239
Tonality, auditory adaptation, 175–176
Tonebursts, short-duration stimuli employed in audiologic tests, 7–8
Tonndorf, J., 18, 19–21, 27, 188
TORCHS, 55
Tos, M., 87, 132
Townsend, T. H., 397
Toxoplasmosis, 55
Trammell, J., 166, 236
Trauma. *See* Head injury
Treacher-Collins syndrome, 57
Trier, T. R., 153
Troost, B. T., 305
Tuck, G., 195

Tumors
  acoustic and site-of-lesion test, 346
  acoustic immittance testing, 108
  acquired and intracranial, 62
  BAEP testing, 283, 285
  see also Acoustic schwannomas
Tuning-fork tests, 26–27
Turner, R. G.
  BAEP and retrochochlear pathology, 342
  high presentation level SISI test, 198
  hit- and false-alarm rates for BCL testing, 208
  site of lesion test and acoustic tumors, 346
  site-of-lesion test evaluation, 333, 334–335, 336–337, 338, 339–340
  suprathreshold adaptation test, 178
Turpin, L. L., 252
Tympanic membrane, 84–85
Tympanometry
  air pressure, 85–86
  infants, 121–122
  low probe-tone frequencies, 92
  static acoustic immittance, 84, 102–103
Tympanosclerosis, 53

Upper respiratory infection, 354, 357
Usher's syndrome, 56
Utriculopetal deviation, 299
Utting, J., 196

Van Campen, L. E., 261
Van Camp, K. J., 76, 78, 83, 89, 91
Van de Heyning, P. H., 91
Van Frank, L., 150
Vanhuyse, V. J., 89, 91, 92, 130, 131
Vanpeperstraete, P. M., 89, 91
Variable intensity pulse–count method, 139
Ventilation, 29
Ventry, I. M.
  Bekesy audiometry, 147
  collapsed ear canals, 27
  Doerfler-Stewart test, 143
  functional hearing loss, 137, 139, 140, 141, 153
  most comfortable loudness (MCL) level, 167
  SRT procedure, 33, 35
  SRT-PTA agreement, 32
  Stenger test, 145, 146
Vertigo, 298, 365
Vestibular system, anatomy and physiology, 298–299, 301
Vestibulo-ocular reflex, 301–305
Veterans
  electrodermal audiometry, 150, 151
  functional hearing loss, 137–138
Visser, S., 267–268
Visual Reinforcement Audiometry (VRA), 17
Von Recklinghausen's disease, 61–62

Waardenburg's syndrome, 56
Wallin, A., 119
Wall, L. G., 35
Walsh, T. E., 33, 158
Ward, W. D., 172
Warren, V. G., 169–170
Waveform, BAEP and abnormal morphology, 283
Weatherby, L. A., 120, 122
Weber, B. A., 17, 281–283, 286, 392
Weber test, 27
Wedenberg, E., 107, 108, 114, 158
Weider, D. J., 283
Weiland, L., 54–55
Weiss, B., 193, 195–196
Weiss, E., 21
Welsh, O. L., 241
Welsh, T., 319
Werbs, M., 281
White noise, 3–4
Whitfield, I., 197
Wilber, L. A., 15–16, 164, 244, 245, 397
Wiley, T. L., 91, 175, 178
Willeford, J. A., 177, 232, 235, 238, 243, 244–245
Williston, H., 158
Williston, J. S., 249
Wilpezeski, C. R., 195–196
Wilson, L. K., 169
Wilson, R., 32, 34–35, 159
Wilson, R. H., 76, 89, 92, 115, 117
Winegar, W. J., 202
Wittich, W. W., 26
Woellner, R. C., 158
Wolfe, J., 316
Woods, R. W., 140
Word lists, abbreviated SRT, 170–171
Work, W. P., 137
Worthington, D. W., 265, 267, 269, 391
Wright, G., 314

Yantis, P. Q., 174, 177, 207
Yes-no method, 139
Ylikoski, J., 188–189
Yoshle, N., 267
Young, I. M.
  Bekesy audiogram modifications, 204, 205
  Bekesy sweep-frequency audiograms and excursion size, 193
  Bekesy tracings and loudness recruitment, 207
  eighth-nerve pathology and tone decay, 173, 177
  SISI scores and presentation level, 194, 195
  tonality versus audibility, 176
Young, L. L., 31
Young, R. R., 256, 283

Zollner, F., 192
Zwislocki, J., 42, 44, 190–191, 192